Healthy, Resilient, and Sustainable

COMMUNITIES
AFTER DISASTERS

Strategies, Opportunities, and
Planning for Recovery

Committee on Post-Disaster Recovery of a Community's Public Health, Medical, and Social Services

Board on Health Sciences Policy

INSTITUTE OF MEDICINE
OF THE NATIONAL ACADEMIES

THE NATIONAL ACADEMIES PRESS
Washington, D.C.
www.nap.edu

THE NATIONAL ACADEMIES PRESS   500 Fifth Street, NW   Washington, DC 20001

NOTICE: The project that is the subject of this report was approved by the Governing Board of the National Research Council, whose members are drawn from the councils of the National Academy of Sciences, the National Academy of Engineering, and the Institute of Medicine. The members of the committee responsible for the report were chosen for their special competences and with regard for appropriate balance.

This study was supported by contracts between the National Academy of Sciences and the U.S. Department of Health and Human Services, Office of the Assistant Secretary for Preparedness and Response (Contract No. HHSO100201200037A and Contract No. 1 HITEP130013-01-00); the U.S. Department of Housing and Urban Development (Contract No. 1 HITEP130013-01-00); and the Robert Wood Johnson Foundation (Contract No. 71003 and Contract No. 72398). Any opinions, findings, conclusions, or recommendations expressed in this publication are those of the author(s) and do not necessarily reflect the views of the organizations or agencies that provided support for the project.

Library of Congress Cataloging-in-Publication Data

Institute of Medicine (U.S.). Committee on Post-Disaster Recovery of a Community's Public Health, Medical, and Social Services, author.
Healthy, resilient, and sustainable communities after disasters : strategies, opportunities, and planning for recovery / Committee on Post-Disaster Recovery of a Community's Public Health, Medical, and Social Services, Board on Health Sciences Policy, Institute of Medicine of the National Academies.
    p. ; cm.
Includes bibliographical references.
ISBN 978-0-309-31619-4 (pbk.) — ISBN 978-0-309-31620-0 (pdf) I. Title.
[DNLM: 1. Community Health Services—organization & administration—United States. 2. Disaster Planning—organization & administration—United States. 3. Health Policy—United States. 4. Public Health Administration—methods—United States. 5. Relief Work--organization & administration—United States. 6. Survivors—United States. WA 546 AA1]
RA971
362.1068—dc23
                                2015029208

Additional copies of this report are available for sale from the National Academies Press, 500 Fifth Street, NW, Keck 360, Washington, DC 20001; (800) 624-6242 or (202) 334-3313; http://www.nap.edu.

For more information about the Institute of Medicine, visit the IOM home page at: www.iom.edu.

Printed and bound in Great Britain by Marston Book Services Ltd, Oxfordshire

The serpent has been a symbol of long life, healing, and knowledge among almost all cultures and religions since the beginning of recorded history. The serpent adopted as a logotype by the Institute of Medicine is a relief carving from ancient Greece, now held by the Staatliche Museen in Berlin.

Suggested citation: IOM (Institute of Medicine). 2015. *Healthy, resilient, and sustainable communities after disasters: Strategies, opportunities, and planning for recovery.* Washington, DC: The National Academies Press.

"Knowing is not enough; we must apply.
Willing is not enough; we must do."
—Goethe

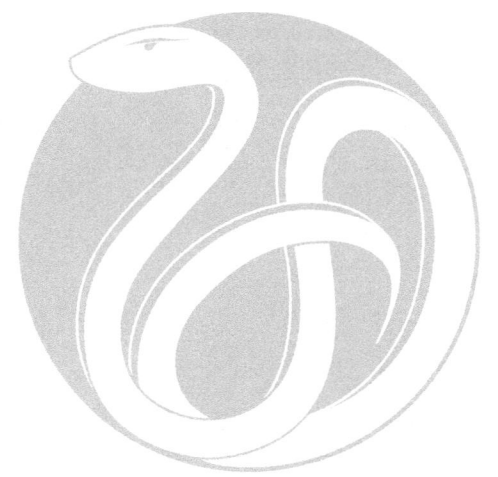

INSTITUTE OF MEDICINE
OF THE NATIONAL ACADEMIES

Advising the Nation. Improving Health.

THE NATIONAL ACADEMIES
Advisers to the Nation on Science, Engineering, and Medicine

The **National Academy of Sciences** is a private, nonprofit, self-perpetuating society of distinguished scholars engaged in scientific and engineering research, dedicated to the furtherance of science and technology and to their use for the general welfare. Upon the authority of the charter granted to it by the Congress in 1863, the Academy has a mandate that requires it to advise the federal government on scientific and technical matters. Dr. Ralph J. Cicerone is president of the National Academy of Sciences.

The **National Academy of Engineering** was established in 1964, under the charter of the National Academy of Sciences, as a parallel organization of outstanding engineers. It is autonomous in its administration and in the selection of its members, sharing with the National Academy of Sciences the responsibility for advising the federal government. The National Academy of Engineering also sponsors engineering programs aimed at meeting national needs, encourages education and research, and recognizes the superior achievements of engineers. Dr. C. D. Mote, Jr., is president of the National Academy of Engineering.

The **Institute of Medicine** was established in 1970 by the National Academy of Sciences to secure the services of eminent members of appropriate professions in the examination of policy matters pertaining to the health of the public. The Institute acts under the responsibility given to the National Academy of Sciences by its congressional charter to be an adviser to the federal government and, upon its own initiative, to identify issues of medical care, research, and education. Dr. Victor J. Dzau is president of the Institute of Medicine.

The **National Research Council** was organized by the National Academy of Sciences in 1916 to associate the broad community of science and technology with the Academy's purposes of furthering knowledge and advising the federal government. Functioning in accordance with general policies determined by the Academy, the Council has become the principal operating agency of both the National Academy of Sciences and the National Academy of Engineering in providing services to the government, the public, and the scientific and engineering communities. The Council is administered jointly by both Academies and the Institute of Medicine. Dr. Ralph J. Cicerone and Dr. C. D. Mote, Jr., are chair and vice chair, respectively, of the National Research Council.

www.nationalacademies.org

Consultants

STEVEN BINGLER, President, Concordia

RONA BRIERE, Senior Editor

MELISSA BRYMER, Director, Terrorism and Disaster Programs, National Center for Child Traumatic Stress, University of California, Los Angeles

MIRIAM DAVIS, Independent Medical Writer

ERIN HAMMERS FORSTAG, Independent Medical Writer

GAVIN SMITH, Executive Director, Department of Homeland Security Coastal Hazards Center of Excellence, Associate Professor, Department of City and Regional Planning, University of North Carolina at Chapel Hill

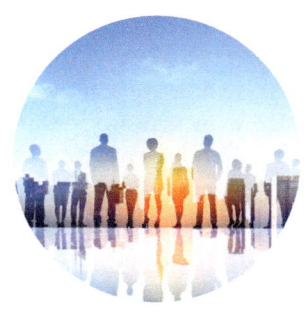

Reviewers

This report has been reviewed in draft form by individuals chosen for their diverse perspectives and technical expertise, in accordance with procedures approved by the National Research Council's Report Review Committee. The purpose of this independent review is to provide candid and critical comments that will assist the institution in making its published report as sound as possible and to ensure that the report meets institutional standards for objectivity, evidence, and responsiveness to the study charge. The review comments and draft manuscript remain confidential to protect the integrity of the deliberative process. We wish to thank the following individuals for their review of this report:

John Agwunobi, Former President Walmart Health and Wellness
Allison Blake, New Jersey Department of Children and Families
Frederick M. Burkle, Jr., Harvard School of Public Health
Anita Chandra, RAND Corporation
C. Robert Cloninger, Washington University School of Medicine
James Craig, Mississippi State Department of Health
Brian W. Flynn, Uniformed Services University of the Health Sciences
Jeffery Hebert, New Orleans Redevelopment Authority
Anthony B. Iton, The California Endowment
Vivian E. Loftness, Carnegie Mellon University
Kevin Massey, Advocate Lutheran General Hospital
Scott M. Needle, Healthcare Network of Southwest Florida
Jan Opper, Opper Strategies & Solutions, LLC
Samantha Phillips, City of Philadelphia
Mary Pittman, Public Health Institute

Although the reviewers listed above provided many constructive comments and suggestions, they were not asked to endorse the report's conclusions or recommendations, nor did they see the final draft of the report before its release. The review of this report was overseen by **Bobbie Berkowitz,** Columbia University, and **Joan B. Rose,** Michigan State University. Appointed by the National Research Council and the Institute of Medicine, they were responsible for making certain that an independent examination of this report was carried out in accordance with institutional procedures and that all review comments were carefully considered. Responsibility for the final content of this report rests entirely with the authoring committee and the institution.

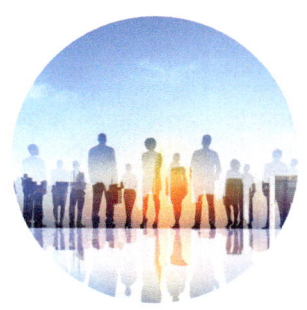

Preface

Healthy, Resilient, and Sustainable Communities After Disasters is intended as both a call to action and an action guide for maximally leveraging the resources associated with disaster planning and recovery toward realizing healthier communities. The report is premised in the study committee's appreciation of the importance of engaging all community stakeholders and available resources thoughtfully, creatively, and appropriately in working synergistically to address the unacceptable reality that the nation's communities, and its people, are less healthy than they can and should be. The report is intended to focus the attention of those individuals and organizations involved in planning for and carrying out disaster recovery activities and those involved in planning for and building healthy communities on leveraging the millions and sometimes billions of dollars associated with disaster events more effectively toward maximizing healthiness. It would seem intuitive that a community confronted by the tragic necessity of rebuilding roads, houses, health care institutions, parks, and other critical elements of its infrastructure would intentionally seek to optimize health status as one of its major priorities. Unfortunately, as documented in this report, creating healthy communities usually is not high on the list of disaster planning or recovery efforts, and too often a significant gulf exists between the nation's dedicated disaster officials and their equally praiseworthy health leader counterparts. In this context, this report is intended to highlight the key opportunities that disaster recovery offers to advance the social goal of maximizing the health of communities, and to provide practical recommendations for how diverse stakeholders can work more collaboratively to realize this goal in the normal course of addressing their specific accountabilities. It is the committee's hope that the disaster professional community and the health professional community both will see this report as relevant to their work and, in the process, be drawn more closely together.

In this report, the committee endorses a comprehensive definition of a healthy community proposed by the National Network of Public Health Institutes:

> A healthy community is one in which a diverse group of stakeholders collaborate to use their expertise and local knowledge to create a community that is socially and physically conducive to health. Community members are empowered and civically engaged, assuring that all local policies consider health. The community has the capacity to identify, address, and evaluate their own health concerns on an ongoing basis, using data to guide and benchmark efforts. As a result, a healthy community is safe, economically secure, and environmentally sound, as all residents have equal access to high quality educational and employment

opportunities, transportation and housing options, prevention and healthcare services, and healthy food and physical activity opportunities.

This vision was important to the committee's work in large measure because of its emphasis on holistic engagement and community-specific strategies. Testimony before the committee consistently emphasized that no "one-size-fits-all" strategy or menu of recommendations will work everywhere or fit every scenario. A consistent lesson learned, however, was the importance of pre-disaster planning that proactively links disaster and health leadership at the community level and that benefits from the accumulated wisdom gleaned from other experiences.

The committee appreciates the thoughtful vision of the study sponsors: the Assistant Secretary for Preparedness and Response (ASPR) at the U.S. Department of Health and Human Services (HHS); the Office of Lead Hazard Control and Healthy Homes at the U.S. Department of Housing and Urban Development (HUD); the Veterans Health Administration at the U.S. Department of Veterans Affairs (VA); and the Robert Wood Johnson Foundation. They all recognized the need for recommendations and guidance that would be useful to local and national leaders who were sensitized to the need to mitigate disaster-related health impacts and optimize the use of rebuilding resources to pursue the goal of creating communities that are healthier and more resilient in a more proactive, deliberate, and thoughtful manner. The committee's work benefited greatly from the exceptional Institute of Medicine staff team, led by study director Autumn Downey and including Bruce Altevogt, Elizabeth Cornett, Jack Herrmann, Rachel Kirkland, Crysti Park, Megan Reeve, and Lauren Shern. We are also indebted to the consultants who contributed substantially to this project. Steven Bingler, Melissa Brymer, and Gavin Smith lent the committee their invaluable expertise, and the report could not have been produced without the technical writing and editing contributions of Rona Briere, Miriam Davis, and Erin Hammers Forstag. Finally, I wish to offer thanks and acknowledgment to my fellow committee members, all of whom gave generously of their time in the undertaking of this important and challenging task.

After 18 months of careful examination of testimony from a wide array of officials and experts, case studies, and the available literature, three compelling impressions remain with the committee members. First are the heartbreaking stories of misery and suffering experienced by so many people who live with or die prematurely from preventable illnesses and the many others who become sickened or injured as a result of experiencing a disaster event. We want better for them. Second is the gratitude that cannot be expressed often enough to the nation's disaster planning and response officials, workers, and volunteers, most of whom labor in anonymity and often are taken for granted. The nation needs more of them, and they deserve more from all Americans. Third, because no community is immune to a devastating event and because no community is maximally healthy, every reader of this report is urged to use this opportunity to contribute immediately to a process of collaborative planning that brings all stakeholders and community residents together to envision a healthy community, assess and prioritize key deficiencies, and then engage the resources and expertise of the disaster community as a key component of the collective effort to achieve an environment in which all people have the opportunity to live maximally healthy lives. It is the committee's hope that the observations and recommendations offered in this report will serve as a call to action and a useful guide for transformative action.

Reed V. Tuckson, M.D., *Chair*
Committee on Post-Disaster Recovery of a Community's
Public Health, Medical, and Social Services

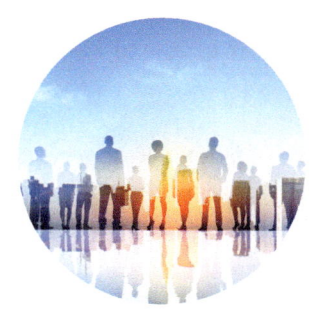

Contents

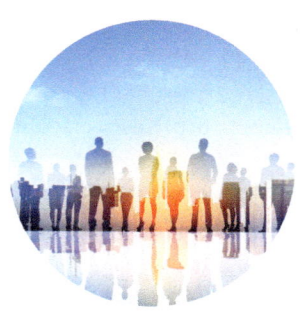

Boxes, Figures, and Tables

BOXES

FIGURES

TABLES

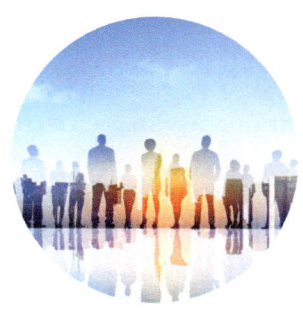

Acronyms and Abbreviations

ACA   Patient Protection and Affordable Care Act
ACF   Administration for Children and Families
ACL   Administration for Community Living
AHRQ   Agency for Healthcare Research and Quality
ASLA   American Society of Landscape Architects
ASPR   Assistant Secretary for Preparedness and Response
ASTHO Association of State and Territorial Health Officials

CAN   Coordinated Assistance Network
CART   Citizens Advisory Recovery Team
CBITS   Cognitive-Behavioral Intervention for Trauma in Schools
CCDF   Child Care and Development Fund
CCP   Crisis Counseling Assistance and Training Program
CDBG   Community Development Block Grant
CDBG-DR Community Development Block Grant for Disaster Recovery
CDC   Centers for Disease Control and Prevention
CDFI   Community Development Financial Institution
CEHD   Center to Eliminate Health Disparities
CERA   Canterbury Earthquake Recovery Authority
CHNA   community health needs assessment
CHW   community health worker
CMS   Centers for Medicare & Medicaid Services
COAD   Community Organizations Active in Disaster
CONOPS Concept of Operations
COOP   continuity of operations
CPCB   Community Planning and Capacity Building

DCMP   Disaster Case Management Program
DHS   U.S. Department of Homeland Security

DMAT   disaster medical assistance team
DMORT   disaster mortuary operational response team
DOT   U.S. Department of Transportation
D-SNAP   Disaster-Supplemental Nutrition Assistance Program

EDA   Economic Development Administration
EMAC   Emergency Management Assistance Compact
EMPG   Emergency Management Performance Grant
EMTALA   Emergency Medical Treatment and Active Labor Act
EPA   U.S. Environmental Protection Agency
ESAR-VHP   Emergency System for Advance Registration of Volunteer Health Professionals
ESF   Emergency Support Function

FEMA   Federal Emergency Management Agency
FHA   Federal Housing Administration
FHWA   Federal Highway Administration
FQHC   federally qualified health center
FTA   Federal Transit Administration

GAO   U.S. Government Accountability Office
GIS   geographic information systems

HAvBED   Hospital Available Beds for Emergencies and Disasters
HDMT   Healthy Development Measurement Tool
HFA   Hyogo Framework for Action
HHS   U.S. Department of Health and Human Services
HIA   health impact assessment
HiAP   Health in All Policies
HIPAA   Health Insurance Portability and Accountability Act
HMGP   Hazard Mitigation Grant Program
HPP   Hospital Preparedness Program
HSGP   Homeland Security Grant Program
HUD   U.S. Department of Housing and Urban Development
HVA   hazard vulnerability assessment

IOM   Institute of Medicine
IRS   Internal Revenue Service
IT   information technology

LACCDR   Los Angeles County Community Disaster Resilience
LEED   Leadership in Energy & Environmental Design
LEED-ND   Leadership in Energy & Environmental Design for Neighborhood Development
LTRC   long-term recovery committee

MAPP   Mobilizing for Action through Planning and Partnerships
MARC   multi-agency resource/relief center
MOA   memorandum of agreement
MPO   metropolitan planning organization
MRC   Medical Reserve Corps

NACCHO   National Association of County and City Health Officials
NDRF   National Disaster Recovery Framework
NEN   Neighborhood Empowerment Network
NEPA   National Environmental Policy Act
NGO   nongovernmental organization
NHSS   National Health Security Strategy
NHTSA   National Highway Traffic Safety Administration
NIH   National Institutes of Health
NRF   National Response Framework

PA   Public Assistance
PAHPA   Pandemic and All-Hazards Preparedness Act
PCCI   Parkland Center for Clinical Innovation
PCMH   patient-centered medical home
PDM   Pre-Disaster Mitigation
PDRP   post-disaster redevelopment plan
PFA   psychological first aid
PHEP   Public Health Emergency Preparedness
PTSD   posttraumatic stress disorder

RSF   Recovery Support Function

SAMHSA   Substance Abuse and Mental Health Services Administration
SBA   Small Business Administration
SCI   Sustainable Communities Index
SERG   SAMHSA's Emergency Response Grant
SFRA   San Francisco Redevelopment Agency
SNAP   Supplemental Nutrition Assistance Program
SPR   skills for psychological recovery
SSBG   Social Services Block Grant
SSBG-DR   Social Services Block Grant for Disaster Recovery

TAC   Technical Advisory Committee
TF-CBT   trauma-focused cognitive-behavioral therapy
THIRA   threat and hazard identification and risk assessment
TIF   tax increment financing
TIGER   Transportation Investment Generating Economic Recovery

UNISDR   United Nations International Strategy for Disaster Reduction
USDA   U.S. Department of Agriculture

VA   U.S. Department of Veterans Affairs
VOAD   Voluntary Organizations Active in Disaster

WHO   World Health Organization
WIC   Special Supplemental Nutrition Program for Women, Infants, and Children

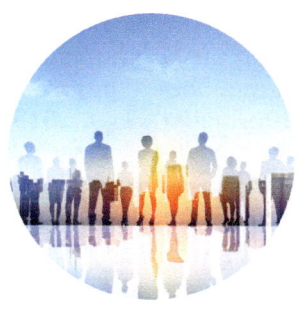

Glossary

Community health assessment[1]	A systematic examination of the health status indicators for a given population that is used to identify key problems and assets in a community. The ultimate goal of a community health assessment is to develop strategies to address the community's health needs and identified issues. A variety of tools and processes may be used to conduct a community health assessment; the essential ingredients are community engagement and collaborative participation (PHAB, 2013, p. 10).
Disaster	A serious disruption of the functioning of a community or a society involving widespread human, material, economic or environmental losses and impacts, which exceeds the ability of the affected community or society to cope using its own resources (United Nations, 2009).
Hazard mitigation	Cost-effective action taken to prevent or reduce the threat of future damage to a facility (FEMA, 2007, p. 24).
Health impact assessment	A systematic process that uses an array of data sources and analytic methods and considers input from stakeholders to determine the potential effects of a proposed policy, plan, program, or project on the health of a population and the distribution of those effects within the population. Health impact assessment provides recommendations on monitoring and managing those effects (NRC, 2011, p. 1).

---

[1] Community health assessment is also sometimes referred to as a community health needs assessment.

Health in All Policies An approach to public policies across sectors that systematically takes into account the health implications of decisions, seeks synergies, and avoids harmful health impacts, in order to improve population health and health equity (WHO, 2013).

Healthy community One in which a diverse group of stakeholders collaborate to use their expertise and local knowledge to create a community that is socially and physically conducive to health. Community members are empowered and civically engaged, assuring that all local policies consider health. The community has the capacity to identify, address, and evaluate their own health concerns on an ongoing basis, using data to guide and benchmark efforts. As a result, a healthy community is safe, economically secure, and environmentally sound, as all residents have equal access to high quality educational and employment opportunities, transportation and housing options, prevention and health care services, and healthy food and physical activity opportunities (HRIA, 2013).

Population health The health outcomes of a group of individuals, including the distribution of such outcomes within the group (Kindig and Stoddart, 2003).

Resilience The ability to prepare and plan for, absorb, recover from, and more successfully adapt to adverse events (NRC, 2012, p. 1).

Social determinants of health The conditions in which people are born, grow, live, work, and age. These circumstances are shaped by the distribution of money, power, and resources at global, national, and local levels (WHO, 2014).

Sustainability The ability of communities to consistently thrive over time as they make decisions to improve the community today without sacrificing the future (McGalliard, 2012).

REFERENCES

FEMA (Federal Emergency Management Agency). 2007. *Public assistance guide*. Washington, DC: FEMA.

HRIA (Health Resources in Action). 2013. *Defining healthy communities*. http://hria.org/uploads/catalogerfiles/defining-healthy-communities/defining_healthy_communities_1113_final_report.pdf (accessed October 21, 2014).

Kindig, D., and G. Stoddart. 2003. What is population health? *American Journal of Public Health* 93(3):381.

McGalliard, T. 2012. Reframing the sustainability conversation from what to how. *Public Management* 94:2.

NRC (National Research Council). 2011. *Improving health in the United States: The role of health impact assessment*. Washington, DC: The National Academies Press.

NRC. 2012. *Disaster resilience: A national imperative*. Washington, DC: The National Academies Press.

PHAB (Public Health Accreditation Board). 2013. *PHAB acronyms and glossary of terms version 1.5*. http://www.phaboard.org/wp-content/uploads/FINAL_PHAB-Acronyms-and-Glossary-of-Terms-Version-1.5.pdf (accessed October 30, 2014).

Rudolph, L., J. Caplan, K. Ben-Moshe, and L. Dillon. 2013. *Health in All Policies: A guide for state and local governments*. Washington, DC, and Oakland, CA: American Public Health Association and Public Health Institute.

United Nations. 2009. *UNISDR terminology on disaster risk reduction*. Geneva, Switzerland: United Nations Office for Disaster Risk Reduction.

WHO (World Health Organization). 2013. *Health in All Policies*. http://www.healthpromotion2013.org/health-promotion/health-in-all-policies (accessed December 4, 2014).

WHO. 2014. *Social determinants of health*. http://www.who.int/social_determinants/en (accessed October 30, 2014).

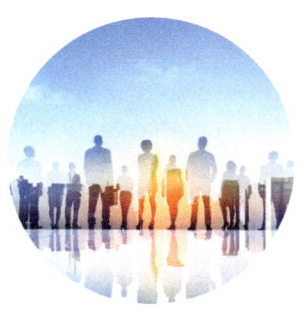

Abstract

Disasters often impact fundamental elements of a community—physical infrastructure, health and social services, social connectedness—that affect the health of its residents. Accordingly, the recovery period, with its attendant influx of resources and synchronization of planning processes, presents an important opportunity to redesign physical and social environments in a manner that will improve a community's long-term health status while simultaneously reducing its vulnerability to future hazards. In response to concerns that health considerations are not adequately incorporated into disaster recovery decision making, the Institute of Medicine assembled an ad hoc committee to develop recommendations and guidance on strategies for mitigating disaster-related health impacts and optimizing the use of recovery resources and pursue more deliberately and thoughtfully the goal of healthier and more resilient and sustainable communities.

The committee found that, although there is growing emphasis on incorporating resilience-building efforts into the recovery process, such efforts tend to focus on hardening critical infrastructure and not on strengthening the health and resiliency of individuals and communities. Unfortunately, the idea of using disaster recovery efforts to enhance the health of communities and their residents is not widespread. The committee noted few communities taking this forward-looking and synergistic approach; as a result, important opportunities are being missed.

Recognizing that disaster recovery is a process of community strategic planning and that communities can build on prior strategic planning initiatives and cross-sector collaborations, the committee developed a framework for integrating health considerations into recovery decision making. Each step in the strategic planning process presents opportunities for this integration:

- **Visioning**—Recovery is viewed as an opportunity to advance a shared vision of a healthier and more resilient and sustainable community.
- **Assessment**—Community health assessments and hazard vulnerability assessments provide data that show the gaps between the community's current status and desired state and inform the development of goals, priorities, and strategies.
- **Planning**—Health considerations are incorporated into recovery decision making across all sectors. This integration is facilitated by involving the health sector in integrated planning activities and by ensuring that decision makers are sensitized to the potential health impacts of all recovery decisions.

- **Implementation**—Recovery resources are used in creative and synergistic ways so that the actions of the health sector maximize health outcomes and the actions of other sectors yield co-benefits for health. A learning process is instituted so that the impacts of recovery activities on health and well-being are continuously evaluated and used to inform iterative decision making.

In this report, the committee presents 12 recommendations, along with sector-specific guidance, that provide strategies for leveraging each of these opportunities. Success, however, will depend on breaking down the barriers to cross-sector collaboration, thereby enabling community planners, emergency managers, health professionals, and other key governmental and nongovernmental stakeholders to come together around a shared goal, with each sector bringing its resources (knowledge, tools, funding streams) to bear. The end result will be a community that is a healthier, more livable place in which current and future generations can grow and thrive, and one better prepared for future adversities.

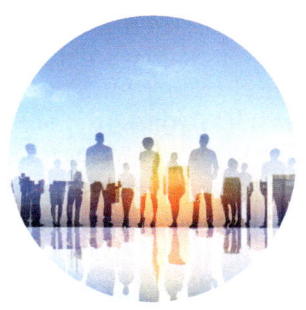

Summary

Disasters are by their very nature devastating to communities,[1] often having significant and long-lasting individual- and population-level effects on physical, mental, and social well-being in communities where health in many cases already is suboptimal. In addition to the tragic loss of human life and devastating health consequences for survivors, disasters often necessitate billions of dollars in public, private, and philanthropic expenditures for recovery assistance. Depending on the nature of the disaster and its impact, these expenditures may support strategic planning and decision making on resource allocation; rebuilding of critical public infrastructure, homes, and businesses; workforce development; provision of health and human services; and restoration of care delivery systems. Given the poor health status characterizing so many American communities and the associated financial and societal costs, the traditional characterization of disaster recovery as a process that restores a community to pre-disaster conditions is shortsighted. This report illustrates how the process of preparing for disasters and the comprehensive array of short- and long-term recovery activities represent a continuum of opportunities that, if exploited thoughtfully, can advance the long-term health, resilience, and sustainability of a community and its residents. Pursuit of this underrealized social goal begins with a vision of a healthy, resilient, and sustainable community and requires a recovery approach that incorporates health considerations into every step of the planning process, informed by an assessment of community health and vulnerability.

STUDY CHARGE AND SCOPE

Disaster recovery is a developing discipline that is creating an experiential-based fund of knowledge with insights into community strategic planning and redevelopment, economic revitalization, and health and human services delivery, among other fields. The collective body of knowledge stemming from these continuously learning laboratories represents an invaluable resource to recovering communities and the local officials who must make difficult decisions in the face of uncertainty, armed only with the best information available. Accordingly, there is a need to make lessons learned from past disasters available to guide

---

[1] Community can be defined in multiple ways—for example, as a population of individuals that share a geographic area, a culture, religious beliefs, or self-defined interests. For communities defined by geographic area, the scale varies from the macro (e.g., the national level) to the hyperlocal (the neighborhood or even block level). For the purposes of this report, the term "community" refers to a community of place at the city or county level, unless otherwise indicated.

those decisions and for leaders at all levels to act on them. Recognizing a need for better dissemination of this knowledge and evidence to enable communities to build capacity and to support more informed decision making, the Office of the Assistant Secretary for Preparedness and Response (ASPR) at the U.S. Department of Health and Human Services (HHS), the Office of Lead Hazard Control and Healthy Homes at the U.S. Department of Housing and Urban Development (HUD), the Veterans Health Administration at the Department of Veterans Affairs, and the Robert Wood Johnson Foundation requested that the Institute of Medicine convene the committee that conducted this study. The committee was charged with developing recommendations and guidance on how local and national leaders can mitigate disaster-related health impacts and optimize use of disaster resources—which inevitably must be spent in rebuilding—to pursue more proactively, deliberately, and thoughtfully the goal of creating communities that are healthier and more resilient (see Box S-1).

This report is organized into three parts: Part I sets forth the committee's strategic framework for building healthier and more resilient and sustainable post-disaster communities, while Part II provides operational-level guidance on sector-specific strategies for achieving this goal. Part III provides the report appendixes. The scope of the report is intentionally broad, with the aim of fostering the integration of health considerations into recovery decision making across a range of disciplines and stakeholder groups. The committee's recommendations and guidance, therefore, are not specific to any particular disaster scenarios but are meant to be tailored for relevance to local realities and the nature and scale of the incident.

AUDIENCES FOR THIS REPORT

This report is directed at several key audiences that fall into two groups—those individuals and organizations involved in planning for and carrying out disaster recovery activities and those involved in planning for and building healthy communities. Through this report, the committee endeavors to bring these two stakeholder groups together so that a health lens is applied to disaster recovery planning, and the menu of tools and resources for health improvement planners is expanded to include those associated with disaster planning and recovery activities. The constituents of these two groups include

- state, local, tribal, and territorial[2] elected and public officials who typically hold leadership roles in emergency management and strategic planning (i.e., governors, mayors, city managers and council members, emergency managers, disaster recovery coordinators);
- state, local, tribal, and territorial public health officials;
- infrastructure support professionals such as those in the fields of urban and regional planning, housing, transportation, and public works;
- federal agency stakeholders;
- health care delivery professionals and organizational leaders;
- social services professionals;
- community support (including faith-based) organizations and nongovernmental organizations;
- schools and education sector leaders;
- private-sector stakeholders; and
- empowered community members.

A FRAMEWORK FOR INTEGRATING HEALTH INTO DISASTER RECOVERY

Disaster recovery is a process of strategic community planning similar to that which takes place in communities throughout the country every day, except for the tremendous challenges of time compression—planning processes that would have occurred over decades are compressed into a relatively brief period of

---

[2] Throughout this report, the phrase "state and local" is used for the purposes of brevity but should be inferred to include tribal and territorial leaders.

BOX S-1
Statement of Task for the Committee on Post-Disaster Recovery of
a Community's Public Health, Medical, and Social Services

An ad hoc committee will conduct a study and issue a report on how to improve the short-, intermediate-, and long-term health outcomes and public health impact for individuals in a community of place (as contrasted with communities of faith, identity, etc.). The committee will investigate and identify key activities that impact health and public health outcomes in a community of place recovering from a disaster, and develop recommendations for their implementation. In doing so, the committee will consider the determinants of health and how various activities could leverage those determinants to improve health in the post-disaster setting, including the needs of at-risk populations.

The committee will do this by identifying (based in part on a literature review of domestic and international disasters) and recommending a series of recovery practices and novel programs most likely to impact overall community public health and contribute to resiliency for future incidents in the short-, intermediate-, and long-term period during disaster response and following incident stabilization. Specifically the committee will:

- Examine existing guidance and frameworks, peer-reviewed literature, and case studies from post-disaster response and recovery operations;
  - Characterize and identify key determinants of pre- and post-disaster public health, medical, and social services that may serve as indicators for the affected population's long-term recovery, from various perspectives amongst the different levels of government and nongovernment actors generally located within a community of place;
  - Ascertain which other sectors are responsible for, or have the organizational interest and capacity for, directly affecting the identified determinants, and identify opportunities for collaborative engagement or support amongst those sectors;
- Identify practical guidance for recovery practices and programs for each sector that will benefit community post-disaster health and public health outcomes in the short-, intermediate-, and long-term.
  - Consider how community needs may be integrated into health recovery efforts.
  - Consider any key determinants, differences, and similarities in recovery between rural and urban communities; among household-income strata; among single-family, low-rise multifamily, and high-rise multifamily housing, among households receiving government assistance and unassisted households, etc.
  - Consider how long-term gains for health may be achieved through investments in community, housing, and other non-traditional health infrastructures.
- Identify areas of research that should be explored to answer key questions about where to direct resources before, during, and after an event occurs.

time. Beginning the process before a disaster and leveraging the products of other steady-state community planning processes (as shown in Figure S-1) can make post-disaster recovery planning more efficient but also ensure that opportunities for community betterment (including health improvement) are not missed.

Unfortunately, the committee found that the model that currently predominates is one whereby the development of community comprehensive plans,[3] health improvement plans, hazard mitigation plans, sustainability plans, and disaster recovery plans occurs largely in isolation. The general structure of such planning processes is similar. An initial period of laying the groundwork often is followed by a visioning

---

[3] The comprehensive plan, also known as the general plan, is the product of a community's comprehensive planning process, which is used to determine community goals and aspirations for future community development.

process and an assessment of community status and needs, assets, and contextual factors (e.g., the political environment). The results of these two processes are used to establish goals and set priorities by comparing the findings of the assessment against the community's vision to identify gaps between the community's current status and desired state. Strategies are developed to close the gaps through stakeholder (including public) input and analysis of alternatives. These strategies are incorporated into a plan, and implementation partnerships (or operational structures) are developed. Finally, the plan is implemented. Resources are identified and applied, and ideally, progress is continuously measured using preestablished benchmarks. Thus, the process of implementation feeds into a continuous cycle of assessment, planning, and implementation. This strategic planning process offers a framework for integrating health considerations into recovery—each of the steps in the cycle presents opportunities:

Visioning: Recovery is viewed as an opportunity to advance a shared vision of a healthier, more resilient, and sustainable community.

Assessment: Community health assessments and hazard vulnerability assessments provide data that show the gaps between the community's current status and desired state and inform the development of goals, priorities, and strategies.

Planning: Health considerations are incorporated into recovery decision making across all sectors. This integration is facilitated by involving the health sector in integrated planning activities and by ensuring that decision makers are sensitized to the potential health impacts of all recovery decisions.

Implementation: Recovery resources are used in creative and synergistic ways so that the actions of the health sector maximize health outcomes and the actions of other sectors yield co-benefits for health. A learning process is instituted so that the impacts of recovery activities on health and well-being are continuously evaluated and used to inform iterative decision making.

A HEALTHY, RESILIENT, SUSTAINABLE COMMUNITY RECOVERY VISION

Disasters, although unquestionable tragedies, can provide communities access to previously unavailable resources and opportunities for transformation to advance a vision of a healthier and more resilient and sustainable community. However, leveraging the disaster recovery process to this end necessitates an understanding of the diverse determinants that influence health and healthy communities. It is increasingly understood that health is influenced largely by the locally specific built, natural, and social environments within communities—the social determinants of health, defined by the World Health Organization as "the conditions in which people are born, grow, live, work, and age. These circumstances are shaped by the distribution of money, power, and resources at global, national, and local levels" (WHO, 2014). For the purposes of this report, the committee adopted the following definition of a healthy community proposed by the National Network of Public Health Institutes:

> A healthy community is one in which a diverse group of stakeholders collaborate to use their expertise and local knowledge to create a community that is socially and physically conducive to health. Community members are empowered and civically engaged, assuring that all local policies consider health. The community has the capacity to identify, address, and evaluate their own health concerns on an ongoing basis, using data to guide and benchmark efforts. As a result, a healthy community is safe, economically secure, and environmentally sound, as all residents have equal access to high quality educational and employment opportunities, transportation and housing options, prevention and healthcare services, and healthy food and physical activity opportunities. (HRIA, 2013, p. 24)

Emerging from this definition are underlying themes of equity, resilience, and sustainability. Health, equity, resilience, and sustainability are interdependent and mutually reinforcing—part of the same vir-

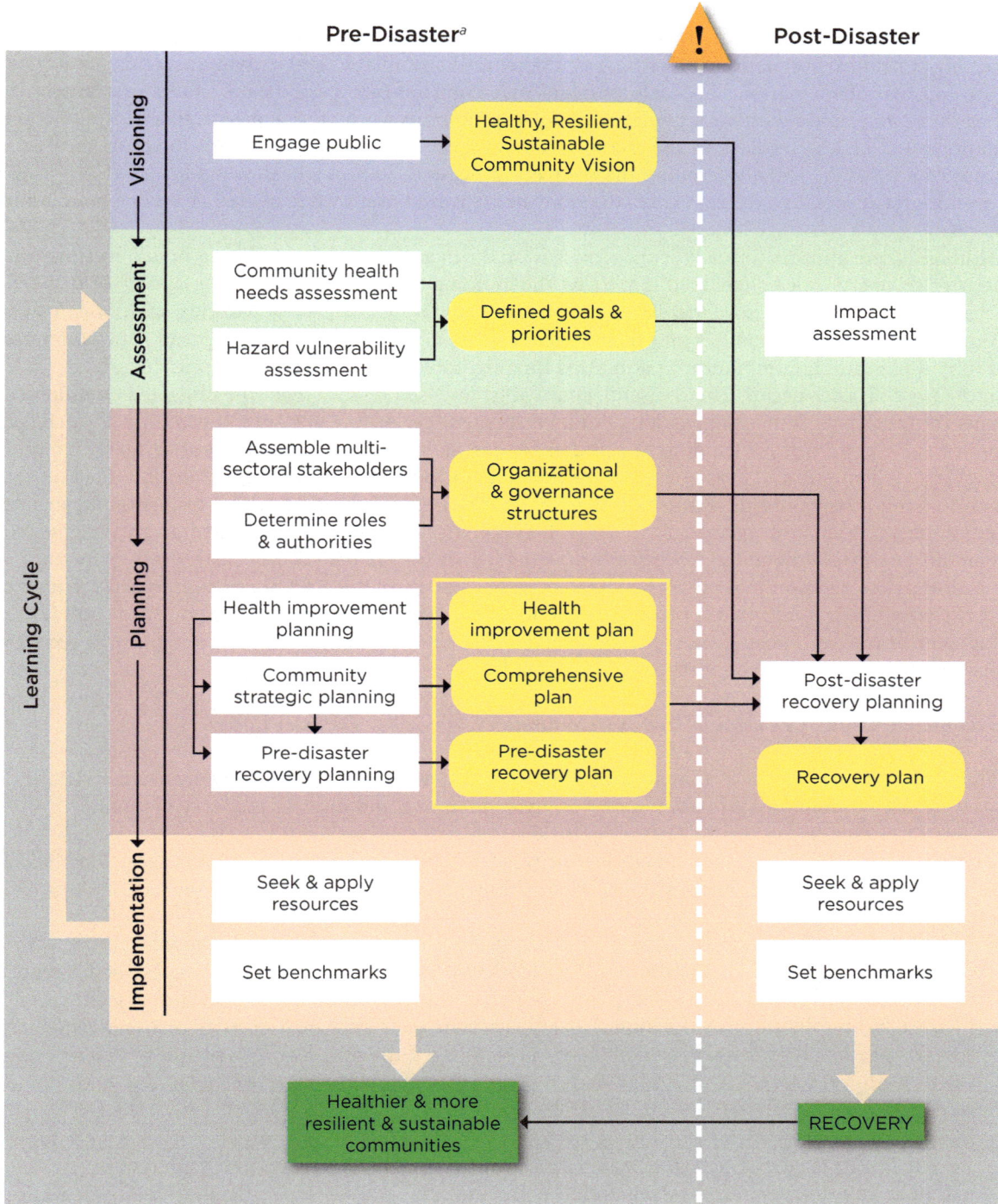

FIGURE S-1 Leveraging the products of pre-disaster planning processes to support a healthy community approach to disaster recovery.

a Although the committee strongly encourages communities to undertake these activities in the pre-disaster period to maximize opportunities for leveraging the post-event recovery process to create healthier and more resilient and sustainable communities, there is still benefit to incorporating them into post-disaster recovery planning if they have not been undertaken beforehand.

tuous cycle. As a result of this interdependence, initiatives that reduce inequities will yield ancillary or co-benefits for population health, as will efforts to strengthen a community's sustainability or resilience. Conversely, a healthy population is a critical component of sustainable and thriving economic and social systems and a resilient nation. The determinants that contribute to poor health status are largely the same as those associated with social vulnerability. A community with large concentrations of vulnerable populations will be less resilient in the face of social and economic disruption and slower to recover in the event of a disaster. Thus, leveraging the recovery process to improve health and health equity is not only an important social goal and a cost containment measure but also a means of achieving community health resilience—a national strategic priority.

Although there appears to be growing emphasis on the incorporation of resilience-building efforts into the disaster recovery process (spurred in part by the looming threat of climate change), such efforts tend to focus on critical infrastructure instead of people. Unfortunately, the idea of working simultaneously to enhance the health of communities and their residents does not appear to be widespread. The committee noted only a handful of communities taking this forward-looking and synergistic approach.

In the post-disaster period, there is, understandably, intense pressure from the impacted community's residents to return to a state of normalcy as quickly as possible. As a result, attempts to address deficiencies in pre-event conditions (including health deficiencies and disparities) through post-disaster planning alone will be challenging and may not be successful. Integration of health considerations into the recovery decision-making process for all sectors will depend on a shared vision of a healthy, resilient, and sustainable community. What this means for an individual community needs to be defined as an integral part of community strategic planning processes conducted before an event so that a clear vision is in place to drive post-disaster decision making as new resources become available and opportunities arise. Unfortunately, the committee found that a healthy, resilient, and sustainable community vision rarely guides the development of pre- and post-disaster recovery plans; as a result, a health lens is not applied to recovery decision making, and unique opportunities are missed.

Recommendation 1: *Develop a Healthy Community Vision for Disaster Recovery.*

The committee recommends that state and local elected and public officials incorporate a vision for a healthy community into community strategic planning and disaster recovery planning.

Implementation of this recommendation will require action at the state and local as well as federal levels. Specifically, at the state and local levels, the following actions should be taken:

- Public health leaders should enhance health improvement planning through engagement with a comprehensive group of community stakeholders (representing each of the audiences for this report, as outlined above) and ensure that plans are based on the community's needs and assets.
- Elected and public officials, including emergency managers and local disaster recovery managers, should together lead relevant stakeholders in risk-based disaster recovery planning that develops the procedures, processes, and administrative arrangements to be used for integrated, coordinated recovery.
- Elected and public officials, including emergency managers and local disaster recovery managers, should integrate public health officials and health improvement plans into community strategic planning and disaster recovery planning before and after a disaster. To facilitate that integration, the community's needs and plans for health improvement should be reflected in disaster recovery priorities.

At the federal level, a coordinated, interagency effort is needed to support state and local stakeholders in the development of recovery plans that ensure that communities build back stronger. To this end, the committee believes that aligned grant guidance and technical assistance are essential motivators. Alignment is key to promoting synergy and ensuring that opportunities are not missed. Federal agencies should use existing grant programs to enhance the capacity of state and local stakeholders to plan for and implement a healthy community perspective in disaster recovery. Specifically, federal agencies should take the following actions:

- HHS, HUD, the U.S. Department of Transportation (DOT), the U.S. Environmental Protection Agency (EPA), and other federal agencies should use aligned grant guidance and technical assistance for existing and future grant programs to incentivize preparedness, community health, and community development grantees to collaborate on the integration of local health improvement goals into comprehensive plans and disaster recovery plans.
- The Centers for Disease Control and Prevention (CDC) and ASPR should revise preparedness grant guidance related to the recovery capability to include greater focus on long-term recovery and opportunities for using recovery to advance healthier and more resilient and sustainable communities.
- The Federal Emergency Management Agency (FEMA) should incentivize emergency management preparedness program grantees to incorporate health considerations into recovery planning by providing grant guidance and technical assistance aligned with HHS guidance.

A HEALTH IN ALL POLICIES APPROACH TO DISASTER RECOVERY

Intentional consideration of health, including health equity, is needed during recovery to mitigate the negative effects of disasters and seize opportunities to advance population health and well-being. Health in All Policies (HiAP) is "an approach to public policies across sectors that systematically takes into account the health implications of decisions, seeks synergies, and avoids harmful health impacts, in order to improve population health and health equity" (WHO, 2013). Motivation for a HiAP approach comes from understanding that health is essential to achieving a strong economy and a vibrant society, but that health outcomes are influenced by social and physical environments shaped by decisions made outside of the health sector. The committee asserts not only that the aftermath of a disaster is a prime opportunity to apply a HiAP approach but also that there is in fact an acute need for such an approach. The health sector acting alone cannot be successful in addressing the complex population health challenges faced by communities, particularly after a disaster. As a result of the failure to apply a HiAP approach more broadly, the health sector, like many others involved in disaster recovery, has tended to act in isolation rather than as part of a coordinated multidisciplinary group. HiAP in the disaster recovery context is about (1) creating organizational structures that optimally enable the coordination of efforts and the creation of synergies where core missions of other sectors align with healthy community objectives, and (2) ensuring that information on the potential health impacts of recovery decisions is available to the decision makers within those structures.

Organizing for an Integrated Approach

The HiAP concept is compatible with the "whole-community" approach to integrated disaster recovery now being promoted by FEMA and others. In a whole-community approach, government, the nonprofit sector, and the private sector work together as partners. Success depends on (1) the development of organizational and governance structures that create efficient and informed networks for decision making, and (2) a robust engagement process that encourages the participation of all community stakeholders (governmental and nongovernmental), including the community's residents.

Establishing Organizational and Governance Structures

Communities are complex systems in which decision making is distributed and myriad cross-sector interdependencies exist. Organizational structures influence the siloing of related services and functions, which can impede potential synergies and co-benefits. As a result, successful recovery requires a governance structure that promotes integration across the full range of stakeholder groups, both horizontally and vertically, so that capabilities and resources, both public and private, are leveraged in a coordinated manner to achieve the best outcome for the community as a whole. All communities have structures and processes in place during steady-state periods to support multisector approaches to strategic decision making regarding investments and prioritization. Among these structures and processes are ongoing collaborations inclusive of governmental and nongovernmental organizations that address a community's health and social service needs. The task for decision makers in the development of recovery governance structures is to ensure that collaborative arrangements operating prior to a disaster are added to the list of organizational assets and incorporated into the recovery planning effort.

The National Disaster Recovery Framework (NDRF), released in 2011, guides the establishment of an overarching multistakeholder coordination structure and may provide a means of integrating existing health-related community collaborations into a recovery governance structure, although optimal arrangements for doing so have not yet been elucidated (FEMA, 2011). Health and social services are represented prominently as one of six Recovery Support Functions (RSFs) defined in the NDRF. However, since the activities of all sectors will impact health during recovery, either positively or negatively, the committee concludes that health impacts need to be considered in disaster recovery decisions related to each of the other RSFs.

> **Recommendation 2:** *Integrate Health Considerations into Recovery Decision Making Through the National Disaster Recovery Framework.*
>
> **The committee recommends that the Federal Emergency Management Agency (FEMA) and the five other federal agencies that represent coordinating agencies for the Recovery Support Functions take steps to further develop and promote the National Disaster Recovery Framework (NDRF) as the basis for a locally defined organizing structure for disaster recovery at the state and local levels to promote information sharing and alignment of funding streams. Further, to ensure that health considerations are integrated into all recovery operations, FEMA, in consultation with the U.S. Department of Health and Human Services (HHS), should update the NDRF to explicitly include health implications for the activities of all Recovery Support Functions.**
>
> **State and local elected and public officials should establish a steering committee to guide the development of an operational structure that incorporates the organizing principles of the NDRF— including a disaster recovery coordinator and the Recovery Support Functions—and builds on existing collaborative municipal and civic structures, authorities, and initiatives.**

Engaging the Whole Community in Recovery Planning

Successful recovery and the post-disaster rebuilding of healthier and more resilient and sustainable communities require the coordinated efforts of a broad multidisciplinary group of stakeholders from health and nonhealth sectors (i.e., a whole-community approach). Yet many of these stakeholders are unaccustomed to working in the emergency management context and unfamiliar with its processes, terminology, and resources. Following a review of the federal grey literature related to recovery and hearing testimony from experts at the federal, state, and local levels, the committee was concerned by how difficult it is for key stakeholders outside of (and even within) the emergency management field to understand the relationships among the array of federal, state, and local resources that must be mobilized after a disaster; how they interrelate; and who is accountable at each level. The committee concludes that the federal government needs to make information on federal recovery resources and the processes by which they are mobilized available in a simplified and more accessible manner to facilitate maximum involvement by all stakeholders. Further, those leading recovery planning need to be sensitized and trained on the importance of engaging all relevant stakeholder groups, including the health and human services sectors, through robust outreach efforts. Key stakeholders themselves similarly need to be educated on the importance of their participation and mechanisms by which they should engage proactively in the disaster recovery process.

Recommendation 3: *Facilitate the Engagement of the Whole Community in Disaster Recovery Through Simplified and Accessible Information and Training.*

To facilitate the engagement of the whole community in building healthier communities after disasters, the Federal Emergency Management Agency should lead an interagency effort centered on increasing the accessibility and coherence of information related to disaster recovery and the provision of relevant training.

Priorities should include

- the development of educational materials, including a single overarching federal document that serves as a primer on the recovery process and is easily accessible on the Web regardless of the pathway by which a stakeholder seeks to enter the recovery planning process;
- the development of companion guidance documents for state, local, and nongovernmental stakeholders for each of the Recovery Support Functions, providing more detailed descriptions that facilitate stakeholder understanding of available resources, best practices, and the pathways by which they can engage in the pre- and post-disaster recovery planning processes; and
- the development of coordinated training programs for stakeholders and their professional societies that raise awareness of threats and opportunities related to health and promote broad stakeholder participation in recovery planning under the NDRF.

Training programs should

- sensitize stakeholders to the importance of short-term health protection concerns and long-term opportunities to build healthier communities during recovery, highlighting the critical role of each sector in advancing community health, resilience, and sustainability;
- strengthen connections among emergency management, public health, community development, community planning, human services, and other stakeholder organizations to better prepare them to work together within the structure of the NDRF to increase the chances that recovery resources will be used for creating healthier communities; and
- raise awareness of steady-state community planning processes and administrative structures (partnerships and municipal and civic structures) and mechanisms for leveraging these existing processes and structures by identifying key partnerships and professional resources/sources of technical assistance.

The involvement of informed and empowered community members through an authentic and robust outreach and engagement process is nearly universally recognized as a factor that determines the success of any community planning endeavor, including disaster recovery. Using an inclusive process that leverages existing community organizations and social networks builds trust, creates a sense of ownership, and ensures that recovery decisions align with the community's vision. After disasters, community planning initiatives that utilize equitable processes and increase interaction among residents also can build social capital—the social ties that are an integral feature of a community—promoting healing, restoring the social fabric of the community, and strengthening resilience. Local governments, by partnering with schools, neighborhood associations, community groups, and private businesses, can help foster the collaborative potential and sense of community ownership that are critical to optimal community health improvement and recovery planning.

Recommendation 4: *Enhance and Leverage Social Networks in Community Health Improvement and Recovery Planning.*

Local elected and public officials should develop and support programs designed to strengthen social networks and deepen trust among community members before and after disasters, thereby increasing resilience. Strategies for enhancing and preserving social networks should be specifically included in community health improvement and disaster recovery plans. Before and after a disaster, existing social networks, such as neighborhood associations, should be leveraged to enhance mechanisms for integrating the community into recovery planning.

Informing Recovery Decision Making Through Health Information

Organizational structures provide the necessary scaffolding to support decision-making processes but by themselves are not sufficient. The effectiveness of an integrated planning and recovery approach is greatly enhanced by shared information. At the same time that operational structures for recovery are being developed and exercised, pathways for sharing information, including health information, need to be evaluated and delineated. To this end, a pre-disaster investment in infrastructure—and in some cases, data-sharing agreements—is required. Continuous evaluation of health and recovery indicators through a learning system approach enables decision makers to evaluate progress toward a healthy, resilient, and sustainable community vision and adapt future recovery management strategies as needed.

Recommendation 5: *Establish Pathways by Which Health Information Can Inform Recovery Decision Making.*

State and local elected and public officials should ensure that clear pathways for integration and dissemination of health information are established, including mechanisms that enable concerns and priorities of community members to be transmitted to disaster recovery decision makers. Additionally, a continual feedback process should be established to allow for updating to reflect changes in conditions and measured progress toward recovery. Thus, indicators for measuring progress and success should be (1) developed, (2) incorporated into pre-disaster recovery plans, and (3) updated after a disaster based on its health impact.

Several kinds of information can be used to support the incorporation of health considerations into the recovery decision-making process to improve health outcomes after a disaster. These include (1) knowledge of the potential health impacts of alternatives being considered; (2) historical knowledge from past disaster experiences and, in particular, information on effective (and ineffective) practices; (3) knowledge of available resources; and (4) up-to-date information on health status and human needs. Reliable sources of each of these kinds of information should be identified in advance of a disaster as part of pre-event planning. Sources of such information include

- health impact assessments;
- guidance, training, and technical assistance; and
- health information systems.

Leveraging Recovery Resources to Improve Health, Resilience, and Sustainability

Although a diverse set of resources (federal, state, private, philanthropic) becomes available after a disaster to support the rebuilding of community features and the restoration of services that impact health, these resources often are not mobilized with the conscious goal of advancing a vision of a healthier and more resilient and sustainable community. The committee concludes that communities are missing opportunities during the post-disaster recovery process to maximize the health benefits that can be derived from the resources applied by nonhealth sectors in the course of achieving their sector-specific goals. Funders need to take steps to ensure that recovery decision makers use financial resources more effectively to achieve such synergies. To this end, it will be necessary to apply a coordinated approach and remove impediments that restrict the flow of funds across vertical hierarchies and their creative use to address multiple priorities simultaneously.

Recommendation 6: *Leverage Recovery Resources in a Coordinated Manner to Achieve Healthier Post-Disaster Communities.*

Federal agencies (the Federal Emergency Management Agency [FEMA], the U.S. Department of Housing and Urban Development [HUD], the U.S. Department of Health and Human Services [HHS], the U.S. Department of Transportation [DOT], and other federal partners) providing funding for recovery, including pre-event recovery planning, should lead and promote an integrated recovery approach by

- aligning technical requirements and guidance for federal recovery funding opportunities within and across agencies around identified core needs;
- including a requirement and financial incentives for grantees to demonstrate how health considerations will be incorporated into short- and long-term recovery planning conducted using those funds; and
- identifying and removing disincentives that impede the coordination of efforts and the combining of different funding streams to support a healthy community approach to recovery.

Working with private and philanthropic organizations, elected and public officials should ensure that state and local funding regulations and guidelines are consistent with these federal integration efforts.

SECTOR-SPECIFIC STRATEGIES

Part II of this report presents the committee's recommendations and operational-level guidance for specific sectors, focusing on (1) health and human services strategies to support human recovery—the processes by which the physical and psychological health and social functioning of a community are restored; and (2) place-based recovery strategies that promote and protect health through alteration of a community's interconnected physical and social environments.

Health and Human Services Strategies

Activities of the health and human services sectors can improve post-disaster health outcomes in a number of ways. Key among these are (1) the delivery of services to meet the public health, medical, behavioral health, and social service needs of disaster survivors; and (2) the collection, assessment, and dissemination of health information to inform decision making during recovery. The three recommendations below represent strategic priorities necessary to support health and human services stakeholders at the state and local levels in carrying out these two key functions.

The best way to ensure that health information is available after a disaster is to ensure that the necessary infrastructure and expertise are in place beforehand. Thus, the threat of disaster provides an additional motivating factor for the establishment of health information technology infrastructure. In the event that such systems are not in place before a disaster, however, the recovery process can be leveraged to advance both infrastructure and plans for its use to ensure continuity of care and ongoing community health improvement after an event. The committee found that current information technology systems do not adequately support post-disaster coordination of health and human services at the individual and community levels.

Recommendation 7: *Ensure a Ready Health Information Technology Infrastructure.*

State and local governmental officials should ensure the necessary leadership and accountability to support establishment of the interconnected data systems and analytic capacity that are essential to the continuity of health care and social services delivery across the continuum of disaster response and recovery. To this end, coordination of efforts will be required among local and regional public health, health care, health insurance plans, private-sector information technology innovators and vendors, and regulatory and governmental stakeholders at all levels.

At the federal level, the Office of the National Coordinator for Health Information Technology should build on its current efforts and develop a 3-year implementation plan for health information technology integration. This plan should be designed to facilitate data sharing and portability of individual health records across health care settings in support of pre- and post-disaster recovery health care planning and optimal recovery of essential infrastructure for medical and behavioral health care, public health, and social services.

A disaster both increases human needs in a community and, as a result of disruption to the public health, health care, behavioral health, and social services systems that collectively support human recovery, diminishes a community's capacity to help individual community members and families recover. The committee observed significant gaps, siloing, and fragmentation in the systems needed to support human recovery. Clear, accountable leadership and a national strategy or framework for meeting these human recovery needs are notably lacking.

Recommendation 8: *Develop a National Disaster Behavioral Health Policy.*

The U.S. Department of Health and Human Services and the Federal Emergency Management Agency should engage state and local governments, as well as private- and nonprofit-sector stakeholders, in the development of a national disaster behavioral health policy. This policy should delineate the roles, responsibilities, and authorities of the federal government for optimal integration of behavioral health services across the continuum of health care, public health, social services, and all other sectors (e.g., housing, public safety, education) before, during, and after a disaster or other emergency.

To support the implementation of this recommendation, the following steps should be taken at the federal level:

- Federal agencies responsible for funding and developing behavioral health policy should support and collaborate with behavioral and other health professional societies to enhance national understanding of the importance of behavioral health to the realization of healthy communities so that this agenda will be included more effectively in general community health planning.
- HHS should use its preparedness funding requirements and currently existing collaborative bodies (e.g., Disaster Behavioral Health Preparedness Forum, Federal Community Health Resilience Coalition), as well as other mechanisms, to overcome the fragmentation of disaster behavioral health services and stimulate their coordination and integration with health care, social support, emergency management, and information technology services.
- HHS should commission a study to analyze current federal behavioral health programs and generate recommendations for efforts at the federal level to address the long-term behavioral health needs of individuals and communities after a disaster or other emergency.

At the state and local levels, the following steps should be taken:

- State and local government disaster preparedness, response, and recovery officials should make the necessary efforts to ensure that behavioral health professionals at all levels are included in disaster preparedness planning and in emergency operations centers after a disaster.
- State and local government public health and mental health officials, supported by federal preparedness funding from the Hospital Preparedness Program (HPP) and Public Health Emergency Preparedness (PHEP) cooperative agreements, should work together and with other key community stakeholders, including state and local emergency managers, to integrate behavioral health into efforts to build community resilience and enhance planning for long-term behavioral health recovery. Opportunities to leverage other funding sources, such as the Substance Abuse Prevention and Treatment Block Grant, Community Mental Health Services Block Grant, and Social Services Block Grant, should be evaluated.
- Given the scale and range of mental health consequences associated with disasters and the need for local capacity to support long-term behavioral health recovery, the adequacy of the behavioral health workforce to meet disaster-related needs should be enhanced. Efforts to this end should include pre-disaster identification of trained professionals; training and exercising of support personnel; attention to licensure and credentialing requirements; and coordination of government mental health care systems, community- and faith-based organizations, and for-profit provider companies.

Recommendation 9: *Develop an Integrated Social Services Recovery Framework.*

The U.S. Department of Health and Human Services should lead the development of an integrated post-disaster social services framework that more effectively meets human services needs during recovery.

The following steps should be taken to enable the development of the framework:

- ASPR should commission a study to analyze federal programs related to disaster recovery social services and to generate recommendations for decreasing duplication and fragmentation, streamlining processes, and optimally meeting the needs of the affected populations.
- Based on the results of this study, ASPR should work with federal and nonfederal partners—including but not limited to FEMA, HHS (including the Administration for Children and Families, the Substance Abuse and Mental Health Services Administration, and the Health Resources and Services Administration), HUD, the U.S. Department of Agriculture, the U.S. Department of Education, the U.S. Department of Veterans Affairs, the American Red Cross, and other appropriate nongovernmental organizations—to create a framework linking current and future funding sources, policies, and regulations to the recommended strategies for optimizing social services after disasters.
- The multiple federal agencies and nongovernmental organizations that provide day-to-day funding for human services and funding to support social services during recovery (including those agencies cited above) should condition funding on the creation by each state or municipality (in cases where large municipalities receive funding directly) of an integrated strategy for social services delivery. This strategy should be designed to facilitate the accessibility of these services through such means as collocation of services and data portability for disaster survivors.
- Departments responsible for human/social services within states and municipalities should serve as the coordinators for operationalizing the above strategy and for coordinating faith-based and other nongovernmental organizations as well as related state agencies that are implementing the post-disaster social services framework.

Place-Based Recovery Strategies

Disasters often necessitate significant efforts to restore the physical infrastructure of a community, including repair of roads and bridges, reconstruction of housing and other buildings, repair of public works, and restoration of natural resources. Rather than rebuilding to a prior state, the recovery process offers a unique opportunity to mitigate against future hazards and create environments intentionally designed to support health through healthier housing and community features that enhance active lifestyles and improve equitable access to critical goods (e.g., healthy food), community services (e.g., medical care), and amenities (e.g., libraries, schools, recreational/physical fitness facilities). A well-planned recovery also attends to the economic vitality of the affected area, seeking commercial revitalization, industrial and business development, and greater employment opportunities, thereby improving financial prospects for both residents and businesses. To ensure that these opportunities are not missed, professionals from diverse fields, including planning and design, housing, community development, environmental management, and public health, need to be engaged in the development of pre- and post-disaster recovery strategies, which should tie back to community plans to improve health and social well-being developed in advance of a disaster. Communities that have plans in hand when a disaster strikes are equipped to transition to recovery more quickly with a long-term objective of health, resilience, and sustainability. Given that the pool of resources for recovery is limited, creative uses of funds that meet multiple objectives simultaneously can improve the efficiency of recovery and the opportunities to integrate health considerations. Such opportunities deserve special attention in disaster recovery plans.

> **Recommendation 10:** *Design for Healthy Post-Disaster Communities.*
>
> **State and federal agencies (the Federal Emergency Management Agency, the U.S. Department of Transportation, the U.S. Department of Housing and Urban Development, the U.S. Environmental Protection Agency, the U.S. Department of Health and Human Services, and others), acting alone or as components of the federal Partnership for Sustainable Communities, should ensure through funding requirements that the use of federal community development and disaster recovery and preparedness funds optimizes the built environment in support of healthy communities by creating places that protect against health threats, promote good health, and address unmet social needs.**
>
> **Local and state planning entities should develop a team-based approach to integrated recovery planning aligned with the policies and processes of the Partnership for Sustainable Communities so as to maximize efficiency in the use of federal resources to enhance smart growth, equity, hazard mitigation, resilience, sustainability, and other elements necessary to the creation of healthy communities. Priority areas for funding should specifically address the following essential health-enhancing requirements that are pertinent to the community's needs as laid out in pre- and post-disaster health improvement and comprehensive plans:**
>
> - **physical activity-enhancing infrastructure that includes trails, bike paths, sidewalks, and parks and recreational spaces, as well as walkable, mixed-use neighborhood designs; and**
> - **comprehensive transportation infrastructure and land use policies that ensure the accessibility of healthy food retail outlets, employment, health and social services, schools, and community amenities such as libraries and community centers for all residents.**

Optimal health, social well-being, and safety are dependent on avoiding or reducing the impacts of disasters by using best practices of hazard mitigation, including both structural and nonstructural (e.g., zoning and land use) standards and strategies. Forward-looking strategic plans, improved infrastructure, and stronger construction codes need to be used in combination to address identified community vulnerabilities, thereby reversing the nation's trend toward higher disaster losses and the attendant human misery and social and economic costs, as well as preparing the nation for the potential effects of climate change.

Recommendation 11: *Mitigate Against Future Health Hazards.*

Building on the National Mitigation Framework, federal agencies, led by the Federal Emergency Management Agency, should immediately intensify their efforts, undertaken collectively and supported by aligned funding eligibility requirements, to ensure that all critical infrastructure and facilities—such as hospitals (public and private), nursing homes, fire stations, and public utilities—constructed after a disaster are designed and built with a level of protection that better ensures post-disaster safety and functionality essential to protecting health and recovering more quickly. When feasible, they should be located outside of known hazard zones. Additionally, requirements should ensure that existing critical infrastructure and facilities restored with federal recovery funds are upgraded to the new standards.

Housing meets some of people's most basic needs (shelter from the elements, privacy, a place of respite, and socialization). Disasters can compromise living conditions, making rapid and appropriate provision of housing after a disaster essential for health and well-being. However, it is also critical to ensure that the urgency of post-disaster housing reconstruction does not give rise to practices that compromise health and preclude opportunities to promote long-term housing affordability, resiliency, and sustainability.

Recommendation 12: *Ensure Healthy and Affordable Post-Disaster Housing.*

To reduce housing-related health risks, federal, state, and local governmental housing agencies should require that new residential construction and substantial rehabilitation of existing residences financed with public funds after disasters comply fully with Enterprise Green Communities standards or their equivalent and with the minimum requirements set forth in the National Healthy Housing Standard. Federal and state funding agencies should tie these requirements to recovery funds, and private funders should consider incentivizing compliance with these standards. Additionally, multiple affordable housing options should be considered during redevelopment to ensure that people of all income levels can remain in the community.

CONCLUSION

The committee's recommendations are designed to provide practical strategies to assist disaster-impacted communities in making key decisions relevant to realizing a healthy, resilient, and sustainable community vision. These recommendations call for multiple and coordinated actions at a variety of levels by a wide range of governmental and nongovernmental actors. Box S-2 provides key recovery strategies for each sector that, if implemented, would support the implementation of the committee's recommendations. Given the broad scope and complexity of the subject matter, it is expected that this initial product will prompt further work, providing the opportunity for deeper analysis and elucidation of the influences and relationships that will advance the nation's sophistication in the process of disaster recovery, one critical aspect of which is health.

Table S-1 shows those stakeholders whose coordinated actions are needed to lead the implementation of each of the committee's recommendations. If acted upon in a coordinated and comprehensive manner, these recommendations will enable *all* stakeholders involved in the pre-disaster and immediate- and long-term post-disaster strategic planning processes to be engaged, empowered, and supported in maximizing the opportunities to transform an unfortunate crisis into long-term benefit in the form of healthier communities and individuals.

BOX S-2
Summary of Key Health Recovery Strategies by Sector

PUBLIC HEALTH SECTOR

- Leverage existing relationships and networks (e.g., coalitions, collaboratives) to integrate public health and other community partners into recovery planning.
- Identify opportunities for alignment between ongoing public health improvement processes (e.g., accreditation prerequisites of community health assessments and community health improvement plans) and recovery planning.
- Educate nonhealth sectors and the community on why health is integral to recovery and how recovery activities impact health outcomes.
- Use and expand health technology infrastructure for data collection and analysis to facilitate data sharing, evidence-based decision making, and continual evaluation of progress toward an optimally healthy community.

HEALTH CARE SECTOR

- Use multidisciplinary team-based care strategies to meet multifaceted health care needs.
- Ensure continuity of access to health care services.
- Use health information technology to drive decision making for individual and community health and to inform future planning.
- Leverage health care coalitions and other relationships with local care providers for strategic decision making on health care services and alignment of clinical resources.

BEHAVIORAL HEALTH SECTOR

- Integrate behavioral health activities and programming into other sectors (e.g., education, health care, social services) to reduce stand-alone services, reach more people, foster resilience and sustainability, and reduce stigma.
- Provide a spectrum of behavioral health services and use an approach based on stepped care (from supportive intervention to long-term treatment).
- Maximize the participation of the local affected population in recovery planning with respect to behavioral health, and identify and build on available resources and local capacities and networks (community, families, schools, and friends) in developing recovery strategies.
- Promote a sense of safety, connectedness, calming, hope, and efficacy at the individual, family, and community levels.

REFERENCES

FEMA (Federal Emergency Management Agency). 2011. *National disaster recovery framework*. Washington, DC: FEMA.

HRIA (Health Resources in Action). 2013. *Defining healthy communities*. http://hria.org/uploads/catalogerfiles/defining-healthy-communities/defining_healthy_communities_1113_final_report.pdf (accessed October 21, 2014).

SOCIAL SERVICES SECTOR

- Build on existing relationships and establish comprehensive plans for collaboration among social services funders and providers, nongovernmental and faith-based organizations, and advocates to ensure coordinated social services delivery through all phases of disaster planning and recovery.
- Integrate social services recovery plans into other disaster recovery services.
- Create compatible structures, policies, and procedures to promote the flow of funding and information across federal, state, and local systems.
- Provide support to reunite families and promote resilience through community programming designed to strengthen social support networks.
- Focus on restoring normalcy through key community services/activities, such as child care, elder care, foster care, behavioral health services, schools, housing, jobs, and transportation.
- Enhance efforts to increase accessibility and reach the most vulnerable populations to provide needed social services.
- Promote ongoing evaluation and continuous learning to advance social services efforts in achieving health community goals.

URBAN AND REGIONAL PLANNING, TRANSPORTATION, ENVIRONMENTAL MANAGEMENT, AND COMMUNITY DEVELOPMENT SECTORS

- Reduce health disparities and improve access to essential goods, services, and opportunities.
- Preserve and promote social connectedness.
- Use a systems approach to community redevelopment that acknowledges the connection among social, cultural, economic, and physical environments.
- Seek holistic solutions to socioeconomic disparities and their perverse effects on population health through place-based interventions.
- Rebuild for sustainability and resilience.
- Capitalize on existing planning networks to strengthen recovery planning, including attention to public health, medical, and social services, especially for vulnerable populations.

HOUSING SECTOR

- Protect survivors and recovery workers from health hazards associated with unhealthy or unsafe housing.
- Preserve and promote social connectedness in plans for immediate response, short-term housing, and long-term rebuilding.
- Consider needs for access to health and social services during all phases of housing recovery.
- Incentivize the use of healthy and/or green criteria for the rebuilding of homes, buildings, and neighborhoods.
- Engage community members, including representatives of and advocates for vulnerable populations, in the development of post-disaster housing plans to ensure that the needs of all community members are met.

WHO (World Health Organization). 2013. *Health in All Policies*. http://www.healthpromotion2013.org/health-promotion/health-in-all-policies (accessed December 4, 2014).

WHO. 2014. *Social determinants of health*. http://www.who.int/social_determinants/en (accessed October 30, 2014).

TABLE S-1 Key Stakeholders Involved in Leading the Implementation of the Committee's Recommendations

Committee Recommendation	Federal Gov.	State Gov.	Local Gov.	Nonprofit/ Faith-based	Private Sector	Community Members
1 Develop a Healthy Community Vision for Disaster Recovery	✓ MULTᵃ	✓	✓	✓	✓	✓
2 Integrate Health Considerations into Recovery Decision Making Through the National Disaster Recovery Framework	✓ DHS (FEMA)/ HHS	✓	✓			
3 Facilitate the Engagement of the Whole Community in Disaster Recovery Through Simplified and Accessible Information and Training	✓ DHS (FEMA)					
4 Enhance and Leverage Social Networks in Community Health Improvement and Recovery Planning			✓	✓	✓	
5 Establish Pathways by Which Health Information Can Inform Recovery Decision Making		✓	✓			
6 Leverage Recovery Resources in a Coordinated Manner to Achieve Healthier Post-Disaster Communities	✓ MULT	✓	✓	✓	✓	
7 Ensure a Ready Health Information Technology Infrastructure	✓ HHS	✓	✓		✓	
8 Develop a National Disaster Behavioral Health Policy	✓ DHS (FEMA)/ HHS	✓	✓	✓	✓	
9 Develop an Integrated Social Services Recovery Framework	✓ HHS	✓	✓	✓		
10 Design for Healthy Post-Disaster Communities	✓ MULT	✓	✓	✓	✓	
11 Mitigate Against Future Health Hazards	✓ DHS (FEMA)	✓	✓		✓	
12 Ensure Healthy and Affordable Post-Disaster Housing	✓ HUD	✓	✓	✓	✓	

ᵃ MULT = Indicates multiple federal agencies will need to work cooperatively to implement the recommendation. Depending on the recommendation, these may include but are not limited to the Federal Emergency Management Agency (FEMA) at the U.S. Department of Homeland Security (DHS), the U.S. Department of Health and Human Services (HHS), the U.S. Department of Housing and Urban Development (HUD), the U.S. Department of Transportation (DOT), the U.S. Environmental Protection Agency (EPA), the U.S. Department of Agriculture (USDA), the U.S. Department of the Interior, the U.S. Department of Commerce, the U.S. Department of Education, and the U.S. Department of Veterans Affairs (VA).
Gov. = Government.

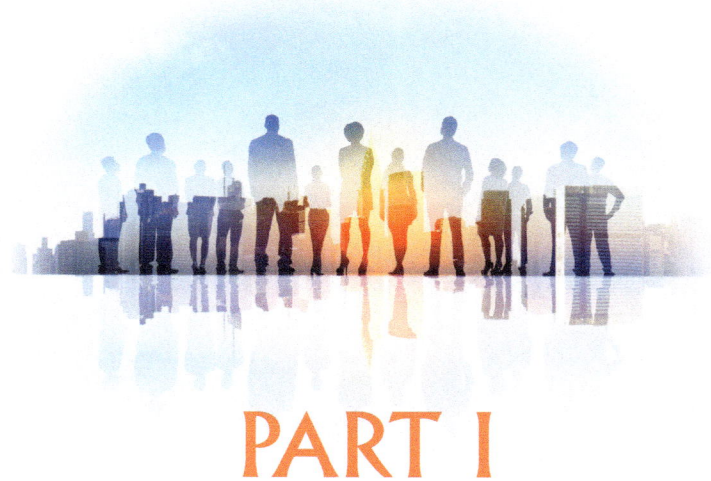

PART I

A HEALTHY COMMUNITY APPROACH
TO DISASTER RECOVERY

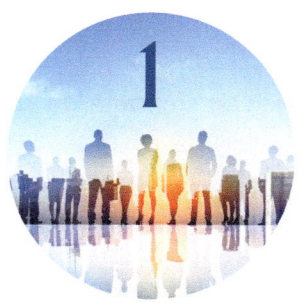

Introduction

"Every American should have the opportunity to be as healthy as he or she can be. Every community should be safe from threats to its health. And all individuals and families should have a high level of services that protect, promote, and preserve their health, regardless of who they are or where they live."

—Trust for America's Health (TFAH, 2013b)

The above quote from Trust for America's Health is indicative of the widely shared social and civilizing ethic that people should live in communities[1] that maximize opportunities to be healthy[2] and minimize preventable misery and suffering from disease. Disasters are by their very nature devastating to communities, often having significant and long-lasting effects on the physical, mental, and social well-being of the impacted population that compromise the realization of a healthy community (see Box 1-1). Further, disaster-related effects may be experienced differentially within a community as a result of the disproportionate vulnerability of certain subpopulations (see Box 1-2). Each year the nation experiences approximately 60 presidentially declared major disasters[3] and a far greater number that do not receive such a declaration.[4] Not only do they result in tragic loss of human life and have devastating health consequences for survivors; they also often require the expenditure of billions of dollars in public, private, and philanthropic funds for recovery (see Figure 1-1). Depending on the nature of the disaster and its impact,

---

[1] Community can be defined in multiple ways—for example, as a population of individuals that share a geographic area, a culture, religious beliefs, or self-defined interests. For communities defined by geographic area, the scale varies from macro (e.g., national level) to hyperlocal (neighborhood or even block level). For the purposes of this report, the term "community" refers to a community of place at the city or county level, unless otherwise indicated.

[2] Health, as defined by the World Health Organization (WHO, 1948) is "a state of complete physical, mental, and social well-being and not merely the absence of disease or infirmity."

[3] This number was derived from Federal Emergency Management Agency (FEMA) data available at https://www.fema.gov/disasters/grid/year. Major disaster declarations are made by the President of the United States following a request from the governor of an affected state that is submitted through the regional FEMA office.

[4] According to estimates from FEMA, less than 10 percent of all disasters in the United States receive a presidential disaster declaration (FEMA, 2010).

BOX 1-1
Disaster Impacts on Health

The impact of a disaster on the health of a community is complex to predict, difficult to measure, and heavily influenced by both health- and nonhealth-related preexisting factors, including

- the level of pre-disaster planning,
- community demographics,
- social and economic conditions,
- community health status,
- community cohesion and cultural practices,
- geography, and
- any history of previous disaster events.

Disasters have direct and indirect impacts on physical and/or mental health that may manifest in the short-, intermediate-, and long-term post-disaster periods. These effects are worse for vulnerable populations in particular. Indirect effects occur through the disruption of access to health-sustaining goods and services and deterioration of living conditions immediately following a disaster and, in some cases, for extended periods of time thereafter. In many cases, disasters exacerbate preexisting health conditions at the individual and community levels.

Impacts on Short-Term Health Outcomes

- *Physical and mental trauma and illness*: Direct causes of morbidity and mortality vary by disaster type. Examples of physical health impacts include lacerations, punctures, and trauma caused by debris or falling objects; drowning; burns; and infections (epidemics). Accidents after disasters (e.g., during debris removal or reconstruction) are another common cause of physical trauma. While most disaster survivors display remarkable resilience and experience only short periods of shock, some develop immediate symptoms of psychopathology, such as acute stress disorder or posttraumatic stress disorder (PTSD).
- *Lack of access to life-sustaining resources and medications*: In the early post-disaster period, lack of access to safe food, clean water, shelter, and critical medications may contribute to additional disaster-related morbidity and mortality. Deaths and illnesses may occur from dehydration, consumption of contaminated food or water, exposure to the elements, carbon monoxide poisoning (from incorrect use of heaters and generators), and heatstroke. Loss of power may be catastrophic for those dependent on medical devices powered by electricity, such as individuals undergoing dialysis.
- *Impacts from disruption of critical emergency and medical services and infrastructure*: During the disaster response phase, the predominant focus is on saving lives through search and rescue operations and the provision of emergency medical care. These critical services may be directly impacted (e.g., by infrastructure loss), or access to the services may be hindered by the disaster's effects on transportation systems (e.g., responders cannot access certain areas, or community members cannot reach medical facilities). Furthermore, limited resources may necessitate a transition from conventional standards of

---

strategic planning and resource allocation decisions must be made; public works, roads, homes, and businesses must be rebuilt; and medical services must be provided and care delivery systems restored. The committee that conducted this study explicitly rejected the traditional characterization of disaster recovery as a process that restores a community to pre-disaster conditions. When viewed through a health lens, this formulation is shortsighted given the general state of suboptimal health status that characterizes so many American communities and the associated economic and societal costs. Although the United States spends

care to contingency or crisis standards of care (IOM, 2012a). In such cases, otherwise preventable morbidity (e.g., infection of wounds) and mortality (e.g., victims succumbing to injuries) may occur.

Intermediate- and Long-Term Health Outcomes

- *Effects of trauma and chronic stress on behavioral health*: The psychosocial impacts of a disaster may not manifest in survivors until weeks, months, or even years later and may include changes in emotional, physical, cognitive, and interpersonal conditions (Landesman, 2005). These effects may be brought on by the trauma of the disaster itself or by secondary causes such as disruption of social networks, bereavement and loss, and chronic stress associated with the challenges of recovery. The effects of chronic stress on health worsen as recovery time increases. In addition to PTSD, depression and anxiety disorders are serious post-disaster mental health sequelae. Trauma and stress also may induce behaviors that negatively impact health, such as substance abuse and other risky behaviors, as well as violence and abuse.
- *Effects of physical stress*: The physical demands of recovery can have minor (e.g., musculoskeletal strains) and serious (e.g., acute myocardial infarction or heart attack) health effects. Increased incidence of heart attack after a disaster may persist for years and may be associated with chronic stress (Peters et al., 2014).
- *Impacts from degraded capacity of or access to health and human services*: Following the disaster response phase, increased demand for primary care services can be associated with, for example, the need for chronic disease management and follow-up care for those who sustained acute injuries during or immediately after the disaster. Chronic illnesses are exacerbated by conditions during the early recovery period (lack of nutritious food, impeded access to medications, stress) (Mensah et al., 2005). Preventable morbidity and mortality result when disrupted health systems are unable to meet this secondary surge or when community members cannot access primary care services (Runkle et al., 2012). Disruption of social services that ensure access of vulnerable populations to resources for disease management further contributes to negative health outcomes.
- *Exposure to pollutants and degradation of environmental conditions*: Disasters can cause a number of environmental public health concerns. For example, sanitation problems can give rise to infectious diseases such as food and waterborne illnesses and skin infections. Exposure to mold and endotoxins associated with microbial growth in water-damaged buildings may exacerbate asthma and contribute to other acute and chronic respiratory disorders. Exposure to pollutants (e.g., industrial chemicals) in water, food, sediment, or air can result in acute toxic effects, development or exacerbation of chronic health conditions (e.g., respiratory disorders), and cancer (Brandt et al., 2006).
- *Impacts on social determinants of health*: Major disasters impact many of the conditions known collectively as social determinants of health, such as employment opportunities, the quality and affordability of housing, schooling and child care, and transportation access to essential goods and services. Job loss, displacement, and transportation disruption are common after a disaster. Disparities in these social and economic conditions are correlated with health disparities (e.g., rates of malnutrition, obesity-related chronic diseases, infant mortality, and cancer), which are exacerbated by disproportionate effects of disasters on already vulnerable populations (see Box 1-2).

more on health care than does any other country in the world, the health of its citizens is worse than that in many peer nations that spend less, as evidenced by key health status indicators such as lower average life expectancy (see Figure 1-2) and higher incidence of preventable diseases[5] (Bradley et al., 2011; NRC

---

[5] In the United States, chronic diseases account for 7 of the 10 leading causes of mortality and affect almost 50 percent of Americans (CDC, 2011). Annual health care spending in the United States has grown to approximately $2.7 trillion, more than 75 percent of which goes to management of preventable chronic diseases (IOM, 2012b; KFF, 2012; RWJF, 2014; TFAH, 2013a).

BOX 1-2
Vulnerable Populations

Vulnerable, or at-risk, populations are, as defined by the U.S. Department of Health and Human Services, those individuals and groups that "[b]efore, during, and after an incident ... may have additional needs in one or more of the following functional areas: communication, medical care, maintaining independence, supervision, and transportation. In addition to those individuals specifically recognized as at-risk in the Pandemic and All-Hazards Preparedness Act (i.e., children, senior citizens, and pregnant women), individuals who may need additional response assistance include those who have disabilities, live in institutionalized settings, are from diverse cultures, have limited English proficiency or are non-English speaking, are transportation disadvantaged, have chronic medical disorders, and have pharmacological dependency" (HHS, 2009a, p. 37).

As the community transitions into recovery, vulnerable populations often are the most difficult to reach and/or experience complications and worsening health status as a result of delays in seeking and receiving treatment, provider scarcity and overload, and limited supplies. These populations are at higher risk for negative outcomes after a disaster, including mortality, and may require more time and effort to recover (O'Sullivan et al., 2014).

Although there is no one accepted list of all vulnerable subpopulations, most fall into one or more of the following broad categories that confer vulnerability:

- economic disadvantage;
- language and literacy barriers;
- medical condition or disability (physical, mental, cognitive, or sensory);
- isolation (cultural, geographic [e.g., rural] or social); and
- age (children and the elderly) (CDC, 2010).

Disasters and the conditions left in their wake also may create newly vulnerable populations, thus increasing the scope of the problem during the recovery period. These individuals and families can be difficult to reach and link to services because they have not accessed support services in the past and may be reticent to ask for help. Examples of the newly vulnerable include but are not limited to

- individuals and families previously above the poverty line who may be ineligible for some services because their income level exceeds the cutoff, but who end up destitute as a result of disaster-related costs;
- individuals that develop physical or mental health conditions as a direct or indirect result of the disaster; and
- newly homeless, isolated, or displaced individuals.

Despite clear evidence demonstrating the special needs of vulnerable populations during and after a disaster, these populations continue to be excluded from emergency management planning in some jurisdictions (Sherry and Harkins, 2011). However, recent legislative and judicial proceedings have established some accountability for ensuring that their needs are met. The repercussions of not meeting the needs of at-risk individuals were demonstrated on a national scale after Hurricane Sandy when a federal court found that New York City violated the Americans with Disabilities Act by not adequately protecting the vulnerable disabled population during that disaster (DRA, 2013). This was the first case of its kind in the country, and it has far-reaching implications for emergency planning at the state and local levels. There now is greater focus on vulnerable populations at the federal level as well. The Pandemic and All Hazards Preparedness Act (reauthorized in 2013) requires that the Secretary of Health and Human Services consider the public health and medical needs of at-risk individuals during public health emergencies and, more specifically, "oversee an advisory committee on at-risk persons and disseminate novel and best practices on outreach to and care of the at-risk before, during, and after public health emergencies" (ASTHO, 2012).

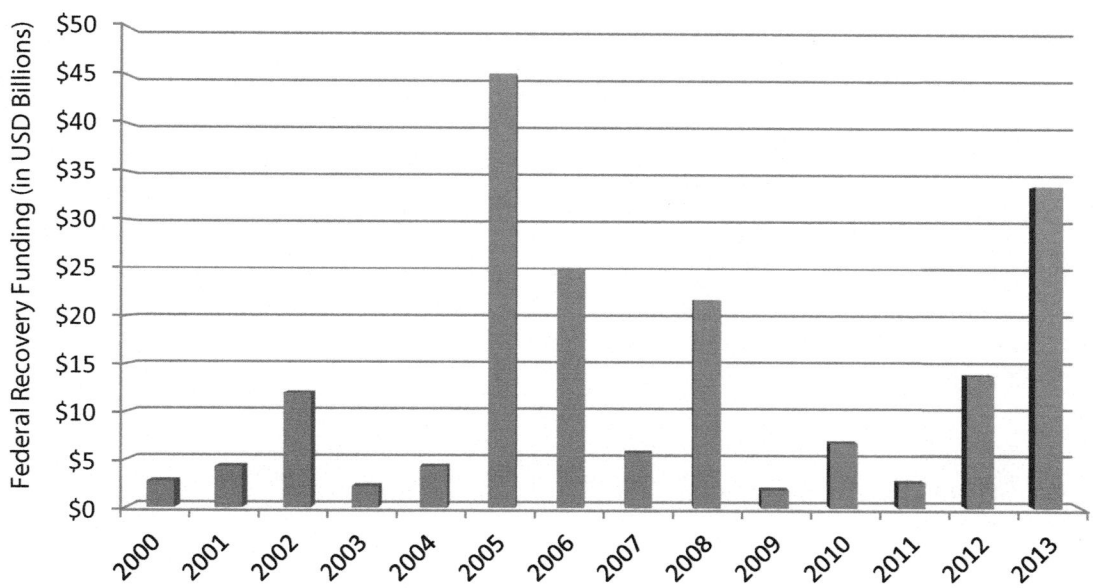

FIGURE 1-1 Federal expenditures on disaster recovery over the past decade.
NOTE: There is no single source for tracking all federal expenditures on recovery assistance. Federal recovery funding estimates in this figure are derived from just three of the largest sources: Federal Emergency Management Agency (FEMA) disaster relief funds, U.S. Department of Housing and Urban Development (HUD) Community Development Block Grant Disaster Recovery funds and Social Services Block Grant Disaster Recovery funds. These estimates are likely underestimates of the total amount of federal recovery assistance from all agencies (Weiss and Weidman, 2013). SOURCE: Data from CRS (2014) and HUD (2014a).

and IOM, 2013; OECD, 2013). In comparison with other nations, expenditures in the United States are disproportionately directed at health care services (see Figure 1-3), despite evidence that a higher ratio of social services to health care spending is significantly associated with better health outcomes (Bradley and Taylor, 2013; Bradley et al., 2011).

It is clear that the process of community planning in the United States has not fully addressed the fundamental elements necessary to protect and enhance health. However, there is growing recognition of the need to leverage the essential health-advancing opportunities presented by the ways in which communities are built and designed; how people live, work, are educated, and play; the social relationships among individuals and the resiliency that results (Aldrich, 2012); and how health and medical care services are organized and financed—all of which, taken together, ultimately determine the health of a community. Several definitions of a healthy community have been advanced, but for the purposes of this report, the committee adopted the following definition proposed by the National Network of Public Health Institutes:

> A healthy community is one in which a diverse group of stakeholders collaborate to use their expertise and local knowledge to create a community that is socially and physically conducive to health. Community members are empowered and civically engaged, assuring that all local policies consider health. The community has the capacity to identify, address, and evaluate their own health concerns on an ongoing basis, using data to guide and benchmark efforts. As a result, a healthy community is safe, economically secure, and environmentally sound, as all residents have equal access to high quality educational and employment opportunities, transportation and housing options, prevention and healthcare services, and healthy food and physical activity opportunities. (HRIA, 2013, p. 24)

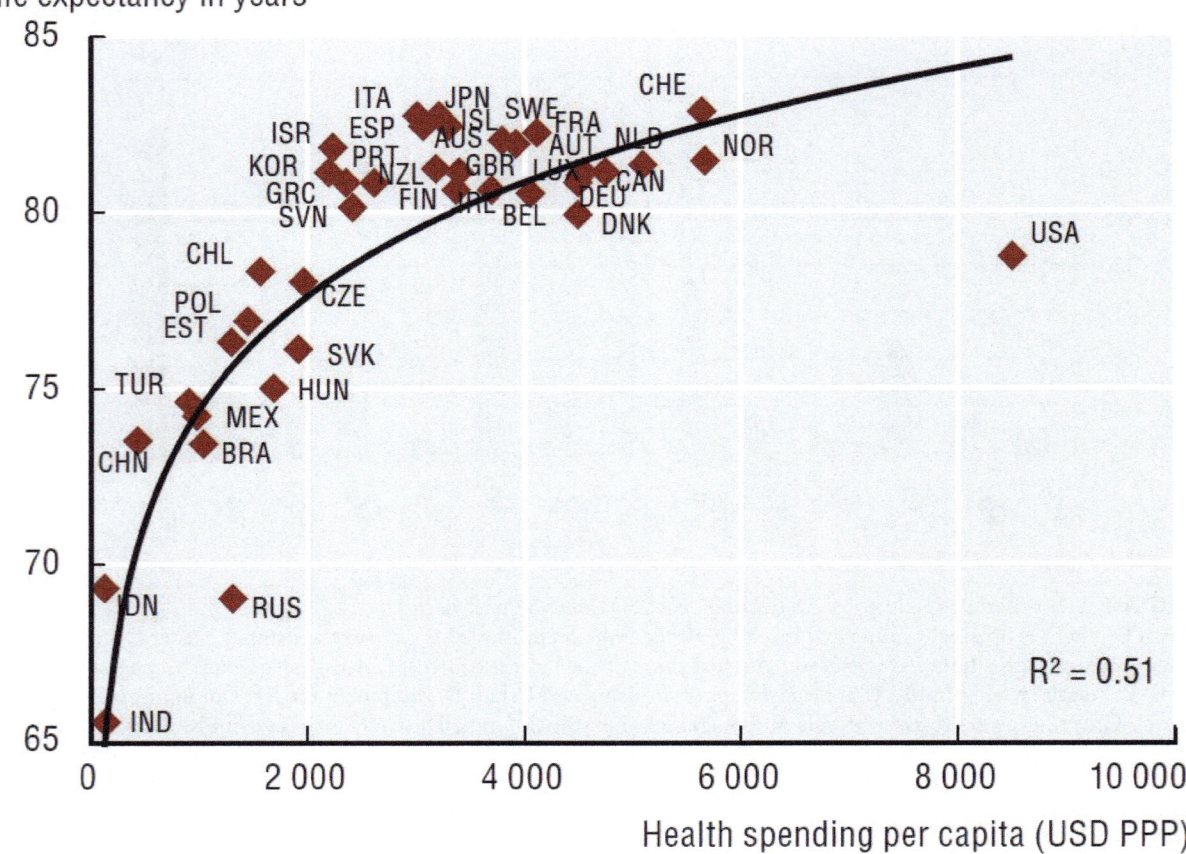

FIGURE 1-2 Average life expectancy as a function of spending on health care.
SOURCE: OECD (2013), *Health at a Glance 2013: OECD Indicators*, OECD Publishing. http://dx.doi.org/10.1787/health_glance-2013-en.

This definition conveys the concept that a healthy community is one in which the broad array of factors that impact community well-being are addressed, including social, environmental, political, economic, cultural, and health (physical, emotional, and developmental) components. One cannot expect communities to become healthier without understanding the complex interplay among these factors and designing comprehensive strategies to address this complexity. Furthermore, the above definition stresses the importance of a focus on individuals, recognizing that individual and community characteristics reinforce one another. It is the central thesis of this report that optimizing the health of the nation and its communities will require, in large measure, greater attentiveness to the full range of elements that encompass community design and social life and their essential interactions. The process of preparing for disasters and the comprehensive array of immediate and long-term recovery activities represent a continuum of opportunities that, if leveraged thoughtfully, can advance the long-term goal of creating healthy communities.

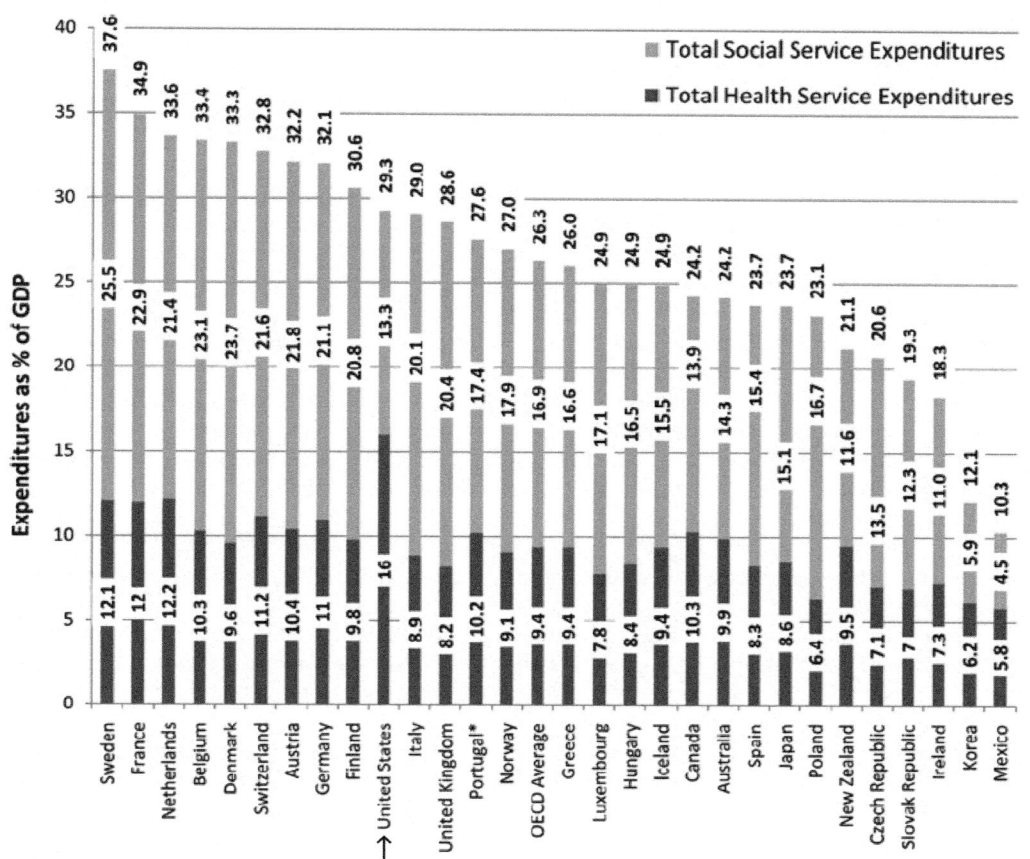

FIGURE 1-3 Relative expenditures on health care and social services in the United States in the context of other peer nations.
SOURCE: Reproduced from *BMJ Quality and Safety*, Bradley, E. H., B. R. Elkins, J. Herrin, and B. Elbel, 20, p. 828, 2011 with permission from BMJ Publishing Group Ltd.

CHARGE TO THE COMMITTEE

This report was commissioned by the Office of the Assistant Secretary for Preparedness and Response (ASPR) within the U.S. Department of Health and Human Services (HHS), the Office of Lead Hazard Control and Healthy Homes within the U.S. Department of Housing and Urban Development (HUD), the Veterans Health Administration within the U.S. Department of Veterans Affairs, and the Robert Wood Johnson Foundation. Initiation of this study was spurred by concerns that too often, absent from discussions on recovery is the critical importance of health—including the roles of the health (public health, medical, and social services) and nonhealth sectors in ensuring that health considerations are incorporated into recovery decision making and activities. In the field of disaster and emergency management, the United States has made substantial progress in the preparedness and response arena, but the prevailing approach to recovery remains ad hoc and fragmented (Fossett, 2013). Additionally, guidance on recovery frequently focuses on the restoration of previously extant physical or economic systems within a community; little information is available to aid communities in developing post-disaster recovery approaches that address the physical, social, and economic dimensions of community life with the deliberate intent of improving health and promoting overall well-being.

Communities that have been through a disaster represent a cohort of "learning laboratories." The

---

BOX 1-3
Statement of Task for the Committee on Post-Disaster Recovery of
a Community's Public Health, Medical, and Social Services

An ad hoc committee will conduct a study and issue a report on how to improve the short-, intermediate-, and long-term health outcomes and public health impact for individuals in a community of place (as contrasted with communities of faith, identity, etc.). The committee will investigate and identify key activities that impact health and public health outcomes in a community of place recovering from a disaster, and develop recommendations for their implementation. In doing so, the committee will consider the determinants of health and how various activities could leverage those determinants to improve health in the post-disaster setting, including the needs of at-risk populations.

The committee will do this by identifying (based in part on a literature review of domestic and international disasters) and recommending a series of recovery practices and novel programs most likely to impact overall community public health and contribute to resiliency for future incidents in the short-, intermediate-, and long-term period during disaster response and following incident stabilization. Specifically the committee will:

- Examine existing guidance and frameworks, peer-reviewed literature, and case studies from post-disaster response and recovery operations;
  - Characterize and identify key determinants of pre- and post-disaster public health, medical, and social services that may serve as indicators for the affected population's long-term recovery, from various perspectives amongst the different levels of government and nongovernment actors generally located within a community of place;
  - Ascertain which other sectors are responsible for, or have the organizational interest and capacity for, directly affecting the identified determinants, and identify opportunities for collaborative engagement or support amongst those sectors;
- Identify practical guidance for recovery practices and programs for each sector that will benefit community post-disaster health and public health outcomes in the short-, intermediate-, and long-term.
  - Consider how community needs may be integrated into health recovery efforts.
  - Consider any key determinants, differences, and similarities in recovery between rural and urban communities; among household-income strata; among single-family, low-rise multifamily, and high-rise multifamily housing, among households receiving government assistance and unassisted households, etc.
  - Consider how long-term gains for health may be achieved through investments in community, housing, and other non-traditional health infrastructures.
- Identify areas of research that should be explored to answer key questions about where to direct resources before, during, and after an event occurs.

---

collective body of knowledge stemming from those experiences represents an invaluable resource for recovering communities and the local officials who must make difficult decisions in the face of uncertainty, armed only with the best information available. There is an ethical and moral obligation for lessons learned from past disasters to be made available to guide those decisions and for leaders at all levels to act on them (CommonHealth ACTION, 2007). Recognizing the need for better dissemination of the knowledge and evidence from past disaster recovery experiences both in the United States and abroad to enable communities to build capacity and to support more informed decision making, the sponsors of this study requested that the Institute of Medicine (IOM) convene a committee to develop guidance and recommendations on how local and national leaders can mitigate disaster-related health impacts and optimize the use of resources—which inevitably must be spent in rebuilding—to pursue more proactively, deliberately, and thoughtfully the goal of creating communities that are healthier and more resilient. The full charge to the committee is presented in Box 1-3.

APPROACH TO ADDRESSING THE CHARGE

Scope of the Study

Disasters are variable: they come in many forms, from many causes, with different magnitudes of severity, and they trigger different levels of response and recovery effort. They also are context-specific—an event may rise to the level of disaster in one community but not another. Desiring this report to be of maximum utility to decision makers at all levels, the committee decided not to use a set of specific scenarios as the basis of its approach but chose to look at disasters more generally as events causing a community's status to deteriorate at a level that exceeds its capacity to remedy without outside assistance (see Box 1-4 for the complete definition of a disaster adopted by the committee). Given this broad definition, the committee recognizes that no one set of guidance and recommendations could apply to every disaster scenario. For example, guidance related to behavioral health may be applicable following a pandemic, but guidance on healthy approaches to reconstruction of physical infrastructure may not. The committee's objective was to provide a set of recommendations for key stakeholders that could be tailored for relevance to local realities and the scale of an incident and would be of practical use during pre-disaster planning and post-disaster recovery to facilitate the building of healthier communities. Local adaptation, innovation, and initiative will be key to success.

BOX 1-4
Defining Disaster

For the purposes of this report, the committee adopted the following definition from the United Nations International Strategy for Disaster Reduction:

Disaster: A serious disruption of the functioning of a community or a society involving widespread human, material, economic or environmental losses and impacts, which exceeds the ability of the affected community or society to cope using its own resources.

Comment: Disasters are often described as a result of the combination of: the exposure to a hazard; the conditions of vulnerability that are present; and insufficient capacity or measures to reduce or cope with the potential negative consequences. Disaster impacts may include loss of life, injury, disease and other negative effects on human physical, mental and social well-being, together with damage to property, destruction of assets, loss of services, social and economic disruption and environmental degradation. (UNISDR, 2009)

It should be noted that a hazardous event that results in a disaster declaration also can be declared separately as a public health emergency "when its health consequences have the potential to overwhelm routine community capabilities to address them" (Nelson et al., 2007, p. S9). Such hazardous events might include an infectious disease outbreak; natural disaster; or chemical, biological, or nuclear event (HHS, 2015b). Public health emergency declarations are made by the Secretary of Health and Human Services and enable the Secretary to take measures to respond to the emergency and support states and local communities.

Consistent with the committee's charge, the language of this report focuses largely on health; socio-economic components often are discussed as mechanisms for improving health outcomes. However, the committee recognizes that in a healthy community, broader community well-being is the real objective. In a sense, the nation cannot seek health improvements after a disaster without addressing the other aspects of well-being for its people. This report provides a new perspective on the special relationships between healthy communities and recovery from disasters. The study also is about knowledge transfer, blending fields of professionalism and expertise that have not been united before. Given the breadth of scope and the complexity of the subject matter, the committee expects that this initial product will prompt further work, providing the opportunity for deeper analysis and greater elucidation of the influences and relation-ships that can advance the nation's sophistication in dealing with disaster recovery, one critical aspect of which is health. This is more than a call for further research, however; it is a recognition that synergies of many sorts are probable when a community's socioeconomic systems undergo adjustment after a disaster, aided by the infusion of new resources and potentially by surge staffing and outside expertise. Going forward from this initial inquiry oriented to the role of health in post-disaster recovery, it will be time to take advantage of research, knowledge, and best practices focused on achieving more holistic community well-being, thereby linking the full range of socioeconomic endeavors for a more inclusive scope of post-disaster recovery.

Report Audiences

The audiences for the committee's guidance and recommendations and the report as a whole include

- state, local, tribal, and territorial[6] elected and public officials who typically hold leadership roles in emergency management and strategic planning (i.e., governors, mayors, city managers and council members, emergency managers, disaster recovery coordinators);
- state, local, tribal, and territorial public health officials;
- infrastructure support professionals, such as those responsible for urban and regional planning, housing, transportation, and public works;
- federal agency stakeholders;
- health care delivery professionals and organizational leaders;
- social services professionals;
- community support (including faith-based) organizations and nongovernmental organizations;
- schools and education sector leaders;
- private-sector stakeholders; and
- empowered community members.

Study Approach

The committee's approach was four-pronged. First, we developed a shared vision of a healthy commu-nity and defined the elements necessary to realize it. Next, we identified the various ways in which disasters impact health in the short-, intermediate-, and long-term periods following an event. We then examined the opportunities and resources existing uniquely in a post-disaster environment that are relevant to the elements necessary to achieving a healthy community. Finally, we explored the processes and mechanisms that determine how the relevant resources are deployed. Specifically, we examined

- the availability of post-disaster resources,

---

[6] Throughout this report, the phrase "state and local" is used for the purposes of brevity but should be inferred to include tribal and territorial leaders.

- the processes by which resources are mobilized to meet the immediate and long-term demands of a disaster,
- the elements that affect prioritization for the use of resources, and
- the broad range of expertise that must come together.

In this regard, we examined in some detail the availability and flow of financial assistance resources that are mobilized from federal, state, local, private, and philanthropic sources. To support these efforts, we commissioned a paper describing the sources of recovery funding and the pathways for disseminating those resources to localities (see Appendix B). We reviewed the appropriate federal statutes and executive agency authorizing documents and developed case studies from recent experiences with disaster recovery, both domestically and abroad; these case studies are presented throughout the report. Additional information was gathered from a review of the peer-reviewed and grey literature, as well as interviews with key stakeholders from federal, state, and local agencies; elected officials with firsthand experience in disaster recovery; human services organizations; and academic researchers (agendas from the seven public meetings held for this study are available in Appendix G).

A notable challenge for the committee was the paucity of published research and findings connecting recovery practices and approaches with health or social well-being outcomes. Further, as a result of the length of the recovery period and the inevitable delays associated with research and publication, the scientific literature that is available generally pertains to events that occurred nearly a decade ago (Hurricane Katrina) or more. Lessons learned from Hurricane Katrina and legislation subsequent to that disaster (the Post-Katrina Emergency Management Reform Act[7]) substantially altered the nation's approach to all aspects of emergency management, including recovery. However, research on more recent disasters is still under way, and available information is primarily anecdotal in nature. Collecting this kind of information in a systematic way requires extensive interviewing, which the committee did not have sufficient time or resources to conduct. Instead, we relied on invited testimony from decision makers representing multiple sectors (e.g., emergency management, public health, city management) whose communities had recently been struck by a disaster.

Guiding Principles

The following guiding principles informed the committee's guidance for recovery and its recommendations:

- Because most communities do not enjoy optimal health prior to a disaster, a crisis presents important opportunities to rebuild to a more optimal state of health post-recovery that should not be squandered.
- The guidance and recommendations of this committee should build on successful planning infrastructures and collaborative frameworks to promote an integrated recovery approach, rather than reinventing wheels.
- They should enhance flexibility and innovation at the local level and facilitate local community buy-in.
- They should focus on people, optimizing the opportunities for each person to achieve maximum health.
- They should encourage and facilitate collaboration across administrative, bureaucratic, political, and professional discipline boundaries because the actions of each of these sectors will impact health, either positively or negatively.
- They should recognize the value of nonmonetary resources such as social and cultural capital, community resiliency, leadership, community dynamics, and volunteerism.

---

[7] Post-Katrina Emergency Management Reform Act of 2006, 109th Cong., S.3721 (October 4, 2006).

- They should emphasize the importance of pre-disaster planning and capacity building.
- They should recognize that pre-disaster planning and post-disaster recovery are part of an ongoing cyclical process of community improvement involving assessment, planning, and implementation.

DISASTER RECOVERY IN THE CONTEXT OF COMPREHENSIVE RISK MANAGEMENT

Disaster recovery is "the phase of the emergency management cycle that begins with stabilization of the incident and ends when the community has recovered from the disaster's impacts" (i.e., achieves a new normal) (Lindell et al., 2006, p. 313). The Federal Emergency Management Agency (FEMA) defines recovery as "those capabilities necessary to assist communities affected by an incident to recover effectively, including, but not limited to, rebuilding infrastructure systems; providing adequate interim and long-term housing for survivors; restoring health, social, and community services; promoting economic development; and restoring natural and cultural resources" (FEMA, 2011, p. 81). The recovery process often is broken down into a series of phases that are not discrete, but represent a continuum of activities (see Figure 1-4). Although this taxonomy is useful for the purposes of discussion, it must be recognized that there will be considerable overlap between phases and that different communities will move through phases at different paces depending on the nature of the disaster-related damage and the capacity within the community. The phases are as follows:

- Pre-disaster preparedness—The phase of the disaster management cycle prior to a disaster focused on mitigation, response and recovery planning, and capacity and resilience building (not part of the recovery process itself, but ongoing).
- Short-term recovery—The phase of recovery that entails addressing health and safety needs beyond rescue; assessing the scope of damages and needs; restoring basic infrastructure; and mobilizing recovery organizations and resources, including restarting and/or restoring essential services. The short-term recovery phase should begin immediately after a disaster, running parallel to response activities.
- Intermediate recovery—The phase of recovery that involves returning individuals, families, critical infrastructure, and essential government or commercial services to a functional, if not pre-disaster, state.
- Long-term recovery—The phase of recovery that includes complete redevelopment and revitalization of the impacted area; rebuilding or relocation of damaged or destroyed social, economic, natural, and built environments; and the transition to self-sufficiency, sustainability, and resilience. Long-term recovery may continue for months or years after the event.

A crucial element of Figure 1-4 is the explicit inclusion of the pre-disaster planning phase, which includes planning for recovery. In the United States, pre-event preparedness has been focused heavily on preparation for the response phase (Leonard and Howitt, 2010). A more comprehensive approach to managing disaster risks requires that the United States expand its focus beyond crisis management to consider the longer-term aspects of recovery, as well as prevention and mitigation efforts that should be undertaken well in advance of any disaster (Leonard and Howitt, 2010). Within a comprehensive risk management framework, there are three stages during which actions can be taken to preserve—and ideally, to improve—social welfare (inclusive of health) following a disaster:

- **Prior to a disaster,** prevention and mitigation efforts are aimed at eliminating or reducing the probability that a hazardous event will occur or reducing the harm caused should a disaster take place. In addition, interventions undertaken in advance of an event such as pre-event response planning and building of recovery infrastructure limit damage from disasters that do occur and accelerate the recovery process.

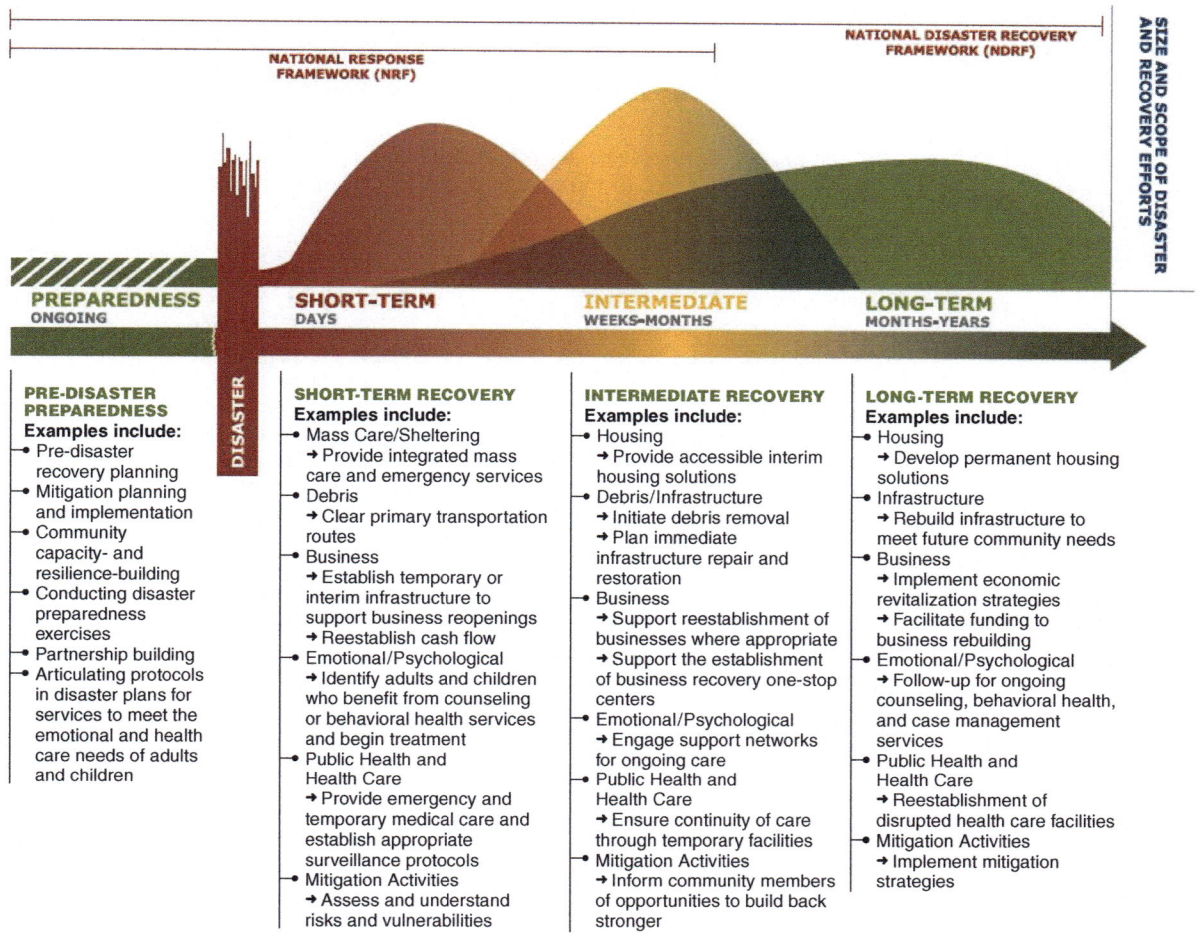

FIGURE 1-4 The recovery continuum: Description of activities by phase.
SOURCE: FEMA, 2011.

- **During and immediately after a disaster,** crisis management is aimed at limiting damage.
- **After a disaster,** recovery efforts are aimed at restoring social welfare quickly, and if undertaken thoughtfully, at improving it beyond pre-disaster levels (Leonard and Howitt, 2010).

As is the case for emergency response, disaster recovery is facilitated if communities anticipate the most significant recovery demands and plan for them in advance (Rubin, 1991; Rubin et al., 1985). The committee recognizes that the extent to which a community should undertake disaster recovery planning needs to be based on a comprehensive analysis of risks. Minimally, however, communities should ensure that a vision is in place and organizational arrangements have been laid out that will enable a coordinated approach to recovery planning. Pre-event recovery planning allows communities to think carefully about the obstacles that will be encountered during recovery, when there will be great pressure to act quickly, and, importantly, to identify opportunities to approach redevelopment in ways that enhance the health, resilience, and sustainability of the community. Pre-event recovery planning should be used to

---

BOX 1-5
Emergency Managers as Risk Management Practitioners

The following, extracted from the report *Principles of Emergency Management*, identifies some of the principles of emergency management that relate to the role of emergency managers as practitioners of risk management:

Emergency managers generally employ risk management principles such as hazard identification and risk analysis to identify priorities, allocate resources and use resources effectively.... Setting policy and programmatic priorities is therefore based upon measured levels of risk to lives, property, and the environment. The National Fire Protection Association (NFPA) 1600 states that emergency management programs should identify and monitor hazards, the likelihood of their occurrence, and the vulnerability to those hazards of people, property, the environment, and the emergency program itself. The Emergency Management Accreditation Program (EMAP) Standard echoes this requirement for public sector emergency management programs.... Emergency managers are seldom in a position to direct the activities of the many agencies and organizations involved in emergency management. In most cases, the people in charge of these organizations are senior to the emergency manager, have direct line authority from the senior official, or are autonomous. Each stakeholder brings to the planning process their own authorities, legal mandates, culture and operating missions. The principle of coordination requires that the emergency manager, or other actors responsible for risk management and increasing resilience, gain agreement among these disparate agencies as to a common purpose, and then ensure that their independent activities help to achieve this common purpose.

SOURCE: Excerpted from NRC, 2012, p. 31.

- build relationships among stakeholders and plan and exercise administrative structures for decision making so that coordination and collaboration both horizontally (across sectors) and vertically (across levels of government) are enhanced during recovery (discussed further in Chapter 3);
- develop strategies and identify needed resources for addressing critical issues likely to arise early in the recovery phase that can impede the progress of recovery and impact health/quality of life for survivors (e.g., get children back into schools and daycare, address mental health needs);
- identify opportunities to build resilience, mitigate hazards, address unmet needs, promote health during long-term recovery, and deal with expected barriers to seizing these opportunities (e.g., controversial issues such as private property rights); and
- identify and adopt a shared vision developed as part of ongoing community strategic planning.

Finally, although disaster management is a primary function of emergency managers, a comprehensive approach to managing disaster risks will require the engagement of the whole community (see Box 1-5).

THE CURRENT POLICY CONTEXT FOR HEALTH-FOCUSED RECOVERY: WHY NOW?

This report was developed in the context of the convergence of two shifting policy landscapes: (1) a disaster policy environment that increasingly reflects a growing emphasis on incorporating health considerations into resilience building and recovery efforts, and (2) a shift in the U.S. approach to population health to support greater emphasis on prevention. It is the committee's belief that this convergence, while still evolving, is bringing unprecedented attention to the interconnectedness of health, resilience, and sustainability, thereby creating a social and policy context that will support the call for a healthy community approach to disaster recovery that is the central theme of this report. Brief descriptions of key domestic and international policies in these two areas are provided below.

The Changing Disaster Policy Landscape

The increasing focus on the health implications of disasters, in terms of both challenges and opportunities, can be seen in a number of domestic and international disaster-related policies, including the National Health Security Strategy; domestic preparedness and disaster recovery policy, including the National Preparedness System and the recent National Disaster Recovery Framework; international disaster risk reduction policy; and climate change policy. Each of these is described briefly below; a more comprehensive description of recovery-related legislation and policies can be found in Appendix A.

The National Health Security Strategy

The Pandemic and All-Hazards Preparedness Act[8] of 2006 called for the development of a National Health Security Strategy (NHSS),[9] the first version of which was released by ASPR in December 2009. The second version, released in 2015, presents a vision for the nation's health security to guide action over the next 4 years (HHS, 2015a).[10] The new NHSS defines and will support five strategic objectives:

1. Build and sustain healthy, resilient communities.
2. Enhance the national capability to produce and effectively use both medical countermeasures and non-pharmaceutical interventions.
3. Ensure comprehensive health situational awareness to support decision making before incidents and during response and recovery operations.
4. Enhance the integration and effectiveness of the public health, health care, and emergency management systems.
5. Strengthen global health security (HHS, 2015a).

Unlike the original NHSS, which identified health recovery as an independent objective, the new version integrates recovery into each of the above strategic objectives. Of particular interest to this committee is the increased focus on building community health resilience—"the ability of a community to use its assets to strengthen public health and healthcare systems and to improve the community's physical, behavioral, and social health to withstand, adapt to, and recover from adversity" (HHS, 2015a, p. 10)— and acknowledgment of the multisector nature of this important endeavor. Key priorities for community health resilience include (1) encouraging social connectedness; (2) enhancing coordination of health and human services; and (3) building a culture of resilience through physical, behavioral, and social health, as well as leveraging health and community systems and increasing access to information and training to empower individuals to assist their communities after incidents (HHS, 2015a). The committee notes that these are all themes that run throughout this report.

Domestic Preparedness and Disaster Recovery Policy

Domestic disaster policy is framed by the architecture of the National Preparedness System, which outlines the process by which the whole community works toward achieving the National Preparedness Goal—"a secure and resilient nation with the capabilities required across the whole community to prevent,

---

[8] Pandemic and All-Hazards Preparedness Act, Public Law 109-417, 109th Cong., S.3678 (December 19, 2006).

[9] As defined by the NHSS, national health security is "a state in which the Nation and its people are prepared for, protected from, and resilient in the face of health threats or incidents with potentially negative health consequences" (HHS, 2009b, p. 3).

[10] HHS is required to submit an updated version of the NHSS every 4 years.

protect against, mitigate, respond to, and recover from the threats and hazards that pose the greatest risk" (FEMA, 2014, p. 1). The National Planning Frameworks,[11] which are part of the National Preparedness System, establish the strategy and doctrine for building, sustaining, and delivering the core capabilities identified in the National Preparedness Goal. They describe the roles, responsibilities, and coordinating structures for the whole community—individuals, nongovernmental entities, the private sector, and governments at all levels. Of particular relevance to this report is the National Disaster Recovery Framework (NDRF), released in 2011, which serves as a guide to facilitate recovery at the community level (FEMA, 2011). Health and social services are featured prominently in the NDRF as one of six recovery support functions[12] with a mission of helping locally led recovery efforts restore and improve public health, health care, and social services networks, thereby promoting community resilience, health, independence, and well-being. The NDRF is discussed in more detail in Chapter 3.

The growing national focus on disaster recovery has been accompanied by increasing integration of sustainability and resilience agendas into recovery efforts, with significant implications for health. A 2010 memorandum of agreement between FEMA and the U.S. Environmental Protection Agency's Office of Sustainability was developed to identify and leverage opportunities to incorporate sustainability and smart growth principles into long-term disaster recovery and hazard mitigation activities (DHS and EPA, 2010). Additionally, HUD has become a major player in disaster recovery as its Community Development Block Grant (CDBG) program has increasingly been used as a vehicle for funding post-disaster redevelopment, either through reprogramming of previously awarded funds or through supplemental appropriations from Congress. The CDBG program, with its focus on helping low- and moderate-income individuals, has historically addressed affordable housing, community development, and employment opportunities, all of which are social factors that influence health (HUD, 2014b). As discussed in more depth later in this report, requirements and guidance associated with recent supplemental appropriations for disaster recovery (i.e., CDBG-Disaster Recovery [DR] funds for Hurricane Sandy recovery) are being used to promote broader goals of community resilience and sustainability. Further, in 2014, President Obama announced the National Disaster Resilience Competition, which offers communities that have recently experienced a natural disaster the opportunity to compete for funds that would enable them to rebuild in ways that would increase resilience to future disasters (White House Office of the Press Secretary, 2014). Although the funds for this competition came from a one-time supplemental appropriation, it is spurring a national conversation about resilience and sustainability that may lead to further investment and legislation supporting resilience and sustainability at all levels, ultimately yielding benefits for health as well.

International Disaster Risk Reduction Policy

Internationally, greater emphasis on incorporating health considerations into resilience building and recovery is evident in recent efforts surrounding the second Hyogo Framework for Action (HFA-2), titled "Building the Resilience of Nations and Communities to Disasters" (Burkle et al., 2014). The first Hyogo Framework for Action (HFA-1) came about in 2005 at the request of the United Nations General Assembly and served as a 10-year international disaster risk reduction plan (UNISDR, 2015a). Disaster risk reduction refers to the "concept and practice of reducing disaster risks through systematic efforts to analyse and reduce the causal factors of disasters," such as by minimizing hazard exposure, reducing the vulnerability of people and property, and improving preparedness (UNISDR, 2015b). Investment in disaster risk reduction stems from the recognition that a disaster is a consequence of the choices societies make for their populations and environments (e.g., how they grow food, where and how they build homes, what

---

[11] There are five National Planning Frameworks—one for each of the core mission areas under the National Preparedness System, which are Prevention, Protection, Mitigation, Response, and Recovery (FEMA, 2014).

[12] The six recovery support functions are (1) Community Planning and Capacity Building, (2) Economic, (3) Health and Social Services, (4) Housing, (5) Infrastructure Systems, and (6) Natural and Cultural Resources (FEMA, 2011).

kind of government they have, how their financial system works). Every decision and action can make communities more vulnerable to—or more resilient to—disasters.

The United Nations International Strategy for Disaster Reduction (UNISDR) led the implementation of HFA-1, which emphasized ensuring the priority of disaster risk reduction, enhancing early warning, working to build a culture of safety and resilience at all levels, reducing underlying risk factors, and strengthening disaster preparedness for effective response (UNISDR, 2005). The original HFA, however, failed to identify health as a priority in disaster risk reduction and management. Since 2005, there has been widespread recognition of and emphasis on the need to make community health, resilience, and well-being, beyond just saving lives, an explicit focus. UNISDR recently reviewed HFA-1 and consulted on the development of HFA-2, a post-2015 framework for disaster risk reduction. At the Third World Conference on Disaster Risk Reduction, which took place in March 2015 in Sendai, Japan, conference representatives from U.S. and international organizations developed a post-2015 framework (Burkle et al., 2014; UNISDR, 2015a). The Sendai Framework for Disaster Risk Reduction 2015-2030 outlines the following goal: to "prevent new and reduce existing disaster risk through the implementation of integrated and inclusive economic, structural, legal, social, health, cultural, educational, environmental, technological, political and institutional measures that prevent and reduce hazard exposure and vulnerability to disaster, increase preparedness for response and recovery, and thus strengthen resilience" (WCDRR, 2015, p. 7). Such efforts are part of a growing recognition that disaster response is costly, whereas mitigation and preparedness initiatives, particularly those that address community health and resilience, save money and lives in the long run (Burkle et al., 2014).

The core mission areas of the U.S. National Preparedness System—prevention, protection, mitigation, response, and recovery—are consistent with a comprehensive approach to disaster risk reduction. Nonetheless, alignment of terminology and greater emphasis on addressing social determinants of health and reducing poverty as key strategies for reducing disaster risk could better harmonize U.S. policy with international efforts.

Climate Change Policy

The growing emphasis in the United States and internationally on increasing resilience is particularly important in the context of the emerging threat of climate change and scientists' predictions on how it may contribute to future disasters. Climate change is expected to lead to higher global temperatures, the secondary effects of which include increased sea levels, reduced snow cover, and changes in rainfall patterns (van Aalst, 2006). Experts project that the global warming observed in the last century will accelerate in the coming decades, likely increasing the frequency and severity of future natural disasters (Schipper and Pelling, 2006). Key determinants of health—water, air, food—are affected by changes in climate. The Fifth Assessment Report of the Intergovernmental Panel on Climate Change states with very high confidence that the health of human populations is sensitive to shifts in weather patterns and other aspects of climate change. This sensitivity is expected to manifest as exacerbations of existing health problems, disproportionately impacting vulnerable populations, such as the poor (O'Brien et al., 2006). With regard to health, the most effective measures for reducing vulnerability in the near term are programs that implement and improve such basic public health functions as providing clean water, sanitation, and essential health care; alleviating poverty; and increasing disaster preparedness capacity (Smith et al., 2014).

Both in the United States and internationally, it is recognized that disaster recovery planning should integrate the projected impacts of climate change with respect to future disasters. The United States has begun to take steps in this direction through President Obama's Climate Action Plan, released in June 2013. This plan not only commits to reducing U.S. carbon pollution and leading international efforts to combat global climate change but also outlines the importance of preparing the nation for the impacts of climate change by reducing vulnerabilities. Areas of focus within this key pillar include directing agencies to support local climate-resilient investments, working to create resilient and sustainable health care institutions, building on the new flood risk reduction standard for the region affected by Hurricane Sandy, and piloting strategies in that region to strengthen those communities against future extreme weather (White House Office of the Press Secretary, 2013).

The Changing Health Policy Landscape

This is a time of major change in the organization and financing of health care services, with increased focus on patient-centered medical homes, accountable care organizations, and outcome-based payment methodologies being driven by public- and private-sector initiatives to improve quality while decreasing costs. The Patient Protection and Affordable Care Act[13] (ACA) demonstrates clear support from the nation's top leadership for an approach to health that favors prevention (e.g., health promotion, access to primary care). This changing health policy landscape is an important factor in the opportunities communities have to achieve optimal health through recovery planning and execution. For example, the ACA includes provisions requiring nonprofit hospitals in the United States to conduct a community health needs assessment and adopt an implementation strategy for meeting identified community health needs. This information represents a valuable resource to inform recovery planning.

There is also increasing recognition that health is not just the responsibility of those working in the health sector (public health, medical system). Other examples of a shifting paradigm in population health are the adoption of a health-in-all-policies approach—"a collaborative approach to improving the health of all people by incorporating health considerations into decision-making across sectors and policy areas"—and the increasing use of health impact assessments to inform policy development (Rudolph et al., 2013, p. 5; WHO, 2014).

Despite the advances described above, there is a clear disconnect between the increasing understanding of how the health of communities can be improved through changes in policies, services, and environments and the approaches taken to community redevelopment after a disaster. It is the committee's premise that the growing prevention-based and all-sectors approach to health needs to be incorporated into disaster planning and recovery efforts.

HOW THIS REPORT IS INTENDED TO BE USED

As detailed earlier, this report is directed at several key audiences. These audiences fall essentially into two groups: those individuals and organizations involved in planning for and carrying out disaster recovery activities (see Figure 1-5) and those involved in planning for and building healthy communities. Through this report, the committee hopes to bring these two stakeholder groups together so that a health lens is applied to disaster recovery planning and the menu of tools and resources for health improvement planners is expanded to include those associated with disaster planning and recovery activities. The committee emphasizes that it does not consider health to be more important than other recovery support functions; in fact, it considers each area as critical to the building of healthy communities. The committee merely asserts that impacts on health outcomes should be one of the many priorities factored into decision making on recovery strategies and allocation of resources.

A particular focus of this report is key leadership involved in disaster recovery activities as they control the processes and resources that are mobilized in the pre- and post-disaster planning process. These leaders include elected officials such as governors, mayors, county and city managers, emergency managers, and disaster recovery coordinators. Following a disaster, pressure for urgent action is intense, and the decisions that must be made are inherently complex. Without prior sensitization, therefore, the longer-term health agenda can too easily be ignored, resulting in missed opportunities. Worse, inadequate attention to critical health protection functions can exacerbate long-standing health challenges or create new ones.

This report also is focused on sensitizing and educating leaders engaged in building healthier communities, who, the committee observed, generally are unaware of the opportunities and mechanisms associated

---

[13] The Patient Protection and Affordable Care Act, Public Law 111-148, 111th Cong., H.R.3590 (March 23, 2010).

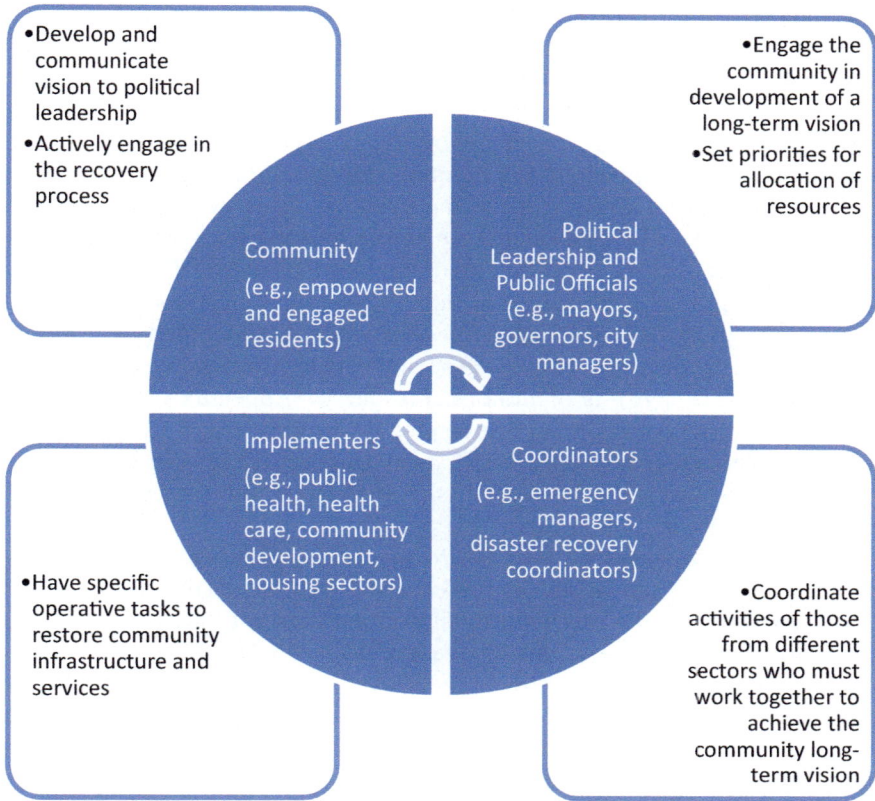

Community
(e.g., empowered and engaged residents)

Political Leadership and Public Officials
(e.g., mayors, governors, city managers)

Implementers
(e.g., public health, health care, community development, housing sectors)

Coordinators
(e.g., emergency managers, disaster recovery coordinators)

- Develop and communicate vision to political leadership
- Actively engage in the recovery process

- Engage the community in development of a long-term vision
- Set priorities for allocation of resources

- Have specific operative tasks to restore community infrastructure and services

- Coordinate activities of those from different sectors who must work together to achieve the community long-term vision

FIGURE 1-5 Key stakeholders in the disaster recovery process.

with disaster recovery. Disasters can catalyze bold changes that would not otherwise have been possible or that would have progressed at a much slower pace. Although there is a growing awareness that the way communities and service delivery systems have been designed has resulted in suboptimal health outcomes, healthy community initiatives often are impeded by a scarcity of resources. By bringing awareness of the opportunities presented during the recovery planning process to advance the goals of those working across multiple sectors to promote community well-being, the committee hopes to elicit their increased engagement in that process—both before and after a disaster.

To facilitate maximum utility for the wide array of audiences from various sectors, the report is organized in a modular format so that key operational guidance and recommendations, as well as their supporting background and evidence, are easily accessible. Part I of the report, which includes Chapters 1 through 4, establishes the framework for a healthy community approach to disaster recovery. These chapters define the concept of healthy communities and detail the comprehensive components that are pertinent to their realization. They also describe the financial and other resources that support disaster recovery and the allocation process by which those resources are mobilized. Some of the information presented in this first part of the report will be rudimentary to audiences who are well experienced in the complexities of recovery planning, financing, and governance. However, a key goal of this work is to present this information in a manner that is comprehensible to stakeholders who are not familiar with disaster management but whose engagement is critical to achieving healthy communities. Furthermore, the committee does not intend for this report to serve as a comprehensive guide to the recovery process and available recovery-related resources. In keeping with its charge, the committee focuses its description on those aspects of the recovery process relevant to the protection and promotion of the health of the affected community.[14]

The committee's operational-level guidance for individual sectors is presented in Part II. Chapters 5 through 8 provide guidance and supporting background regarding the opportunities to enhance human recovery through health and social services, including medical, behavioral and public health, and social support services. Chapters 9 and 10 provide guidance and supporting background regarding the opportunities to use place-based strategies[15] (i.e., coordinated interventions targeted to specific geographic areas) to rebuild the physical, social, and economic environments in a health-enhancing manner.

The final part of the report contains appendixes that include a detailed description of the federal policy environment influencing disaster recovery (Appendix A), a commissioned paper on financial assistance for recovery (Appendix B), a listing of additional resources (Appendix C), a description of measures and tools for evaluating healthy communities (Appendix D), a summary of the research needs identified throughout the chapters of this report (Appendix E), a key to select terms used to describe primary actors and key partners in Chapters 5 through 10 checklists (Appendix F), meeting agendas (Appendix G), and biographical sketches of the committee members (Appendix H).

Although this report was designed in a modular format with a number of sector-specific chapters, the committee emphasizes its intent that the report not contribute to the all too common problem of siloed engagement. As is noted throughout this report, all sectors have a role in creating communities that maximize the opportunities for their residents to live healthy and fulfilled lives. Accordingly, the reader will observe from time to time across different chapters a redundancy intended to advance an integrated perspective. Further, the committee strongly urges readers to consult not only the chapters specifically related to their own sector or field of practice but also those related to others. Reading the report in this way should provide a more holistic picture of the health-related impacts and opportunities associated with disasters and reveal complementary efforts, shared challenges, and abundant opportunities for synergy. With a strong belief that there is an ethical imperative to use every available opportunity to engage all available resources in the fight for health, **the committee concludes that *all* stakeholders involved in the pre-disaster and immediate- and long-term post-disaster strategic planning process need to be engaged, empowered, and supported in maximizing the opportunities to transform an unfortunate crisis into long-term benefit in the form of healthier communities and individuals.** What follows in the subsequent chapters is the committee's vision and recommendations for how this goal can be achieved.

REFERENCES

Aldrich, D. P. 2012. *Building resilience: Social capital in post-disaster recovery.* Chicago, IL: University of Chicago Press.
ASTHO (Association of State and Territorial Health Officials). 2012. *Pandemic and All-Hazards Preparedness Act fact sheet.* http://astho.org/Programs/Preparedness/Public-Health-Emergency-Law/Emergency-Authority-and-Immunity-Toolkit/Pandemic-and-All-Hazards-Preparedness-Act-Fact-Sheet (accessed October 10, 2014).
Bradley, E. H., and L. A. Taylor. 2013. *The American health care paradox: Why spending more is getting us less.* New York: Public Affairs.

---

[14] A broader selection of resources is available from FEMA's Community Recovery Management Toolkit, "a compilation of guidance, case studies, tools, and training to assist local communities in managing long-term recovery following a disaster." The toolkit can be accessed at http://www.fema.gov/national-disaster-recovery-framework/community-recovery-management-toolkit (accessed October 21, 2014). Additional resources are listed in Appendix C.

[15] "Place-based policies leverage investments by focusing resources in targeted places and drawing on the compounding effect of well-coordinated action. Effective place-based policies can influence how rural and metropolitan areas develop, how well they function as places to live, work, operate a business, preserve heritage, and more. Such policies can also streamline otherwise redundant and disconnected programs" (The White House, 2009, p. 1).

Bradley, E. H., B. R. Elkins, J. Herrin, and B. Elbel. 2011. Health and social services expenditures: Associations with health outcomes. *BMJ Quality and Safety* 20(10):826-831.

Brandt, M., C. Brown, J. Burkhart, N. Burton, J. Cox-Ganser, S. Damon, H. Falk, S. Fridkin, P. Garbe, M. McGeehin, J. Morgan, E. Page, C. Rao, S. Redd, T. Sinks, D. Trout, K. Wallingford, D. Warnock, and D. Weissman. 2006. Mold prevention strategies and possible health effects in the aftermath of hurricanes and major floods. *Morbidity and Mortality Weekly Report Recommendations and Reports* 55(RR08):1-27.

Burkle, F. M., S. Egawa, A. G. MacIntyre, Y. Otomo, C. W. Beadlin, and J. T. Walsh. 2014. The 2015 Hyogo Framework for Action: Cautious optimism. *Disaster Medicine and Public Health Preparedness* 8(3):191-192.

CDC (Centers for Disease Control and Prevention). 2010. *Public health workbook: To define, locate, and reach special, vulnerable, and at-risk populations in an emergency.* Atlanta, GA: CDC.

CDC. 2011. *Healthy communities: Preventing chronic disease by activating grassroots change at a glance 2011.* http://www.cdc.gov/chronicdisease/resources/publications/aag/healthy_communities.htm (accessed October 10, 2014).

CommonHealth ACTION. 2007. *Katrina and social determinants of health: Toward a comprehensive community preparedness approach.* http://commonhealthaction.org/PDF/CHA_KatrinaSocialDet.pdf (accessed March 27, 2015).

CRS (Congressional Research Service). 2014. *FEMA's disaster relief fund: Overview and selected issues.* Washington, DC: CRS, Library of Congress.

DHS (U.S. Department of Homeland Security), and EPA (U.S. Environmental Protection Agency). 2010. *Memorandum of agreement between the Department of Homeland Security (DHS), Federal Emergency Management Agency (FEMA) and the Environmental Protection Agency (EPA).* http://www.epa.gov/dced/pdf/2011_0114_fema-epa-moa.pdf (accessed March 17, 2015).

DRA (Disability Rights Activists). 2013. *Federal judge rules New York City's inadequate disaster plans discriminate against hundreds of thousands of New Yorkers with disabilities.* http://www.dralegal.org/pressroom/press-releases/federal-judge-rules-new-york-citys-inadequate-disaster-plans-discriminate (accessed March 4, 2015).

FEMA (Federal Emergency Management Agency). 2010. *Flood insurance dollars and sense.* https://www.fema.gov/news-release/2010/09/29/flood-insurance-dollars-and-sense (accessed February 24, 2015).

FEMA. 2011. *National disaster recovery framework.* Washington, DC: FEMA.

FEMA. 2014. *Overview of the national planning frameworks.* Washington, DC: FEMA.

Fossett, J. W. 2013. *Let's stop improvising disaster recovery.* http://www.rockinst.org/observations/fossettj/2013-07-09-Improvising_Disaster_Recovery.aspx (accessed June 5, 2014).

HHS (U.S. Department of Health and Human Services). 2009a. *HHS/ASPR/ABC fact sheet on at-risk individuals.* http://www.phe.gov/Preparedness/planning/abc/Documents/abc_listening_session.pdf (accessed March 4, 2015).

HHS. 2009b. *National health security strategy of the United States of America.* Washington, DC: HHS.

HHS. 2015a. *National health security strategy and implementation plan: 2015-2018.* Washington, DC: HHS.

HHS. 2015b. *Public health and social services emergency fund.* http://www.hhs.gov/budget/fy2015/fy2015-public-health-social-services-emergency-budget-justification.pdf (accessed March 17, 2015).

HRIA (Health Resources in Action). 2013. *Defining healthy communities.* Boston, MA: Health Resources in Action. http://hria.org/uploads/catalogerfiles/defining-healthy-communities/defining_healthy_communities_1113_final_report.pdf (accessed October 21, 2014).

HUD (U.S. Department of Housing and Urban Development). 2014a. *CDBG-DR active disaster grants and grantee contact information.* https://www.hudexchange.info/cdbg-dr/cdbg-dr-grantee-contact-information (accessed March 31, 2015).

HUD. 2014b. *Community Development Block Grant Disaster Recovery program.* https://www.hudexchange.info/cdbg-dr (accessed March 23, 2015).

IOM (Institute of Medicine). 2012a. *Crisis standards of care: A systems framework for catastrophic disaster response.* Washington, DC: The National Academies Press.

IOM. 2012b. *For the public's health: Investing in a healthier future.* Washington, DC: The National Academies Press.

KFF (The Henry J. Kaiser Family Foundation). 2012. *Health care costs: A primer.* http://kff.org/health-costs/issue-brief/health-care-costs-a-primer (accessed October 9, 2014).

Landesman, L. Y. 2005. *Public health management of disasters: The practice guide.* Washington, DC: American Public Health Association.

Leonard, H. B., and A. M. Howitt. 2010. Acting in time against disasters: A comprehensive risk-management framework. In *Learning from catastrophes: Strategies for reaction and response*, edited by H. Kunreather and M. Useem. Upper Saddle River, NJ: Wharton School Publishing. Pp. 18-40.

Lindell, M. K., W. C. Nicholson, C. S. Prater, and R. W. Perry. 2006. *Fundamentals of Emergency Management*. Washington, DC: FEMA.

Mensah, G. A., A. H. Mokdad, S. F. Posner, E. Reed, E. J. Simoes, M. M. Engelgua, and Chronic Diseases and Vulnerable Populations in Natural Disasters Working Group. 2005. When chronic conditions become acute: Prevention and control of chronic disease and adverse health outcomes during natural disasters. *Preventing Chronic Disease* 2(A04).

Nelson, C., N. Lurie, J. Wasserman, and S. Zakowski. 2007. Conceptualizing and defining public health emergency preparedness. *American Journal of Public Health* 97(Suppl. 1):S9-S11.

NRC (National Research Council). 2012. *Disaster resilience: A national imperative*. Washington, DC: The National Academies Press.

NRC and IOM. 2013. *U.S. health in international perspective: Shorter lives, poorer health*. Edited by S. H. Woolf and L. Aron. Washington, DC: The National Academies Press.

O'Brien, G., P. O'Keefe, J. Rose, and B. Wisner. 2006. Climate change and disaster management. *Disasters* 30(1):64-80.

OECD. 2013. *Health at a glance 2013: OECD indicators*. http://www.oecd-ilibrary.org/docserver/download/8113161e. pdf?expires=1426695435&id=id&accname=guest&checksum=0897D47D81D49EBEA66A34DE4EBC02CF (accessed October 9, 2014).

O'Sullivan, T. L., C. E. Kuziemsky, W. Corneil, L. Lemyre, and Z. Franco. 2014. The EnRiCH Community Resilience Framework for High-Risk Populations. *PLoS Currents Disasters* Oct 2. Edition 1.

Peters, M. N., J. C. Moscona, M. J. Katz, K. B. Deandrade, H. C. Quevedo, S. Tiwari, A. R. Burchett, T. A. Turnage, K. Y. Singh, E. N. Fomunung, S. Srivastav, P. Delafontaine, and A. M. Irimpen. 2014. Natural disasters and myocardial infarction: The six years after hurricane Katrina. *Mayo Clinic Proceedings* 89(4):472-477.

Rubin, C. B. 1991. Recovery from disaster. In *Emergency management: Principles and practice for local governments*. Washington, DC: International City Management Association, Municipal Management Series. Pp. 224-259.

Rubin, C. B., M. D. Saperstein, and D. G. Barbee. 1985. *Community recovery from a major natural disaster*. Monograph No. 41. Boulder, CO: Program on Environment and Behavior, Institute of Behavioral Science, University of Colorado.

Rudolph, L., J. Caplan, K. Ben-Moshe, and L. Dillon. 2013. *Health in All Policies: A guide for state and local governments*. Washington, DC, and Oakland, CA: American Public Health Association and Public Health Institute. http://www.phi.org/uploads/files/Health_in_All_Policies-A_Guide_for_State_and_Local_Governments.pdf (accessed November 18, 2014).

Runkle, J. D., A. Brock-Martin, W. Karmaus, and E. R. Svendsen. 2012. Secondary surge capacity: A framework for understanding long-term access to primary care for medically vulnerable populations in disaster recovery. *American Journal of Public Health* 102(12):e24-e32.

RWJF (Robert Wood Johnson Foundation). 2014. *Time to act: Investing in the health of our children and communities*. Princeton, NJ: RWJF. http://www.rwjf.org/content/dam/farm/reports/reports/2014/rwjf409002 (accessed October 9, 2014).

Schipper, L., and M. Pelling. 2006. Disaster risk, climate change and international development: Scope for, and challenges to, integration. *Disasters* 30(1):19-38.

Sherry, N., and A. Harkins. 2011. Leveling the emergency preparedness playing field. *Journal of Emergency Management* 9(6):11-16.

Smith, K. R., A. Woodward, D. Campbell-Lendrum, D. D. Chadee, Y. Honda, Q. Liu, J. M. Olwoch, B. Revich, and R. Sauerborn. 2014. Human health: Impacts, adaptation, and co-benefits. In *Climate change 2014: Impacts, adaptation, and vulnerability. Part A: Global and sectoral aspects. Contribution of working group II to the fifth assessment report of the intergovernmental panel on climate change*, edited by C. B. Field, V. R. Barros, D. J. Dokken, K. J. Mach, M. D. Mastrandrea, T. E. Bilir, M. Chatterjee, K. L. Ebi, Y. O. Estrada, R. C. Genova, B. Girma, E. S. Kissel, A. N. Levy, S. MacCracken, P. R. Mastrandrea, and L. L. White. Cambridge, United Kingdom and New York: Cambridge University Press. Pp. 709-754.

TFAH (Trust for America's Health). 2013a. *A healthier America 2013: Strategies to move from sick care to health care in the next four years*. Washington, DC: TFAH.

TFAH. 2013b. *Our vision for a healthier America*. http://healthyamericans.org/assets/files/VisionHealthierAmerica. pdf (accessed October 9, 2014).

UNISDR (United Nations International Strategy for Disaster Reduction). 2005. *Summary of the Hyogo framework for action 2005-2015: Building the resilience of nations and communities to disasters (Hyogo framework)*. Geneva, Switzerland: UNISDR.

UNISDR. 2009. *Terminology.* http://www.unisdr.org/we/inform/terminology (accessed February 27, 2015).

UNISDR. 2015a. *Post-2015 framework for disaster risk reduction.* http://www.unisdr.org/we/coordinate/hfa-post2015 (accessed February 13, 2015).

UNISDR. 2015b. *What is disaster risk reduction?* http://www.unisdr.org/who-we-are/what-is-drr (accessed March 17, 2015).

van Aalst, M. K. 2006. The impacts of climate change on the risk of natural disasters. *Disasters* 30(1):5-18.

WCDRR (World Conference on Disaster Risk Reduction). 2015. *Sendai framework for disaster risk reduction 2015-2030.* http://www.wcdrr.org/uploads/Sendai_Framework_for_Disaster_Risk_Reduction_2015-2030.pdf (accessed March 23, 2015).

Weiss, D. J., and J. Weidman. 2013. Disastrous spending: Federal disaster-relief expenditures rise amid more extreme weather. *Center for American Progress.* https://cdn.americanprogress.org/wp-content/uploads/2013/04/Weiss DisasterSpending-1.pdf (accessed March 22, 2015).

The White House. 2009. *Developing effective place-based policies for the FY 2011 budget.* http://www.whitehouse. gov/sites/default/files/omb/assets/memoranda_fy2009/m09-28.pdf (accessed March 4, 2015).

White House Office of the Press Secretary. 2013. *Fact sheet: President Obama's climate action plan.* https://www. whitehouse.gov/the-press-office/2013/06/25/fact-sheet-president-obama-s-climate-action-plan (accessed February 27, 2015).

White House Office of the Press Secretary. 2014. *Fact sheet: National disaster resilience competition.* https://www. whitehouse.gov/the-press-office/2014/06/14/fact-sheet-national-disaster-resilience-competition (accessed March 17, 2015).

WHO (World Health Organization). 1948. *Preamble to the constitution of the World Health Organization.* Geneva, Switzerland: WHO.

WHO. 2014. *Health Impact Assessment (HIA).* http://www.who.int/hia/en (accessed March 25, 2014).

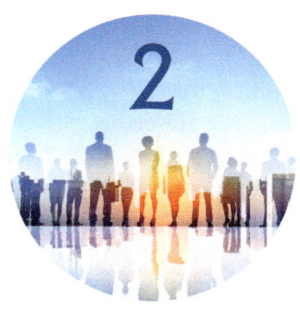

2

Post-Disaster Opportunities to Advance Healthy, Resilient, and Sustainable Communities

A strong category 2 hurricane makes landfall on a small island in the Gulf Coast (NOAA, 2008). Winds estimated at more than 100 mph and a storm surge of more than 10 feet result in significant flooding and damage to the island's physical infrastructure—more than 70 percent of the buildings on the island are damaged or destroyed, including large concentrations of public housing. Much of the island, including the interior of remaining homes and structures, is covered in a layer of sediment contaminated with heavy metals and other toxic residues from an industrial area that was in the path of the storm surge. Residents are displaced for weeks and in some neighborhoods, for months. Many never return. Those that do face enormous challenges. Many of the businesses that supported the economy of the island are closed for months, including the large academic center that represents the largest employer in the area. Jobs are lost as a result of these closures but also because parents are unable to find safe places to leave their children while they work. Most people are not adequately prepared to provide the documentation and paperwork (e.g., proof of home ownership, proof of insurance, medical prescriptions) needed to access critical benefits and resources. The local housing authority experiences a five-fold increase in demand for housing assistance (Nolen et al., 2010). The trauma and stress of this situation exact a toll on the health of the population, especially those with preexisting conditions such as chronic disease or mental illness. At the 1-year mark, more than 10 percent of the population meet criteria for a probable mental health disorder diagnosis (Ruggiero et al., 2012).

As the recovery process proceeds, it becomes clear that disadvantaged individuals and neighborhoods face additional challenges that delay recovery. Many of the most severely damaged neighborhoods are in low-lying areas of the island characterized by large concentrations of impoverished and low-income populations (Nolen et al., 2010). Disruption of public transit in these areas poses great challenges for residents that lack cars, a problem exacerbated by the closure of many neighborhood amenities such as grocery stores. A "not in my backyard" mentality impedes the timely rebuilding of public housing, which was torn down before former residents were allowed to retrieve any remaining belongings. Many former public housing occupants who have been unable to return to the island because of the lack of affordable housing have no voice in the recovery planning process as a result of restrictions that limit participation to current residents. Such cor-

47

rosive social dynamics build distrust among neighbors and further distress the vulnerable. Five years after the storm, public housing still has not been rebuilt (Rice, 2014).

The scenario above is not hypothetical, but describes the impact of Hurricane Ike on the island of Galveston, Texas, in 2008. This example demonstrates how disasters can alter the status of many of the fundamental elements that affect the health of a community—the availability of housing, including public housing for low-income individuals; social networks; environmental quality; economic stability and the availability of employment; transportation access to essential goods and services; safe places for children to play and learn; access to nutritious food; and continuity of medical care. Not only did the disaster add stress for already vulnerable populations and amplify existing health disparities; its effect on the population as a whole was to cause the long-standing suboptimal health of the community to deteriorate further. Even prior to Hurricane Ike, Galveston ranked below the Texas state and national averages with regard to such key health status indicators as mortality from cardiovascular disease, lung cancer, and suicide (GCHD, 2001).

For Galveston, and communities like it, recovery from a disaster can provide a mechanism for addressing many of the factors that contribute to poor health status and vulnerability. Disasters, although unquestionably tragic, create new resources and opportunities to advance the design and realization of healthy communities. One such opportunity is the synchronization of strategic planning across multiple disciplines and sectors that occurs during disaster recovery (Nolen, 2014), providing a mechanism for engaging the whole community in the redesign process. The sudden destruction of physical infrastructure and disruption of systems may in some cases enable significant reorganization of facilities, services, and organizational structures to create more optimal arrangements and dispense with obsolete ones that may have been impeding communities from reaching their full potential. Additionally, an array of resources, scaled appropriately to the nature of the event, are mobilized with the specific purpose of assisting communities in addressing many of the fundamental factors that are important to health, by, among other things,

- restoring public health, medical, and social service systems to meet the needs of the impacted populations;
- supporting safety, psychosocial well-being, and social connections; and
- rebuilding physical infrastructure such as housing, transportation systems, and critical public works systems.

It should be recognized, however, that there is no such thing as a blank slate after a disaster. To varying degrees, all communities are constantly amending their circumstances through a variety of programs and plans. A disaster is an influence on those ongoing practices, a temporary detour. The question becomes how to seize the opportunities of reinvestment to address long-standing and perplexing problems that compromise the health and overall welfare of a community.

Across the world, communities are already working to improve their own health status from the ground up by engaging community members and organizations in all aspects of projects, from setting initial priorities to evaluating outcomes—a phenomenon known as the healthy communities movement (Norris, 2013; Pittman, 2010). Acknowledging that the starting point for individual communities varies widely, the committee emphasizes that disaster recovery offers a unique opportunity to further these efforts. In this chapter, the committee outlines the elements of a healthy, resilient, and sustainable community and explains why an integrated approach is essential to enable the realization of that shared goal.

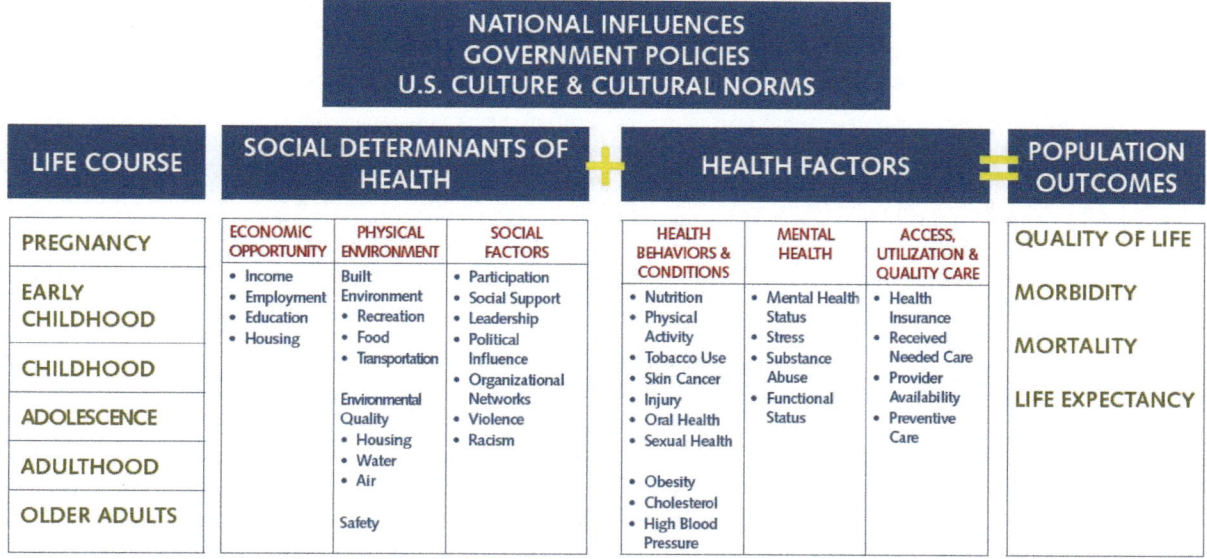

FIGURE 2-1 Model for the combinatorial effects of health determinants on population health outcomes.
SOURCE: Data provided by the Colorado Department of Public Health and Environment, https://www.colorado.gov/pacific/sites/default/files/HealthEquityModel.pdf (accessed April, 4, 2015).

WHAT IS A HEALTHY COMMUNITY?

Leveraging the disaster recovery process to advance the health of a community necessitates an understanding of the diverse determinants that influence health and specific healthy community elements relevant to the post-disaster period. These are described in the sections below.

Determinants of Health

As shown in Figure 2-1, population health outcomes (e.g., life expectancy, morbidity, quality of life) result from a number of different factors. Interventions to improve population health[1] have historically placed significant emphasis on changing health-related behavioral choices of individuals and the quality of public health and health care delivery systems. Although these remain important determinants of health, there is growing awareness that the locally specific built, natural, and social environments—now understood to be social determinants of health (see Box 2-1)—also are prominent influences on health outcomes. As is increasingly understood, "place matters" to health. As expressed by one set of authors, "Your zip code is a powerful predictor of how healthy you are and how long you are likely to live" (Standish and Ross, 2014, p. 31). Such factors as the presence of safe places to be physically active, access to healthy and nutritious food, a clean environment, quality educational systems, accessible social services, and strong systems for community support can make a big difference in the health of an individual, as well as the health of a community. Yet a large number of communities in the United States lack even these basic features. According to the Robert Wood Johnson Foundation Commission to Build a Healthier America, "nearly a fifth of all Americans live in unhealthy neighborhoods that are marked by limited job opportu-

---

[1] The term "population health" describes "the health outcomes of a group of individuals, including the distribution of such outcomes within the group" (Kindig and Stoddart, 2003, p. 380).

BOX 2-1
What Are the Social Determinants of Health?

"The social determinants of health are the circumstances in which people are born, grow up, live, work and age, and the systems put in place to deal with illness. These circumstances are in turn shaped by a wider set of forces: economics, social policies, and politics" (WHO, 2014b).

---

nities, low-quality housing, pollution, limited access to healthy food, and few opportunities for physical activity" (RWJF Commission to Build a Healthier America, 2014, p. 10).

Geographic variation in factors that influence health creates significant differences in health outcomes across segments of the population (i.e., health inequities). Within a single city, for example, life expectancy can vary by as much as 15 to 25 years depending on the neighborhood (Standish and Ross, 2014). Many of the factors that contribute to this observed effect of place are systemic, with roots in the nation's historical social policies, such as segregation (e.g., racially restrictive zoning) and other policies related to civil rights that have created barriers to meaningful civic participation (IOM, 2014). Thus, the physical and social environments are inextricably linked, and targeted, place-based interventions aimed at changing those environments in ways that better promote health and address socioeconomic disparities could have a large impact on population health outcomes.

Elements of a Healthy Community

In Chapter 1, a healthy community is defined as

> one in which a diverse group of stakeholders collaborate to use their expertise and local knowledge to create a community that is socially and physically conducive to health. Community members are empowered and civically engaged, assuring that all local policies consider health. The community has the capacity to identify, address, and evaluate their own health concerns on an ongoing basis, using data to guide and benchmark efforts. As a result, a healthy community is safe, economically secure, and environmentally sound, as all residents have equal access to high quality educational and employment opportunities, transportation and housing options, prevention and healthcare services, and healthy food and physical activity opportunities. (HRIA, 2013, p. 24)

Inherent in this definition is the premise that a healthy community is not a fixed entity but results from continual efforts to create and improve physical and social environments that allow community members to support each other in carrying out the day-to-day functions of living and achieving their full potential. To increase awareness among stakeholders regarding their role in shaping the conditions that affect health, a better understanding of what makes a healthy community is needed. The committee found a wealth of sources that describe elements of healthy communities, with significant overlap. One of the most comprehensive lists was developed by the California Health in All Policies[2] Task Force as a healthy community framework (California Health in All Policies Task Force, 2010; Rudolph et al., 2013a). The committee adapted that framework to derive the list of healthy community elements in Box 2-2. Communities can use such resources to develop their own locally relevant healthy community vision and goals. More detailed discussion of the link between health and many of the elements listed in Box 2-2 is included in the sector-specific chapters of this report (Chapters 5-10).

---

[2] Health in All Policies is defined as "a collaborative approach to improving the health of all people by incorporating health considerations into decision-making across sectors and policy areas" (Rudolph et al., 2013a, p. 5).

BOX 2-2
Elements of a Healthy Community

A healthy community encompasses the following elements:

A safe, healthy, and aesthetically pleasing physical environment, including:
- All features of complete and livable communities (quality schools, recreational areas and facilities, child care, libraries, financial services, and other daily needs)
- Clean (i.e., free of toxins) indoor and outdoor environments, including air, soil, surfaces, and water
- Affordable and sustainable energy use
- Parks and green spaces, including a healthy tree canopy and agricultural lands
- A regional transportation grid featuring street connectivity and safe, sustainable, accessible, and affordable active and public transportation options
- Facilities and recreational areas for safe, affordable physical activity and policies that promote equitable access to those areas
- Accessible locations at which to obtain affordable and nutritious foods
- Affordable, high-quality, and location-efficient housing that meets national healthy housing criteria
- Building construction that incorporates universal design principles to support access for all community members
- Land use policies that help mitigate against known hazards
- Safe, functional, and resilient critical infrastructure

An inclusive, supportive social environment, including:
- A whole-community approach to strategic planning and problem solving, involving robust civic participation by empowered residents and leadership from community organizations and public officials
- An emphasis on data-driven decision making and ongoing quality improvement in all sectors
- Inclusive, supportive, respectful community social bonds, from the neighborhood to the regional level
- Resiliency to adapt to changing environments and emergencies
- Quality educational opportunities accessible to all residents
- Living-wage, safe, and healthy job opportunities for all residents and a thriving economy
- Safe communities, free of violence, crime, bullying, racism, and discrimination
- Integrated and accessible social and community services to address the spectrum of human needs efficiently and effectively
- Support for healthy development of children and adolescents
- Opportunities for engagement with arts, music, and culture

A high-quality, comprehensive health system, including:
- Affordable, accessible, high-quality, and patient-centered preventive health services and health care
- Emphasis on individual and family health literacy, capacity building, and empowerment
- A robust public health system that provides the essential public health services

SOURCE: Adapted from California Health in All Policies Task Force, 2010.

From the list in Box 2-2, several cross-cutting themes for healthy communities emerge:

- **Equity**—The World Health Organization defines equity as "the absence of avoidable or remediable differences among groups of people, whether those groups are defined socially, economically, demographically, or geographically" (WHO, 2014a). Health inequity denotes health disparities that result from "systemic, avoidable and unjust social and economic policies and practices that create barriers to opportunity" (Rudolph et al., 2013a, p. 135).

- **Resilience**—Resilience is the ability to prepare and plan for, absorb, respond to, recover from, and adapt more successfully to adverse events. No person or place is immune from disasters or disaster-related losses. "Enhanced resilience allows better anticipation of disasters and better planning to reduce disaster losses" (NRC, 2012, p. 1). Although the term often is associated with disasters and climate change, the concept of resilience also applies to everyday challenges in communities, such as gradual economic decline.
- **Sustainability**—Building on the Brundtland Commission's definition of sustainable development,[3] sustainability can be described as "the ability of communities to consistently thrive over time as they make decisions to improve the community today without sacrificing the future" (McGalliard, 2012, p. 2).

Health, equity, resilience, and sustainability are interdependent and mutually reinforcing—part of the same virtuous cycle. As a result of this interdependence, initiatives that reduce inequities will yield benefits for population health, as will efforts to strengthen the sustainability or resilience of a community. Conversely, a healthy population is a critical component of sustainable and thriving economic and social systems (Rudolph et al., 2013b).

EQUITY, RESILIENCE, SUSTAINABILITY, AND HEALTH IN THE POST-DISASTER CONTEXT

Equity, resilience, and sustainability are all relevant to post-disaster efforts to build healthier communities. To better clarify these linkages, each is described below in the context of health and disaster recovery.

Equity

Equity is integral to a healthy, resilient, and sustainable community; conversely, policies and practices that are exclusionary and promote inequality undermine a community's long-term viability. In an equitable society, differences in the conditions and successes of individuals are not strongly linked to categories such as ethnicity, race, gender, or disability status (ICMA, 2014). Unfortunately, too many communities are characterized by significant variability in access to essential goods, services (including health care), amenities, and opportunities (e.g., education, employment, and other social determinants of health) across subgroups (RWJF, 2008). This unequal distribution of resources often manifests as geographic clusters of poverty, crime, and poor health status. The World Health Organization has declared addressing the underlying inequities resulting from "poor social policies and programmes, unfair economic arrangements, and bad politics" an ethical imperative (CSDH, 2008, p. 1).

Disasters tend to expose and exacerbate preexisting inequities. Past experiences have shown that the impacts of disasters are not experienced equally across a community, and recovery proceeds at different rates for different groups. People with fewer resources (financial and social) struggle to recover more than their more affluent and connected peers do. Health disparities also can be exacerbated by disasters, resulting in poorer health outcomes for those already dealing with preexisting conditions such as chronic disease (Davis et al., 2010). In effect, the social determinants of health are also the determinants of social vulnerability (see Box 2-3). This is an important point not only at the individual level but also at the community level: a community with large concentrations of vulnerable populations will be less resilient in the face of social and economic disruption and slower to recover. Thus, addressing equity issues before a disaster is also a means of overcoming system weaknesses or vulnerabilities. Although the importance of addressing social vulnerability through comprehensive disaster risk reduction strategies (discussed in

---

[3] The Brundtland Commission defined sustainable development as "development that meets the needs of the present without compromising the ability of future generations to meet their own needs" (World Commission on Environment and Development, 1987).

BOX 2-3
Social Vulnerability to Disasters

Disasters can be viewed as a result of the interaction between a hazardous event and a vulnerable community. "Vulnerability is place-based and context-specific" (NRC, 2012, p. 97), linked to both the physical environment (e.g., where communities are built, the strength of buildings) and social environments, inclusive of a variety of economic, political, and cultural conditions. The concept of social vulnerability refers to "the characteristics of a person or group and their situation that influence their capacity to anticipate, cope with, resist and recover from the impact of a natural hazard" (Wisner et al., 2003, p. 11), and stratification in this capacity is observed across groups of people as a result of inequalities. As a result, disaster impacts are experienced differently among and within communities. The inverse relationship between social vulnerability and resilience (discussed in the following section) is apparent from the congruence in their definitions, with resilience having been defined as the ability to prepare and plan for, absorb, respond to, recover from, and adapt more successfully to adverse events (NRC, 2012).

Chapter 1) is increasingly being acknowledged, the connection between efforts to address social vulnerability and activities aimed at reducing disparities in social determinants of health has not been widely recognized (Few, 2007; Lindsay, 2003), and this represents a missed opportunity to achieve synergy among different professional sectors with shared goals.

After a disaster, there may be new opportunities to address inequities and related social vulnerability issues through recovery efforts. However, leveraging these opportunities requires careful planning in which equity is intentionally included as an objective, and special attention is given to accessibility, affordability, and inclusiveness as the community rebuilds. Recovery practices that intentionally or unintentionally exclude marginalized groups can instead deepen inequities. The committee heard in testimony that "not in my backyard" attitudes can arise during recovery and create significant tension within communities, potentially driving displacement of low-income and other underserved groups (disaster-related gentrification). For example, rebuilding of public housing became a hotly debated and highly politicized topic in Galveston, Texas, after Hurricane Ike (Nolen, 2014). However, discussions on health and creating healthy communities provided a pathway for overcoming these "not in my backyard" concerns and polarizing issues such as public housing. When these concerns and issues are presented in the context of the health and well-being of the whole community, common ground can be found (Nolen, 2014). Indeed, health and well-being have previously been described as foundations for expanding social equity initiatives (ICMA, 2014).

Examples of efforts that promote both social equity and health that may be relevant to post-disaster recovery include but are not limited to

- supporting development of affordable housing,
- providing housing options well suited to the elderly and disabled,
- developing transportation programs specifically for low-income residents and expanding bus routes,
- building community centers that offer educational and recreational programs designed to bring all members of a community together,
- ensuring access to information technology/the Internet for all residents (which helps ensure inclusiveness since digital forms of communication are increasingly being used),
- developing energy reduction programs to assist low-income residents,
- creating workforce development programs for underserved groups to increase economic stability among vulnerable populations, and
- developing initiatives to address food deserts (ICMA, 2014).

To be optimally effective, however, communities require complementary investments targeted to areas of greatest need (data-driven), leveraging cross-sector collaborations and aligned funding streams.

Resilience

Resilience is multifaceted, and it can refer to infrastructure, individuals, environmental or economic systems, and organizations. Growing concerns regarding climate change and experiences from recent disasters such as Hurricanes Katrina and Sandy and the Deepwater Horizon oil spill have prompted greater attention to resilience among the emergency management, health, environmental, and public policy sectors. Such initiatives as 100 Resilient Cities—pioneered by the Rockefeller Foundation—are enabling cities around the world to learn from each other and develop a road map for becoming more resilient to the physical, social, and economic challenges resulting from sudden events (e.g., disasters such as hurricanes and earthquakes), as well as chronic stresses that weaken the fabric of a community (e.g., unemployment, an overtaxed or inefficient public transportation system, community violence, food and water shortages) (100 Resilient Cities, 2014).

Health status and resilience (or inversely, vulnerability) are intimately linked at both the individual and community levels. As stated by LTG Russell Honoré, Commander, Joint Task Force, Katrina, "The health of a community before any crisis has a direct correlation to the magnitude of the health crisis after the event" (Honoré, 2008, p. S6). Unhealthy individuals suffer more severe consequences when routine health system functions and social networks are disrupted and may require more time and resources to recover. For example, chronic diseases are exacerbated as routine disease management services are interrupted and access to nutritious food and medications is impeded (Davis et al., 2010).

Resilience-building efforts generally are aimed at reducing the impacts of future disasters,[4] including impacts on health and the length of the recovery period. At the same time, however, actions that can be taken to make communities less vulnerable, and thus more resilient, also benefit the community in the everyday context through improvements in community health and well-being—for example, by addressing social determinants of health that create social vulnerability. This point is of paramount importance because in a fiscally constrained environment, investment in resilience (i.e., the future) is easier to justify when there are co-benefits to the community and its well-being beyond the disaster context (i.e., today). Community health resilience then emerges within this dual opportunity space that represents the intersection of community health promotion and emergency preparedness and provides a mechanism for alignment (Chandra, 2014). The process of building community health resilience has been described as a "reframing of long-standing approaches to improve community well-being" (Plough et al., 2013, p. 1190). Under this aligned framework, coalitions and partnerships developed for purposes of emergency preparedness and resilience can be leveraged for health promotion and disease prevention initiatives and vice versa (Plough et al., 2013). The resulting efficiency should have broad appeal as funding for both public health emergency preparedness and community health promotion continues to decline.

Like health status, social connectedness is a human characteristic that affects resilience at both the individual and the population level. Social networks are formed from the connections among community residents, as well as residents' connections with individuals and organizations outside of their community (Bourdieu, 1986; Coleman, 1988; Granovetter, 1973). Previous experience has shown that communities with high levels of social connectedness (often referred to as social capital) display resilience that serves them well during post-disaster recovery (Aida et al., 2013; Aldrich and Sawada, 2014; Cutter et al., 2003; Nakagawa and Shaw, 2004). Individuals and communities with shared norms and strong ties can better connect to critical resources and mobilize to overcome problems that arise during a crisis through collective action (Adeola and Picou, 2012; Aldrich and Crook, 2008; Hurlbert et al., 2000; Kawachi et al., 2008). Following a disaster, many of the standard providers of resources and services—such as medical,

---

[4] It should be noted that resilience-strengthening activities undertaken during the disaster response/early recovery stages can improve the efficiency of recovery (shorten recovery time) in addition to providing protection against future disasters (Chandra, 2014).

retail, and child care—are shut down for days, if not weeks. These resources and services may be available only through friends, family, and neighbors, and they can be better accessed by individuals with stronger connections following a catastrophe (Hurlbert et al., 2000).

A number of the challenges faced by communities following a disaster occur at the neighborhood or block level, not the individual level. When a disaster strikes, and many times beforehand, social networks help organize evacuations. After a disaster, social capital continues to help communities mobilize as a collective. If only a single homeowner decides to clean up disaster debris, for example, the property values of that and the neighbors' homes will not stabilize, but when all members of a neighborhood work together, they can improve the appearance of the whole area. Social ties to an area are important to its recovery because for many without such ties, the high costs of returning, including financial, opportunity, and psychological burdens, may overwhelm the benefits, and they may choose to start life anew elsewhere.

Like other forms of capital, social capital can be deliberately created. Double-blind field experiments have demonstrated that deliberate interventions can deepen existing bonds in a community regardless of its socioeconomic status or level of homogeneity (Brune and Bossert, 2009; Pronyk et al., 2008). Ideally, such efforts should be undertaken before a disaster as a component of resilience-building initiatives and may entail either top-down or bottom-up approaches (see the examples in Box 2-4).

Sustainability

Disaster recovery can be viewed as a special case of the ongoing sustainable community development process, with the benefit of linking recovery to existing sustainability planning activities in many communities[5] (Natural Hazards Center, 2005). In sustainable development, values related to physical, economic, and social environments are balanced so that contemporary communities can thrive without compromising future generations (ICMA, 2014). The achievement of that balance results in communities that are livable (built in a way that allows residents to live the lives they want to live), equitable (such that the burdens and benefits of policy decisions are distributed evenly across a community), and viable (with policies and practices being flexible enough to adapt to changing needs and not compromising future generations).[6] Needs related to these same three environments (physical, social, and economic) must be addressed holistically during recovery.

Although health and well-being are implicit in these concepts, there has been increased attention recently to addressing health issues strategically in the context of sustainability (Mishkovsky, 2010). When health is integrated into ongoing sustainability planning efforts, accountability extends beyond the public health agency to the broader local government. Because development decisions made by local government policy makers shape so many aspects of the physical, social, and economic environments that impact health, there is growing consensus that these leaders should work more consciously and deliberately to achieve public health goals (Mishkovsky, 2010).

U.S. sustainability policy leapt forward in 2009 with the development of the Partnership for Sustainable Communities—a joint initiative of the U.S. Department of Housing and Urban Development (HUD), the U.S. Department of Transportation (DOT), and the U.S. Environmental Protection Agency (EPA)—and its six principles for livability (see Box 2-5). Over the past 5 years, HUD, DOT, and EPA have improved coordination and collaboration to better align federal policies and investments, reducing duplication and facilitating comprehensive and integrated solutions to the complex and interrelated economic, environmental, and social challenges that impede the realization of healthy communities (Partnership for Sustainable Communities, 2014). With increasing support from federal leadership, communities nationwide

---

[5] Although the term "sustainability" may for some denote only efforts to address long-term environmental problems (e.g., climate change) or issues of financial affordability, the committee uses it in its broadest sense to include dimensions of environmental integrity, economic viability, and social equity (ICMA, 2014).

[6] In some communities, strategic planning focuses on these three core values rather than an explicit commitment to sustainability, which is a more politically charged term (ICMA, 2014).

BOX 2-4
Building Social Capital to Strengthen Communities:
Examples of Top-Down and Bottom-Up Approaches

Top-Down Approaches to Building Social Capital

Following the 2011 New Zealand earthquakes, the central government set up the Canterbury Earthquake Recovery Authority (CERA) to coordinate recovery efforts; among its core interests was strengthening social capital in the area by building efficacy and community connectedness. CERA has worked to use funds collected from the lottery to support the Community Organisation Grants Scheme by streamlined application processes. Through this program, volunteers can receive funds to support the development of local community and non-governmental organizations. Further, CERA tracks various indicators of social capital in the area, including volunteering rates and sense of belonging, to track how its programs are impacting local community members. Through these top-down programs, the central government has strengthened the resilience of the community (CERA, 2013a,b).

Bottom-Up Approaches to Building Social Capital

San Francisco, California

In recognition of the value of strong community bonds and social networks to a region, a collaborative was formed in 2007 in San Francisco, California. This initiative brought together city agencies, business associations, corporations, community organizations, nonprofit and faith-based institutions, foundations, and academic centers around the mission of empowering their neighborhoods with the capacity to build resiliency. This collaborative, known formally as the Neighborhood Empowerment Network (NEN), has focused on using a grassroots approach to design tools and resources for use in all stages of community organization (NEN, 2014a).

NEN has established programs in several areas—including public safety, education, infrastructure, and emergency management—focused on building social capital in San Francisco neighborhoods. One such program, Resilientville, is a role-playing exercise aimed at developing awareness of the benefits of problem solving at the neighborhood level and strengthening the ability of residents to respond collectively to a wide variety of unforeseen challenges and opportunities by encouraging community members to focus first on daily issues

are integrating smart growth, environmental justice,[7] and equitable development approaches to create the healthy, equitable, and sustainable communities that Americans have shown they want (Partnership for Sustainable Communities, 2014). In the post-disaster environment, sustainable redevelopment efforts often focus on hazard mitigation, but this focus reflects a narrow view of sustainability. As discussed in Chapter 1, increasing involvement of federal agencies, including HUD and EPA, with broader sustainability agendas is focusing more attention on interrelated economic, environmental, and public health outcomes.

The Need for an Explicit Focus on Health

The concept of capitalizing on the unique opportunities to reshape a community after a disaster is not a novel one, and sustainability and (more recently) resilience are common goals in recovery efforts focused

---

[7] EPA defines environmental justice as "the fair treatment and meaningful involvement of all people regardless of race, color, national origin, or income with respect to the development, implementation and enforcement of environmental laws, regulations and policies" (EPA, 2014). Environmental justice concerns have arisen primarily in response to empirical data showing that minority, tribal, and low-income groups are disproportionately exposed to environmental health hazards.

(SFDEM et al., 2015). Other events include parties, door-knocking events, and festivals, along with community planning meetings and block captain nominations.

In the low-income neighborhood of Bayview, for example, residents from a variety of age and demographic groups now meet regularly to implement a Resilience Action Plan (NEN, 2014c). Many of the participants had little connection to each other or city decision makers before these meetings began, but the increased communication, participation, and trust among residents enable them to participate collectively in problem solving and in planning for future disasters (NRC, 2012).

NEN also has launched a pilot initiative, the Empowered Communities Program, which is focused solely on building the neighborhood engagement that could make the difference for communities following a disaster or emergency. Modeled after the core tenets of the Federal Emergency Management Agency's (FEMA's) Whole Community Approach, this program "supports communities as they work to achieve a pre-event condition that will allow them to perform at the highest level in times of stress" (NEN, 2014b). The program includes forming partnerships with organizations that are not traditionally identified as disaster preparedness institutions (i.e., schools, civic groups), as well as focusing on building the social capital characteristics of trust, ownership, and cooperation within a community.

Lyttelton, New Zealand

Well before major earthquakes struck New Zealand in 2010 and 2011, the community of Lyttelton had established a time-banking program to develop local cohesion and build trust among residents. In 2005, the community of some 3,000 people set up a time bank whereby residents exchanged skills and earned credits for doing work for others that were traded for services. In exchange for transporting a neighbor to the doctor, for example, one could earn on hour of gardening on one's property. Community currencies and other time-banking programs have been shown to increase levels of social capital and trust (Richey, 2007). Having this program in place well before the earthquakes struck allowed local residents in Lyttelton's various organizations to work together in a nonemergency situation and build trust and experience. When the disaster struck, emergency providers worked seamlessly following the event and had various focal points, including local cafés and recreation centers, that served as hubs for recovery programs (Jefferies, 2012). The community's cohesion allowed it to develop its own vision for development and to move more effectively toward recovery (Ozanne, 2010). For more information, see Lyttelton Harbour Timebank, available at http://www.lyttelton.net.nz/timebank (accessed April 4, 2015).

on "building back better." It is clear from the above descriptions that equity, resilience, and sustainability are inextricably linked and that, ultimately, the community's health and welfare are drivers of each. Nonetheless, the committee strongly believes there is still a critical need for both health and non-health sectors to include an explicit focus on health in recovery planning to ensure that recovery activities do not have unintended negative impacts on health, that opportunities to create healthier communities are not lost, and that health outcomes are tracked and used as measures of program success. At the same time, however, it is also critical that a healthy community approach to recovery not be presented as an alternative to post-disaster resilience and sustainability initiatives. Separate efforts that fail to recognize the links among these concepts dilute resources, cause confusion, and perpetuate silos.

The measurement and evaluation of recovery strategies focused on health improvement has been a sorely neglected area of research. Evaluation of programs or projects during recovery is conducted primarily in terms of process measures (e.g., numbers of individuals served) rather than outcome measures (e.g., changes in health status indicators). Consequently, the committee found a paucity of data on the return on investment from post-disaster investments in health improvement strategies. However, experience from healthy community initiatives outside the disaster context suggests that investing in health-promoting

---

BOX 2-5
Six Livability Principles of the Partnership for Sustainable Communities

The Partnership for Sustainable Communities is an interagency partnership among the U.S. Department of Housing and Urban Development, the U.S. Department of Transportation, and the U.S. Environmental Protection Agency's Office of Sustainable Communities. Its six livability principles are as follows:

1. **Provide more transportation choices.**
   Develop safe, reliable, and economical transportation choices to decrease household transportation costs, reduce our nation's dependence on foreign oil, improve air quality, reduce greenhouse gas emissions, and promote public health.

2. **Promote equitable, affordable housing.**
   Expand location- and energy-efficient housing choices for people of all ages, incomes, races, and ethnicities to increase mobility and lower the combined cost of housing and transportation.

3. **Enhance economic competitiveness.**
   Improve economic competitiveness through reliable and timely access to employment centers, educational opportunities, services, and other basic needs by workers, as well as expanded business access to markets.

4. **Support existing communities.**
   Target federal funding toward existing communities—through strategies like transit-oriented, mixed-use development and land recycling—to increase community revitalization and the efficiency of public works investments and safeguard rural landscapes.

5. **Coordinate and leverage federal policies and investment.**
   Align federal policies and funding to remove barriers to collaboration, leverage funding, and increase the accountability and effectiveness of all levels of government to plan for future growth, including making smart energy choices such as locally generated renewable energy.

6. **Value communities and neighborhoods.**
   Enhance the unique characteristics of all communities by investing in healthy, safe, and walkable neighborhoods—rural, urban, or suburban.

SOURCE: Excerpted from Partnership for Sustainable Communities, 2013.

---

measures during recovery will yield benefits at the individual and community levels and may also result in significant downstream savings in health-related and other societal costs (see Box 2-6).

THE NEED FOR AN INTEGRATED APPROACH

The concept of vulnerability, discussed above, creates an interface for two fields that both are developing more proactive approaches to ameliorating the elements that contribute to vulnerability but have been "doing so along parallel paths" (Lindsay, 2003, p. 292). Disaster management professionals from a variety of sectors (e.g., emergency management, urban planning) have shifted their focus away from the hazardous event itself to minimizing the event's negative impact on the community. Accordingly, greater emphasis has been placed on understanding the factors that make communities vulnerable. The health

---

BOX 2-6
Why Invest in Healthy, Resilient, and Sustainable Communities?

- **Improve quality of life**—Health has a significant impact on quality of life. Many steps that improve the physical and social environments of a community also improve quality of life by making communities more livable and reducing the chronic stresses associated with inadequate access to basic needs.
- **Reduce health-related costs**—Poor health comes at a significant cost for individuals, communities, and the nation. Annual health care spending in the United States has grown to approximately $2.7 trillion, more than 75 percent of which goes to the management of preventable, chronic diseases (IOM, 2012; KFF, 2012; RWJF Commission to Build a Healthier America, 2014). Changes to the physical and social environments that promote health and prevent disease will reduce the unsustainable costs associated with the treatment of disease.
- **Stimulate economic vitality**—Beyond health care–related costs, unhealthy communities are bad business more generally. Failure to attend to the social determinants of health (employment, education, food access) can lead to high human service costs and a vicious cycle of disinvestment and depopulation. Healthy, livable communities attract residents and businesses, spurring improvement in economic vitality (Cornett, 2014).
- **Reduce vulnerability to hazardous events**—As discussed earlier in this chapter, social vulnerability and deficiencies in physical health increase the susceptibility of individuals and communities to the negative effects of a hazardous event. Disasters are associated with a variety of significant societal and financial costs that can be reduced through health improvement and resilience initiatives that bolster the ability of individuals and communities to cope with adversity.

---

sector simultaneously has been moving away from a reactive, treatment-focused approach to a population health model. As a result, it has been working to understand and address the upstream causes of the suboptimal health status observed within and across the nation's communities. However, a health-focused approach to pre- and post-event (i.e., recovery-related) mitigation that addresses social vulnerabilities has been largely neglected; great benefit can potentially be achieved by bringing these paths together (Lindsay, 2003).

The committee notes with optimism a national policy context for achieving this goal. As noted in Chapter 1, the National Health Security Strategy places unprecedented emphasis on community health resilience—"the ability of a community to use its assets to strengthen public health and healthcare systems and to improve the community's physical, behavioral, and social health to withstand, adapt to, and recover from adversity" (HHS, 2015, p. 10). It proposes the following vision for building and sustaining healthy, resilient communities:

> The nation will create a robust culture of health resilience, promoting physical and behavioral health and well-being, connecting communities, and championing volunteers. Across the nation, communities, organizations, and individuals will all contribute through their unique resources and capabilities. A culture of resilience will equip them not only to address daily challenges, but also to prevent, prepare for, mitigate, respond to, and recover from large-scale emergencies. Individuals and households will know how to improve health and will act on that knowledge. They will be engaged with the healthcare system and understand how to support their neighbors and community. Households and communities will work together, with the support of local organizations, and will engage in training and planning that prepare them to fulfill their roles in health security. Communities will promote health in part by supporting community infrastructure, including secure housing, economically viable neighborhoods, quality healthcare facilities, and spaces for

gathering and exercise. Public health, healthcare, behavioral health, and social service organizations will understand the needs of the people they serve and be ready to meet those needs before, during, and after an incident. As individuals and organizations become more health-resilient and build robust social networks, whole-community resilience will thrive. (HHS, 2015, p. 10)

Of critical importance is the acknowledgment in this national policy document that this vision cannot be achieved by the actions of any one sector; a wide variety of capabilities and partners must be brought together (HHS, 2015). The health sector can work to reduce the vulnerability of its own facilities and programs, and it can advocate for measures that reduce the vulnerability of communities and their residents by strengthening community systems and addressing social determinants of health. However, every resident and organization within the community has a role to play and a responsibility to help break the negative cycle by which disasters exacerbate preexisting vulnerabilities. Leveraging the opportunities afforded by recovery to advance this health-focused approach to community resilience and ultimately the creation of healthier communities will require an understanding of the nature of a community as a complex system and a mechanism for incorporating health considerations across all elements of that system.

Communities as Systems

To contemplate options for building healthier and more resilient and sustainable communities after disasters, the community is best viewed from a systems perspective (see Box 2-7 and Figure 2-2). According to Duhl (2000, p. 116), "cities must be looked at as interrelated complex ecological organisms in which

---

BOX 2-7
The Community as a System:
Interdependence Among Sectors Influences Recovery

A community is not simply a collection of buildings and inhabitants; it represents a complex "system of systems." A sharp distinction often is made between infrastructure and systems, with systems viewed as encompassing the combination of human needs and human services, but such a distinction fails to capture the critical interdependencies among sectors.

This point is illustrated by the example of Greensburg, Kansas, which received global attention for its investment in sustainability after a tornado in 2007 demolished 90 percent of the small rural town. The town made the choice to rebuild and to rebuild greener. Greensburg now has wind turbines providing power to the town and a plethora of energy-saving Leadership in Energy & Environmental Design (LEED) Platinum buildings (ULI, 2014). What it does not have (in adequate supply), however, is affordable housing stock. A three-bedroom home that would have cost $50,000 or $60,000 before the tornado is now priced at upwards of $160,000. The town lost about 50 percent of its population after the storm (Montgomery, 2014). Although population loss is common after a major disaster when displaced residents decide not to return, the lack of affordable housing serves as a barrier to drawing in new residents. Decisions regarding the recovery of the housing sector affect not only the overall economic recovery of the town but also other sectors in less expected ways. For example, Greensburg now has the first critical access hospital to reach LEED Platinum status. However, according to Mary Sweet, hospital administrator for Kiowa County Memorial Hospital, a number of the current staff live outside the town, and recruiting new staff has been a challenge because of the now relatively high cost of living in this small rural town (personal communication, Mary Sweet, Kiowa County Memorial Hospital, September 10, 2014). In the event of an emergency, this means that few of the local medical personnel will be nearby during off-duty hours to provide assistance, impeding the capacity of the medical system.

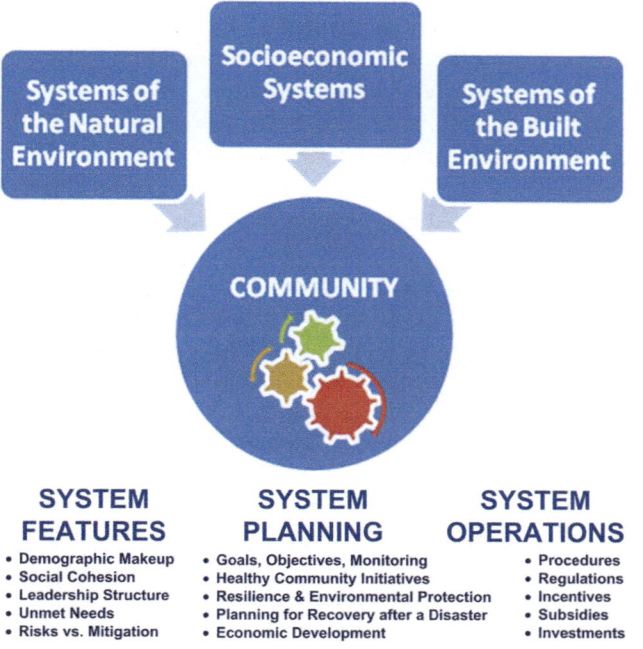

FIGURE 2-2 Illustration of the systems perspective of a community when contemplating options after a disaster.
SOURCE: B. Hokanson/PLN Associates.

housing, transport, city planning, economic development, and many other facets interact with health and medical issues." During recovery planning, interdependencies among components of the system need to be understood so that opportunities for synergy can be identified and unintended consequences can be avoided (see Box 2-7).

Community systems operate through a range of public and private initiatives. Some components of the overall community system are extensively planned and programmed, with established protocols, methodologies, budgeting, and subsidies. Transportation and land use planning, for example, are routine functions of communities and metropolitan areas, representing among the most highly organized influences on the configuration of community systems. Personal investments in housing and transportation are heavily influenced by public systems such as roads, development controls, utility lines, and public services. Commerce and government serve the population with education, employment, and the distribution of goods and services. There are gaps in these systems, however, causing unemployment, poverty, and hardship, with additional consequences affecting the health and well-being of families and individuals. In many cases, these social dysfunctions are concentrated in areas of blight and deterioration with high crime, low educational attainment, and unhealthy living environments.

All communities have processes in place to try to remediate these gaps through both place- and people-focused interventions. For example, community development programs attempt to address social dysfunction in communities through job training and a combination of public and private investment in neighborhood revitalization. The social services sector offers early childhood interventions and food access programs. Public health agencies may offer health services to the most vulnerable members of communities through a safety net system. In many cases, these programs and activities will target the same geographic regions and populations within a community, utilizing a systems approach to achieve synergies through coordinated investments. Because disasters create dysfunction similar in nature to that which already exists in communities (although a disaster will increase the magnitude of the problem), these ongoing community remediation processes are important assets that can and should be augmented and leveraged to address post-disaster community needs and improve health outcomes.

In the course of its research, the committee found examples of forward-looking communities that, recognizing the connections among system components (economic opportunity, social cohesion and stability, the conditions of the built and natural environments, and health), are developing strategic approaches that employ an array of diverse but coordinated place-based initiatives to address the complex and interrelated challenges posed by concentrated poverty, crime, blight, and economic decline. In Washtenaw County, Michigan, for example, cooperative agreements were used to create a collaborative organizational structure and a single, coordinated funding process to facilitate investment by county and municipal governments, local nonprofits, and foundations in human services initiatives related to safety net health services, hunger relief, homelessness, the elderly, children and youth, affordable housing, parks and recreation amenities, and workforce development (ICMA, 2014). In King County, Washington, persistent health disparities and unsustainable health care costs are spurring the implementation of a transformation plan that will facilitate the integration of health, human services, and community-based prevention (see Box 2-8) (King County, 2013). Similar efforts are under way in nearby Thurston County, Washington (see Box 2-9).

These initiatives are in many cases being driven by health sector stakeholders with the support of public and elected community leaders (with federal and state incentives) who are sensitized to the substantial social and economic costs associated with these chronic challenges, including significant health care–related costs arising from the association between poverty and poor health. Such initiatives, which are designed to yield improved health and social outcomes, as well as cost containment and economic vibrancy, require alignment of funding and collaborative efforts across a number of departments and nongovernmental entities, including health and human services, community development, education, law enforcement, economic development, housing, and urban planning. The process of developing and implementing these kinds of initiatives is a valuable asset that can be leveraged during disaster recovery since disaster-related deterioration of social, economic, and physical environments creates an end result similar to that of declines that take place over a much longer period of time. Moreover, as discussed further in Chapter 3, the same stakeholder groups that are involved in these initiatives should be engaged in the disaster recovery process.

A Health in All Policies Approach to Disaster Recovery

As discussed earlier in this chapter, intentional consideration of health, including health equity, is necessary during recovery to mitigate the negative effects of a disaster and seize opportunities to advance population health and well-being. Although disasters have direct impacts on health in the short term, negative effects on health also arise in the long term through the impacts of the disaster on social determinants of health, often exacerbating preexisting health inequities. Optimizing post-disaster health outcomes involves addressing acute conditions but also finding synergies to help overcome chronic health problems, thus advancing the achievement of a healthy, resilient, and sustainable community.

Since a community's social and physical environments are shaped largely by the decisions and actions of nonhealth sectors, those sectors must be sensitized to the potential impacts of their activities on health outcomes and should be actively engaged in efforts to protect and promote health throughout the recovery period. The integration of health considerations into decision making across all sectors has been termed Health in All Policies (HiAP). The World Health Organization has put forth the following definition of HiAP:

> Health in All Policies is an approach to public policies across sectors that systematically takes into account the health implications of decisions, seeks synergies, and avoids harmful health impacts, in order to improve population health and health equity. (WHO, 2013)

BOX 2-8
Health and Human Services Transformation in King County, Washington

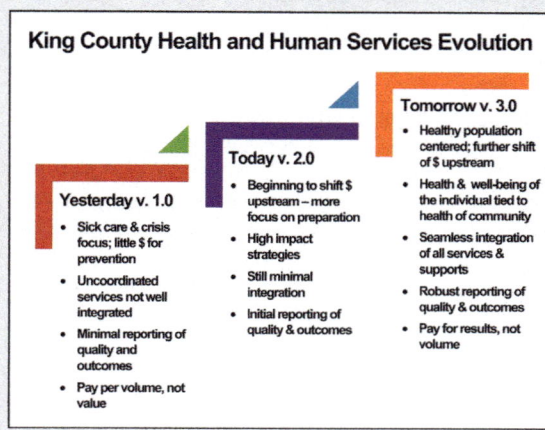

"Our region's health and human services delivery system is fragmented, focused more on providing costly late-stage care than on preventing crises from happening in the first place, and has not adapted to demographic trends that call for a shift in how and where services are delivered. With our partners, King County is working to create a system that is responsive, customer friendly, and focused on prevention and the social and health outcomes that support healthy and vibrant people and communities."

—King County Executive
Dow Constantine (King County, 2014)

While King County is on average one of the healthier counties in the nation, behind the averages lie large disparities in health and unequal access to opportunities and choices. Among different zip codes in the county, for example, life expectancy varies by almost 10 years, obesity rates range from 8 percent to 35 percent, and the rate of uninsured residents ranges from 3 percent to 30 percent. To address these disparities, as well as the high costs of health care, the Metropolitan King County Council passed Motion 13768 in 2012, requesting that the county executive create a plan for integrating the systems of health, human services, and community-based prevention (King County, 2013).

The Health and Human Services Transformation Plan, accepted by the Council in 2013, charts a course for improving health and well-being by shifting "from a costly, crisis-oriented response to health and social problems, to one that focuses on prevention, embraces recovery, and eliminates disparities by providing access to services that people need to realize their full potential" (King County, 2013, p. 6). The plan, fueled by a vision that all people in the county should have "the opportunity to thrive and reach their full potential," is focused on improving and integrating systems at two levels—individual/family and community (King County, 2013, p. 20). The plan lays out a whole-person approach that acknowledges that social and health conditions are intertwined, and that a person's care must be holistic, seamless, and extend across multiple domains (e.g., housing, health promotion, clinical services, employment). At the community level, the plan focuses on improving the conditions in the community (e.g., education, food security, access to parks), recognizing that a person's health is determined in large part by the community in which he or she lives (King County, 2013). Thus King County is applying both people- and place-based strategies for improving the lives of its community members.

The planning and implementation of this initiative have brought together stakeholders from social services, health care, government, and nonprofits whose focus ranges from housing to developmental disabilities. The initiative has broken down silos by integrating social services, community development, health prevention, and health care, allowing for more holistic, efficient, and effective care for individuals and communities. After any disaster, sectors are forced to work together to respond to the myriad needs of affected individuals and communities. Thus by establishing this integrated system with input from multiple stakeholders *before* a disaster strikes, King County may be better prepared in the event of a disaster. The communication, collaboration, and integration that are the backbone of the Transformation Plan have the potential to result in more organized and successful disaster response and recovery.

SOURCE FOR FIGURE: King County, 2013. *Health and Human Services Transformation Plan.* King County, Washington. p. 19. Available at http://www.kingcounty.gov/elected/executive/health-human-services-transformation/background.aspx.

BOX 2-9
Thurston Thrives:
An Example of Integrating Health and Social
Services Across the Broader Community

Thurston Thrives is an initiative developed to unite a wide range of community partners from within Thurston County, Washington, around the shared goal of making Thurston a healthy and safe place to live. One of the main focuses of the project is on aligning public health and social services efforts to promote health and social well-being in the community more effectively by addressing many of the social determinants of health through policy decisions. The program was initiated by the Thurston Board of Health but aimed to engage leaders from across numerous stakeholder groups. Thus, the 13-member Advisory Council for Thurston Thrives comprises representatives from the governmental, nonprofit (e.g., United Way and Habitat for Humanity), and private sectors and includes professionals from the fields of health, housing, economic development, education, planning, and social services. Thurston Thrives is using action teams to develop targets and strategies for achieving those targets for the following nine major areas that affect the health of the community:

- Child/youth resilience
- Clinical care and emergency care
- Community design
- Community resilience
- Economy
- Education
- Environment
- Food
- Housing

Each of these action areas would be relevant to the post-disaster environment. Thus, great efficiencies could be achieved by leveraging these preestablished transdisciplinary teams in disaster recovery planning.

SOURCE: Thurston County Board of Health, 2015.

A HiAP approach is founded on health-related rights and obligations. It emphasizes the consequences of public policies on health determinants and aims to improve the accountability of policy makers for health impacts at all levels (WHO, 2013). Motivation for a HiAP approach comes from understanding that "good health is fundamental for a strong economy and vibrant society, and that health outcomes are largely dependent on the social determinants of health, which in turn are shaped primarily by decisions outside the health sector" (Rudolph et al., 2013b, p. 1). Adoption of HiAP by all levels of government has been recommended by several organizations, including the Institute of Medicine (IOM, 2011), the National Association of County and City Health Officials (NACCHO, 2012), and the Association of State and Territorial Health Officials (ASTHO, 2013).

The committee asserts that not only is the aftermath of a disaster a prime opportunity to apply a HiAP approach; it in fact poses an acute need for this approach. Governmental public health agencies are an essential component of the diverse web of entities that make up the health system responsible for providing the health-related, population-based services required to create conditions in which people can be healthy. However, governmental public health acting alone cannot be successful in addressing the complex population health challenges faced by communities, particularly after a disaster. Partnering with other governmental and nongovernmental organizations brings

- new opportunities to influence policy (outside of the health sector) and spur system-level changes, and
- a means of yielding improved health outcomes from funds being spent in other sectors.

However, as indicated to the committee by James Blumenstock, chief program officer of ASTHO's public health practice division, the connection between disaster recovery and HiAP has not been adequately made. Referring to ASTHO materials on HiAP, Blumenstock said that "while everything in writing is relevant to post-disaster recovery, there is absolutely no reference to post-disaster recovery as an opportunity or an issue or a circumstance where health in all policies needs to apply. No examples, no case studies, no verbiage basically linking the two" (Blumenstock, 2014). In point of fact, the committee found only two examples of the application of HiAP to disaster recovery operations. In New Zealand, the HiAP approach to recovery was government led, and the recovery process was recognized as an opportunity to advance HiAP efforts already under way by local health agencies (Stevenson et al., 2014). As a result of early successes, HiAP has become more institutionalized, with regular public health input into major policies (see Box 2-10). In the second case, an academic organization, the Center to Eliminate Health Disparities at University of Texas Medical Branch, championed a HiAP approach to recovery in Galveston after the devastating effects of Hurricane Ike (see Box 2-11). The Galveston case study demonstrates the challenges of applying a HiAP approach to disaster recovery without adequate pre-disaster investment in building cross-sector relationships (such as that illustrated by the King County and Thurston County examples described in Boxes 2-8 and 2-9, respectively) and support for creating healthier communities.

The HiAP concept is compatible with the "whole-community" approach to integrated disaster recovery now being promoted by the Federal Emergency Management Agency (FEMA) and others (described in Chapter 3). As a result of the failure to apply a HiAP approach more broadly, the health sector, like many

---

BOX 2-10
Advancing Health in All Policies After Disasters: A Case Study from New Zealand

In 2010 and 2011, a series of earthquakes struck Canterbury, New Zealand (see also Box 2-4); the most severe aftershock occurred on February 22, 2011, in the city of Christchurch. It caused mass destruction in the central city, leading to 185 deaths and more than 65,000 injuries and destroying more than 6,000 residential properties (Stevenson et al., 2014). Prior to the earthquake, the Canterbury District Health Board had been working on a health impact assessment on urban development programs as part of a broader Health in All Policies (HiAP) initiative, under which the multi-agency Canterbury Health in All Policies Partnership was formed. The local Public Health Unit leadership team, involved in these prior efforts, "recognised that this was an opportunity to 'leapfrog' to the HiAP approach and consequently, immediately after the February earthquake, the unit was reconstructed in order to prioritize HiAP and support staff to utilise a determinants framework in all areas of their work" (Stevenson et al., 2014, p. 125). Federal grants were allocated from the Ministry of Health to mobilize a HiAP team within the Public Health Unit, focused on post-disaster recovery issues. One particular area of focus was the promotion of health-centered urban designs in the Canterbury communities. The HiAP team also has provided input to local and regional policy makers on such issues as air quality, water quality, and building standards and ensured that local public health officials and community members are included in the recovery planning cycle. According to Stevenson and colleagues (2014, p. 126), "The HiAP team continues to lead major interagency collaborative projects with the result that public health input into major policy is now routinely sought at an early stage by our local and regional government partners."

BOX 2-11
A Health in All Policies Approach to Disaster Recovery:
A Case Study of Galveston, Texas, After Hurricane Ike

Hurricane Ike struck the island of Galveston, Texas, in September 2008. The city's population of 50,000 faced pervasive devastation, largely from flooding, with 70 percent of city buildings being destroyed or badly damaged. According to Dr. Alexandra Nolen, director of the University of Texas Medical Branch Center to Eliminate Health Disparities (CEHD), the city's health and safety network was essentially wiped out, as was its communication and social infrastructure. While Hurricane Ike brought significant challenges for all residents of the ravaged island, the city's disproportionately high number of low-income residents, with their poor health and social indicators, faced an even more uncertain recovery. But amidst the chaos, Dr. Nolen and her center envisioned an opportunity to tap into the investment dollars flowing in for Galveston's recovery to rectify health disparities and create a model healthy community.

Funded by two grants beginning in October 2009, Dr. Nolen and her center sought to increase the evidence base for post-disaster recovery planning through informed policy making related to the social determinants of health. She was driven by the hypothesis that post-disaster environments afford opportunities for local planners to address health disparities through the lens of Health in All Policies (HiAP).

The strategy behind CEHD's efforts centered on three pillars of action: (1) assembling an evidence base on local challenges related to social determinants of health, (2) raising community awareness and knowledge of social determinants of health through education and engagement, and (3) partnering with decision makers and planners to incorporate evidence-based recommendations into the planning process.

To assemble evidence on local health challenges, CEHD adapted the Sustainable Communities Index (also known as the Healthy Development Measurement Tool, or HDMT) to a post-disaster context, tested its applicability, and drew lessons more generally on using this tool to improve health in a post-disaster planning environment. The HDMT was originally developed by the San Francisco Department of Public Health for the purpose of improving community health through urban development projects. The National Institutes of Health (NIH) grant to CEHD also funded geographic information systems (GIS) mapping of 125 health-related indicators from the HDMT, including indicators of environmental stewardship, sustainable and safe transportation,

---

others involved in disaster recovery, has tended to act in isolation rather than as part of a coordinated, multidisciplinary group. HiAP in the recovery context is about (1) creating organizational structures that optimally enable the coordination of efforts and the creation of synergies whereby core missions of other sectors align with healthy community objectives, and (2) ensuring that information on potential health impacts of recovery decisions is available to the decision makers within those structures. These processes are discussed further in Chapter 3, but roles for health professionals in facilitating a HiAP approach to disaster recovery can include

- assembling the evidence base (data) on local challenges,
- raising community awareness (in the public but also among other sectors) regarding the myriad factors that affect health, and

social cohesion, public infrastructure/access to goods and services, adequate and healthy housing, and healthy economy. The GIS mapping showed that the hurricane adversely affected the social determinants of health: it left more concentrated poverty and segregation, fewer grocery stores, quick recovery of low-nutrition fast-food restaurants, greater environmental hazards from toxins in the sediment, higher residential proximity to truck routes, fewer infant and child care centers, and lack of geographically distributed primary care facilities.

Despite significant educational and advocacy efforts by CEHD in areas spanning social services, housing, comprehensive planning, health care, food security, and environmental health, a number of challenges remain in Galveston, particularly for the most vulnerable. For example, the hurricane reduced access to healthy food after several full-service grocery stores were flooded. Although Dr. Nolen and her colleagues documented the problem, especially for poor people, explored options with local community economic development groups, and highlighted the problem in the media, the problem remains unresolved. Public housing also remains an unresolved issue and has become a flashpoint for the community. Galveston's public housing was badly damaged by the flooding and has yet to be rebuilt, despite CEHD's advocacy regarding the benefits of mixed-income, mixed-use neighborhoods as an alternative to segregated neighborhoods. With rebuilding of public housing in limbo, the slower return of lower-income residents also appeared to impact overall recovery, including recovery of the local economy.

In terms of lessons learned, Dr. Nolen observed that one of the biggest problems is that recovery programs were not necessarily designed so as to have a positive impact on health. It was also difficult to coordinate funding streams for recovery. There were too many players at the table with divergent interests and not enough focus on healthy communities. Another important lesson was the value of preestablished relationships on which a HiAP approach should be built. CEHD was too new to have standing or a recognized role in the community when Ike struck the island. It took 2 years of frequent presentations at local planning meetings before the concept of a healthy community began to gain traction to the extent that community groups began seeking input from CEHD. Thus, pre-disaster planning and relationship building are essential to accelerating recovery and supporting a HiAP approach.

SOURCE: Nolen, 2014.

- partnering with decision makers and planners to incorporate evidence-based recommendations into the planning process by applying a health lens to the programs and services of other sectors (see Figure 2-3).

RESEARCH NEEDS

A primary barrier to the integration of health improvement strategies into the recovery process is the lack of data on return on investment. In the course of future disaster recovery efforts, it will be important to measure impacts on health outcomes.

A HiAP approach is ideally suited to ensuring that health considerations are incorporated into the recovery decision-making process across all sectors. However, further research is needed to better understand the facilitators of and barriers to a HiAP approach in the disaster recovery context.

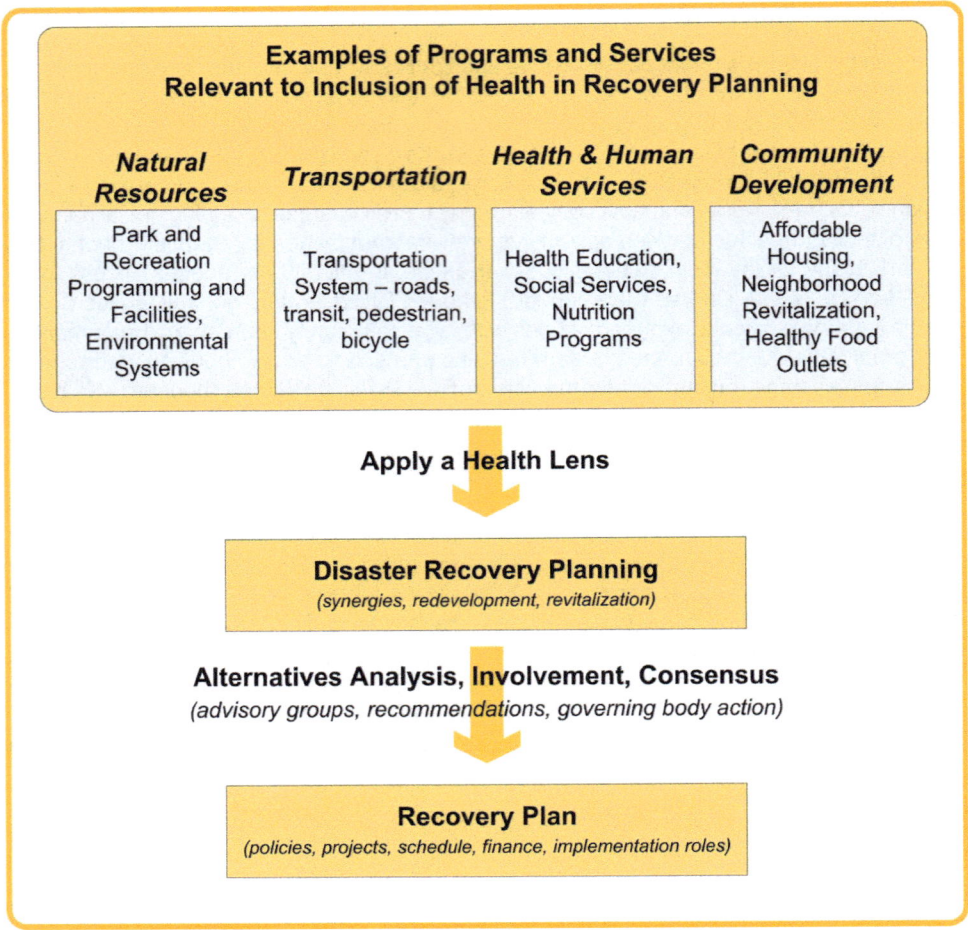

FIGURE 2-3 Application of a health lens across sectors during the recovery planning process. In this way, health considerations are included in the weighing of alternatives and prioritization processes that ultimately generate a cohesive recovery plan with coordinated strategies that, in addition to other objectives, address community health needs. SOURCE: B. Hokanson/PLN Associates.

SUMMARY OF FINDINGS

The process of recovery from a disaster is well recognized to be a long one, often taking years. It is also a unique opportunity to address systemic issues that have multiple negative effects on communities in such areas as health, economic viability, and vulnerability. Although there appears to be growing emphasis on the incorporation of resilience-building efforts into the recovery process (spurred in part by the looming threat of climate change), the idea of simultaneously working to enhance the health of communities and their residents does not, unfortunately, appear to be widespread. Despite a growing healthy community movement outside of the disaster context, the committee noted only a handful of communities taking this forward-looking and synergistic approach to recovery. There are a number of reasons why the committee believes this approach should be adopted in a far more systematic way.

First, addressing the inequities that contribute to disparities in health is an ethical imperative. As stated by the World Health Organization's Commission on the Social Determinants of Health, "social injustice is killing people on a grand scale" (CSDH, 2008, p. 26). The disruption caused by disasters may offer an opportunity to change the physical, social, and economic environments that have stemmed from a legacy of unfair and discriminatory social policies. Beyond this ethical reason, however, is a national security reason: poor health and the social determinants of health contribute to social vulnerability in the disaster context. Disasters are unquestionably tragedies, but they are also an enormous burden for the communities they affect and the nation in which those communities reside. This burden manifests not only as financial but also social costs (e.g., the tearing of a community's social fabric). Working to improve health and social well-being after a disaster needs to receive greater attention as a hazard mitigation process. This concept has much more weight outside of the United States in the context of disaster risk reduction. Finally, there is the issue of economic viability. Poor health indicators tend to cluster with other troubling and systemic problems for communities—issues such as blight, crime, and poverty. All can contribute to a negatively reinforcing cycle of disinvestment and economic decline, with rising, unsustainable health care and social service costs. Recovery offers an opportunity to infuse new vigor into declining communities. More livable and vibrant cities, towns, and neighborhoods will draw residents and businesses alike.

Although there are a number of challenges to wider adoption of this healthy community approach, the committee believes the first step is simply to put health on the radar for recovery. In this chapter, the committee has presented its rationale for using the recovery period, and the resources that will necessarily be allocated to the recovery process, to synergistically improve health and social well-being. Chapter 3 lays out a framework for how this can be achieved, building on the integrative concept of HiAP. It is the committee's hope that an integrated approach to recovery driven by a vision of a healthy, resilient, and sustainable community can help break down the barriers to cross-sector collaboration and enable planners, emergency managers, health advocates, and other relevant stakeholders to come together around shared goals, with each sector bringing its resources (knowledge, tools, funding streams) to bear. The end result will be a community that is a healthier, more livable place for current and future generations to grow and thrive, and one better prepared for future adversities.

REFERENCES

100 Resilient Cities. 2014. *About us.* http://www.100resilientcities.org/pages/about-us (accessed December 1, 2014).

Adeola, F. O., and J. S. Picou. 2012. Race, social capital, and the health impacts of Katrina: Evidence from the Louisiana and Mississippi Gulf Coast. *Human Ecology Review* 19(1):10-24.

Aida, J., K. Kondo, I. Kawachi, S. V. Subramanian, Y. Ichida, H. Hirai, N. Kondo, K. Osaka, A. Sheiham, G. Tsakos, and R. G. Watt. 2013. Does social capital affect the incidence of functional disability in older Japanese? A prospective population-based cohort study. *Journal of Epidemiology and Community Health* 67(1):42-47.

Aldrich, D. P., and K. Crook. 2008. Strong civil society as a double-edged sword: Siting trailers in post-Katrina New Orleans. *Political Research Quarterly* 61(3):379-389.

Aldrich, D. P., and Y. Sawada. 2014. *The physical and social determinants of mortality in the 3.11 tsunami.* https://www.purdue.edu/discoverypark/climate/assets/pdfs/Aldrich%20Sawada%20WP%20April%202014.pdf (accessed October 20, 2014).

ASTHO (Association of State and Territorial Health Officials). 2013. *Health in All Policies position statement.* http://www.astho.org/Policy-and-Position-Statements/Position-Statement-on-Health-in-All-Policies (accessed December 4, 2014).

Blumenstock, J. 2014. *Coordination among state and local government agencies.* Paper presented at IOM Committee on Post-Disaster Recovery of a Community's Public Health, Medical, and Social Services: Meeting Three, April 28-29, Washington, DC.

Bourdieu, P. 1986. The forms of capital. In *Handbook of theory and research for the sociology of education*, edited by J. C. Richardson. New York: Greenwood Press. Pp. 241-258.

Brune, N., and T. Bossert. 2009. Building social capital in post-conflict communities: Evidence from Nicaragua. *Social Science and Medicine* 68:885-893.

California Health in All Policies Task Force. 2010. *Report to the Strategic Growth Council.* http://sgc.ca.gov/docs/HiAP_Task_Force_Report-_Dec_2010.pdf (accessed November 3, 2014).

CERA (Chartered Enterprise Risk Analyst). 2013a. *Canterbury wellbeing index: Social connectedness.* http://cera.govt.
    nz/sites/default/files/common/2013-06-26-canterbury-wellbeing-index-14-social-connectedness.pdf (accessed
    October 20, 2014).
CERA. 2013b. *Community in mind.* http://cera.govt.nz/sites/default/files/common/community-in-mind-background-
    document.pdf (accessed October 20, 2014).
Chandra, A. 2014. *Considerations for community health in disaster recovery.* Paper presented at IOM Committee
    on Post-disaster Recovery of a Community's Public Health, Medical, and Social Services: Meeting Three, April
    28-29, Washington, DC.
Coleman, J. S. 1988. Social capital in the creation of human capital. *American Journal of Sociology* 94:S95-S120.
Cornett, M. 2014. *Investing in health: Pre- and post-disaster experiences from Oklahoma City.* Paper presented at
    IOM Committee on Post-Disaster Recovery of a Community's Public Health, Medical, and Social Services:
    Meeting Four, June 13, Washington, DC.
CSDH (Commission on Social Determinants of Health). 2008. *Closing the gap in a generation: Health equity through
    action on the social determinants of health. Final report of the Commission on Social Determinants of Health.*
    Geneva, Switzerland: WHO.
Cutter, S. L., B. J. Boruff, and W. L. Shirley. 2003. Social vulnerability to environmental hazards. *Social Science
    Quarterly* 84(2):242-261.
Davis, J. R., S. Wilson, A. Brock-Martin, S. Glover, and E. R. Svendsen. 2010. The impact of disasters on populations
    with health and health care disparities. *Disaster Medicine and Public Health Preparedness* 4(1):30-38.
Duhl, L. J. 2000. Healthy communities: A young movement that can revolutionize public health. A short history and
    some acknowledgments. *Public Health Reports* 115(2-3):116-117.
EPA (U.S. Environmental Protection Agency). 2014. *What is environmental justice?* http://www.epa.gov/environmen-
    taljustice (accessed December 1, 2014).
Few, R. 2007. Health and climatic hazards: Framing social research on vulnerability, response and adaptation. *Global
    Environmental Change* 17(2):281-295.
GCHD (Galveston County Health District). 2001. *Galveston County health status indicator report.* http://gchd.org/
    epidemiology/HSTAT01b.pdf (accessed October 20, 2014).
Granovetter, M. 1973. The strength of weak ties. *American Journal of Sociology* 78:1360-1380.
HHS (U.S. Department of Health and Human Services). 2015. *National health security strategy and implementation
    plan: 2015-2018.* Washington, DC: HHS.
Honoré, R. L. 2008. Health disparities: Barriers to a culture of preparedness. *Journal of Public Health Management
    and Practice* 14(6):S5-S7.
HRIA (Health Resources in Action). 2013. *Defining healthy communities.* Boston, MA: HRIA. http://hria.org/uploads/
    catalogerfiles/defining-healthy-communities/defining_healthy_communities_1113_final_report.pdf (accessed
    October 21, 2014).
Hurlbert, J. S., V. A. Haines, and J. J. Beggs. 2000. Core networks and tie activation: What kinds of routine networks
    allocate resources in nonroutine situations? *American Sociological Review* 65:598-618.
ICMA (International City/County Management Association). 2014. *Local governments, social equity, and sustainable
    communities: Advancing social equity goals to achieve sustainability.* Washington, DC: ICMA. http://icma.org/
    en/results/sustainable_communities/projects/advancing_social_equity_goals_to_achieve_sustainability (accessed
    October 21, 2014).
IOM (Institute of Medicine). 2011. *For the public's health: Revitalizing law and policy to meet new challenges.* Wash-
    ington, DC: The National Academies Press.
IOM. 2012. *For the public's health: Investing in a healthier future.* Washington, DC: The National Academies Press.
IOM. 2014. *Applying a health lens to decision making in non-health sectors: Workshop summary.* Washington, DC:
    The National Academies Press.
Jefferies, M. 2012. *Lyttelton: A case study.* http://fleeingvesuvius.org/2012/02/27/lyttelton-a-case-study (accessed
    October 20, 2014).
Kawachi, I., S. V. Subramanian, and D. Kim. 2008. Social capital and health: A decade of progress and beyond. In
    Social capital and health, edited by I. Kawachi, S. V. Subramanian, and D. Kim. New York: Springer. Pp. 1-26.
KFF (The Henry J. Kaiser Family Foundation). 2012. *Health care costs: A primer.* http://kff.org/health-costs/issue-brief/
    health-care-costs-a-primer (accessed October 9, 2014).
Kindig, D., and G. Stoddart. 2003. What is population health? *American Journal of Public Health* 93(3):380-383.

King County. 2013. *HHS transformation plan and process.* http://www.kingcounty.gov/exec/HHStransformation/plan. aspx (accessed December 4, 2014).

King County. 2014. *2014 state of the county: Building a shared and sustainable prosperity.* http://www.google.com/url? sa=t&rct=j&q=&esrc=s&source=web&cd=1&ved=0CCEQFjAA&url=http%3A%2F%2Fwww.kingcounty.gov %2F~%2Fmedia%2Felected%2Fexecutive%2Fequity-social-justice%2F2014%2FPolicy_Brief_-_Building_a_ Shared_and_Sustainable_Prosperity_2014-02-10.ashx%3Fla%3Den&ei=sXLvVJSTG6fesASv74Aw&usg= AFQjCNHzwKyvI75JL1XQVLPfRijMrwFv0w&bvm=bv.86956481,d.cWc (accessed February 26, 2015).

Lindsay, J. 2003. The determinants of disaster vulnerability: Achieving sustainable mitigation through population health. *Natural Hazards* 28(2-3):291-304.

McGalliard, T. 2012. Reframing the sustainability conversation from what to how. *Public Management* 94:2.

Mishkovsky, N. 2010. Building sustainability on a healthy foundation. *Public Management* 92(2).

Montgomery, R. 2014. Greensburg, Kan., rebuilds from 2007 tornado—now it just needs more people. *Emergency Management.* http://www.emergencymgmt.com/disaster/Greensburg-Kan-Rebuilds-from-2007-Tornado.html (accessed December 4, 2014).

NACCHO (National Association of County and City Health Officials). 2012. *Statement of policy: Implementing Health in All Policies through local health department leadership.* http://www.naccho.org/advocacy/positions/ upload/12-01-health-in-all-policies.pdf (accessed December 4, 2014).

Nakagawa, Y., and R. Shaw. 2004. Social capital: A missing link to disaster recovery. *International Journal of Mass Emergencies and Disasters* 22(1):5-34.

Natural Hazards Center. 2005. *2005 annual report.* http://www.colorado.edu/hazards/about/annualreport/ 05annualreport.pdf (accessed October 21, 2014).

NEN (Neighborhood Empowerment Network). 2014a. *About us.* http://empowersf.org/about-us (accessed February 26, 2015).

NEN. 2014b. *Empowered communities program.* http://empowersf.org/ecp (accessed February 26, 2015).

NEN. 2014c. *Resilient bayview.* http://empowersf.org/resilientbayview (accessed February 26, 2015).

NOAA (National Oceanic and Atmospheric Administration). 2008. *Hurricane Ike: Storm surge estimates from damage surveys.* http://www.srh.noaa.gov/hgx/?n=projects_ike08_storm_surge_overview (accessed October 20, 2014).

Nolen, A. 2014. *A Health in All Policies approach to disaster recovery: Lessons from Galveston.* Paper presented at IOM Committee on Post-disaster Recovery of a Community's Public Health, Medical, and Social Services: Meeting Four, June 13, Washington, DC.

Nolen, A., C. Bezold, J. Prochaska, M. Masel, J. Sullivan, and J. Ward. 2010. *Galveston hurricane and healthy neighborhood scenarios.* http://www.utmb.edu/CEHD/Documents/ScenariosWkbook/UTM%20-CEHD-Hurricane-Scenarios-and-Maps%20Workbook.pdf (accessed December 1, 2014).

Norris, T. 2013. Healthy communities at twenty-five. *National Civic Review* 102(4):4-9.

NRC (National Research Council). 2012. *Disaster resilience: A national imperative.* Washington, DC: The National Academies Press.

Ozanne, L. K. 2010. Learning to exchange time: Benefits and obstacles to time banking. *International Journal of Community Currency Research* 14:A1-16.

Partnership for Sustainable Communities. 2013. *Livability principles.* http://www.sustainablecommunities.gov/mission/ livability-principles (accessed October 21, 2014).

Partnership for Sustainable Communities. 2014. *Five years of learning from communities and coordinating federal investments.* http://www2.epa.gov/sites/production/files/2014-08/documents/partnership-accomplishments-report-2014.pdf (accessed November 18, 2014).

Pittman, M. A. 2010. Multisectoral lessons from health communities. *Preventing Chronic Disease* 7(6):A117. http:// www.cdc.gov/pcd/issues/2010/nov/10_0085.htm (accessed December 1, 2014).

Plough, A., J. E. Fielding, A. Chandra, M. Williams, D. Eisenman, K. B. Wells, G. Y. Law, S. Fogleman, and A. Magaña. 2013. Building community disaster resilience: Perspectives from a large urban county department of public health. *American Journal of Public Health* 103(7):1190-1197.

Pronyk, P. M., T. Harpham, J. Busza, G. Phetla, L. A. Morison, J. R. Hargreaves, J. C. Kim, C. H. Watts, and J. D. Porter. 2008. Can social capital be intentionally generated? A randomized trial from rural South Africa. *Social Science & Medicine* 67(10):1559-1570.

Rice, H. 2014. Rebuilding begins for Galveston public housing 6 years after Ike. *Houston Chronicle* 12. http:// www.houstonchronicle.com/news/houston-texas/texas/article/Rebuilding-begins-for-Galveston-public-housing-6-5746823.php (accessed October 20, 2014).

Richey, S. 2007. Manufacturing trust: Community currencies and the creation of social capital. *Political Behavior* 29(1):69-88.

Rudolph, L., J. Caplan, K. Ben-Moshe, and L. Dillon. 2013a. *Health in All Policies: A guide for state and local governments.* Washington, DC, and Oakland, CA: American Public Health Association and Public Health Institute. http://www.phi.org/uploads/files/Health_in_All_Policies-A_Guide_for_State_and_Local_Governments. pdf (accessed November 18, 2014).

Rudolph, L., J. Caplan, C. Mitchell, K. Ben-Moshe, and L. Dillon. 2013b. *Health in All Policies: Improving health through intersectoral collaboration.* Discussion Paper. September 18, 2013. http://iom.edu/~/media/Files/Perspectives-Files/2013/Discussion-Papers/BPH-HiAP.pdf (accessed December 1, 2014).

Ruggiero, K. J., K. Gros, J. L. McCauley, H. S. Resnick, M. Morgan, D. G. Kilpatrick, W. Muzzy, and R. Acierno. 2012. Mental health outcomes among adults in Galveston and Chambers counties after Hurricane Ike. *Disaster Medicine and Public Health Preparedness* 6(1):26-32.

RWJF (Robert Wood Johnson Foundation). 2008. *Overcoming obstacles to health.* Princeton, NJ: RWJF. http://www. rwjf.org/content/dam/farm/reports/reports/2008/rwjf22441 (accessed November 5, 2014).

RWJF Commission to Build a Healthier America. 2014. *Time to act: Investing in the health of our children and communities.* Princeton, NJ: RWJF. http://www.rwjf.org/content/dam/farm/reports/reports/2014/rwjf409002 (accessed October 9, 2014).

SFDEM (San Francisco Department of Emergency Management), NEN, and American Red Cross Bay Area Chapter. 2015. *Resilientville.* http://thrivingearthexchange.org/wp-content/uploads/2015/01/Resilientville.pdf (accessed February 26, 2015).

Standish, M. B., and R. K. Ross. 2014. Transforming communities for health. *National Civic Review* 102(4):31-33.

Stevenson, A., A. Humphrey, and S. Brinsdon. 2014. A Health in All Policies response to disaster recovery. *Perspectives in Public Health* 134(3):125-126.

Thurston County Board of Health. 2015. *Thurston thrives!* http://www.co.thurston.wa.us/health/thrives/docs/ Overview-ThurstonThrives.pdf (accessed February 26, 2015).

ULI (Urban Land Institute). 2014. *Housing in America: Integrating housing, health, and resilience in a changing environment.* Washington, DC: Urban Land Institute.

WHO (World Health Organization). 2013. *Health in All Policies.* http://www.healthpromotion2013.org/health-promotion/health-in-all-policies (accessed December 4, 2014).

WHO. 2014a. *Health systems: Equity.* http://www.who.int/healthsystems/topics/equity/en (accessed December 1, 2014).

WHO. 2014b. *Social determinants of health: Key concepts.* http://www.who.int/social_determinants/thecommission/ finalreport/key_concepts/en (accessed December 1, 2014).

Wisner, B., P. Blaikie, T. Cannon, and I. Davis. 2003. *At risk: Natural hazards, people's vulnerability and disasters.* 2nd ed. London: Routledge.

World Commission on Environment and Development. 1987. *Our common future.* Oxford, New York: Oxford University Press.

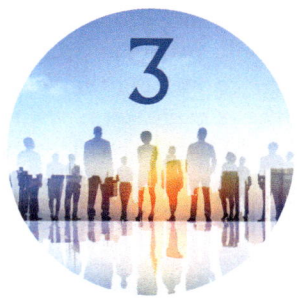

A Framework for Integrating Health into Recovery Planning

"Long-term recovery planning is an opportunity to improve a community's quality of life and disaster resiliency. It has the potential to inspire communities to set goals beyond restoration of the status quo."

—Boyd, 2014, p. 3

Disaster recovery is a process of strategic community planning, similar to that which takes place in communities throughout the country every day, except that it entails the enormous challenges of time compression: a process that would normally occur over decades must be carried out within a relatively short period of time (Olshansky, 2014). Beginning the recovery planning process before a disaster and leveraging the products of other community planning efforts can make post-disaster recovery planning more efficient and also better ensure that opportunities for community betterment (including health improvement) are not missed. In this chapter, the committee uses the strategic planning process as a framework for describing the opportunities and mechanisms for incorporating health considerations into the recovery planning process, both before and after a disaster. It should be emphasized that the intent here is not to provide a comprehensive description of the recovery planning process; such a description is beyond the scope of this study and has been provided elsewhere.[1]

THE STRATEGIC PLANNING PROCESS AS A FRAMEWORK

In strategic planning, quantifiable data and a process of systematic analysis are used to develop goals, identify alternatives, and establish criteria for decision making. Although there are slight variations and differences in terminology, the general structure of such planning processes (whether developing a comprehensive plan, health improvement plan, or disaster recovery plan) is similar. After an initial period

---

[1] Of note, in 2014 the American Planning Association released *Planning for Post-Disaster Recovery: Next Generation*, an update of its 1998 report on recovery planning (APA, 2014). The committee suggests this report as a useful resource for those desiring a more detailed description of the disaster recovery planning process. The report is available online at: https://www.planning.org/research/postdisaster (accessed March 13, 2015).

of laying the groundwork, there is often a visioning process and an assessment of community status and needs, assets, and contextual factors (e.g., political environment). The results of these two processes are used to establish goals and set priorities by comparing the findings of the assessment against the community's vision to identify gaps between the current status within the community and the desired state. Strategies are developed to close the gaps through input from stakeholders (including the public) and analysis of alternatives. These strategies are incorporated into a plan, and implementation partnerships (or operational structures) are developed. Finally, the plan is implemented. Resources are identified and applied, and progress is continuously measured using preestablished benchmarks. Even if it is not possible to tackle each priority area initially, a prioritized list makes it possible to evaluate future opportunities to determine how they can be leveraged to achieve the community's shared vision. Thus, the process of implementation feeds into a continuous cycle of assessment, planning, and implementation.

The strategic planning process, if successful, creates new channels for communication and builds consensus on the community's greatest needs going forward. This consensus building is critical to keep decision makers focused on long-term strategic objectives rather than on reactionary responses to the crisis of the day. Thus, obtaining buy-in from leadership is an essential step in ensuring that the plan is acted upon.

In the context of integrating health into the disaster recovery planning process, each of the steps in the strategic planning cycle presents opportunities. These are summarized below and then described in more detail throughout this chapter. It should be emphasized that, although the process is presented as sequential for purposes of exposition, in reality the order of steps may be varied, and some may be undertaken simultaneously. For example, visioning may occur before, simultaneously with, or after an assessment process, and because the process is a continuous cycle, the implementation step feeds into a new assessment used to evaluate the impact of the activities undertaken.

- **Visioning:** Recovery is viewed as an opportunity to advance a shared vision of a healthier and more resilient and sustainable community.
- **Assessment:** Community health assessments and hazard vulnerability assessments provide data that show the gaps between the community's current status and desired state and inform the development of goals, priorities, and strategies.
- **Planning:** Health considerations are incorporated into recovery decision making across all sectors. This integration is facilitated by involving the health sector in integrated planning activities and by ensuring that decision makers are sensitized to the potential health impacts of all recovery decisions.
- **Implementation:** Recovery resources are used in creative and synergistic ways so that the actions of the health sector maximize health outcomes and the actions of other sectors yield co-benefits for health. A learning process is instituted so that the impacts of recovery activities on health and well-being are continuously evaluated and used to inform iterative decision making.

Building on Previous Strategic Planning Processes

Rationale for the Integration of Planning Processes

In the post-disaster period, there is intense pressure from the residents of the community to return to a state of normalcy. As a result, attempts to address deficiencies in pre-event conditions (including health deficiencies and disparities) through post-disaster planning alone will be challenging and may not be successful. Thus, pre-disaster recovery planning is critical to seizing opportunities for improving community conditions beyond the pre-disaster state. After a disaster, the resources that become available to support recovery can then be evaluated against the preestablished goals for improvement of health and social vulnerability, and relationships developed through the planning process can be leveraged in developing strategies for achieving the community's preestablished vision of a healthy, resilient, and sustainable community.

In most cases, communities (cities, counties, towns) that have been struck by a disaster already have strategic plans in place that were created to guide decision making related to long-term development and investment. It follows that these plans would be consulted in the process of developing a recovery strategy so that the recovery process can help the community advance toward a previously agreed-upon vision and set of goals. Figure 3-1 shows how products from previous planning processes—including a shared vision, assessments, and plans—are optimally leveraged and built upon to guide the disaster recovery planning process.

Relevant to the purposes of this report, a community's comprehensive plan,[2] health improvement plan, sustainability plan, and mitigation plan—and, in some cases, its regional development plan—can yield health-related goals and investment strategies to inform the recovery planning process. Ideally, the community health improvement plan (following from a community health assessment) will have informed the development of the comprehensive plan. The decisions and strategies that are the domain of the comprehensive planning process—land use, transportation, housing—determine the nature of the physical and social environments in which people live. Planning decisions over the past century have had enormous impacts on some of the nation's most intractable public health challenges, such as obesity, chronic respiratory diseases, health disparities, and mental health (Dannenberg et al., 2003; Frumkin et al., 2004; Ricklin et al., 2012). Consequently, the comprehensive planning process is an important mechanism for enacting change in arenas beyond the direct influence of the health sector, such as the design of the built environment (APA, 2006a).

The integration of a health-focused community vision and health improvement goals into the community strategic planning process and the comprehensive plan itself helps ensure buy-in from leadership (since these plans must be formally adopted by the community's governing body) and subsequently the incorporation of these elements into recovery strategic planning. According to the American Planning Association (Schwab et al., 1998, p. 238), "Post-disaster recovery plans should be a specific application of the relevant portions of the community comprehensive plan, designed to deal with the constraints and opportunities posed by disaster conditions." Thus, a community that has undertaken this integration before a disaster is likely to be better equipped to address health considerations during recovery. Similar approaches are being promoted for the purposes of resilience. The Federal Emergency Management Agency (FEMA) now recommends the integration of hazard mitigation planning into the comprehensive plan as a means of ensuring that resilience is established as a community value and that hazard vulnerability is considered during all future development (FEMA, 2013a). According to the American Planning Association, "hazard mitigation works best as a policy objective of local planning when it is so completely integrated into the comprehensive plan that it becomes a normal assumption behind all daily planning activities" (Schwab et al., 1998, p. 61). The committee envisions the same outcome for health and social well-being.

The Current State of Integration of Planning Processes

Unfortunately, the committee found that the predominant model at present is one in which community comprehensive planning, health improvement planning, resiliency and sustainability planning, and disaster recovery planning occur largely in isolation. Barriers to integration noted by both public health and planning professionals include a lack of resources, tools, and guidelines, as well as an absence of qualified personnel able to bridge the two fields (APA, 2006a). In 2010, the American Planning Association surveyed planning departments across the United States to determine how comprehensive plans and sustainability plans are and can be used to protect and promote health. Just over a quarter of the nearly 900 respondents indicated that public health issues were addressed explicitly in their jurisdiction's officially adopted comprehensive plan, either through stand-alone health planning elements or the incorporation of health concerns into other planning elements, such as land use (Hodgson, 2011). Common health topics in the examined plans included physical activity or active living, clean air and other environmental exposures, and public safety. However, there was a notable lack of focus on food and nutrition, health and human services, social

---

[2] The comprehensive plan, also known as the general plan, is the product of a community's comprehensive planning process, which is used to determine community goals and aspirations for future community development.

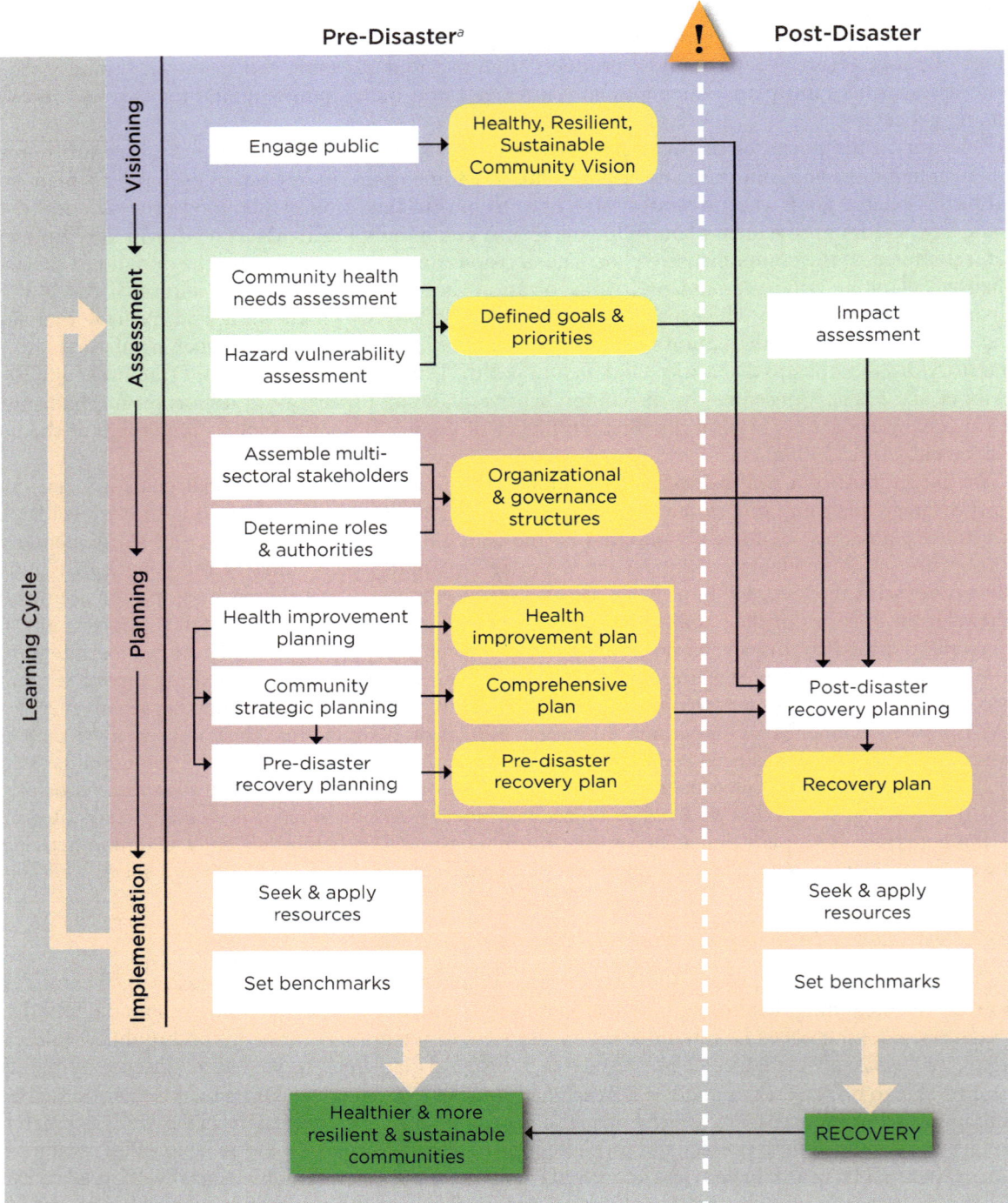

FIGURE 3-1 Leveraging the products of pre-disaster planning processes to support a healthy community approach to disaster recovery.

a Although the committee strongly encourages communities to undertake these activities in the pre-disaster period to maximize opportunities for leveraging the post-event recovery process to create healthier and more resilient and sustainable communities, there is still benefit to incorporating them into post-disaster recovery planning if they have not been undertaken beforehand.

cohesion, and mental health (Ricklin and Kushner, 2013). A 2010 International City/County Management Association survey found that although many communities have a range of sustainability activities that address social equity (e.g., affordable housing, preschool programs, workforce development initiatives), only about one-third of the approximately 2,100 responding local governments considered social justice a priority, and few were organizing and resourcing sustainability-related programs in a coordinated way or incorporating them into the comprehensive plan (ICMA, 2014). The two studies together indicate that the social aspects of health are not yet a focus for most local governments and that much greater effort is needed to integrate all determinants of health into comprehensive plans.

Similarly, the committee found little evidence of integration of a healthy community vision and long-term health improvement goals into pre-disaster recovery plans. Unfortunately, few communities have taken a proactive approach to the development of comprehensive pre-disaster recovery plans (Community Planning Workshop, 2010; Smith, 2011b). Two recent publications highlight cases in which pre-disaster planning for recovery was undertaken (City of Seattle, 2013; Community Planning Workshop, 2010), both concluding that few models were available to guide communities in the development of such plans. This paucity of pre-disaster recovery plans is due in part to the lack of incentives for communities to undergo what can be a complex, time-consuming, and controversial process (Community Planning Workshop, 2010). To better understand the degree to which community health improvement goals have been incorporated into pre-disaster recovery planning, the committee reviewed available pre-disaster recovery plans and sought testimony from public health, emergency management, and city management representatives. These information gathering processes yielded the following findings:

- Approximately three-quarters of the roughly two dozen pre-disaster recovery plans examined[3] explicitly address health considerations to some degree but are focused almost exclusively on short- and intermediate-term recovery activities (e.g., reopening and restoring health facilities; retaining medical personnel; ensuring access to pharmaceuticals; meeting the needs of vulnerable populations; providing mental health assistance; handling mass casualties; controlling disease outbreaks; and preventing exposure to unsafe materials such as debris, mold, and chemicals).
- Pre-disaster recovery plans that are more operational in nature (lay out organizational structures, roles, and responsibilities) focus primarily on short- and intermediate-term recovery activities with discussion of long-term recovery being limited to a return to pre-incident conditions/normal operations. Although these plans address increasing resilience through recovery activities (e.g., through hazard mitigation processes), the committee found no references to using the recovery process as an opportunity to build healthier communities. Plans that are more visionary in nature[4] are more likely to reference opportunities to use the recovery process to create healthier post-disaster communities, although none of the plans examined mentions leveraging the community's health improvement process. However, several plans recommend incorporating the vision and goals of the comprehensive plan, reinforcing the importance of integrating health improvement and comprehensive planning prior to a disaster (Hillsborough County Government, 2010; Pinellas County, 2012).
- Testimony of public health officials from jurisdictions that have been through a disaster was focused largely on short- and intermediate-term needs (e.g., restoring health care operations, ensuring access to pharmaceuticals), although testimony from the former health commissioner of New Orleans did include considerable discussion of strategies undertaken in that city to rebuild both public health

---

[3] It should be noted that the vast majority of these plans were from Florida counties. Florida has led the development of pre-disaster redevelopment plans, spurred in part by a statute requiring all coastal communities to have them (Section 163.3177(6)(g), Florida Statutes; Section 163.3178(2), Florida Statutes). The state developed a planning guide, the Web link to which can be found in Appendix C.

[4] The redevelopment plans of Hillsborough County (Hillsborough County Government, 2010) and Pinellas County (Pinellas County, 2012) in Florida were found to be good models for ensuring that health and social well-being considerations are incorporated into diverse aspects of recovery planning. Links to these plans are available in Appendix C.

and health care systems in a way that would improve the health of the community (DeSalvo, 2013). The testimony of urban and regional planners was more likely to include discussion of opportunities to build the community back in a way that promotes health—perhaps reflecting growing interest in health within the urban and regional planning and design fields since many of the opportunities to change the physical and social environments of a community fall under the purview of planning professionals.

- Health departments find leveraging the recovery process for long-term health improvement challenging because of their intense mission focus on response activities, the lack of funding to support long-term recovery projects, their lack of engagement in community long-term recovery planning, and the perception that a discussion of such topics as long-term health improvement strategies would not be well received by a community still dealing with significant acute post-disaster needs (Beardsley, 2014; Clements, 2014; Zucker, 2014).
- Although federal preparedness funds available from both the Centers for Disease Control and Prevention (CDC) and the Office of the Assistant Secretary for Preparedness and Response within the U.S. Department of Health and Human Services (HHS) are eligible for use to support recovery planning, there is currently little emphasis on using the recovery process for long-term community health improvement (Blumenstock, 2014; Shah, 2014).
- Nearly all communities in the nation are recipients of federal community development funding, and a large proportion of these local governments are using the targeted funds to revitalize troubled neighborhoods and address the needs of residents—efforts essentially similar to those of disaster recovery. Nonetheless, there is low awareness of pre-existing community development endeavors during the preparation of pre-disaster recovery and hazard mitigation plans.

In summary, based on the testimony of a diverse set of stakeholders, including the public health community, and a review of available recovery plans, the committee finds that a healthy community vision rarely guides the development of pre-disaster and post-disaster recovery plans. As a result, a health lens is not applied to the process of decision making regarding the allocation of recovery resources, and unique opportunities are being missed. The following four gaps impede the development of plans to "build back better," and specifically in ways that contribute to an overall healthier community:

- inadequate pre-disaster community health improvement planning (not being done at all, or not using a process that engages the full range of community stakeholders in addressing the comprehensive physical and social determinants of health);
- inadequate integration of health improvement planning and the community comprehensive (strategic) planning process used to set priorities and allocate funds;
- lack of integration of health improvement planning and disaster recovery planning;
- insufficient awareness across all sectors of the health-related threats and opportunities posed by disasters and of the benefits to be gained from integrating community health improvement objectives and priorities into comprehensive and disaster recovery plans to achieve shared goals.

In some cases, these gaps reflect long-standing silos within and among institutional arrangements and staffing structures. Enhanced collaboration across sectors offers an opportunity to align planning processes around a shared vision and goals so as to optimize community health and social service outcomes during recovery. Table 3-1 illustrates potential roles for diverse community stakeholders in this integrative process. For the most vexing problems, however, especially where large-scale community revitalization is at stake, solutions may require significant leadership investment to achieve organizational readiness and the capacity for synergistic, multisector health-sensitive disaster recovery planning.

TABLE 3-1 Collaborative Roles of Sector and Community Stakeholders in the Integration of Strategic Planning Processes[a] to Achieve Healthier and More Resilient and Sustainable Post-Disaster Communities

	Visioning	Assessment	Planning	Implementation
Task	Educate community on elements of healthy, resilient, and sustainable communities	Conduct community health assessments, ensuring that Internal Revenue Service (IRS)-required hospital Community Health Needs Assessments (CHNA) are integrated	Develop health improvement plan based on health assessment	Exercise pre-disaster recovery plan by practicing organizational arrangements suited to hypothetical disasters
Lead(s)	Public health, emergency management, urban and regional planning	Public health, health care	Public health	Emergency management
Partners	All sectors, all stakeholders, community members	Social services, behavioral health	All sectors	All sectors
When[b]	❶ ❸	❶ ❸	❶ ❸	❶
Task	Conduct community visioning process	Assess vulnerability of critical infrastructure	Develop comprehensive plan, ensuring inclusion of all relevant plans (e.g., hazard mitigation, health improvement, economic, redevelopment)	Adopt regulations, incentives, programs, budgets, and community outreach to achieve community vision and goals
Lead(s)	Urban and regional planning, public health	Public health, public works, emergency management, facility management, planning	Urban and regional planning	Chief executive, community managers, elected governing body
Partners	All other sectors	Management, finance, budget	Public health, emergency management, other local agencies	All implementing agencies and organizations
When[b]	❶ ❸	❶ ❷ ❸	❶ ❸	❶ ❷ ❸
Task	Incorporate community vision into comprehensive planning process	Identify areas with large socially vulnerable populations	Plan organizational structures for post-disaster coordination of activities	Seek methods for making optimum use of technology and information systems for both public outreach and pre-disaster policy analysis
Lead(s)	Urban and regional planning, public health, environmental health, social services	Public health, urban and regional planning, emergency management, social services	Emergency management	Emergency management, public health, urban and regional planning

continued

TABLE 3-1 Continued

	Visioning	Assessment	Planning	Implementation
Partners	All sectors, plus management, finance, budget offices	Research organizations, community groups, neighborhood associations, health and medical system partners	All sectors	All sectors
When[b]	❶ ❸	❶ ❸	❶	❶ ❸
Task	Ensure that pre-disaster recovery plan incorporates community-developed vision of healthy, resilient, sustainable community	Periodically assess effectiveness of institutional arrangements that promote cross-sector collaborations and joint mitigation activities	Develop pre-disaster recovery plan	Establish joint communications center; facilitate information exchange on community recovery needs
Lead(s)	Emergency management, urban and regional planning	Emergency management, urban and regional planning, public health	Urban and regional planning, economic development agency, emergency management	Emergency management, public officials
Partners	Public health and other agencies	Education system, health and medical system partners, business representatives	All sectors	Public health, health care, behavioral health, social services
When[b]	❶	❶ ❸	❶ ❸	❷
Task	Periodically revisit community vision statements for relevance in light of changing conditions and altered vulnerabilities	Assess unmet social needs, pre- and post-disaster	Conduct health impact assessments to inform recovery planning	Develop recovery finance strategy, determine funding eligibility, apply for funds, administer grants
Lead(s)	Urban and regional planning, public health, emergency management	Social services	Public health	Designated recovery manager
Partners	All sectors, plus management, finance, budget offices	Public health, behavioral health, emergency management	All sectors	All sectors
When[b]	❶	❶ ❸	❸	❸
Task	Monitor economic development and community development initiatives that may strengthen the community, add resilience, create sustainability	Conduct post-disaster assessment of disaster impact on infrastructure and systems	Develop post-disaster recovery plan	Carry out recovery projects and programs; arrange project and program management

TABLE 3-1 Continued

	Visioning	Assessment	Planning	Implementation
Lead(s)	Urban and regional planning, public health, emergency management	Emergency management	Emergency management, urban and regional planning	All sectors
Partners	All sectors, plus management, finance, budget offices	Urban and regional planning, public works, public health, management	All sectors	Management departments such as budget, finance, legal services
When[b]	❶	❸	❸	❸

^a The processes to be integrated include community comprehensive planning, health improvement planning, mitigation/resilience planning, and disaster recovery planning.

^b 1 = pre-disaster; 2 = response and short-term recovery; 3 = long-term post-disaster recovery. Coloring of the symbols indicates urgency: red = priority; black = possibility.

A HEALTHY, RESILIENT, SUSTAINABLE COMMUNITY VISION FOR DISASTER RECOVERY

Disasters, although devastating, create an opportunity through the recovery process to advance a shared vision of a healthier and more resilient and sustainable community. In Chapter 2, the committee describes the elements of a healthy community and its linkages with the concepts of equity, resilience, and sustainability. How these elements are incorporated into the shared vision for an individual community needs to be defined as an integral part of community strategic planning processes conducted before an event, so that a clear vision is in place to drive post-disaster decision making as new resources become available and opportunities arise. Otherwise, pressure to rebuild quickly after a disaster may result in missed opportunities.

The Critical Role of a Vision

A common vision for recovery is highlighted by FEMA (2011c) as one of eight major components of a successful recovery in *Lessons in Community Recovery*, a 2011 report that presents lessons learned from 7 years of experience with the long-term community recovery emergency support function. A vision provides a "beacon for decision makers and some framework within which decisions will be taken" (Schwab et al., 1998, p. 47). Without an overall vision, goals and objectives often are disconnected from each other and from a larger purpose. A community's vision becomes the foundation for subsequent policies and regulatory changes, and investments. A visioning process also can drive enthusiasm and provide a foundation for creative collaboration. It is not surprising, then, that many planning processes, including disaster recovery planning, begin with a visioning process that defines a desired future state.

The Importance of Having a Vision and Goals in Place Before a Disaster

Visioning is a common early step in the recovery planning process after a disaster. As the committee learned through testimony from disaster recovery experts and from a review of case studies, however, a community that has already gone through the process of envisioning its future and setting measurable goals and priorities before a disaster is in a better position to converge on a plan for recovery quickly after such an event (see Box 3-1). The urgency of the post-disaster period poses a significant challenge to the development of recovery plans that meet a community's long-term needs. Governments facing the complex

---

BOX 3-1
The Value of Pre-Disaster Visioning and Planning: A Tale of Two Cities

The New Orleans Experience

The flooding of New Orleans that resulted from levee failure after Hurricane Katrina struck the Gulf Coast in 2005 is among the most catastrophic disasters in U.S. history. The recovery process in New Orleans continues today and was significantly impeded by disputes over processes and goals for reconstruction, with tensions arising from conflicting desires to quickly rebuild the familiar or to create a safer and more sustainable and equitable city (Kates et al., 2006). In many cases, ideas for reducing the size of the city and increasing green space were viewed as efforts to get rid of predominantly African American and low-income neighborhoods (Colten et al., 2008). Although the recovery planning process was initiated shortly after the flood, it took nearly 2 years and multiple rounds of planning initiated independently by the state and city to develop an officially accepted plan (the Unified New Orleans Plan). Despite these delays, the city of New Orleans has seized on the opportunities presented by disaster recovery to build back better. A 2010 update of the city's comprehensive plan, *Plan for the 21st Century: New Orleans 2030*, includes as goals livability, opportunity, and sustainability (Collins, 2011).

The Cedar Rapids Experience

On June 13, 2008, the Cedar River, which flows through Cedar Rapids, Iowa, rose a record-setting 30+ feet, causing significant flooding in the city. Although no deaths resulted, the flood caused widespread destruction of the city's physical infrastructure and resulted in the displacement of more than 10,000 residents. Fortuitously, the city council and city manager had initiated a broad community engagement effort just months before the flood to develop a shared vision for the community's future (CARRI and CaRES, 2013). This existing engagement process, the resultant community vision, and a related effort to adopt a systems approach to government operations all enabled the community to come together quickly after the flood around a plan for what their new community would look like. The recovery plan, which incorporated input from thousands of residents, included such goals as encouraging active, healthy lifestyles; ensuring equitable redevelopment; building resource-efficient and resilient buildings; and protecting the city against future floods by rebuilding outside of flood-prone areas (ULI, 2014). Cedar Rapids has been recognized for its success by the U.S. Army Corps of Engineers, the American Planning Association, and the International Downtown Association, and it is touted as a model for other communities because of its ability to rapidly develop a publicly supported recovery plan that will create a better, safer future for all of its residents (CARRI and CaRES, 2013).

---

process of reconstruction after a disaster must balance two competing priorities—speed and deliberation (Johnson and Olshansky, 2013). Tensions inevitably arise between the need to restore infrastructure and a sense of normalcy as quickly as possible and the desire to leverage the recovery process as an opportunity for community betterment. Without a preexisting vision and associated goals, reactive decision making early in the recovery period may severely limit the range of options for betterment during later recovery phases. Accordingly, the phrase "window of opportunity" often is associated with the short period of time immediately after a disaster. As expressed by Jennifer Pratt, assistant director of planning services for the city of Cedar Rapids, Iowa, "One thing we heard from other communities that had suffered natural disasters was that it was important to have a plan rather quickly, because people naturally become nostalgic and just say, 'Well, I want it the way it was before'" (ULI, 2014, p. 21).

Communities undertake a number of planning processes that yield a shared vision for the future that could be incorporated into pre- and post-disaster recovery planning efforts. A disaster should not change the long-term vision for a community, just the steps for achieving it. Plans that should be examined (if available) include a community's comprehensive plan, health improvement plan, and sustainability plan. If a holistic vision for a healthy, resilient, sustainable community is lacking, however, the pre-disaster recovery planning process can be used to build on previous visioning efforts. Using the shared vision as a guide, action plans can be developed after a disaster based on the new social, economic, and environmental conditions of the community (ASTHO, 2007).

Creating a Shared Vision as a First Step in Engaging the Public in Disaster Recovery

The involvement of informed and empowered individuals and communities through an authentic community engagement process is nearly universally recognized as a factor in the success of any community planning endeavor, including healthy community planning and disaster recovery (FEMA, 2011c; Love and Vallance, 2014). Community engagement has been defined as "the process of working collaboratively with and through groups of people affiliated by geographic proximity, special interest, or similar situations to address issues affecting the well-being of those people" (CDC, 1997, p. 9). "With and through" are the key words in this definition. Community engagement entails more than extracting information from residents about their needs and wants. True engagement integrates the affected community into every aspect of a project, from identifying needs to selecting priorities to implementing programs. Thus, there should be an "ongoing dialogue among residents to build relationships and a shared vision of what the community is, what it should be, and how to get there" (Norris and Pittman, 2000, p. 121).

The visioning process is an opportunity for communities to begin to rectify a legacy of exclusion that has contributed to the significant disparities apparent across U.S. communities today. Consequently, it is essential that groups representative of *all* members of the community—including the most vulnerable populations—be involved in the planning process, thus ensuring that the voices, perspectives, and needs of all segments of the community are addressed. Vulnerable populations often have special needs during and after a disaster, but they continue to be excluded from disaster planning processes (Sherry and Harkins, 2011). For example, low-income residents displaced by a disaster may not be able to return to the community as easily as their higher-income neighbors. Because of their absence, their voices are not heard at meetings and their perspective is not taken into account when rebuilding is being planned. In Galveston, Texas, this scenario led to a harsh outcome for low-income residents (Nolen, 2014). After 569 public housing units on the island were demolished following Hurricane Ike, many locals, including city council members, fought vigorously not to rebuild them. Community advisory committees that were providing input on recovery plans were limited to residents who were living in Galveston after the disaster, thus excluding anyone who had not yet returned. It took state and federal intervention to finally spur rebuilding of the units, a full 6 years after the hurricane struck (Rice, 2014). Had there been an attempt to include the displaced low-income residents in the crafting of the recovery plan, their voices would have been heard, and the public housing might have been rebuilt much more quickly.

Means of engaging the community in visioning often include town hall meetings, public workshops, surveys, and charrettes.[5] Some activities undertaken while laying the groundwork for planning can help ensure the success of the visioning process. These activities may include but are not limited to

- identifying and engaging local health champions (from health and nonhealth sectors) to facilitate discussions;
- identifying other previous efforts and experiences that are relevant; and
- conducting health literacy efforts and educating the community on the elements of and benefits to healthy, resilient, and sustainable communities.

---

[5] A charrette is an iterative process that is often used to exchange ideas between urban and regional planners/designers and the community, resulting in an evolving series of designs (APA, 2006b).

ASSESSMENTS TO INFORM RECOVERY PLANNING

An assessment process is undertaken to inform the strategic approach to community planning. This process can be used to identify the needs, assets, and capacities of the community; prioritize interventions; and provide a baseline against which change can be measured. Three common assessments of relevance to disaster recovery planning are community health assessments, threat and hazard identification and risk assessments, and disaster impact assessments (see also the discussion of health impact assessments later in this chapter).

Community Health Assessments

A community health assessment (sometimes referred to as a community health needs assessment) is "a systematic examination of the health status indicators for a given population that is used to identify key problems and assets in a community" (PHAB, 2011, p. 8). Community health assessments are part of a strategic planning process for health improvement, such as that described by the Mobilizing for Action through Planning and Partnerships (MAPP) framework (Lenihan, 2005). MAPP was developed to enable communities to "seek to achieve optimal health by identifying and using their resources wisely, taking into account their unique circumstances and needs, and forming effective partnerships for strategic action" (NACCHO, 2014c). Communities that use MAPP carry out a six-phase process: organizing, visioning, assessments, strategic issues, goals/strategies, and action cycle (NACCHO, 2014d). Although the collection of traditional health status indicators (e.g., obesity rates, numbers of uninsured) is an important part of the assessment process, it is necessary to adopt a more holistic approach. Other information relevant to a community health assessment may include community perceptions regarding health and quality of life, the performance of the local health system, and an evaluation of factors influencing health in the community (e.g., policies). Conducting a more comprehensive community health assessment to include these additional elements will provide a more complete understanding of the factors that influence community health (NACCHO, 2014b). Another valuable tool for community health assessment is the Community Health Needs Assessment Toolkit from Community Commons, an online tool that consolidates data from multiple sources and enables users to create maps and reports of health indicators (Community Commons, 2014).

Many local health departments, as well as nonprofit hospitals, are conducting community health assessments and leveraging them in the development of community health improvement plans. Health improvement planning is a requirement for public health agency accreditation, and under the Patient Protection and Affordable Care Act (ACA), the Internal Revenue Service (IRS) requires nonprofit hospitals to conduct a community health needs assessment (CHNA) at least once every 3 years as a condition for retaining tax-exempt status.[6,7] Data from the *2013 National Profile of Local Health Departments* indicate that within the past 5 years 70 percent of local health departments conducted a community health assessment, and more than half (56 percent) completed a community health improvement plan (NACCHO, 2014a). While the committee found these data encouraging, it is unclear how many of these plans have been successfully implemented. The suboptimal status of nationwide health statistics indicates that despite these increased planning initiatives, problems with implementation remain. Further, there is little evidence to suggest that these plans are aligned with broader community strategic planning processes such as those associated with the development of comprehensive or sustainability plans. As a result, the goals developed in those planning processes may not be sufficiently understood by the key community leaders and officials who are typically responsible for managing disaster recovery and, thus, may not be identified as priorities or leveraged during the recovery planning process.

---

[6] Under a final regulation effective as of December 29, 2014, a charitable hospital must (1) define the community it serves; (2) assess the health needs of that community; (3) take into account input from representatives of the community, including those with expertise in public health; (4) document the community health needs assessment in a written report; and (5) make that report available to the public (See 79 F.R. 78953, Dec. 31, 2014.)

[7] 79 F.R. 78953, Dec. 31, 2014.

Threat and Hazard Identification and Risk Assessments

Disaster recovery planning should be based on an assessment of locally specific risks. The threat and hazard identification and risk assessment process (described in Box 3-2) is a valuable tool for communities, helping them answer the following key questions as part of the pre-disaster planning process: "What do we need to prepare for, what sharable resources are required in order to be prepared, and what actions could be employed to avoid, divert, lessen or eliminate a threat or hazard?" (FEMA, 2014d). The assessment process is a community-wide initiative that emphasizes anticipation prior to assessment. As part of this process, community members themselves identify threats and hazards of concern and place them in the context of the greater community (FEMA, 2013b). The community then assesses each risk in context, developing capability targets and estimating the resources needed to achieve these targets for each of the core capabilities identified in the National Preparedness Goal. The use of community-level assessments, as opposed to traditional top-down assessments, reflects the fact that disasters and their impacts are unique to a given community and results in a more specific and informative assessment process overall. Internationally, the use of such community-level assessments has resulted in accelerated response and recovery (Reaves et al., 2014). Australia, for example, has expanded community-level input to its hazard anticipation and assessment as part of its Prepared Community model (Reaves et al., 2014).

Included among the capabilities under the National Preparedness Goal is Health and Social Services, as well as numerous other capabilities that impact a community's health, such as Community Resilience, Long-Term Vulnerability Reduction, Risk and Disaster Resilience Assessment, Environmental Response/Health and Safety, and Mass Care and Infrastructure Services. The Health and Social Services capability focuses on the ability to "restore and improve health and social services networks to promote the resilience, independence, health (including behavioral health), and well-being of the whole community" (FEMA, 2014a). Consequently, a community health assessment may inform the Threat and Hazard Identification and Risk Assessment process, particularly with regard to social vulnerability (discussed in Chapter 2), and there may be benefit to better integrating these two processes. Similarly, health care organizations are required to conduct a hazard vulnerability analysis as part of the accreditation process. These analyses help health care stakeholders prioritize risks so that appropriate planning, prevention, response, and recovery actions can be taken (The Joint Commission, 2005). The hazard vulnerability analysis provides an interface between the health care and emergency management sectors and should be complementary to the Threat and Hazard Identification and Risk Assessment process.

BOX 3-2
The Threat and Hazard Identification and Risk Assessment Process

1. Identify Threats and Hazards of Concern: Based on a combination of experience, forecasting, subject matter expertise, and other available resources, identify a list of the threats and hazards of primary concern to the community.
2. Give the Threats and Hazards Context: Describe the threats and hazards of concern, showing how they may affect the community.
3. Establish Capability Targets: Assess each threat and hazard in context to develop a specific capability target for each core capability identified in the National Preparedness Goal. The capability target defines success for the capability.
4. Apply the Results: For each core capability, estimate the resources required to achieve the capability targets through the use of community assets and mutual aid, while also considering preparedness activities, including mitigation opportunities.

SOURCE: Excerpted from FEMA, 2013b.

Disaster Impact Assessments

In the aftermath of a disaster, a disaster impact assessment can help determine what damage the disaster has caused, providing public officials and emergency management with information about the needs of an affected community. The assessment includes not just damage to infrastructure but all of the needs of the community. As part of this assessment, interview teams comprising staff and volunteers from state, local, and regional health departments conduct community-specific surveys. Officials can then use this information to identify what resources are needed and to target specific warnings to affected residents (IOM and NRC, 2005).

The disaster impact assessment helps identify unmet health needs. It is important that such assessments be conducted periodically throughout the response and recovery process following a disaster. Such reassessment provides real-time information about the status of various health-related factors such as housing, mental health, and utilities services. As response and recovery activities progress, the health needs of a community may change, especially if migration of families takes place into or out of an affected community (IOM and NRC, 2005). Conducting a disaster impact assessment immediately after a disaster and then reassessing throughout the recovery process enables continuous monitoring of how a disaster has impacted and continues to impact the health of a community.

PLANNING FOR RECOVERY

Among the keys to successful community recovery identified by FEMA are preparing (establishing roles and responsibilities) and actively planning (FEMA, 2014b). As emphasized throughout this report, depending on the nature of the disaster, recovery initiatives present a multitude of opportunities to build the community back better (healthier and more resilient and sustainable). But arranging the planning process itself is complicated, and the inclusion of public health, medical, and social services requires that additional consideration and effort be devoted to crafting creative solutions that meet multiple needs. Resources must be harnessed in a coherent fashion matched to the situation in the community, incorporating both the current status and the prior developments that will be the foundation for future progress. Blending new features into community systems after a disaster, including consideration of socioeconomic and physical environments, is a significant design challenge: creative solutions and synergistic perspectives are required in deciding what can be rearranged, identifying institutional resources to accompany this redesign, building stronger, mitigating hazards, and incorporating an emphasis on health and social services for better outcomes. The goal is better recovery by all measures, a more vital community where resilience and stability add to overall well-being—a healthy community in the fullest sense.

In Chapter 2, the committee describes Health in All Policies as "an approach to public policies across sectors that systematically takes into account the health implications of decisions, seeks synergies, and avoids harmful health impacts, in order to improve population health and health equity" (WHO, 2013), and it presents a rationale for the relevance of this approach to the recovery context. Operationalizing Health in All Policies in the disaster recovery context entails (1) creating organizational structures that optimally enable the coordination of efforts and the creation of synergies whereby core missions of non-health sectors align with healthy community objectives, and (2) ensuring that information on the potential health impacts of recovery decisions is available to the decision makers within those structures. Each of these requirements is described in the sections below.

Organizing for an Integrated Approach

Communities are complex adaptive systems[8] where decision making is distributed and myriad cross-sector interdependencies exist (Olshansky, 2014). Organizational structures influence the siloing of related

---

[8] Complex adaptive systems (1) are nonlinear and dynamic, (2) are composed of independent agents whose goals and behaviors may conflict, (3) are self-organizing, learning systems, and (4) have no single point of control (Rouse, 2000).

services and functions that can impede potential synergies and co-benefits. Despite the clear importance of an integrated approach (as discussed in Chapter 2), the committee consistently learned, through testimony (Nolen, 2014) and its review of the disaster literature (Johnson and Olshansky, 2013), about the inefficiencies and challenges during recovery related to a lack of coordination. As a result, resources are not used effectively and people suffer unnecessarily, especially those who were most vulnerable prior to the disaster. The resulting delays in individual and community recovery impact all facets of community life, including the health of the population, social cohesion, and economic viability. The committee concludes that disaster recovery and ultimately the health of the community would be improved by the development of organizational structures that support

- integrating horizontally across sectors and agencies;
- integrating vertically from the federal to the local level;
- integrating across phases of the disaster continuum, from pre-event planning to long-term recovery; and
- integrating health considerations into recovery planning and practices.

The new national framework describing a governance structure for disaster recovery—the National Disaster Recovery Framework (NDRF)—if implemented effectively, provides a structure for addressing all four of these dimensions of integration. As discussed below, however, some challenges remain.

The National Disaster Recovery Framework: A Structure for Integration

The NDRF, released in 2011, provides a guide for the federal government to facilitate effective recovery at the community level (FEMA, 2011d). The NDRF grew out of recognition of the failure to plan for recovery after Hurricane Katrina, the failure to link local needs with available resources, and the failure to plan for the actions of multiple parties to address disagreements about resource allocation (Smith, 2011a). In 2006, Congress passed the Post-Katrina Emergency Management Reform Act,[9] which mandated the development of a national recovery strategy by the federal government. Spearheaded by FEMA and its federal partners, the NDRF is not an explicit plan; rather, it is a framework document that defines how federal agencies should organize and operate during recovery to support states, tribes, and localities. It defines "core recovery principles; roles and responsibilities of recovery coordinators and other stakeholders; a coordinating structure that facilitates communication and collaboration among all stakeholders; guidance for pre- and post-disaster recovery planning; [and] the overall process by which communities can capitalize on opportunities to rebuild" what the NDRF asserts are "stronger, smarter, and safer" communities (FEMA, 2011d, p. 1). As discussed below, the NDRF is intended for a wide audience of governmental, nongovernmental, and private organizations with expertise spanning all sectors.

Recovery roles and responsibilities under the NDRF The NDRF supports a whole-community approach to disaster recovery. Emergency management has historically been a strongly government-led enterprise. However, there has been increasing recognition that a solely government-driven approach cannot adequately meet the complex and unique needs of an individual community preparing for, responding to, and recovering from a disaster (FEMA, 2011a). Nongovernmental partners play critical roles in the restoration of the "social and daily routines and support networks" that promote health, well-being, and resilience after disasters (Chandra and Acosta, 2009, p. ix). However, these roles have been poorly represented in state and federal policy, and inadequate attention has been paid to the impacts of policy and guidance issued by federal agencies on nongovernmental entities. Within the past 5 years, FEMA has sought to foster a new philosophical approach based on the "whole community" (FEMA, 2011b). Through stakeholder engagement processes, the agency identified three core principles that drive its whole-community approach:

---

[9] Post-Katrina Emergency Management Reform Act of 2006, 109th Cong., S.3721 (October 4, 2006).

- Understand and meet the actual needs of the whole community.
- Engage and empower all parts of the community.
- Strengthen what works well in communities on a daily basis (FEMA, 2011a, pp. 4-5).

The objective is to perform emergency management functions in a manner that integrates needs, capabilities, and resources across the whole community and to empower the community—government, the nonprofit sector, and the private sector—to work together as partners (CDC and CDC Foundation, 2013). Roles for specific groups are outlined below.

- **Individuals and households:** The NDRF envisions that individuals and households need to be prepared to sustain themselves immediately after a disaster by carrying adequate insurance; holding essential supplies of medication, food, and water; and listening to public information announcements on the recovery process.
- **Local government:** Local government plays a central role in planning and managing all phases of a community's recovery. When local governments are overwhelmed by their responsibilities, they seek the services of state and federal governments. Local governments also galvanize the preparation of hazard mitigation and recovery plans, raise hazard awareness, and educate the public prior to and during the recovery process.
- **State government:** The states are central players in coordinating recovery activities, including the provision of financial and technical assistance. One type of financial assistance entails issuing bonds for building critical infrastructure. States often manage federal resources and are conduits to local and tribal governments.
- **Federal government:** The central role of the federal government is to facilitate the efforts of state and local governments to leverage needed resources to rebuild communities. The federal government can use the NDRF to recruit and engage available department and agency capacities to promote local recovery. Federal support must be scalable and adaptable to meet community needs.
- **The nonprofit sector:** The nonprofit sector encompasses faith-based and other volunteer community organizations, charities, foundations and philanthropies, professional associations, and academic institutions. Major roles of the nonprofit sector include case management, volunteer coordination, behavioral health and psychological support, housing repair, and construction. Nonprofits tend to fill the gaps when governmental services and support do not meet a community's comprehensive needs. Nonprofits often conduct advocacy for community members.
- **The private sector:** The private sector plays an essential role by retaining and providing employment and a stable tax base. It also owns and operates much of the country's infrastructure, including electrical power, financial, and telecommunications systems. The private sector, including utilities, banks, and insurance companies, can foster mitigation and encourage community resilience. Public–private partnerships are critical resources during recovery and facilitate the coordinated leveraging of funding from multiple sources (FEMA, 2011d).

Recovery support functions Similar to the Emergency Support Functions (ESFs) defined by the National Response Framework,[10] the NDRF defines six Recovery Support Functions (RSFs): Community Planning and Capacity Building; Economic; Health and Social Services; Housing; Infrastructure Systems; and Natural and Cultural Resources (described in more detail in Box 3-3). The RSFs help define an organizational

---

[10] The National Response Framework (NRF), also produced by FEMA, directs how the nation responds during the immediate period following all types of disasters and emergencies, ranging from "those that are adequately handled with local assets to those of catastrophic proportion that require marshaling the capabilities of the entire Nation" (FEMA, 2013c, p. 4). It "describes the principles, roles and responsibilities, and coordinating structures for delivering the core capabilities required to respond to an incident and further describes how response efforts integrate" with those of other related areas. Its objectives "define the capabilities necessary to save lives, protect property and the environment, meet basic human needs, stabilize the incident, restore basic services and community functionality, and establish a safe and secure environment moving toward the transition to recovery" (FEMA, 2013c, p. i).

structure for recovery operations that can promote vertical integration if aligned with structures created by state and local governments[11] (see Figure 3-2). For each RSF, the NDRF specifies a federal coordinating agency, primary agencies, and supporting organizations. The coordinating agency furnishes leadership, coordination, and oversight. The primary agencies bring significant authorities, capabilities, roles, or resources to bear, but to a lesser extent than the coordinating agency. Supporting organizations, some of which are nongovernmental organizations, have specific capabilities or resources that complement those of the primary agencies. It should be noted that not all RSFs will be activated for all presidentially declared disasters; rather, decisions on RSF activation will be based on a post-disaster assessment of damage and needs. Existing pre-event recovery plans that delineate clear operational structures consistent with the NDRF, such as those of Fairfax County, Virginia, and Pinellas County, Florida, may be useful models (see Appendix C for links to these documents).

As the response period abates, emergency support functions will transition operations over to the RSFs, facilitating integration across disaster management phases. For example, responsibility for health and medical functions will transition from ESF #8 (Public Health and Medical Services) to the Health and Social Services RSF. Although there may be overlap in required expertise in the transition from response to early recovery, later recovery phases will necessitate the involvement of RSF representatives with different expertise, consistent with a transition from emergency functions to long-term reconstruction and community betterment activities. For example, transportation sector representatives supporting the Infrastructure Systems RSF should be those familiar with long-range transportation planning. For the health sector, the Health and Social Services RSF should include representatives working on an everyday basis to create healthier communities through community health improvement and social services activities. It is important to have clear plans in place for this transition and mechanisms for bringing in those trained in long-term community planning.

The NDRF also calls for three new leadership positions to monitor and coordinate disaster recovery through both the pre-disaster and the post-disaster period:

- A *local disaster recovery manager* who, among his/her many responsibilities, organizes the recovery planning process; ensures inclusiveness; develops and implements recovery progress measures; and communicates and coordinates with state, federal, and community stakeholders.
- A *state disaster recovery coordinator* leads statewide agencies by managing the recovery and by providing support for local initiatives. The state disaster recovery coordinator coordinates state, tribal, and federal funding streams; identifies gaps; and works collaboratively with recovery leadership at all levels to ensure a well-coordinated, timely, and well-executed recovery.
- A *federal disaster recovery coordinator* is responsible for facilitating recovery coordination and collaboration among all stakeholders. He/she monitors state and local decision making, evaluating the need for additional assistance. During the transition from response to recovery, coordination responsibilities will transition from the federal coordinating officer (who operates under the National Response Framework) to the federal disaster recovery coordinator.

The local disaster recovery manager, state disaster recovery coordinator, and federal disaster recovery coordinator facilitate vertical integration from the local to the federal level (FEMA, 2011c).

---

[11] Substate, regional organizations (e.g., Councils of Government, Metropolitan Planning Organizations, Regional Planning Commissions, Economic Development Districts) should also be considered in alignments with the federal NDRF structure since many states are organized into regional districts that are defined by a unified geography—established by state legislation—for diverse functions, both as regional entities with governing boards and as operating units of state agencies. These intergovernmental structures are key to organizing effective post-disaster community recovery. One example of a regional social service organization is an Area Agency on Aging. Such operations are often managed by Councils of Government or Regional Planning Commissions, offering a wide range of support services to senior citizens—who are often particularly vulnerable to the effects of disasters—including nutrition (Meals on Wheels, for example), transportation, and access to community programs.

BOX 3-3
Recovery Support Functions

Community Planning and Capacity Building
Coordinating Agency: DHS/FEMA
Primary Agencies: DHS/FEMA, HHS
    The mission of this RSF is to promote and build recovery capacity and community planning resources for managing and implementing disaster recovery activities. This RSF assists States in developing pre- and post-disaster systems of support for local communities. This can be achieved in part by providing technical assistance and planning support to aid all levels of government to integrate sustainability principles—such as adaptive reuse of historic properties, mitigation considerations, smart growth principles, and sound land-use—into recovery decisions.

Economic
Coordinating Agency: DOC
Primary Agencies: DOC, DHS/FEMA, DOL, SBA, Treasury, USDA
Supporting Organizations include HHS
    The mission of the Economic RSF is to help state, local, and community stakeholders to sustain and/or rebuild businesses and employment, as well as to develop economic opportunities that yield sustainable and economically resilient communities. This mission is achieved by leveraging federal resources, information, and leadership. The key is to encourage private investment and facilitate private sector lending and borrowing for restoring vital markets and economies.

Health and Social Services
Coordinating Agency: HHS
Primary Agencies: HHS, CNCS, DHS (FEMA, NPPD, CRCL), DOI, DOJ, DOL, ED, EPA, VA
Supporting Organizations: DOT, SBA, Treasury, USDA, VA, ARC, National VOAD
    The mission of the Health and Social Services RSF is to help local-led recovery efforts in restoring public health, health care, and social services. The integration of these services promotes community resilience, health, independence, and well-being. (The term "health" subsumes public health, behavioral health, and medical services.) Among the many responsibilities of this RSF is to identify and coordinate with stakeholders an assessment of food, animal, water, and air conditions to ensure safety. Other responsibilities are to coordinate and leverage federal resources for health and social services, and to promote self-sufficiency and continuity of care of affected individuals, especially vulnerable populations. The NDRF envisions specific activities for the Health and Social Services RSF, including encouragement of behavioral health systems to meet the behavioral health needs of affected individuals, response and recovery workers, and the community; the reconnecting of displaced populations with essential health and social services; and the promotion of clear communications and public health messaging to provide accurate and accessible information that is available in multiple mediums, multi-lingual formats, alternative formats and is accessible to underserved populations.

Current limitations of the NDRF A comprehensive analysis of the challenges related to recovery and the utility of the NDRF for addressing them is beyond the scope of this report. Through its information gathering process, however, the committee noted several issues that will ultimately influence the effectiveness of the NDRF as a mechanism for integrating health into the recovery process and thus warrant discussion here.

First, although the NDRF promotes pre-event planning in principle, the framework is not accompanied by any funding to support such planning or capacity building for recovery. The reluctance of federal, state, and local governments to invest in these two critical functions in advance of a disaster has been described as one of the greatest barriers to achieving disaster resilience (Smith, 2011b). As discussed in Chapter 2,

Housing

Coordinating Agency: HUD
Primary Agencies: HUD, DHS/FEMA, DOJ, USDA
Supporting Organizations include HHS

The mission of the housing RSF is to facilitate delivery of federal resources to rehabilitate and reconstruct destroyed or damaged housing and to procure new, accessible permanent housing. This mission can be achieved in part by building accessibility, resilience, sustainability, and mitigation measures into housing recovery in as timely a manner as possible.

Infrastructure Systems

Coordinating Agency: DOD/USACE
Primary Agencies: DOD/USACE, DHS (FEMA and NPPD), DOE, DOT
Supporting Organizations include HHS

The mission of the Infrastructure RSF is to facilitate federal support to local, state, and tribal governments and other infrastructure owners and operators. The scope of this RSF includes energy, water, dams, communications, transportation systems, agriculture, government facilities, utilities, sanitation, engineering, and flood control. This RSF encourages rebuilding infrastructure in a manner that will reduce vulnerability to future disasters.

Natural and Cultural Resources

Coordinating Agency: DOI
Primary Agencies: DOI, DHS/FEMA, EPA
Supporting Organizations do not include HHS

The mission of this RSF is to channel federal assets and capabilities to assist state and local government and communities to address long-term environmental and cultural resource recovery. The key is to protect natural and cultural resources through recovery actions that preserve, conserve, rehabilitate, or restore them. This RSF works to leverage federal resources and available programs to meet local recovery needs.

NOTES: ARC = American Red Cross; CNCS = Corporation for National and Community Service; CRCL = Civil Rights and Civil Liberties; DHS = U.S. Department of Homeland Security; DOC = U.S. Department of Commerce; DOD = U.S. Department of Defense; DOE = U.S. Department of Energy; DOI = U.S. Department of the Interior; DOJ = U.S. Department of Justice; DOL = U.S. Department of Labor; DOT = U.S. Department of Transportation; ED = U.S. Department of Education; EPA = U.S. Environmental Protection Agency; FEMA = Federal Emergency Management Agency; HHS = U.S. Department of Health and Human Services; HUD = U.S. Department of Housing and Urban Development; NPPD = National Protection and Programs Directorate; SBA = U.S. Small Business Administration; USACE = U.S. Army Corps of Engineers; USDA = U.S. Department of Agriculture; VA = U.S. Department of Veterans Affairs; VOAD = Voluntary Organizations Active in Disaster.

SOURCE: FEMA, 2011d.

pre-disaster recovery planning is critical to seizing opportunities for health improvement during recovery. Further, lack of capacity can result in a protracted recovery process and associated negative health effects as community members languish under suboptimal living conditions and experience chronic, toxic stress.

Second, the committee noted incongruence of the NDRF with major federal funding sources that drive community planning at the state and local levels, both during steady-state times and after disasters. During steady state, grants and policies of the U.S. Department of Housing and Urban Development (HUD) and the U.S. Department of Transportation (DOT)—now collaborating along with the U.S. Environmental Protection Agency (EPA) under the banner of the Partnership for Sustainable Communities—are major drivers of urban and regional planning practices. As discussed in Chapter 2, the sustainability practices

Recovery Support Functions Under the Federal NDRF Structure

	Community Planning and Capacity Building	Economic	Health and Social Services	Housing	Infrastructure Systems	Natural and Cultural Resources
Federal Coordinating Agency	FEMA	DOC	HHS	HUD	USACE	DOI
Other Federal Primary Agencies (as indicated in the NDRF)	• HHS	• FEMA • DOL • SBA • Treasury • USDA	• CNCS • DHS (FEMA, NPPD, CRCL) • DOI • DOJ • DOL • Ed • EPA • VA	• FEMA • DOJ • USDA	• DHS (FEMA, NPPD) • DOE • DOT	• FEMA • EPA
Possible Aligned Entities at the State Level	• Planning • Community Development • Economic Development	• Planning • Community Development • Economic Development • Housing Finance Agency	• Planning, Community Development • Economic Development • Social Welfare, Child, and Family Services • Health Department • State mental health authority • Education Department	• Housing Finance Agency • Planning, Community Development • Economic Development	• Department of Environmental Protection • Department of Transportation	• Department of Environmental Protection • Health Department • Natural Resources, Fish/Wildlife, and Parks
Possible Aligned Entities at the Regional Level	• MPOs • RPCs • COGs • RTPOs • EDDs	• RPCs • COGs • RTPOs • EDDs	• RPCs • COGs • EDDs • Health care coalitions	• RPCs • COGs • EDDs	• RTPOs • MPOs • COGs • RPCs	• RPCs • COGs
Possible Aligned Entities at the City and County Levels	• Planning, Community Development, Economic Development, Building Codes • Emergency Management	• Planning, Community Development, Economic Development, Building Codes	• Health Department (Public Health, Environmental Health, Mental Health Authority) • Social Services/ Children and Family Services (WIC, Head Start), Aging, Homeless Services, • School districts	• Housing Authority (HOPE VI, Section 8, Senior housing)	• Transportation (Highway, Transit, Airport) Public Works, Utilities and Engineering	• Parks and Recreation • Libraries

Channels Through Which Federal Agencies Assist in Recovery Plan Development

FIGURE 3-2 Model for aligning organizations and programs with the federal National Disaster Recovery Framework (NDRF) structure.

NOTES: Although the committee shows here an example in which state and local structures are identical to the federally defined recovery support functions, this need not be the case. Depicted here is a level between state and local—the regional planning level—which should also be considered in alignment with the federal NDRF structure.

CNCS = Corporation for National and Community Service; COG = Council of Governments; CRCL = Civil Rights and Civil Liberties; DHS = U.S. Department of Homeland Security; DOC = U.S. Department of Commerce; DOE = U.S. Department of Energy; DOI = U.S. Department of the Interior; DOJ = U.S. Department of Justice; DOL = U.S. Department of Labor; DOT = U.S. Department of Transportation; ED = U.S. Department of Education; EDD = economic development district; EPA = U.S. Environmental Protection Agency; FEMA = Federal Emergency Management Agency; HHS = U.S. Department of Health and Human Services; HUD = U.S. Department of Housing and Urban Development; MPO = metropolitan planning organization; NDRF = National Disaster Recovery Framework; NPPD = National Protection and Programs Directorate; RPC = regional planning commission; RTPO = regional transportation planning organization; SBA = U.S. Small Business Administration; USACE = U.S. Army Corps of Engineers; USDA = U.S. Department of Agriculture; VA = U.S. Department of Veterans Affairs; WIC = Special Supplemental Nutrition Program for Women, Infants, and Children.

(e.g., affordable housing, transportation choices) promoted by the Partnership yield significant co-benefits in terms of health outcomes, and the committee sees great benefit to incorporating the Partnership's livability principles (see Box 2-5 in Chapter 2) into recovery planning, as encouraged by HUD after Hurricane Sandy. Furthermore, HUD-funded community development (e.g., Community Development Block Grant) programs are a major element of community planning and have significant potential to impact the social determinants of health, but they appear to be unlinked to the NDRF structure. Neither HUD nor DOT is included even as a primary agency (both are listed as supporting organizations) for the Community Planning and Capacity Building RSF (FEMA is the coordinating agency).[12] This appears inconsistent with the NDRF definition of primary agencies—those having "significant authorities, roles, resources or capabilities for a particular function within an RSF" (FEMA, 2011d, p. 39). Although HUD is the coordinating agency for the Housing RSF, that area of expertise is separate from the agency's urban planning and community development role. Moreover, after a disaster HUD can have a significant influence on recovery planning at the state and local levels as a funding agency if Congress passes a supplemental appropriation through the HUD Community Development Block Grant for Disaster Recovery (CDBG-DR) vehicle (described in more detail in Chapter 4). After Hurricane Sandy, CDBG-DR funds to support recovery surpassed FEMA disaster relief funds (Donahue, 2014). It is not clear to the committee how CDBG-driven planning is integrated into the NDRF framework. Better incorporation of federal urban planning and community development expertise into the Community Planning and Capacity Building RSF could help address this apparent incongruence.

Finally, testimony provided to the committee revealed that the NDRF, released more than 3 years ago, has not yet been widely adopted and implemented at the state and local levels (Lockwood, 2014; Walsh and Schor, 2014). During a recent study on long-term recovery in which semi-structured interviews were used to collect data on training needs for community leaders in health-related functional roles, the National Center for Disaster Medicine and Public Health found that few respondents who had been actively involved in the recovery from Hurricane Sandy[13] were familiar with the NDRF. Those who were familiar felt that its implementation had been problematic because of a lack of guidance, as well as conflicts with existing community recovery plans.[14]

Current limitations in integration of health into the NDRF The NDRF describes recovery as a continuum of coordinated processes, many concurrent, by which the community

- minimizes and overcomes the physical, emotional, and environmental impacts of a disaster;
- reestablishes an economic and social base that instills confidence in the community members and businesses regarding community viability;
- rebuilds by integrating the functional needs of all residents and reducing the community's vulnerability to all hazards it faces; and
- demonstrates a capability to be prepared, responsive, and resilient in dealing with the consequences of disasters (FEMA, 2011d, p. 13).

This description clearly conveys the notion that community recovery is not just a "bricks and mortar" process of restoring physical infrastructure; rather, it entails the regeneration of all community systems, functions, and social structures in a way that addresses the full range of needs of the affected community members and ensures that the community has the capacity to meet its future needs. This represents a critical paradigm shift in the nation's approach to disaster recovery, which has been criticized in the past

---

[12] The committee did hear that a memorandum of agreement between FEMA and the U.S. Environmental Protection Agency is currently used as a mechanism to bring sustainability expertise into the recovery planning process when state and local partners express interest.

[13] The NDRF was released approximately 1 year before Hurricane Sandy.

[14] Memorandum, K. Schor, Acting Director, National Center for Disaster Medicine and Public Health, to A. Downey, Institute of Medicine, May 28, 2014.

for its focus on physical infrastructure and lack of attention to meeting broader human recovery needs such as psychological and social well-being (Chandra and Acosta, 2010). Psychological and emotional recovery is among the core principles laid out in the NDRF, which acknowledges that community recovery is dependent on the recovery of individuals and families (FEMA, 2011d) and that health and social well-being are essential to recovery at all levels.

The committee was encouraged to see that Health and Social Services is one of the six RSFs in the NDRF, thus helping to institutionalize the role of health in recovery and to draw attention to the opportunities for improving population health and health systems beyond pre-disaster levels. As indicated in the description of responsibilities for this RSF given in Box 3-3, however, the Health and Social Services RSF is focused narrowly on restoration and delivery of public health, medical, behavioral health, and social services. Although these are unarguably functions critical to protecting and promoting short- and long-term health, they do not capture the full spectrum of factors that affect health within a community or the pathways to health discussed in this and the previous chapter (e.g., collaborations with nonhealth sectors such as urban planning and community development). Since the activities of all sectors will impact health during recovery, either positively or negatively, it is critical that health not be siloed but integrated with all other recovery functions, which should operate cohesively through a systems approach.

Table 3-2, although not comprehensive, illustrates how the activities of the other five RSFs have health implications. As shown in this table, HHS is associated with nearly all of these other RSFs, providing a mechanism for approaching health during recovery in a more holistic way, if RSFs are operationalized with this intent. Making HHS a supporting organization for the Natural and Cultural Resources RSF as well might better enable HHS and its component agencies to infuse health across the full spectrum of RSFs and promote a broader vision for the role of health in recovery. Although the Office of the Assistant Secretary for Preparedness and Response provides the coordinating function for the Health and Social Services RSF on behalf of the HHS Secretary, greater involvement of other HHS agencies and most notably the CDC, which is a major funder of both community health improvement and community resilience building efforts, might facilitate a healthy community approach to recovery. The CDC supports diverse community development planning initiatives with co-benefits for population health, such as transit-oriented development; programming of parks, open spaces, and trails; and nutrition strategies aimed at overcoming food deserts. The CDC is a policy leader in such initiatives nationally, taking a science-based approach to health disparities and low health status in many populations.

Building on a Foundation of Existing Organizational Structures and Initiatives

The path by which a community undertakes the long and complex process of recovery is dependent on the characteristics of the disaster—the type of event (e.g., tornado, flood) and the scale (amount) and pattern of damage (features of the community that were damaged)—as well as the prevailing organizational and governance structures utilized by elected and public officials. Consequently, decisions on how to structure recovery planning after a disaster must be locally driven, taking into consideration the different needs for local and regional events (see Box 3-4). The choices facing community leaders at the beginning of the recovery planning process are not about the content of the recovery plan; they are about assembling the resources (including human capital) and agendas for the work ahead. Because institutions often work in some degree of isolation, community leaders sometimes are unaware of the key stakeholders that should be integrated into the recovery planning process. The task after a disaster is to ensure that prior collaborations are added to the list of organizational assets and then to incorporate those personnel and groups into the recovery planning effort. As discussed earlier in this chapter, the committee observed that the dimensions of health and social services are not adequately integrated into disaster recovery planning, particularly in the long-term phase. More intentional efforts are needed to integrate health considerations into recovery planning and decision making.

All communities have in place structures and processes for strategic decision making regarding investments that will be made and projects that will be prioritized. As discussed in Chapter 2, strategies often

TABLE 3-2 Health Implications of Nonhealth Recovery Support Functions

Recovery Support Function	HHS Association	Example Health Implications
Community Planning and Capacity Building	Primary agency	Community design influences physical activity, risk of injury, exposure to toxins, and access to goods (e.g., healthy food) and services (e.g., health care) essential to health. Community redevelopment investments can have significant impacts on social determinants of health.
Economic	Supporting organization	Social and economic factors (e.g., poverty) are among the greatest influences on health outcomes. Job training initiatives are complementary to other community development approaches that address social determinants of health.
Housing	Supporting organization	The quality of the indoor and outdoor housing environments affects health. Affordability of housing is a social determinant of health.
Infrastructure Systems	Supporting organization	Lifeline utilities such as water treatment and power systems are essential to health and hygiene. Transportation systems ensure access to goods (e.g., healthy food) and services (e.g., health care) essential to health.
Natural and Cultural Resources	None	Healthy environments and ecosystems are essential to healthy populations. Parks, trails, and other natural resources provide opportunities for recreation and physical activity.

NOTE: HHS = U.S. Department of Health and Human Services.

are sought that use complementary investments to achieve synergies, reduce costs, and meet multiple objectives, thus maximizing benefits. Multisector approaches to strategic planning also reduce inefficiencies arising from duplication of effort. These mechanisms for everyday problem solving are well suited to envisioning recovery strategies, and collective priority setting for everyday problems equips a community with the systematic analysis and decision processes needed to address the complexities of a new set of physical, social, and economic problems in neighborhoods after a disaster. Although changes are made to decision-making structures within a community during the response phase of a disaster to enable decisive action that will save lives and protect property, the recovery phase sees a return to long-standing strategic planning processes used to prioritize investments. Most communities, for example, have ongoing community development initiatives designed to address the social and economic problems that degrade health and contribute to social vulnerability to disasters (although improved health may not always be an explicit goal of such efforts). Because of the complexity of these challenges, such initiatives are of necessity multisectoral in nature. Community development[15] initiatives to meet the needs of low-income community members and address such issues as blight often utilize collaborative strategies involving charitable, nonprofit, and faith-based groups (the United Way, for example, often participates in local community development collaboratives). Leveraging local community development institutions during disaster recovery will have the effect of improving health outcomes. Given the magnitude of health disparities related to social equity issues, the potential health benefits of integrated approaches to place-based strategies for

---

[15] Community development is a category of planning and service delivery funded largely by HUD that supports the development of "stronger and more resilient communities through an ongoing process of identifying and addressing needs, assets, and priority investments" (HUD, 2014).

BOX 3-4
Recovery Planning on a Regional Scale

When people convene to conduct community disaster recovery planning, their perspective typically is drawn to the community in which they live or perhaps the community they serve. That makes sense, as most disasters are local. However, it is important to recognize that regional and national disasters also occur, some would say with increasing frequency. Experience shows that disaster recovery is different when entire regions are impacted, and the approach that communities take to community disaster recovery planning must differ accordingly.

Regional and local events differ in many ways. First, the expanded scale and scope of a regional disaster serve to magnify known deficiencies in the capacity and capabilities of public health, medical, and social service systems and may expose new challenges. Second, regional disasters encompass a multitude of jurisdictions, each with its own set of laws, regulations, policies, and norms. These differences complicate disaster recovery planning and recovery processes. Third, while disasters expose the disproportionate vulnerability of certain segments of a community, regional disasters demonstrate that these disproportionate vulnerabilities are not distributed proportionally: some communities are more vulnerable and are impacted more severely than others.

While regional disasters can be characterized by many more differences, those cited above are sufficient to support the need for a different approach to the management of regional recovery operations. First, the best-informed decisions come from decision makers who are best informed. That dictum, although obvious, points to the recurrent challenges of ensuring that federal, state, and local officials have access to the necessary channels of health-related information and are able to prioritize, implement, and adjust as needed. Second, the multitude of jurisdictions involved in a regional disaster brings a wider array of players, perspectives, and priorities, all of which need to be incorporated into the decision-making process and harmonized around an integrated strategy and inclusive set of objectives. And third, disasters that span an entire region also are likely to cross political boundaries that may well bring an intensity of interest and beneficial level of visibility.

Community leaders will want to be mindful of the possibility of a region-wide disaster as they develop their vision for improving health outcomes in a post-disaster environment, assess the comprehensiveness of their social networks, and conduct disaster recovery planning. The National Disaster Recovery Framework and its Recovery Support Functions (RSFs) (detailed in Box 3-3) were designed in part to assist communities in planning for just this type of scenario. The inclusion of every federal agency with a role in disaster recovery within the RSF structure provides a channel for their involvement in coordinating the grant processes and funding streams that will be needed to improve health outcomes after a disaster. The linkages among the Federal Emergency Management Agency, the U.S. Department of Health and Human Services, the U.S. Department of Housing and Urban Development, and other departments and agencies and their routine engagement with state and local public health officials can form the foundation for community awareness and set the stage for the collaboration and cooperation that are essential to full-scale recovery at a regional scale.

---

addressing employment, education, crime prevention, sustainability, and revitalization during post-disaster recovery could be substantial. Vulnerability to disasters also tends to coincide with the same socioeconomic indicators that relate to both populations and at-risk geographic areas.

Intersectoral collaboration to support Health in All Policies depends not only on a shared vision and goals but also on relationships built on trust (Rudolph et al., 2013). As highlighted in the Health in All Policies case study from Galveston, Texas, discussed in Chapter 2 (see Box 2-11), there are significant benefits to developing these relationships in advance of a disaster. According to Dr. Alexandra Nolen, former director of the Center to Eliminate Health Disparities—the organization championing the Health in All Policies approach in Galveston—it took 5 years after the 2008 hurricane to reach the early stages of cross-sector collaboration because no such relationships were in place before the hurricane struck (Nolen, 2014). Thus, a community that is working across sectors to achieve improved population health during steady-state times is inherently better suited to recovering from a disaster. The organizational structures and participatory mechanisms used for health improvement during steady-state times can be leveraged after a disaster in developing a recovery strategy and determining priorities. Importantly, though, the benefits of improved organizational arrangements for community problem solving will accrue to the community during times other than disasters.

Organizational approaches such as those in Thurston County, Washington; Washtenaw County, Michigan; and King County, Washington (see Chapter 2) appear to hold promise for supporting Health in All Policies during both disaster recovery and steady-state times. Nonetheless, the committee believes additional research is needed to determine the comparative efficacy of alternative organizational structures for recovery operations. Pilot or demonstration projects could help elucidate best practices for organizational arrangements that could then be incentivized through federal grant funds. The committee is hopeful that such efforts would yield a road map that communities could use in developing disaster recovery arrangements among local institutions under the overarching structure of the NDRF to achieve improved post-disaster health outcomes. What is needed is not a one-dimensional hierarchy but a sophisticated set of participatory mechanisms customized to work in the context of the unique arrangements of a community's pre-disaster agencies and work programs and its policy, technical, operational, and database assets.

Engaging the Whole Community in Recovery Planning

Successful recovery and the post-disaster rebuilding of healthier and more sustainable and resilient communities require the coordinated efforts of an extremely broad, multidisciplinary group of stakeholders (i.e., a whole-community approach). Yet many of these stakeholders are not accustomed to working in the emergency management context and are not familiar with the salient processes, terminology, or resources. Following an extensive review of the federal grey literature related to recovery and hearing testimony from experts at the federal, state, and local levels, the committee was concerned about how difficult it is for key stakeholders outside (and even within) the emergency management field to understand the relationships among the array of federal, state, and local resources that must be mobilized after a disaster; how they interrelate; and who is accountable at each level. The committee found no single federal-level document that provides a clear overarching review of the interconnections among the key legislation, directives, national-level strategies, and frameworks relevant to recovery—one designed to be understood by those outside the emergency management field and describing processes by which stakeholders can engage in the recovery planning process—both before and after a disaster—and leverage recovery resources.

Further, the committee noted inconsistencies among existing federal documents. For example, FEMA's 2014 *Overview of the National Planning Frameworks* describes the eight core capabilities in the NDRF as Planning, Public Information and Warning, Operational Coordination, Economic Recovery, Health and Social Services, Housing, Infrastructure Systems, and Natural and Cultural Resources (FEMA, 2014c, p. 7). The NDRF itself makes no mention of core capabilities but describes the six RSFs discussed earlier: Community Planning and Capacity Building, Economic, Health and Social Services, Housing, Infrastructure Systems, and Natural and Cultural Resources (see Box 3-3). The overabundance of federal documents pertaining to the National Preparedness System (of which recovery is a core mission area) and the inconsistencies among them is confusing and intimidating to those not familiar with the emergency management field. Ambiguous terminology—for example, "planning," which may refer generally to an operational process of coordinating efforts or alternatively to a process by which land use/community design decisions are made—adds further confusion.

To better support a whole-community approach to recovery, the committee has attempted to provide a cogent, high-level description of the processes and resources pertinent to disaster recovery (see Chapter

4 and Appendix A), drawing on a number of federal and nonfederal materials. These materials include but are not limited to

- *National Preparedness Goal* (FEMA, 2011e),
- *National Preparedness System* (FEMA, 2011f),
- *Overview of the National Planning Frameworks* (FEMA, 2014c),
- *National Response Framework* (FEMA, 2013c),
- *National Disaster Recovery Framework* (FEMA, 2011d),
- *National Health Security Strategy* (HHS, 2009, 2015),
- Robert T. Stafford Disaster Relief and Emergency Assistance Act,[16]
- Post-Katrina Emergency Reform Act of 2006,[17]
- Sandy Recovery Improvement Act of 2013,[18] and
- Pandemic and All-Hazards Preparedness Act.[19]

In the face of such complexity, communities often need to hire outside professional consultants to navigate the disaster recovery process. The committee concludes that the federal government needs to make information on federal recovery policy and resources (and the process by which they are mobilized) available in a more accessible and coherent manner to facilitate maximum involvement by all stakeholders. Further, those leading recovery planning need to be sensitized to and trained on the importance of engaging all relevant stakeholder groups through robust outreach efforts. Key stakeholders themselves need to be educated on the importance of their participation and mechanisms by which they should engage proactively in the process.

The Role of Leadership

The effective governance of recovery from a disaster requires strong leadership that harnesses the actions of a broad array of agencies from multiple levels of government, along with the nonprofit and private sectors, to address highly complex and interrelated challenges using an integrated multidisciplinary approach. Several emerging approaches to leadership have particular relevance to the disaster recovery context:

- **Meta-leadership** is an approach to leadership focused specifically on breaking down organizational silos and fostering a spirit of cooperation that motivates people to work together (Marcus et al., 2006). Core to the concept of meta-leadership is the ability to lead by influence, since engaging organizations outside of one's silo necessarily means reaching beyond lines of authority. This ability is particularly crucial during recovery, which has been characterized as "nearly the opposite of command and control" (City of Seattle, 2013, p. 5). A model meta-leadership program was developed by the National Preparedness Leadership Initiative, a joint venture of the Harvard School of Public Health's Division of Policy Translation and Leadership Development and the Harvard Kennedy School's Center for Public Leadership, to build heightened capacity for effective cross-agency coordination of effort through education and training (NPLI, 2013).
- **Distributive leadership** is based on the premise that diffusion of responsibility and authority is needed in situations where a centralized command and control approach cannot adequately meet complex decision-making needs. After a disaster, distributive leadership enables rapid response to changing conditions on the ground through locally informed decisions. "With distributive

---

[16] 42 U.S.C. § 5121 et seq.
[17] Post-Katrina Emergency Management Reform Act of 2006, 109th Cong., S.3721 (October 4, 2006).
[18] Sandy Recovery Improvement Act of 2013, Public Law 113-2, 113th Cong., H.R.152 (January 29, 2014).
[19] Pandemic and All-Hazards Preparedness Act, Public Law 109-417, 109th Cong., S.3678 (December 19, 2006).

leadership, there is a shift from reliance on systems and procedures to an increased capacity to adapt, to change, learn, and innovate" (Usdin, 2014, p.159).

Engaging the Public in a Participatory Planning Process

As discussed earlier in this chapter, community engagement does not end with visioning: the community should be an active participant in every aspect of the recovery process, including the development and implementation of plans. This participation is critical to ensuring that recovery decisions align with the community's vision and that community values are respected in decisions about contested issues. Such conversations may center on short-term issues such as priority setting for access to scarce health resources (IOM, 2012) but also should encompass controversial long-term decisions such as buyouts through eminent domain.

Using an inclusive process that leverages existing community organizations and social networks builds trust, ensures that local needs will be met, and creates a sense of ownership, thereby increasing the likelihood of success (see Box 3-5 for how this was accomplished in Kobe, Japan, after a devastating earthquake). After a disaster, the active engagement of the community in the recovery planning process also promotes healing and strengthens resilience. When the community gathers together to plan and implement a recovery strategy, ties among residents are strengthened, thereby building social networks and empowering residents. Thus, organizational structures for recovery planning must enable bidirectional communication between the community and decision makers. Mechanisms to this end can include (1) partnerships between local government and community organizations and (2) official advisory bodies that act as a link between the community and decision makers and represent the voices and needs of the affected population.

Community partnerships A partnership between local government and community organizations can help foster the collaborative spirit and sense of community ownership that, while not always easily measured, can aid in building community resilience. Partnering with organizations that are already linked to the community can be an essential tool for local governments, helping them communicate with and assist difficult-to-reach populations. Community organizations often play a major role in recovery because of gaps in government-provided services. After Hurricane Sandy struck New York City, for example, many

---

BOX 3-5
Leveraging Social Networks After Disasters

Encouraging or even requiring the solicitation of input from neighborhood-level organizations (e.g., homeowners associations) in a community requiring significant redevelopment after a disaster can help ensure that the people most affected by recovery plans are included in their development. After the 1995 earthquake in Kobe, Japan, neighborhood associations organized into councils (called Machizukuri) that in many cases were recognized by city ordinance. These councils not only provided support to the community (e.g., finding temporary housing, coordinating food distribution, and providing updated information through newsletters) but also were actively engaged in the formulation of neighborhood redevelopment plans (Edgington, 2011). The councils served to balance what had initially begun as a top-down process. Social capital also was strengthened as participants in the council became more civically engaged. Residents in Kobe communities that engaged in this bottom-up planning process that sought to harness citizens' visions for their neighborhoods reported higher satisfaction with the overall process than those with more top-down approaches (Aldrich, 2012; Nakagawa and Shaw, 2004).

residents found relief and assistance in community centers, tenant associations, or faith-based organizations. A survey of public housing residents in New York found that 59 percent accessed such assistance. These organizations have deep and long-standing ties with the community, and when government was slow to respond to residents' needs, they stepped in. However, they did not have the expertise, resources, or capacity to fully meet the needs of the storm-struck residents and were not coordinated with government services. Since Hurricane Sandy, the New York City Housing Authority has proposed partnerships with these community organizations and has suggested using community centers as hubs for communication, counseling, and coordination of volunteers and supplies (The Alliance for a Just Rebuilding et al., 2014).

Advisory bodies Some jurisdictions have opted to create official bodies to engage with the community and obtain input on the recovery process. These bodies act as a link between the community and decision makers, and they should represent the full geographic, cultural, and economic diversity of the community to ensure that the voices and needs of all the affected population are heard. After severe weather caused major flooding in Iowa in 2008, for example, the governor established the Rebuild Iowa Advisory Commission (RIAC), a 15-member independent advisory body made up of a cross-section of Iowans. The RIAC traveled to affected areas of the state, holding town meetings and talking to residents to gain insight into their immediate- and long-term needs, and then developed recommendations for recovery and provided strategic direction to recovery decision makers. The RIAC proved to be an invaluable tool for focusing the recovery effort on the needs of residents and giving Iowans a channel for their feedback on the recovery process (Rebuild Iowa Office, 2011).

Using Health-Related Information to Inform Recovery Decision Making

Organizational structures such as those discussed earlier in this chapter provide essential scaffolding for decision-making processes but by themselves are not sufficient. The effectiveness of an integrated planning and recovery approach is greatly enhanced by shared information. One of the greatest challenges associated with disaster recovery is that decision makers often must take action before the information needed to support those decisions can arrive (Olshansky, 2014). Planning processes that may in normal times have been spaced out over a period of years must now be conducted in a timeframe of just months. Moreover, as discussed in the section on leadership above, decision making is distributed during disaster recovery, creating challenges related to coordination of actions. Recovery proceeds more effectively when the myriad actors involved are aware of each other's actions. Thus, accelerating and broadening the flow of information is crucial to success (Johnson and Olshansky, 2013).

Several kinds of information can be used to support the incorporation of health considerations into the recovery decision-making process to improve health outcomes after a disaster. These include (1) knowledge of the potential health impacts of alternative decisions; (2) knowledge gained from past disaster experiences and in particular, effective (and ineffective) practices; (3) knowledge of available resources; and (4) up-to-date information on the recovery environment (i.e., status). Reliable sources of each of these kinds of information should be identified in advance of a disaster as part of pre-event planning. Sources of such information include

- health impact assessments;
- guidance, training, and technical assistance; and
- information systems, including health information systems.

Each is discussed further in the sections below.

Health Impact Assessments

Health impact assessment (HIA) is a process by which scientific data, professional expertise, and stakeholder input are used to determine the positive and negative public health impacts of a policy, project, plan, or program under consideration[20] (NRC, 2011). HIAs can be used to generate recommendations on how to increase positive benefits and minimize negative impacts to health. According to Health Impact Project[21] data, hundreds of HIAs either have been completed or are in progress in the United States spanning the federal, state, and local levels and covering diverse topics, including transportation, land use, agriculture, education, energy, and natural resources. HIAs are one of the key assets that public health professionals can contribute to community strategic planning by providing data and analytical skills to inform the prioritization of planning policies and to aid in the development of benchmarks for success (Ricklin et al., 2012).

HIAs can be performed on local, state, or federal policies or regulations, and they can be performed by governments, think tanks, academic institutions, nonprofits, or community organizations. The major steps in performing an HIA include screening (determining plans, projects, or policies for which an HIA would be useful); scoping (identifying which health effects to consider); assessing benefits and risks; developing recommendations; reporting; and monitoring and evaluating to determine the effect of the HIA on policy (CDC, 2015).

HIAs enable health professionals to raise awareness of the impact of recovery decisions on health outcomes. Box 3-6 describes how HIA is being used to inform recovery decision making in New Jersey as communities continue rebuilding after the effects of Hurricane Sandy. This tool can potentially be used in prioritizing different recovery initiatives for effective allocation of scarce resources so as to optimize long-term health outcomes. However, additional guidance on using HIA in the disaster recovery context is needed.

Although HIA has gained traction only recently as an important decision-making tool, a model for this kind of impact assessment has been in place in communities for decades. Under the National Environmental Policy Act[22] (NEPA), all development projects funded with federal dollars must undergo a data-driven process of analysis with explicit consideration of alternatives and their respective degrees of environmental impact. As a result of NEPA compliance, this process of analysis of alternatives is well understood and accepted at the municipal level, paving the way for adoption of a similar technique for evaluating impacts on human health.

Guidance, Training, and Technical Assistance

Guidance As discussed earlier, the NDRF supports the idea that recovery goes beyond restoration of a community's physical infrastructure and emphasizes the equal importance of providing adequate care to address the full range of needs of the affected community members and ensuring that the community has the capacity to meet its future needs. However, little guidance is available to support communities in the development of a strategy for restoring and ultimately improving their physical, mental, emotional, and social well-being. As guidance for each of the NDRF RSFs is developed, it will need to include health considerations for the recovery activities of that RSF. Guidance in Chapters 5-10 of this report may inform the development of such guidance initially but updates should reflect ongoing efforts to collect best practices.

For the health sector, it will be important to align current guidance for federal funding programs

---

[20] An HIA is distinct from a community health assessment (discussed earlier in this chapter). Whereas HIA is a process for determining health impacts of a policy, project, plan, or program, community health assessment is a process by which health status indicators for a given population are examined to identify key health problems and assets in a community.

[21] The Health Impact Project, a collaborative effort of the Pew Charitable Trust and the Robert Wood Johnson Foundation, is promoting the use of HIAs as decision-making tools for policy makers. Information on completed and in-progress HIAs can be found at http://www.pewtrusts.org/en/multimedia/data-visualizations/2014/hia-in-the-united-states (accessed February 23, 2015).

[22] National Environmental Policy Act of 1969, Public Law 91-190 (January 1, 1970).

BOX 3-6
Integrating Health Impact Assessment into Recovery
Decision Making and Planning

New Jersey's Rutgers University is leading a project that will utilize health impact assessments (HIAs) to inform disaster decision making and recovery in the aftermath of Hurricane Sandy. Funding for this project, which began in September 2014 and will continue through February 2016, comes from the Health Impact Project, a collaboration of the Robert Wood Johnson Foundation and the Pew Charitable Trusts (Rutgers, 2014). HIA utilizes scientific data, health expertise, and public input to incorporate health considerations into decision making, providing a tool for predicting the frequently overlooked health impacts that may arise from decisions not typically considered related to health. As part of this project, Rutgers will conduct an HIA in two communities—Little Egg Harbor in Ocean County and Hoboken in Hudson County. Additionally, the project will generate a toolkit for use by other municipalities in New Jersey in integrating HIA into their decision making, as well as recommendations on integrating HIA into post-disaster decision making and planning more broadly in the United States (Rutgers, 2014).

In Little Egg Harbor, the HIA will provide officials with information on the potential health outcomes of a decision on whether to support a voluntary buyout strategy for properties in a flood-prone neighborhood. While many residents have responded favorably to the offer of a buyout, some officials remain concerned about the potential loss of tax revenue and the impact on the local economy. The HIA will aid in determining the physical and mental health outcomes associated with a variety of voluntary buyout scenarios (ranging from no buyout to full buyout of the area in question, as originally proposed). In particular, it will address how the program would affect vulnerable populations, household finances, social cohesion, and the municipal budget. It also will address how the buyout program would change the future risks of flooding damage and how the new open space created by buying out these homes would affect the health of the community (Lowrie, 2014).

The HIA in Hoboken is focused on a stormwater management plan for addressing chronic flooding. This HIA will provide information on health impact considerations currently absent from the consulting work and deliberations already under way regarding adoption of a stormwater management plan and ordinance. Persistent flooding and sewer system overflow are serious hazards in Hoboken, as are the resulting health risks. The HIA will focus on these problems to inform Hoboken's City Council about the health risks of flooding and the resulting sewage overflow events, as well as the potential health benefits and risks of implementing green infrastructure solutions as part of the stormwater management plan (Carnegie, 2015).

---

that support the development of a health recovery capability—specifically, the Public Health Emergency Preparedness (PHEP) Cooperative Agreement and the Hospital Preparedness Program (HPP) (discussed in more detail in Chapters 5 and 6, respectively)—with the RSF-specific guidance so that cooperative agreement funds are used effectively. PHEP and HPP represent important opportunities to support incorporation of broad health considerations into an integrated recovery approach. Currently, however, there is a paucity of PHEP and HPP guidance specific to recovery. PHEP guidance, for example, addresses public health, medical, and behavioral health systems all together, with no specifics provided for any of these services. Additionally, although there is some emphasis on utilizing recovery actions to mitigate damage from future events, completely absent from current guidance is any messaging regarding the opportunities to use recovery as a vehicle for creating healthier communities or the need to create a healthy community vision to guide long-term recovery efforts—both of which need to be key messages of RSF-specific as well as PHEP/HPP guidance.

Training Outside of the disaster recovery context, there is increasing awareness of the importance of collaboration among public health, human services, and community planning stakeholders (including transportation and the community development enterprise) to support a coordinated approach for achieving healthy community goals, avoiding duplication of effort, and leveraging synergies among the missions of diverse community organizations. These kinds of connections function outside of the emergency management context and therefore may not be leveraged during recovery planning and implementation. All stakeholders with a role in recovery, and particularly elected and public officials who lead such efforts, need to be sensitized regarding the importance not only of short-term health protection concerns but also of long-term opportunities to create healthier and more resilient and sustainable communities. Training programs need to be developed for this purpose.

Given the need for intra- as well as intersectoral collaboration to support effective disaster recovery and a Health in All Policies approach, cross-training programs are needed to break down silos within sectors, including the health sector. As discussed earlier in this chapter, a healthy community approach to disaster recovery requires that public health professionals with an understanding of the key principles behind healthy communities be engaged in the recovery planning process. Although the public health sector increasingly is being engaged across the full continuum of the emergency management cycle, its representatives generally are those working in the field of public health emergency preparedness. Throughout its information gathering, the committee noted a divide between the public health professionals working in emergency preparedness and in the area of healthy communities (this separation of disciplines was not specific to public health but also was observed within the public management and planning fields). This siloing within public health is due in part to the structure of funding streams (PHII and NACCHO, 2008). In the past 50 years, conditions attached to the receipt of federal funds have institutionalized and reinforced siloing (Turnock and Atchison, 2002), and preparedness planning often is isolated from the expertise and input of other divisions within health departments (Duncan et al., 2007). Because of this siloing across the public health enterprise, public health emergency preparedness personnel may understand short-term health challenges relevant to the response and early recovery phases but not the opportunities for long-term population health improvement after a disaster. Cross-training is a means of bridging this divide so that both groups of professionals have a better understanding of each other's roles in the recovery process and can leverage relationships within their agencies to bring the appropriate public health expertise to bear on strategic planning discussions.

Technical assistance Technical assistance can come from peer organizations that have previously undergone the process of disaster recovery or from state and federal partners (e.g., through ESF and RSF coordinating agencies). Even when there is no major disaster declaration, federal experts at regional- and national-level offices can provide targeted technical assistance to grantees through existing programmatic channels upon request. Technical assistance can be used to

- inform grantees about how to leverage existing programs, including repurposing of current grants;
- educate about waivers and flexibilities;
- disseminate information on best and promising practices;
- connect decision makers with leaders from other localities that have recovered from a disaster; and
- educate on how to meet the needs of specific populations.

Of interest to this committee is a recent (2010) memorandum of agreement (MOA) between FEMA and EPA. This MOA provides a pathway for EPA's Office of Sustainable Communities to provide technical assistance to disaster-impacted communities on rebuilding in ways that protect the environment, reduce vulnerability, strengthen neighborhoods, support long-term economic vitality, and improve quality of life (DHS and EPA, 2010). After an F-5 tornado devastated the town of Joplin, Missouri, in 2012, for example, EPA provided technical assistance on the creation of a "multi-modal transportation corridor that would meet the need for more walkable, bikeable streets and also manage stormwater in a more environmentally friendly manner" (EPA, 2014). Prior to initiating the project, FEMA helped local stakeholders identify long-term community recovery needs and then assisted EPA in matching its sustainable community assistance capabilities with those identified needs. This MOA serves as a model and a point of departure for a broader interagency effort to better coordinate federal assistance to local communities and help them use the post-disaster recovery process as an opportunity to rebuild healthier and more resilient and sustainable communities (DHS and EPA, 2010).

Information Systems, Including Health Information Systems

Recovery decision makers require frequently updated data to maintain situational awareness. This capability requires an investment in infrastructure (including mapping software and expertise) to support the acquisition, synthesis, and distribution of data at multiple scales (the city/county and neighborhood levels being most critical). However, this responsibility need not be carried out directly by government agencies. Those agencies, which often are hampered by the constraints of bureaucracy, also can leverage the assets and agility of nongovernmental organizations that often emerge to fill gaps related to coordination and information. After Hurricane Katrina, for example, the Greater New Orleans Community Data Center, now called The Data Center, a nongovernmental organization supported with philanthropic funds, provided critical and timely data to support recovery decision making across a number of fields and was valued for its independence and transparency (Plyer and Ortiz, 2011). Uses for recovery data such as those supplied by The Data Center include but are not limited to

- informing redevelopment decisions;
- justifying requests for funding;
- targeting services to areas of greatest need;
- providing updates to the public and institutional stakeholders; and
- supporting collaborations (e.g., coordination of services based on measured needs).

With regard to health-related data, in most cases, state, local, tribal, and territorial health departments will be primary resources for informing health sector and nonhealth sector decision makers. To this end, health departments can draw on vital statistics and health records, although nongovernmental organizations, including academic institutions, may help combine these data with other indicators to create a more comprehensive picture of community well-being (relevant data would include crime rates, median household income, and adequacy of affordable housing). Having preestablished systems in place for data aggregation and distribution (e.g., responding to data requests) increases the community's ability to recover quickly and effectively, thus increasing its resilience (Plyer and Ortiz, 2011). Formal data-sharing agreements may be an important part of that infrastructure, with special attention to privacy protections as appropriate (DeSalvo et al., 2014). Ideally, such arrangements would be established before a disaster.

IMPLEMENTATION

Seeking and Applying Recovery Resources

Developing a comprehensive financial strategy is an important component of the recovery planning process. This strategy should consider a community's needs, known sources of recovery resources, and any potential gaps in funding (APA, 2014). It should be guided by the vision for a community's recovery and, through the consideration of short- and long-term needs, serve as a road map by which recovery resources can be applied to restore—and, where possible, improve beyond pre-disaster levels—the community's infrastructure, services, economy, and health. The process of distributing and applying recovery resources is complex, and it requires that a community best match the available resources to its needs. Furthermore, to obtain and implement these resources effectively requires a thorough understanding of the varied sources of funding available, along with the requirements and restrictions associated with each (APA, 2014).

The committee identified a paucity of disaster recovery resources specifically targeted for health protection and promotion. In the case of a major disaster, funding may be available for short-term behavioral health support and for the repair of critical health care infrastructure. In addition, a supplemental appropriation can potentially generate funds for specific social services needs. Largely, though, recovery resources are allocated predominantly to other sectors and services. However, the activities of other sectors can be leveraged in ways that have a positive effect on health outcomes. It is here that health sector stakeholders need to have preestablished relationships with other agencies to ensure integration and coordination of resource allocation to support long-term health, resilience, and sustainability. The use of recovery resources by all sectors represents an opportunity to consider health impacts and to develop complementary strategies whereby these funds can be used to achieve multiple goals, one of which is improved health. Recovery assistance programs and their potential applications for health benefits are discussed in more detail in Chapter 4.

Creating a Learning System

Disasters are relatively rare occurrences, and the success of recovery is based on community context. As a result, the evidence base for interventions is often imperfect, and scientific knowledge is only one of multiple factors that influence decision making during recovery. However, uncertainty cannot deter those responsible for making decisions that will drive the recovery process forward. Leaders must be prepared to act using the best information available and to change course as new information emerges. Consequently, decision-making frameworks need to be built on a learning system approach whereby new knowledge is captured as strategies are implemented and is fed back into the decision-making process to support continuous improvement.

Communities are complex adaptive systems, and an adaptive management approach to disaster recovery is therefore warranted. Adaptive management is an approach that allows community leaders and members to explore alternative ways of achieving disaster recovery objectives, identify potential outcomes, implement one or more methods, and monitor their impacts on the recovery process so that course corrections can be made in the process of iterative decision making. Continuous evaluation of progress toward recovery goals is thus an integral part of the process that needs to be incorporated into pre-event plans so that its results can be used to adjust future recovery management strategies. Evaluation can occur at multiple scales, including the individual organization, sector, and community levels (e.g., through a composite recovery indicator). This learning-based approach to decision making links learning with policy and implementation over time, providing a framework that enables policy planners to make good decisions in the face of uncertainty as outcomes from previous disaster recovery actions become better understood.

An important component of a learning system approach is metrics with which to evaluate progress toward identified goals (i.e., success as locally defined) and to inform strategy adjustments. Defined metrics also are needed to collect relevant baseline information, such as measures of health for a community, to enable comparison with pre-disaster states. The absence of core metrics with which to measure the progress of recovery is a major gap with which communities currently struggle (Chandra, 2014). The committee was not charged with the development of recovery metrics and thus did not undertake to propose a core set. However, the committee notes that several research institutions, including RAND Corporation and the University of North Carolina's Natural Hazards Center, are evaluating recovery and community resilience metrics that, if validated, could be incorporated into future iterations of the NDRF. National-level rollout of a core data set would facilitate not only community-level evaluations but also comparison across disasters.

Evaluation of recovery efforts also requires a preestablished methodology. Although a methodology designed specifically to evaluate the impact of recovery efforts on community health status does not yet exist and further research in this area is needed, examples of existing measures and assessment tools that may help evaluators establish a methodology include

- community health rankings and associated measures such as those provided in *America's Health Rankings*® annual report (United Health Foundation et al., 2014) and the Robert Wood Johnson Foundation's *County Health Rankings* (2015);
- the Sustainable Communities Index, a set of methods for measuring environmental, economic, and social conditions of cities and neighborhoods (previously adapted to measure conditions during disaster recovery; see Appendix D);
- HUD's Healthy Communities Index and Healthy Communities Assessment Tool (being developed to help local communities assess the physical, social, and economic roots of community health and use this assessment to inform evidence-based policies, planning, and development);
- AARP's Livability Index (a Web-based tool in development that scores communities on measures of livability as identified by U.S. residents over age 50);
- the Social Vulnerability Index, used to identify and map risks for geographic clusters of socially vulnerable populations; and
- the National Health Security Preparedness Index™, a new, comprehensive annual measure of health security and preparedness at the federal and state levels.

These measures and tools are described in more detail in Appendix D.

RESEARCH NEEDS

The committee identified four key areas in which additional research could significantly improve the integration of health considerations into recovery planning processes:

- How does integration of health improvement plans with comprehensive plans and pre-disaster recovery plans prior to a disaster support a healthy community approach to disaster recovery?
- What are the optimal organizational arrangements at the state and local levels under the structure of the NDRF that facilitate coordination across sectors, including the often separate health and social services domains?
- What strategies can be used to better integrate the ongoing collaborative initiatives that occur in nearly all communities under the rubric of community development and human services transformation into NDRF-driven organizational and governance structures for recovery?
- What core set of metrics would best enable communities to evaluate the effects of recovery activities on health outcomes and adjust strategic approaches as needed in the context of a learning system?

SUMMARY OF FINDINGS AND RECOMMENDATIONS

The committee was charged with providing recommendations and guidance on actions that could be taken by all sectors to improve health outcomes after disasters. The committee took this charge to mean not just restoring systems to pre-disaster levels of functioning but building back better and in ways that contribute to an overall healthier community. This goal is best accomplished through pre-disaster planning informed by a community's shared vision and a locally driven assessment of community health needs, assets, and risk. Those assessments are an essential component of a health improvement plan. Thus, incorporating health goals from a formal health improvement planning process into disaster recovery planning is a critical mechanism for ensuring improved individual and community health and resilience after a disaster. However, the committee recognizes that health improvement plans are underdeveloped or nonexistent in many communities, and when they do exist, they may be outdated and may not be familiar to or supported by current local leadership (Bennett, 2014). Further, health goals from a health improvement plan need to be integrated into the community's strategic planning process, which is used to set priorities and allocate funds, so that decision making before and after a disaster is guided by a vision of a healthier community. A community that has already integrated health considerations into its strategic planning process and comprehensive plan is better equipped to rebuild infrastructure and systems in ways that promote health, resilience, and sustainability because it is more likely to have leadership buy-in and collaborative structures that include health components. However, it is important to note that even if a healthy, resilient, sustainable community vision and associated goals have not been integrated into a community's pre-disaster community strategic planning processes, this health perspective can still be included in post-disaster recovery planning.

Recommendation 1: *Develop a Healthy Community Vision for Disaster Recovery.*

The committee recommends that state and local elected and public officials incorporate a vision for a healthy community into community strategic planning and disaster recovery planning.

Implementation of this recommendation will require action at the state and local as well as federal levels. Specifically, at the state and local levels, the following actions should be taken:

- Public health leaders should enhance health improvement planning through engagement with a comprehensive group of community stakeholders (representing each of the audiences for this report; see Chapter 1) and ensure that plans are based on communities' needs and assets.
- Elected and public officials, including emergency managers and local disaster recovery managers, should together lead relevant stakeholders in risk-based disaster recovery planning that develops the procedures, processes, and administrative arrangements to be used for integrated, coordinated recovery.
- Elected and public officials, including emergency managers and local disaster recovery managers, should integrate public health officials and health improvement plans into community strategic planning and disaster recovery planning before and after a disaster. To facilitate that integration, the community's needs and plans for health improvement should be reflected in disaster recovery priorities.

At the federal level, a coordinated, interagency effort is needed to support state and local stakeholders in the development of recovery plans that ensure that communities build back stronger. To this end, the committee believes that aligned grant guidance and technical assistance are essential motivators. Alignment is key to promoting synergy and ensuring that opportunities are not missed. Federal agencies should use existing grant programs to enhance the capacity of state and local stakeholders to plan for and implement a healthy community perspective in disaster recovery. Specifically, federal agencies should take the following actions:

- HHS, HUD, DOT, EPA, and other federal agencies should use aligned grant guidance and technical assistance for existing and future grant programs to incentivize preparedness, community health, and community development grantees to collaborate on the integration of local health improvement goals into comprehensive plans and disaster recovery plans.
- The CDC and the Office of the Assistant Secretary for Preparedness and Response should revise preparedness grant guidance related to the recovery capability to include greater focus on long-term recovery and opportunities for using recovery to advance healthier and more resilient and sustainable communities.
- FEMA should incentivize emergency management preparedness program grantees to incorporate health considerations into recovery planning by providing grant guidance and technical assistance aligned with HHS guidance.

Every policy decision made regarding a community's recovery should be seen as an opportunity to improve the health and well-being of the population. Although testimony to the committee from federal agencies representing various RSFs demonstrated progress toward cooperation and even collaboration, the committee did not find evidence that this vision or level of health integration (i.e., Health in All Policies) has been achieved during operationalization of the NDRF at the federal level.

Disasters create and exacerbate unmet human needs that, if not addressed, have significant impacts on long-term health outcomes in a community. Because these unmet needs closely resemble those with which many communities struggle during normal times (i.e., the vulnerable populations before a disaster are also the vulnerable populations after the event), the municipal structures already established for dealing with these challenges represent an important resource that can be tapped to enable integrated, coordinated recovery planning and to facilitate Health in All Policies. In such cases, critical relationships have already been built and barriers to intersectoral collaboration overcome. In developing operational and governance structures under the framework of the NDRF, state and local decision makers should ensure that these collaborative arrangements operating prior to a disaster are added to the list of organizational assets and incorporated into the recovery planning effort.

Recommendation 2: *Integrate Health Considerations into Recovery Decision Making Through the National Disaster Recovery Framework.*

The committee recommends that the Federal Emergency Management Agency (FEMA) and the five other federal agencies that represent coordinating agencies for the Recovery Support Functions take steps to further develop and promote the National Disaster Recovery Framework (NDRF) as the basis for a locally defined organizing structure for disaster recovery at the state and local levels to promote information sharing and alignment of funding streams. Further, to ensure that health considerations are integrated into all recovery operations, FEMA, in consultation with the U.S. Department of Health and Human Services (HHS), should update the NDRF to explicitly include health implications for the activities of all Recovery Support Functions.

State and local elected and public officials should establish a steering committee to guide the development of an operational structure that incorporates the organizing principles of the NDRF— including a disaster recovery coordinator and the Recovery Support Functions—and builds on existing collaborative municipal and civic structures, authorities, and initiatives.

Successful recovery will require a systems approach with integration across the full range of community stakeholder groups, both horizontally and vertically, so that capabilities and resources, both public and private, are leveraged in a coordinated manner to achieve the best outcomes for the community as a whole. Many key stakeholders (including those from the public health, health care, behavioral health, and social services sectors) are not accustomed to working in the emergency management context and are not familiar with the relevant processes, terminology, or resources. Through this report, the committee hopes to facilitate the engagement and support of those stakeholders from both the health and the nonhealth sector whose involvement in recovery planning and implementation is essential to the building of healthier and more resilient and sustainable communities after disasters. This involvement will require (1) access to easy-to-use guidance materials describing the recovery process, including an overview of critical resources that are mobilized and accountable parties; and (2) a clear understanding of mechanisms for stakeholder engagement in the recovery planning process.

Recommendation 3: *Facilitate the Engagement of the Whole Community in Disaster Recovery Through Simplified and Accessible Information and Training.*

To facilitate the engagement of the whole community in building healthier communities after disasters, the Federal Emergency Management Agency should lead an interagency effort centered

on increasing the accessibility and coherence of information related to disaster recovery and the provision of relevant training.

Priorities should include

- the development of educational materials, including a single overarching federal document that serves as a primer on the recovery process and is easily accessible on the Web regardless of the pathway by which a stakeholder seeks to enter the recovery planning process;
- the development of companion guidance documents for state, local, and nongovernmental stakeholders for each of the Recovery Support Functions, providing more detailed descriptions that facilitate stakeholder understanding of available resources, best practices, and the pathways by which they can engage in the pre- and post-disaster recovery planning processes; and
- the development of coordinated training programs for stakeholders and their professional societies that raise awareness of threats and opportunities related to health and promote broad stakeholder participation in recovery planning under the NDRF.

Training programs should

- sensitize stakeholders to the importance of short-term health protection concerns and long-term opportunities to build healthier communities during recovery, highlighting the critical role of each sector in advancing community health, resilience, and sustainability;
- strengthen connections among emergency management, public health, community development, community planning, human services, and other stakeholder organizations to better prepare them to work together within the structure of the NDRF to increase the chances that recovery resources will be used for creating healthier communities; and
- raise awareness of steady-state community planning processes and administrative structures (partnerships and municipal and civic structures) and mechanisms for leveraging these existing processes and structures by identifying key partnerships and professional resources/sources of technical assistance.

When appropriate, existing federal and professional disaster preparedness training programs, such as those for public health emergency preparedness coordinators and the FEMA Emergency Management Institute's classroom and independent study courses for emergency managers (including those for federal disaster recovery coordinators), should be leveraged. However, new training courses may be needed to meet the priorities listed above.

The participation of community members (including representatives from vulnerable populations) in all stages of the recovery process is essential to ensuring that recovery decisions align with the community's shared vision. Achieving this participation will require robust community organizing and extensive outreach. After disasters, community planning initiatives that utilize equitable processes and increase interaction among residents can also build social capital—the social ties that are an integral feature of a community—promoting healing, restoring the social fabric of the community, and strengthening resilience. By partnering with schools, neighborhood associations, community groups, and private businesses, local governments can help foster the collaborative potential and sense of community ownership that are critical to optimal community health improvement and recovery planning. Ideally, these social networks should be developed in advance of a disaster as part of resilience-building efforts.

Recommendation 4: *Enhance and Leverage Social Networks in Community Health Improvement and Recovery Planning.*

Local elected and public officials should develop and support programs designed to strengthen social networks and deepen trust among community members before and after disasters, thereby increasing resilience. Strategies for enhancing and preserving social networks should be specifically included in community health improvement and disaster recovery plans. Before and after a disaster, existing social networks, such as neighborhood associations, should be leveraged to enhance mechanisms for integrating the community into recovery planning.

To support implementation of this recommendation, the committee offers the following suggestions for building social capital in advance of a disaster, preserving it during a disaster, and leveraging it thereafter:

- **Building social capital prior to a disaster**—Examples of successful programs that have enhanced social cohesion include community currency and time-banking programs (as discussed earlier in this chapter) (Richey, 2007); social marketing campaigns; and administrative and financial support for local initiatives and institutions such as faith-based organizations, sport and social clubs, and civil society organizations. An example of a social marketing campaign created as part of preparedness efforts is SF72, a program created by the San Francisco Department of Emergency Management in coordination with city residents that helps San Franciscans expand their social networks (SF72, 2014). The success of these programs can be measured through surveys of levels of social cohesion and civic and neighborhood participation.
- **Preserving social networks during a crisis**—During a disaster, local disaster managers, nongovernmental organizations such as the Red Cross, and federal agencies such as FEMA should ensure that disaster management policies support existing social networks. Following Hurricane Katrina, for example, the random placement of survivors in temporary housing across the country crippled social networks by separating kin and friends (Aldrich, 2012; Underhill, 2008). Despite time pressures, decision makers should do their best to ensure the continuation of social networks after a disaster, even during evacuation and temporary sheltering. Further, once survivors have been placed in shelters (ideally in groups that continue pre-disaster relationships), organizers should ensure that they have access to technologies that connect them with their networks.
- **Leveraging social capital during recovery**—Following a disaster, disaster managers should ensure that recovery plans and neighborhood rebuilding schemes develop through bottom-up and equitable neighborhood processes whereby local citizens, not outsiders, drive visions of the future. This can be achieved by encouraging or even requiring the solicitation of input from neighborhood-level organizations (e.g., homeowners associations) in a community requiring significant redevelopment, and outcomes can be measured through surveys that probe the depth of resident involvement in and satisfaction with planning activities.

The consideration of potential health impacts of recovery decisions in a systematic way necessitates a ready source of health information. Health impact assessments support a Health in All Policies approach and are increasingly being used to inform a wide range of policy decisions. While not yet widely applied to recovery decision making, this technique holds great potential. As operational structures for recovery are being developed and exercised, pathways for sharing information, including health information, should simultaneously be evaluated and delineated. To this end, a pre-disaster investment in infrastructure and, in some cases, data-sharing agreements are required. Continuous evaluation of health and recovery indicators through a learning system approach enables decision makers to evaluate progress toward a healthy, resilient, and sustainable community vision and adapt recovery management strategies as need. This learning process also supports efforts to identify best practices and expand the evidence base for guidance and training (Recommendation 3).

Recommendation 5: *Establish Pathways by Which Health Information Can Inform Recovery Decision Making.*

State and local elected and public officials should ensure that clear pathways for integration and dissemination of health information are established, including mechanisms that enable concerns and priorities of community members to be transmitted to disaster recovery decision makers. Additionally, a continual feedback process should be established to allow for updating to reflect changes in conditions and measured progress toward recovery. Thus, indicators for measuring progress and success should be (1) developed, (2) incorporated into pre-disaster recovery plans, and (3) updated after a disaster based on its health impact.

REFERENCES

Aldrich, D. 2012. *Building resilience: Social capital in post-disaster recovery.* Chicago: University of Chicago Press.

The Alliance for a Just Rebuilding, ALIGN, Community Development Project, Community Voices Heard, Faith in New York, Families United for Racial and Economic Equality, Good Old Lower East Side, Red Hook Initiative, and New York Communities for Change. 2014. *Weathering the storm: Rebuilding a more resilient New York City housing authority post-Sandy.* http://www.rebuildajustny.org/wp-content/uploads/2014/03/Weathering_The_Storm.pdf (accessed October 20, 2014).

APA (American Planning Association). 2006a. *Integrating planning and public health: Tools and strategies to create healthy places.* Chicago, IL: APA.

APA. 2006b. *Planning and urban design standards.* Hoboken, NJ: John Wiley and Sons, Inc.

APA. 2014. *Planning for post-disaster recovery: Next generation.* Chicago, IL: APA.

ASTHO (Association of State and Territorial Health Officials). 2007. *Disaster recovery for public health.* http://www.astho.org/programs/preparedness/disaster-recovery-for-public-health (accessed November 18, 2014).

Beardsley, D. 2014. *Session I: Public health, panel discussion.* Paper presented at IOM Committee on Post-Disaster Recovery of a Community's Public Health, Medical, and Social Services: Meeting Two, February 3, Washington, DC.

Bennett, G. 2014. *Coordination among federal recovery support functions.* Paper presented at IOM Committee on Post-Disaster Recovery of a Community's Public Health, Medical, and Social Services: Meeting Three, April 28-29, Washington, DC.

Blumenstock, J. 2014. *Coordination among state and local government agencies.* Paper presented at IOM Committee on Post-Disaster Recovery of a Community's Public Health, Medical, and Social Services: Meeting Three, April 28-29, Washington, DC.

Boyd, A. 2014. Long-term recovery planning: Goals and policies. In *Planning for post-disaster recovery: Next generation: PAS report 576,* edited by J. C. Schwab. Chicago, IL: APA. Pp. 72-91.

Carnegie, J. 2015. *City of Hoboken, New Jersey proposed stormwater management plan health impact assessment (HIA).* New Brunswick, NJ: Rutgers, The State University of New Jersey.

CARRI (Community and Regional Resilience Institute) and CaRES (Campus Resilience Enhancement System). 2013. *Success stories: The importance of effective community engagement.* http://www.resilientus.org/wp-content/uploads/2013/10/Oct-Success-Stories-Compilation-Community-Engagement.pdf (accessed December 1, 2014).

CDC (Centers for Disease Control and Prevention). 1997. *Principles of community engagement.* Washington, DC: CDC.

CDC. 2015. *Health Impact Assessment.* http://www.cdc.gov/healthyplaces/hia.htm (accessed March 26, 2015).

CDC and CDC Foundation. 2013. *Building a learning community & body of knowledge: Implementing a whole community approach to emergency management.* Atlanta, GA: CDC.

Chandra, A. 2014. *Considerations for community health in disaster recovery.* Paper presented at IOM Committee on Post-Disaster Recovery of a Community's Public Health, Medical, and Social Services: Meeting Three, April 28-29, Washington, DC.

Chandra, A., and J. D. Acosta. 2009. *The role of nongovernmental organizations in long-term human recovery after disaster: Reflections from Louisiana four years after Hurricane Katrina.* Santa Monica, CA: RAND Corporation.

Chandra, A., and J. D. Acosta. 2010. Disaster recovery also involves human recovery. *Journal of the American Medical Association* 304(14):1608-1609.

City of Seattle. 2013. *Toward a resilient Seattle: Post-disaster recovery plan framework.* http://www.seattle.gov/ Documents/Departments/Emergency/PlansOEM/Recovery/SeattleDisasterRecoveryPlanFrameworkJan2013final. pdf (accessed October 20, 2014).

Clements, B. 2014. *Public health and community recovery: Texas' experience.* Paper presented at IOM Committee on Post-Disaster Recovery of a Community's Public Health, Medical, and Social Services: Meeting Two, February 3, Washington, DC.

Collins, R. A. 2011. No more "planning by suprises": Post-Katrina land use planning in New Orleans. In *Resilience and opportunity: Lessons from the U.S. Gulf Coast after Katrina and Rita,* edited by A. Liu, R. V. Anglin, R. M. Mizelle, and A. Plyer. Washington, DC: Brookings Institution Press. Pp. 161-172.

Colten, C. E., R. W. Kates, and S. B. Laska. 2008. Three years after Katrina: Lessons for community resilience. *Environment: Science and Policy for Sustainable Development* 50(5):36-47.

Community Commons. 2014. *Community Health Needs Assessment (CHNA).* http://assessment.communitycommons. org/chna/About.aspx (accessed November 18, 2014).

Community Planning Workshop. 2010. *Pre-disaster planning for post-disaster recovery: Case studies.* Eugene, OR: Community Planning Workshop.

County Health Rankings. 2015. *Our approach.* http://www.countyhealthrankings.org/our-approach (accessed April 1, 2015).

Dannenberg, A. L., R. J. Jackson, H. Frumkin, R. A. Schieber, M. Pratt, C. Kochtitzky, and H. H. Tilson. 2003. The impact of community design and land-use choices on public health: A scientific research agenda. *American Journal of Public Health* 93(9):1500-1508.

DeSalvo, K. B., N. Lurie, K. Finne, C. Worrall, A. Bogdanov, A. Dinkler, S. Babcock, and J. Kelman. 2014. Using Medicare data to identify individuals who are electricity dependent to improve disaster preparedness and response. *American Journal of Public Health* 104(7):1160-1164.

DeSalvo, K. B. 2013. *The Katrina experience: Considerations for health system recovery.* Paper presented at IOM Committee on Post-Disaster Recovery of a Community's Public Health, Medical, and Social Services: Meeting One, November 25, Washington, DC.

DHS (U.S. Department of Homeland Security) and EPA (U.S. Environmental Protection Agency). 2010. *Memorandum of agreement between the Department of Homeland Security (DHS), Federal Emergency Management Agency (FEMA) and the Environmental Protection Agency (EPA).* http://www.epa.gov/dced/pdf/2011_0114_fema-epa-moa.pdf 10 (accessed November 18, 2014).

Donahue, K. 2014. Follow the money: Hurricane Sandy recovery, two years later. *Harvard Political Review.* http://harvard politics.com/united-states/follow-money-hurricane-sandy-recovery-two-years-later (accessed April 1, 2015).

Duncan, W. J., P. M. Ginter, A. C. Rucks, M. S. Wingate, and L. C. McCormick. 2007. Organizing emergency preparedness within United States public health departments. *Public Health* 121(4):241-250.

Edgington, D. W. 2011. *Reconstructing Kobe: The geography of crisis and opportunity.* Vancouver: University of British Columbia Press.

EPA (U.S. Environmental Protection Agency). 2014. *EPA and FEMA partner to help communities prepare for and recover from natural disasters.* http://www.epa.gov/smartgrowth/fema_moa.htm (accessed March 18, 2015).

FEMA (Federal Emergency Management Agency). 2011a. *A whole community approach to emergency management: Principles, themes, and pathways for action.* Washington, DC: FEMA.

FEMA. 2011b. *FEMA strategic plan: Fiscal years 2011-2014.* Washington, DC: FEMA.

FEMA. 2011c. *Lessons in community recovery: Seven years of emergency support function #14 long-term community recovery from 2004 to 2011.* Washington, DC: FEMA.

FEMA. 2011d. *National disaster recovery framework.* Washington, DC: FEMA.

FEMA. 2011e. *National preparedness goal.* Washington, DC: FEMA.

FEMA. 2011f. *National preparedness system.* Washington, DC: FEMA.

FEMA. 2013a. *Building community resilience by integrating hazard mitigation: Integrating hazard mitigation into the local comprehensive plan.* http://www.fema.gov/media-library-data/20130726-1908-25045-9918/factsheet1. pdf (accessed December 1, 2014).

FEMA. 2013b. *Information sheet: Threat and hazard identification and risk assessment.* http://www.fema.gov/ media-library-data/1388146249060-7b2abfe6be10c67c4070ed42deaaadf1/THIRA%20Information%20 Sheet_20131104.pdf (accessed March 18, 2015).

FEMA. 2013c. *National response framework.* Washington, DC: U.S. Department of Homeland Security.

FEMA. 2014a. *Core capabilities.* https://www.fema.gov/core-capabilities (accessed March 26, 2015).

FEMA. 2014b. *Overview of the federal interagency operational plans.* Washington, DC: U.S. Department of Homeland Security.

FEMA. 2014c. *Overview of the national planning frameworks.* Washington, DC: U.S. Department of Homeland Security.

FEMA. 2014d. *Threat and hazard identification and risk assessment.* https://www.fema.gov/threat-and-hazard-identification-and-risk-assessment (accessed December 2, 2014).

Frumkin, H., L. Frank, and R. Jackson. 2004. *Urban sprawl and public health.* Washington, DC: Island Press.

HHS (U.S. Department of Health and Human Services). 2009. *National health security strategy of the United States of America.* Washington, DC: HHS.

HHS. 2015. *National health security strategy and implementation plan 2015-2018.* Washington, DC: HHS.

Hillsborough County Government. 2010. *Post-disaster redevelopment plan.* http://www.hillsboroughcounty.org/index.aspx?nid=1795 (accessed November 18, 2014).

Hodgson, K. 2011. *Comprehensive planning for public health: Results of the planning and community health research center survey.* https://www.planning.org/research/publichealth/pdf/surveyreport.pdf (accessed December 1, 2014).

HUD (U.S. Department of Housing and Urban Development). 2014. *Community development.* http://portal.hud.gov/hudportal/HUD?src=/program_offices/comm_planning/communitydevelopment (accessed December 4, 2014).

ICMA (International City/County Management Association). 2014. *Local governments, social equity, and sustainable communities: Advancing social equity goals to achieve sustainability.* http://icma.org/en/results/sustainable_communities/projects/advancing_social_equity_goals_to_achieve_sustainability (accessed October 21, 2014).

IOM (Institute of Medicine). 2012. *Crisis standards of care: A systems framework for catastrophic disaster response.* Washington, DC: The National Academies Press.

IOM and NRC (National Research Council). 2005. *Public health risks of disasters: Communication, infrastructure, and preparedness—workshop summary.* Washington, DC: The National Academies Press.

Johnson, L. A., and R. B. Olshansky. 2013. The road to recovery: Governing post-disaster reconstruction. *Land Lines*:14-21. https://www.lincolninst.edu/pubs/2259_The-Road-to-Recovery--Governing-Post-Disaster-Reconstruction (accessed October 14, 2014).

The Joint Commission. 2005. *Standing together: An emergency planning guide for America's communities.* Oakbrook Terrace, IL: Joint Commission on Accreditation of Healthcare Organizations.

Kates, R. W., C. E. Colten, S. Laska, and S. P. Leatherman. 2006. Reconstruction of New Orleans after Hurricane Katrina: A research perspective. *Proceedings of the National Academy of Sciences of the United States of America* 103(40):14653-14660.

Lenihan, P. 2005. MAPP and the evolution of planning in public health practice. *Journal of Public Health Management and Practice* 11(5):381-388.

Lockwood, B. 2014. *Coordination among state and local government agencies.* Paper presented at IOM Committee on Post-Disaster Recovery of a Community's Public Health, Medical, and Social Services: Meeting Three, April 28-29, Washington, DC.

Love, R., and S. Vallance. 2014. The role of communities in post-disaster recovery planning: A Diamond Harbour case study. *Lincoln Planning Review* 5(1-2):3-9.

Lowrie, K. 2014. *Mystic Island, New Jersey voluntary buyout scenarios: Health impact assessment.* New Brunswick, NJ: Rutgers, The State University of New Jersey.

Marcus, L. J., B. C. Dorn, and J. M. Henderson. 2006. Meta-leadership and national emergency preparedness: A model to build government connectivity. *Biosecurity and Bioterrorism* 4(2):128-134.

NACCHO (National Association of County and City Health Officials). 2014a. *2013 national profile of local health departments.* Washington, DC: NACCHO.

NACCHO. 2014b. *The assessments.* http://www.naccho.org/topics/infrastructure/mapp/framework/phase3.cfm (accessed March 18, 2015).

NACCHO. 2014c. *MAPP basics: Introduction to the MAPP process.* http://www.naccho.org/topics/infrastructure/mapp/framework/mappbasics.cfm (accessed December 1, 2014).

NACCHO. 2014d. *Visioning.* http://www.naccho.org/topics/infrastructure/mapp/framework/phase2.cfm (accessed August 25, 2014).

Nakagawa, Y., and R. Shaw. 2004. Social capital: A missing link to disaster recovery. *International Journal of Mass Emergencies and Disasters* 22(1):5-34.

Nolen, A. 2014. *A health in all policies approach to disaster recovery: Lessons from Galveston.* Paper presented at IOM Committee on Post-Disaster Recovery of a Community's Public Health, Medical, and Social Services: Meeting Four, June 13, Washington, DC.

Norris, T., and M. Pittman. 2000. The healthy communities movement and the coalition for healthier cities and communities. *Public Health Reports* 115(2-3):118-124.

NPLI (National Preparedness Leadership Initiative). 2013. *Who should apply?* http://npli.sph.harvard.edu/executive-development/who-should-apply (accessed March 26, 2015).

NRC (National Research Council). 2011. *Improving health in the United States: The role of health impact assessment.* Washington, DC: The National Academies Press.

Olshansky, R. 2014. *Post-disaster recovery: How to rebuild cities in compressed time.* Paper presented at IOM Committee on Post-Disaster Recovery of a Community's Public Health, Medical, and Social Services: Meeting Two, February 3, Washington, DC.

PHAB (Public Health Accreditation Board). 2011. *Acronyms and glossary of terms.* http://www.phaboard.org/wp-content/uploads/PHAB-Acronyms-and-Glossary-of-Terms-Version-1.0.pdf (accessed November 18, 2014).

PHII (Public Health Informatics Institute) and NACCHO. 2008. *Taking care of business.* https://phii.org/sites/default/files/resource/pdfs/Taking%20Care%20of%20Business%2006-08.pdf (accessed August 19, 2014).

Pinellas County. 2012. *Pinellas County post-disaster redevelopment plan.* Pinellas County, FL: Pinellas County.

Plyer, A., and E. Ortiz. 2011. Building data capacity to foster resilient communities. In *Resilience and opportunity: Lessons from the U.S. Gulf Coast after Katrina and Rita,* edited by A. Liu, R. V. Anglin, R. Mizelle, and A. Plyer. Washington, DC: Brookings Institution Press. Pp. 187-200.

Reaves, E. J., M. Termini, and F. M. J. Burkle. 2014. Reshaping US Navy Pacific response in mitigating disaster risk in South Pacific Island nations: Adopting community-based disaster cycle management. *Prehospital and Disaster Medicine* 29(1):60-68.

Rebuild Iowa Office. 2011. *Disaster recovery lessons learned.* http://publications.iowa.gov/11080/1/2011-06_Iowa_Disaster_Recovery_Lessons_Learned_final.pdf (accessed October 20, 2014).

Rice, H. 2014. Rebuilding begins for Galveston public housing 6 years after Ike. *Houston Chronicle,* 12. http://www.houstonchronicle.com/news/houston-texas/texas/article/Rebuilding-begins-for-Galveston-public-housing-6-5746823.php (accessed October 20, 2014).

Richey, S. 2007. Manufacturing trust: Community currencies and the creation of social capital. *Political Behavior* 29(1):69-88.

Ricklin, A., and N. Kushner. 2013. *Integrating health into the comprehensive planning process: An analysis of seven case studies and recommendations for change.* Chicago, IL: APA.

Ricklin, A., A. Klein, and E. Musiol. 2012. *Healthy planning: An evaluation of comprehensive and sustainability plans addressing public health.* Chicago, IL: APA.

Rouse, W. B. 2000. Managing complexity. *Information, Knowledge, Systems Management* 2(2):143-165.

Rudolph, L., J. Caplan, C. Mitchell, K. Ben-Moshe, and L. Dillon. 2013. Health in all policies: Improving health through intersectoral collaboration. Discussion Paper. September 18, 2013. http://iom.edu/~/media/Files/Perspectives-Files/2013/Discussion-Papers/BPH-HiAP.pdf (accessed December 1, 2014).

Rutgers. 2014. *Health impact assessment in New Jersey: Assessing health outcomes of post-Sandy decision-making.* http://njhic.rutgers.edu/wp-content/uploads/2014/10/PEW-Project-Overview-9-23.pdf (accessed March 12, 2015).

Schwab, J., K. C. Topping, C. C. Eadie, and R. E. Edyle. 1998. *Planning for post-disaster recovery and reconstruction: PAS Report No. 483/484.* Chicago, IL: APA.

SF72. 2014. *SF72 is San Francisco's hub for emergency preparedness.* http://www.sf72.org/home (accessed December 4, 2014).

Shah, U. 2014. *Coordination among state and local government agencies.* Paper presented at IOM Committee on Post-Disaster Recovery of a Community's Public Health, Medical, and Social Services: Meeting Three, April 28-29, Washington, DC.

Sherry, N., and A. Harkins. 2011. Leveling the emergency preparedness playing field. *Journal of Emergency Management* 9(6):11-16.

Smith, G. 2011a. The national disaster recovery framework: A new vision for recovery. In *Planning for post-disaster recovery: A review of the United States disaster assistance framework.* Fairfax, VA: Public Entity Risk Institute.

Smith, G. 2011b. *Planning for post-disaster recovery: A review of the United States disaster assistance framework.* Fairfax, VA: Public Entity Risk Institute.

Turnock, B. J., and C. Atchison. 2002. Governmental public health in the United States: The implications of federalism. *Health Affairs* 21(6):68-78.

ULI (Urban Land Institute). 2014. *Housing in America: Integrating housing, health, and resilience in a changing environment.* http://uli.org/wp-content/uploads/ULI-Documents/Housing-in-America-2014.pdf (accessed October 21, 2014).

Underhill, R. 2008. *Katrina's displacement: The untold consequences of disaster resettlement in Colorado.* MA Thesis submitted by Megan Ruth Underhill to the Colorado State University Department of Anthropology.

United Health Foundation, APHA (American Public Health Association), and Partnership for Prevention. 2014. *America's health rankings®: A call to action for individuals and their communities.* Minnetonka, MN: United Health Foundation.

Usdin, L. 2014. Building resiliency and supporting distributive leadership post-disaster. *International Journal of Leadership in Public Services* 10(3):157-171.

Walsh, L., and K. W. Schor. 2014. *Education and training opportunities in long-term community recovery: Preliminary observations from the field.* Paper presented at IOM Committee on Post-Disaster Recovery of a Community's Public Health, Medical, and Social Services: Meeting Three, April 28-29, Washington, DC.

WHO (World Health Organization). 2013. *Health in all policies.* http://www.healthpromotion2013.org/health-promotion/health-in-all-policies (accessed December 4, 2014).

Zucker, H. 2014. *Post-disaster recovery: New York State Department of Health experience with Superstorm Sandy.* Paper presented at IOM Committee on Post-Disaster Recovery of a Community's Public Health, Medical, and Social Services: Meeting Two, February 3, Washington, DC.

Leveraging Recovery Resources in a Coordinated Manner to Achieve Healthier Post-Disaster Communities

Building healthier and more resilient and sustainable post-disaster communities is a multifaceted endeavor that requires complementary investments to address interrelated physical, social, and economic environments, not single-purpose projects. Recovery entails a multistage process of applying a set of resources, both financial and human capital, first to restore a community's infrastructure, services, economy, and health and then, where possible, to improve them beyond pre-disaster levels. No single program can meet the complex and diverse recovery needs of a community.

The process of assembling the resources required after a disaster has been likened to the creation of a patchwork quilt: community leaders represent the quilters, who must catalyze the development and realization of a new vision; the pattern for the quilt, representing the recovery plan, is informed by information from existing plans, data repositories, and experts who can provide technical assistance; and the material for the quilt comes from an array of programs providing funding and/or services to realize the vision (Thomas et al., 2011). The quilt is created through the concerted efforts of the whole community—government and the nonprofit and private sectors—all working to stitch the many pieces together. This chapter describes this process to facilitate the participation of the many audiences for this report (as detailed in Chapter 1) in the planning for and realization of a vision for a healthier post-disaster community. Included are summaries and analyses of key funding sources that can be applied to minimizing the impacts of a disaster on health and social services and ultimately creating healthier communities.

RESOURCE IMPLICATIONS OF DISASTER DECLARATIONS

The resources that become available after a disaster will depend on the pattern and extent of damage and whether the crisis results in a presidential declaration of a major disaster, which triggers significant federal assistance. Regardless of whether there is a presidential declaration, however, recovery must occur, and the mobilization of resources from all sources represents an opportunity to create a healthier community.

After a disaster, local officials conduct a visual assessment of the damage and share that information with the state, which then decides whether a state disaster declaration is needed. If it is determined that the damages exceed the state's ability to respond, the governor's office can request, through the regional Federal Emergency Management Agency (FEMA) office, that the President make a federal disaster declaration (CRS, 2014a; Smith, 2011). FEMA then conducts its own damage assessment and compares

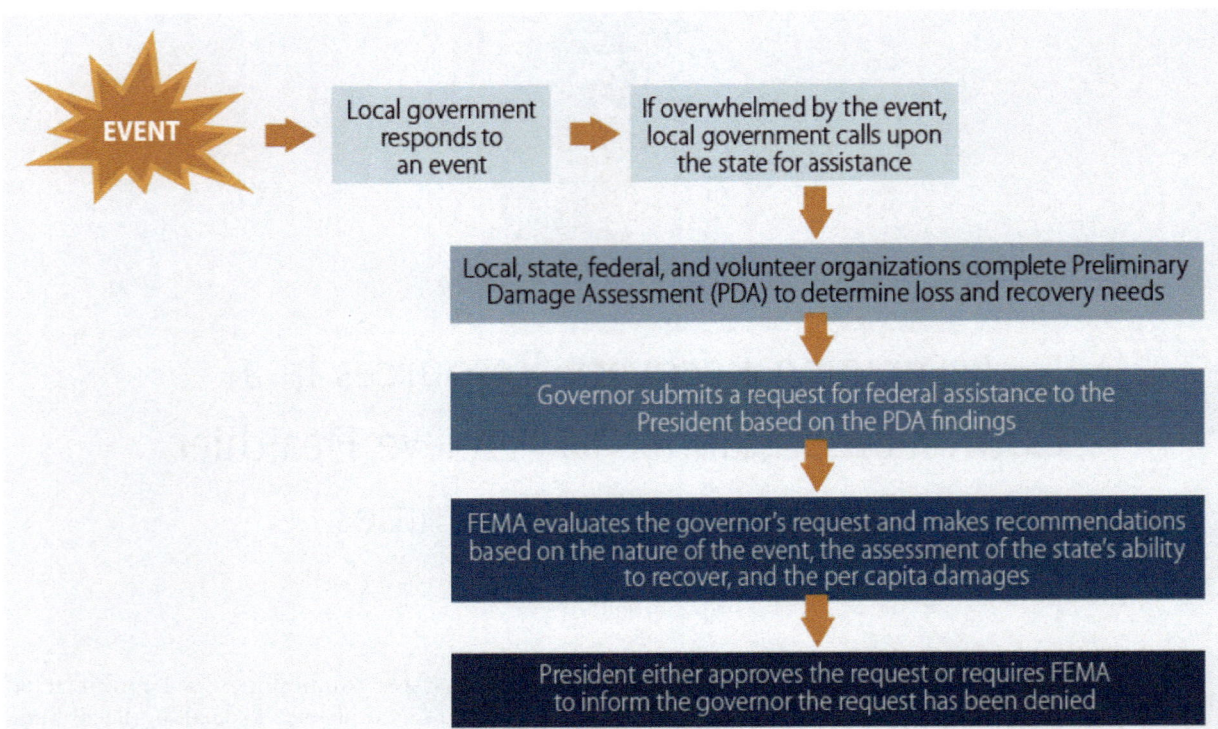

FIGURE 4-1 The Stafford Act process for declaring a major disaster.
SOURCE: CRS, 2014b.

estimated monetary losses with a predetermined per capita threshold. This information is presented to the President along with a recommendation, but ultimately the President decides whether to declare a major disaster (see Figure 4-1). A major disaster is declared when there is a clear need for the President to provide federal disaster assistance under the auspices of the Robert T. Stafford Disaster Relief and Emergency Assistance Act[1] (Stafford Act), which is the traditional federal vehicle through which post-disaster assistance is delivered (CRS, 2014b).

Although funding receives the greatest attention in discussions of disaster assistance resources, Smith (2011) delineates three major resource categories: financial resources, policy, and technical assistance. While there is no question that financial resources are requisite to community recovery efforts, greater attention to the other categories is warranted so that communities understand the full spectrum of assistance that is available. Often, policies and technical assistance will be tied to individual funding programs.

Policy may not commonly be viewed as a resource but can have a major influence on recovery processes and outcomes. Policies can create incentives (or remove disincentives) for rebuilding in smarter, more resilient ways. For example, the Sandy Recovery Improvement Act[2] removed the penalty associated with structural or functional changes made to infrastructure when rebuilding using FEMA Public Assistance funds (described further below).

---

[1] 42 U.S.C. § 5121 et seq.
[2] Sandy Recovery Improvement Act of 2013, Public Law 113-2, 113th Cong., H.R.152 (January 29, 2014).

Technical assistance can encompass education, training, and outreach efforts (Smith, 2011), and it is an important means of sharing knowledge on both lessons learned from previous disasters and resources available to support recovery. It helps build local capacity and expertise and strengthen relationships at the local level so that communities are better able to manage on their own when future disasters fail to elicit a major disaster declaration. The capacity for technical assistance is enabled by assessment processes designed to expand the evidence base for decision making. The practice of conducting after-action evaluations (or hotwashes), for example, has yielded information on best or promising practices, as well as lessons about what has not worked in previous disaster experiences. In some cases, this information is distilled into guidance materials. Examples of databases created to serve as clearinghouses for this information include FEMA's Lessons Learned Information Sharing system and, specific to health information, the U.S. Department of Health and Human Services' (HHS's) Disaster Information Management Research Center (http://disasterinfo.nlm.nih.gov). In most cases, these evaluations have been oriented to the disaster *response phase*, but the information they yield may also be relevant to short-term recovery and may provide valuable methodology or examples.

FEDERAL RECOVERY PROGRAMS AND THEIR APPLICATIONS TO HEALTH RECOVERY

If the President declares a major disaster, a joint field office is established, a federal coordinating officer is named, and an array of federal programs are activated to assist in the response and recovery effort (see Figure 4-2 for a funding timeline and Annex 4-1 at the end of this chapter for a summary of programs). In a major disaster, a federal disaster recovery coordinator also is named, along with a state counterpart. The joint field office includes state partners, including a state coordinating officer, and comprises personnel from federal and state agencies. Staff are organized according to Emergency Support Functions (ESFs) and Recovery Support Functions (RSFs) (described in Chapter 3). Operation plans and project specifications are developed and administered in this office, in some cases supplemented by area field offices in other parts of the state. In coordination with state agencies and the state coordinating officer, federal resources—a combination of grants, loans, and technical assistance—can be used for:

- post-disaster recovery planning,
- debris removal,
- infrastructure repairs,
- financial support to individuals and families,
- services such as crisis counseling and case management,
- economic development, and
- hazard mitigation.

FEMA Funding Programs Authorized Under the Stafford Act

FEMA programs authorized under the Stafford Act include Individual Assistance, the Crisis Counseling Assistance and Training Program, Public Assistance, and the Hazard Mitigation Grant Program, as described briefly below. (For more information on disaster relief funds, see the resource lists in Appendix C.) Not all programs authorized by the Stafford Act are activated after a major disaster. Individual Assistance but not Public Assistance may be offered after some disasters, and vice versa. Damage assessment information, along with other relevant information on need, is used in determining which programs will be activated. In most cases, however, hazard mitigation funds will be offered (FEMA, 2014a).

Individual Assistance comprises a collection of programs designed to provide individuals and families with aid including but not limited to temporary housing, living expenses, limited home repairs (if not covered by insurance), unemployment assistance, legal services, and medical expenses not covered by insurance (CRS, 2012a). For most of these forms of assistance, individuals apply directly to FEMA. Individual Assistance programs support health recovery by providing survivors with financial assistance for

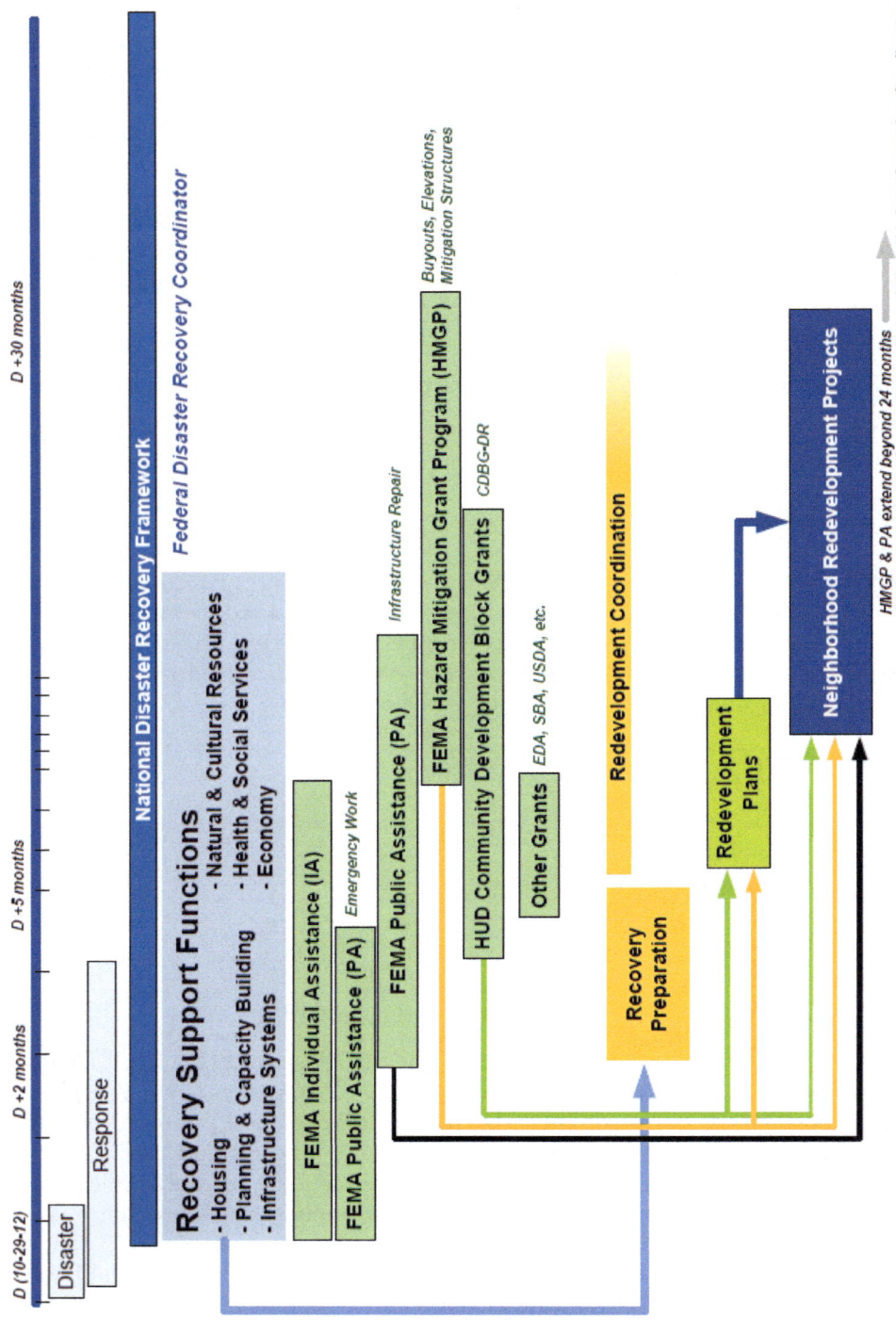

FIGURE 4-2 Recovery planning timeline.
NOTE: The diagram is derived from a combination of various Federal Emergency Management Agency (FEMA) and the U.S. Department of Housing and Urban Development's (HUD's) graphics, based specifically on the post-Sandy recovery initiatives in the state of New York but generalized for all disasters where an element of Community Development Block Grant-Disaster Recovery (CDBG-DR) funding is included. The diagram is not expected to replace the specialized program guidance for funding sources such as FEMA or HUD, rather to illustrate the interrelatedness when viewed from a state or community perspective.
SOURCE: B. Hokanson/PLN Associates.

essential goods (e.g., food), services (e.g., medical services), and shelter (through repair funds or provision for temporary housing costs) during the short-term recovery period (individual and household assistance generally is limited to a period of 18 months).

The **Crisis Counseling Assistance and Training Program** (CCP) is the largest single federal program supporting disaster-related behavioral health services. The U.S. Substance Abuse and Mental Health Services Administration (SAMHSA) operates the CCP with funds provided by FEMA. Authorized under the Stafford Act, CCP grants are available only after a presidential disaster declaration but are not automatic; the affected state must formally apply for CCP funding. The grants are of two types: the Immediate Services Program, with a duration of 60 days, and the Regular Services Program, which lasts 9 months. The main goals of the CCP are to contact a large number of people by face-to-face outreach, to offer basic crisis counseling and connection to community support systems, and to make referrals to traditional mental health services when necessary. The funds cannot be used for formal behavioral health diagnostic and treatment services. The types of services funded by the CCP are individual and group crisis counseling; supportive educational contact; assessment, referral, and resource linkage; and media and public service announcements. These services typically are provided by behavioral health organizations under contract to the state mental health authority (SAMHSA, 2009). The providers of these services are a combination of mental health professionals and paraprofessionals trained in crisis counseling. Training and education of CCP staff also can be undertaken with grant funds. The CCP, as well as challenges related to the program's current design, are discussed further in Chapter 7.

Public Assistance[3] grants generally represent the largest disbursement of federal funds for short- and long-term disaster recovery. They are the primary form of assistance offered by FEMA to state and local governments for debris removal and for the repair, replacement, or restoration of public infrastructure (e.g., roads and bridges, public buildings), including many that support health and safety (police and fire stations, hospitals, schools) and restore the fabric of the community (e.g., libraries, community centers, schools).[4] Certain nonprofit organizations (e.g., hospitals) also are eligible for these grants, but for-profit businesses are not. FEMA obligates funds for Public Assistance projects based on detailed cost estimates derived from damage assessments. There is usually a 25 percent state cost share (FEMA provides 75 percent of estimated costs and states must cover the other 25 percent). However, the President can partially or totally waive these costs to the state, or they can be covered with funds from other federal grant programs, such as the U.S. Department of Housing and Urban Development's (HUD's) Community Development Block Grant for Disaster Recovery (CDBG-DR), which is discussed in more detail below.

Although Public Assistance funds generally have been used to restore facilities to their pre-disaster state and function, hazard mitigation add-on funding (designated as Public Assistance 406 program funds) can be obtained for improvements that strengthen the facility to better resist future hazardous events. Typically, the technical and engineering work of writing specifications and producing cost estimates for repair projects, including additional 406 mitigation, is performed by FEMA personnel or FEMA contractors, subject to approval by the subrecipient and the state. However, 406 proposals must show that the proposed improvements are cost-effective through a cost-benefit analysis. The committee heard testimony that the time requirement for collecting these data and conducting the required analyses can deter making improvements for hazard mitigation purposes during the repair of critical infrastructure, which local governments are under great pressure to restore quickly. It is unclear whether this assertion reflects insuf-

---

[3] This section draws on a paper commissioned by the Committee on Post-Disaster Recovery of a Community's Public Health, Medical, and Social Services on "Disaster Recovery Funding: Achieving a Resilient Future?" by Gavin Smith (see Appendix B).

[4] In the event of a pandemic such as influenza, FEMA may offer direct federal assistance through Public Assistance grants under the Stafford Act if there is a presidential declaration. Such assistance may include, among other things, the provision of emergency medical care and temporary medical facilities; the purchase and distribution of food, water, medicine, and other supplies; management, control, and reduction of immediate threats to public health and safety; and the provision of congregate shelters, mass mortuary services, and security and fencing. However, assistance provided by FEMA may not duplicate assistance provided by HHS or any other federal agency (FEMA, 2009).

ficient surge staffing or other organizational impediments. All costs of project design and development are eligible expenses under the FEMA programs.

Public Assistance funds have historically been among the most restrictive funding sources for recovery because the projects funded under this program generally were limited to restoring pre-disaster conditions (function and structure), with the exception of upgrades to comply with contemporary and applicable codes and standards. Changes to the function or location of facilities can be supported with Public Assistance funds, but in the past, this would result in a reduction in the grant amount (i.e., a penalty). Changes to the Stafford Act brought about by the Sandy Recovery Improvement Act of 2013 not only have streamlined the application processes for Public Assistance funds but also have eliminated disincentives and provided increased flexibility (FEMA, 2013a), thus increasing this program's applicability to the process of creating a healthier and more resilient and sustainable post-disaster communities. For example, the addition of bicycle lanes during the repair of streets previously would have been penalized by a reduction of the costs eligible for coverage, but under alternative procedures authorized by the Sandy Recovery Improvement Act, this penalty has been eliminated. In planning for the use of Public Assistance funds, communities need to be aware of these important changes.

Hazard Mitigation Grant Program funds are used for mitigation activities during recovery designed to reduce impacts and losses associated with future disasters. For example, these funds can be used for elevations and bulkheads (e.g., sea walls) to protect structures in hazard zones or for buyouts to relocate structures out of hazardous areas. In contrast with the Public Assistance 406 program for hazard mitigation discussed above, FEMA does not approve the use of Hazard Mitigation Grant Program funds for individual projects; instead, distribution of these funds to states is formula based (generally 15 percent of estimated aggregate amounts of Stafford Act disaster assistance[5]), and states have wide latitude to determine how the funds will be allocated. Hazard mitigation activities can contribute to healthy, resilient, sustainable communities by reducing the risk of future injury and the significant psychosocial impacts associated with disaster-related losses. These activities are discussed further in Chapter 9 (see Recommendation 11).

One other important FEMA program that provides relief after a disaster is the National Flood Insurance Program. Property owners who have purchased flood insurance through this program can submit claims for flood-damaged properties. Most private insurance does not cover flooding, which has been a large problem for community recovery after a flooding event.

Federal Block Grant Programs for Disaster Recovery

The Stafford Act is the primary means by which federal assistance is provided for recovery, but in the case of a catastrophic disaster, Congress may deem it necessary to provide additional assistance in the form of a supplemental appropriation. In recent decades, two notable grant programs have been used as a vehicle for these supplemental funds: HUD's CDBG-DR program and HHS's Social Services Block Grant (SSBG) program. After Hurricane Sandy, CDBG-DR appropriations exceeded levels of FEMA disaster relief funds (see Figure 4-3).

Community Development Block Grant[6]

Among the largest single sources of supplemental recovery assistance is CDBG-DR. All 50 states and most large cities and counties currently receive an annual appropriation through HUD's CDBG program for such day-to-day activities as funding community centers and fixing roads. After a major disaster, Congress may choose to use this funding mechanism to provide additional support to communities for

---

[5] To incentivize hazard mitigation planning, states with enhanced mitigation plans are eligible to receive 20 percent of estimated disaster assistance disbursements under the Hazard Mitigation Grant Program.

[6] This section draws on a paper commissioned by the Committee on Post-Disaster Recovery of a Community's Public Health, Medical, and Social Services on "Disaster Recovery Funding: Achieving a Resilient Future?" by Gavin Smith (see Appendix B).

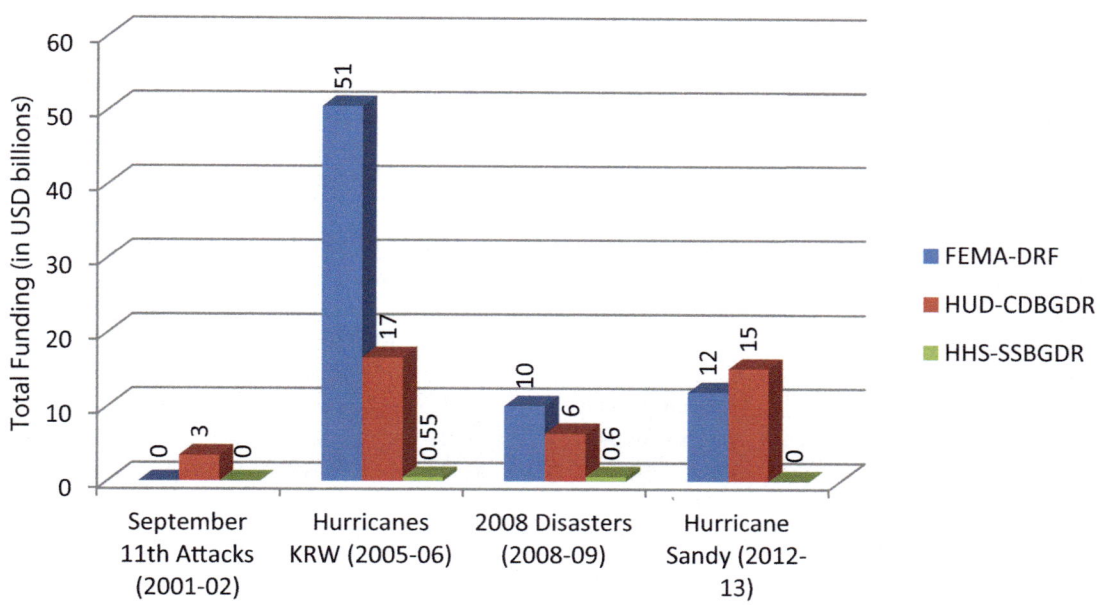

FIGURE 4-3 Comparison of Federal Emergency Management Agency (FEMA), Community Development Block Grant (CDBG), and Social Services Block Grant (SSBG) expenditures for disaster recovery for recent disasters.
NOTES: FEMA-DRF = FEMA Disaster Relief Funds, including Individual Assistance, Public Assistance, and Hazard Mitigation Grant Program funds; HHS-SSBGDR = HHS Social Services Block Grant Disaster Recovery Funds; HUD-CDBGDR = HUD Community Development Block Grant Disaster Recovery funds; KRW = Hurricanes Katrina, Rita, and Wilma.
SOURCES: Data from CRS, 2012b, 2014b; HUD, 2014a

disaster recovery. CDBG-DR funds are targeted to those communities that have demonstrated significant unmet needs not addressed by other grant programs. These funds have three important advantages over Stafford Act funds: flexibility (owing to their nature as a block grant), the ability to address unmet needs, and targeted assistance provided to socially vulnerable populations. At least half of CDBG-DR funds must be used to assist low- and moderate-income people (unless a waiver is granted by the HUD Secretary). The funds can be used for a variety of disaster recovery activities, including

- the acquisition and relocation of flood-damaged housing as a hazard mitigation activity;
- relocation payments for people and businesses displaced by a disaster;
- debris removal not covered by FEMA;
- rehabilitation of homes and buildings damaged by a disaster;
- buying, constructing, or rehabilitating public facilities such as streets and community centers and water, sewer, and drainage systems;
- code enforcement;
- homeownership needs such as down payment assistance, interest rate subsidies, and loan guarantees;
- public services;
- workforce training and development;
- help for businesses in retaining or creating jobs in disaster-impacted areas; and
- recovery planning and administration costs (HUD, 2014b).

Because they are more flexible and available for a broad range of uses, CDBG-DR appropriations create a number of opportunities for communities to make changes to physical and social environments that influence health. "With community development dollars you can address housing, economic recovery as well as social services, bricks and mortar, economic development" (Smith Parker, 2014)—all factors that significantly influence health. All that is needed is vision to utilize the funds in creative ways that meet multiple needs (e.g., multipurpose buildings). However, these funds can be used only for needs that arose as a direct result of a disaster. This restriction can be a challenge for some communities, particularly with regard to health and social service investments, as it can be difficult to demonstrate how a disaster exacerbated homelessness or concerns regarding air pollutants that affect health. Furthermore, given their supplemental nature, CDBG-DR funds are not available in all presidentially declared disasters.

The committee heard about several examples of the use of CDBG-DR funds for health-related purposes. After Hurricane Sandy, New York City invested $183 million CDBG-DR dollars in the restoration of Bellevue and Coney Island Hospitals, along with associated personnel and mobile health service costs. As a result of the lessons learned from Hurricane Katrina, Louisiana invested in the creation of urgent care centers in proximity to other health services (Smith Parker, 2014). (The redesign of the health care delivery system in New Orleans during the recovery from Hurricane Katrina is further discussed in Chapter 6 [see Box 6-7].) While these health care system–focused investments are important to healthy communities, perhaps of even greater importance is the opportunity to use CDBG-DR funds to help communities address some of the upstream or social determinants of health that are often exacerbated after a disaster. For example, these funds can be used for workforce development for residents of disaster-impacted neighborhoods. In Springfield, Massachusetts, CDBG-DR funds were used to finance job training programs for community members from underserved neighborhoods in which the population, which already faced multiple barriers to employment before a tornado struck the town in 2011, was also heavily impacted by the disaster (Leydon, 2014).

HUD has used the CDBG-DR funds to advance a forward-looking agenda that promotes resilience and sustainability (specifically promoting consideration of the six livability principles of the Partnership for Sustainable Communities during rebuilding; see Box 2-5 in Chapter 2). As discussed in Chapter 2, the focus of this agenda will yield co-benefits to health, and from a programmatic standpoint, it may be precedent setting. For example, the most recent CDBG-DR funds for Hurricane Sandy relief included a requirement for grantees to (1) show "sound, sustainable long-term recovery planning informed by a post-disaster evaluation of hazard risk," and (2) "use green rebuilding standards for replacement and new construction of residential housing."

Social Services Block Grant

SSBGs are administered by the Administration for Children and Families (ACF) within HHS (ACF, 2014b). All 50 states, the District of Columbia, and five territories receive these grants (ACF, 2012), which are designed to help states provide residents with "locally relevant social services," such as helping people achieve economic self-support and self-sufficiency to reduce dependence on social services and reducing neglect, abuse, and exploitation of children and adults (ACF, 2013a, 2014b). The money is distributed directly to the states, which then determine what services will be provided and to whom and how the funds will be divided among those services (ACF, 2014c).

Supplemental appropriations through the SSBG program are intended to help meet social service needs linked to a disaster, including social, health, and mental health services for individuals. The funds can be used for

- food cards (ACF, 2013b);
- child care vouchers (ACF, 2013b);
- reimbursement to community agencies that incurred costs in providing services to affected people (ACF, 2013b);
- temporary housing (ACF, 2013b);
- education and training to meet the social service needs of affected people (ACF, 2014a); and
- medication and medical equipment (ACF, 2013b).

The block grant also covers the repair and rebuilding of health care, mental health, child care and other social service facilities, as well as vans or other equipment needed to provide social services. However, the committee heard that SSBG funds are oriented more to supporting individual needs than to addressing social determinants of health at the population level (Nolen, 2014).

Leveraging Block Grant Programs

Regardless of whether a supplemental appropriation is made to provide additional funds beyond those authorized under the Stafford Act, the funds available through annual block grant programs such as CDBG and SSBG generally can be reprogrammed for disaster recovery purposes and used for many of the same functions described above for disaster recovery funds.[7] Because every state and most large cities and counties receive annual funding through the CDBG program for day-to-day purposes, there is broad familiarity with the requirements attached to these federal funds (CRS, 2011). Leveraging this knowledge after a disaster necessitates ensuring that those familiar with these programs are engaged in the recovery planning process. Community development programs in cities and counties are long-term initiatives that address widespread disparities and are connected with diverse organizations concerned about these issues, including advisory committees and community development financial institutions. These organizational resources are key to planning for effective and optimized disaster recovery. Recovery and community development are overlapping initiatives with virtually identical objectives and tools; thus, integrated approaches are essential.

Other Federal Recovery Funding Programs

In addition to FEMA, a number of other federal agencies may offer disaster recovery assistance through a variety of programs:

- Individuals may apply for loans from the Small Business Administration (SBA) that can be used to replace personal property (e.g., furniture) and to restore a creditworthy homeowner's primary residence to its pre-disaster state when the damage is not covered by insurance (the loan can be increased to cover additional costs for hazard mitigation). Similarly, businesses can apply for SBA loans to help cover physical damage and losses, as well as economic losses related to the disaster (CRS, 2012a). SBA loans may be an important source of funding to support recovery for private health care providers who are not eligible for FEMA Public Assistance funds.[8] In hazard areas such as flood plains where buyouts are proposed, SBA plays a crucial role in what is called bridge financing—the temporary arrangements made to help homeowners transition from an existing mortgage on a damaged, unlivable house to a replacement home elsewhere, given the approximately 24-month waiting period for buyout real estate transactions.
- The U.S. Department of Agriculture (USDA) offers a number of housing and rural development programs to support recovery, particularly for rural communities. For example, after a tornado destroyed Kiowa County Memorial Hospital as well as much of the rest of the small town of Greensburg, Kansas, USDA funds were used together with FEMA Public Assistance funds and insurance payouts to help cover the costs of rebuilding the hospital.[9]

---

[7] ACF provides guidance on the use of block grant funds, including CSBGs, SSBGs, and its Child Care and Development Fund, to meet response and recovery needs after a disaster.

[8] Federal Housing Administration (FHA)-insured loans from HUD with up to 90 percent loan-to-value ratios also can be used by hospitals (public and private) for reconstruction.

[9] E-mail communication, M. Sweet, Kiowa County Memorial Hospital, to R. Kirkland, Institute of Medicine, regarding Institute of Medicine study on post-disaster recovery, September 10, 2014.

- Economic Development Agency[10] funds generally are used to support economic recovery. Programming is oriented to job creation or retention projects and initiatives to keep employers from leaving the disaster area. Given the link between economic vitality and the health and well-being of a community, these programs are critical to building healthy communities after a disaster.
- The Federal Highway Administration provides emergency relief assistance for repair and restoration of roads and bridges on the federal-aid highway system (nearly all roads and bridges in the United States are eligible) (CRS, 2014a). These funds can be used for improvements that increase the resilience of the infrastructure if the added cost of the betterment project can be justified based on expected future damages from similar disasters (FHWA, 2013).

Further information on the federal and nonfederal funding programs described in this report, and many others, is available through the National Disaster Recovery Program Database, a web-based tool developed by FEMA to support communities in planning for, responding to, and recovering from disasters. This database can be found at https://asd.fema.gov/inter/ndhpd/public/searchHousingProgramForm.htm.

NONFEDERAL RESOURCES FOR RECOVERY

If there is no presidential declaration of a major disaster, none of the funding programs authorized by the Stafford Act are available to support communities through recovery. As a result, there is little in the way of federal support, although, as discussed earlier, existing federal grant funds received by a community can be reprogrammed after a disaster to yield an additional set of resources, and some federal agencies, such as SBA, USDA, and the Federal Highway Administration, can provide programmatic funding for recovery assistance apart from the funding that is authorized under the Stafford Act. This approach builds local capacity but must be supported by clear guidance and strong vertical integration (e.g., good relationships with federal grant staff).[11] Generally, however, if there is no presidential disaster declaration, communities must look to nonfederal funding opportunities, including private-sector investments; charity from nonprofit and philanthropic organizations; and state and local insurance, cash reserves, and disaster budgets when available.[12] These funding sources, described below, are important contributors to the pool of recovery resources even when a major disaster is declared by the President.

Private-Sector Resources

Funds and other forms of assistance (e.g., goods, facilities) from the private sector are an important component of the disaster assistance framework, and the private sector has an inherent interest in seeing a community recover. Thus, one critical application of private recovery funds is the significant investment made by for-profit organizations—which are rarely eligible to receive federal assistance—in rebuilding their own infrastructure and restoring business operations. As noted earlier, the viability of a community is dependent on its economic vitality (e.g., employment opportunities). Therefore, the decision of local businesses to rebuild within the community has major implications for the ultimate success of recovery in terms of community confidence, employment opportunities, and availability of services, all of which will ultimately affect the health and well-being of the local population.

Businesses also frequently donate funds to nonprofits to support community recovery. For example, Nike provided financial support to the nonprofit design group Architecture for Humanity to support

---

[10] The Economic Development Agency is part of the U.S. Department of Commerce.

[11] This section draws on a paper commissioned by the Committee on Post-Disaster Recovery of a Community's Public Health, Medical, and Social Services on "Disaster Recovery Funding: Achieving a Resilient Future?" by Gavin Smith (see Appendix B).

[12] Cash reserves and disaster budgets are difficult to ensure in current economic times. Some governments levy a tax on certain services to develop this funding source, while others appropriate amounts from their general funds for a disaster account. However, these funds usually are not at a level that can provide the needed recovery assistance and are designed to supplement the expected federal funds (e.g., for cost shares).

the reconstruction of school athletic facilities in New Jersey after Hurricane Sandy (Open Architecture Network, 2014).

One of the most critical sources of funds for rebuilding after a disaster and for accelerating recovery is private insurance. Many homeowners and businesses hold private insurance policies, and payouts are made according to the terms of the contract. Homeowner's policies cover not only the dwelling itself but also the owner's possessions and are usually a condition for obtaining a mortgage. Yet while most homeowner's policies cover the damage from tornadoes, that from floods and earthquakes often is not covered, creating a gap. Flood coverage is available through a separate policy from the National Flood Insurance Program and from some private insurers. Nonetheless, lack of insurance and underinsurance are a major problem for homeowners and businesses, including critical service providers such as hospitals. Moreover, governments often are self-insured, so any expenditures on disaster recovery must come from their overall budget.

Investment firms and private developers will provide funds and human capital used for infrastructure restoration and neighborhood redevelopment, and thus they have a large role to play in a healthy community approach to recovery. The general category of these activities is termed "community development." The scope of these activities, however, is larger than direct federal expenditures, and it entails using such mechanisms as tax credits, community loan funds, and community development financial institutions. Community development corporations, which aid low-income communities with capacity building and planning and development, may invest in micro loans, job creation, affordable housing, and other community amenities that may not otherwise be a priority for developers.[13] Local initiatives are supported by the Community Development Financial Institutions Fund in the U.S. Department of Treasury and the "advent of a new investment tax credit for small business and community facilities, the so-called New Markets Tax Credit" (Erickson and Andrews, 2011, p. 2058). Some types of development have health and social service improvements as explicit goals (Erickson and Andrews, 2011). One study found measurable health benefits to populations served by transit-oriented development and walkable neighborhoods in Charlotte, North Carolina, where a community development organization (Low Income Investment Fund) "was needed to crack the code in assembling favorable capital so that low-income families could share in the benefits of more walkable neighborhoods that have stronger connections to the regional economy" (Erickson and Andrews, 2011, p. 2060). Disaster recovery efforts can tap these diverse resources. In the case of recovery of Joplin, Missouri, from the 2011 tornado, for example, the Missouri Housing Development Commission redistributed its tax credits such that Joplin received 38 percent ($100 million) of the statewide allocation (Novogradac & Company LLP, 2011).

Nonprofit and Philanthropic Resources

Nongovernmental (community-based, faith-based, and national-level) organizations are at the front line of all disaster response and recovery efforts. They provide an array of short- and long-term assistance to fill gaps left by governmental programs that result in unmet needs, including social services and mental health, and thus are essential to health recovery. They are able to respond quickly with funding after a disaster and allow for more flexibility than governmental funding sources; thus, pre-disaster relationships with these organizations at the local level are essential. The programs offered by these organizations are in many situations the first step for an individual's or a family's recovery. Some provide training, and others work directly on restoring the infrastructure of a community, but generally in the realm of assisting in home repairs and/or rebuilding (e.g., Habitat for Humanity), not rebuilding the community's commercial structures or transportation and utility components. Many of these organizations are members of National Voluntary Organizations Active in Disaster (VOAD). Coordination of their activities at the state and local levels occurs through VOAD and/or local Community Organizations Active in Disaster (COAD) (see

---

[13] This section draws on a paper commissioned by the Committee on Post-Disaster Recovery of a Community's Public Health, Medical, and Social Services on "Disaster Recovery Funding: Achieving a Resilient Future?" by Gavin Smith (see Appendix B).

BOX 4-1
Voluntary and Community Organizations Active in Disaster

Voluntary Organizations Active in Disaster (VOAD) are community organizations comprising nonprofit and for-profit organizations that work together to prepare for, respond to, recover from, and mitigate disasters. Rather than providing direct services, VOAD provides a network through which individual organizations can help during a disaster in an efficient manner and with reduced duplication of services (Riverside County VOAD, 2011).

National VOAD is an organization of more than 100 nonprofit and faith-based organizations involved in disaster response and recovery nationwide (NVOAD, 2014). Within National VOAD, each organization/denomination has specialized roles in response and recovery; this system encourages coordinated effort in disasters among members nationwide (VAUMC, 2014).

Community Organizations Active in Disaster (COAD) go by many different names (and are sometimes synonymous with VOAD), but they tend to be local- or regional-level groups that are organized independently but in loose affiliation with state and national VOAD (Missouri SEMA, 2014). COAD works almost exclusively on recovery and can form the core of a long-term recovery group, but there is a growing awareness of the need for their involvement throughout the emergency management cycle. COAD may or may not focus explicitly on health, depending on who is at the table. In Kentucky, for example, the state health department appoints a representative from a county health department to all COAD. COAD emphasizes the building of relationships prior to a disaster, and can facilitate discussion of healthy community goals for recovery.

FEMA's "whole-community" approach acknowledges the critical role of VOAD and COAD, noting that these types of collaborations can leverage existing assets, ensure that recovery efforts meet the actual needs of the community, and make the community more resilient (FEMA, 2011b).

Box 4-1). VOAD and COAD also are often involved in the formation of long-term recovery committees (LTRCs), which can serve as a neutral conduit for recovery funds donated to assist individuals and families. LTRCs comprise representatives from faith-based communities, nonprofit agencies, charities and foundations, and state and local agencies. They are involved in fundraising, organizing volunteers, and providing assistance to those who have unmet needs even after receiving help from government disaster aid programs. FEMA's voluntary agency liaisons and National VOAD can assist communities in setting up LTRCs.[14]

Foundations/philanthropies often become involved in financial assistance during major disasters. Their funds normally are applied to other nonprofit organizations already in the disaster response and recovery arena, or are used specifically to fund LTRCs. As an example of how nonprofit and philanthropic funding can help support improvements in health during recovery, the American Red Cross and the Robert Wood Johnson Foundation funded a mental health infrastructure and training project in New Orleans to address gaps in the capacity to deliver mental health support services after Hurricane Katrina (Meyers et al., 2011).

Academic institutions are another kind of nongovernmental organization that can supply a wide range of resources after a disaster to promote a community's recovery and resilience. Although they are not as likely to be a source of recovery funding as other nongovernmental organizations, these institutions can provide other important resources, such as facilities and training (Dunlop et al., 2014). Yet despite their resources and capacity for community engagement, academic institutions are a source of often untapped potential. Their increased engagement in community recovery may be achieved by establishing formal relationships with emergency management and public health agencies (e.g., contracts, memorandums of understanding, advisory positions) in advance of a disaster (Dunlop et al., 2014).

---

[14] National VOAD has created a manual to support the development of these long-term recovery structures, available at http://www.nvoad.org/wp-content/uploads/2014/05/long_term_recovery_guide_-_final_2012.pdf (accessed April 4, 2015).

State and Local Government Funding Mechanisms

Some states may create rainy day funds that are specifically for or applicable to a disaster situation. A state-level department will administer the grant, and local governments can apply for these funds after a disaster. "Currently, many state grants offer limited funds with extensive administrative requirements and narrowly defined performance expectations. The outcome is that many grant opportunities are prohibitive and ineffective. Efforts are needed to inform and educate policy-makers about these restrictions which impact the intended use of these funds to best meet local community needs" (GCHD, 2007, p. 5).

Taxes and bonds, which are often used to fund capital improvements outside of the disaster context, are another potential source of funding for state and local governments to assist in recovery when there is no presidential declaration of a major disaster or to cover matches and noneligible expenses (e.g., upgrades) under federal grant programs. Bond initiatives allow state and local governments to borrow from investors, usually within their own jurisdictions, and are appealing as a funding vehicle because they often are exempt from federal and state income taxes. These public-purpose bonds are used to improve and rebuild roads, streets, highways, sidewalks, libraries, and government buildings (DOT, 2012). In Joplin, Missouri, where the 2011 tornado destroyed a number of schools, bond financing ($62 million in general-obligation bonds sold by the city's school district) was used to cover some of the rebuilding costs (Niquette, 2013).

FUNDING PATHWAYS[15]

According to Johnson and Olshansky (2013, p. 18), when large sums of public funding become available after a disaster, "the true power over the recovery resides with the level of government that controls the flow of money and how it is acquired, allocated, disbursed and audited." In some cases, a newly established recovery office will hold these powers, but in others, existing legislative and administrative units will assume new responsibilities. Adding to the complexity of the recovery process is the fact that different federal recovery assistance funds may be dispersed to states, local governments, or both.[16] In the case of Hazard Mitigation Grant Program and Public Assistance funds from FEMA, the state (usually the emergency management agency) will be the grantee. However, eligibility of restoration projects for Public Assistance funds is determined by FEMA, and the state acts as a facilitator, working with local governments and institutions that apply for the funds. In contrast, for the Hazard Mitigation Grant Program, the state emergency management agency grantee will make decisions about how the funds are used. In the case of CDBG-DR funds, states and/or local governments can be the grantees, depending on the extent and pattern of damage after the disaster, and the grant often will be administered by an agency responsible for administering the annual CDBG appropriation (i.e., not the emergency management agency). The level of government receiving the funds will control how they are spent (as long as HUD requirements are met). In some cases, a city and the state in which it is located may both receive CDBG-DR funds (as was the case in New York after Hurricane Sandy). In the case of large disasters when there has been a supplemental appropriation, this complexity poses challenges to the coordination of funding both horizontally and vertically (discussed further below).

State grant recipients of Hazard Mitigation Grant Program and CDBG-DR funds can finance recovery activities directly or pass the funds along to local governments. The process by which states determine the localities to fund and the amount of those awards varies. When serving as "pass-through" organizations, states work with both federal agency representatives and local government officials to evaluate a community's needs in the aftermath of a disaster and determine whether damages meet eligibility requirements for federal assistance. State grantees (and local grantees in the case of entitlement communities that receive CDBG-DR funds) are responsible for the development of prioritization (HMGP) or action plans (CDBG-DR). In these plans, the grantee determines which types of projects can be funded, working within

---

[15] This section draws on a paper commissioned by the Committee on Post-Disaster Recovery of a Community's Public Health, Medical, and Social Services on "Disaster Recovery Funding: Achieving a Resilient Future?" by Gavin Smith (see Appendix B).

[16] FEMA Individual Assistance and SBA loans go directly to impacted community members and organizations.

federal guidelines such as "cost-effectiveness" in the case of the Hazard Mitigation Grant Program and providing assistance to a set percentage of low-income disaster recipients in the case of HUD's CDBG-DR.[17] State grantees also set criteria for prioritizing projects when the requests submitted by local governments exceed the available balances. For both HMGP and CDBG-DR activities, planning studies are assumed and encouraged by the federal guidelines, and recipients are expected to spend a portion of the grants (e.g., up to 15 percent) on planning.

CHALLENGES IN APPLYING FUNDING TO THE CREATION OF HEALTHY COMMUNITIES

As discussed earlier, a patchwork quilt approach well describes the process of weaving together various funding sources to meet recovery needs. The complexity of this process is illustrated in Figure 4-4.

A number of challenges related to the funding pathways for disaster recovery impede optimal coordination. Foremost among them is the inadequate investment in pre-event recovery planning and capacity building. Post-disaster challenges include the complicated processes by which funds reach localities and the multiple sets of requirements along the way, as well as the variability in timing of assistance. Further, the considerable burden of administering post-disaster federal assistance programs complicates the recovery process and can impede the ability to plan in the aftermath of a disaster (Smith, 2011).

Limited Pre-Disaster Recovery Planning Resources

The National Disaster Recovery Framework (discussed in detail in Chapter 3) promotes pre-disaster recovery planning, including it as a core principle of the framework, but it is not accompanied by any funding to support state and local governments in such efforts (FEMA, 2011a). There are in fact no dedicated financial resources for pre-disaster recovery planning, which is troubling given the evidence that the timing and success of recovery are greatly enhanced by such investments (CPW, 2010; FEMA, 2011a; Smith, 2011). This national lack of investment in pre-disaster recovery planning contributes to an overemphasis on post-disaster assistance, impeding efforts to plan and develop capacity at the state and local levels before an event.[18] However, several existing grant programs include recovery as a target capability and therefore can be used to support recovery planning. The Public Health Emergency Preparedness (PHEP) Cooperative Agreement and the Hospital Preparedness Program (HPP) (discussed in more detail in Chapters 5 and 6, respectively) provide funds and guidance for health sector recovery planning activities. Other grant programs that similarly include recovery as a supported planning capability are FEMA's Emergency Management Preparedness and Homeland Security grants and Pre-Disaster Mitigation grants; the latter provide states and territories with funds for mitigation planning and activities. By law, hazard mitigation plans must be in place prior to a disaster in order for a community to be eligible for post-disaster mitigation funds, thus providing an incentive for pre-event planning.

Although preparedness programs offer communities an opportunity to fund recovery planning efforts, exploiting this opportunity will require many state and local governments to shift priorities. Determination of how the grant funds are to be applied to the different target capabilities is left to the grantees, so the funds have been applied primarily to preparedness activities related to response capabilities (Lockwood, 2014; Pereira, 2013). If funding from the PHEP Cooperative Agreement and HPP continue to decline, as it has over the past decade,[19] public health departments will be hard-pressed to maintain current capabilities (CDC, 2011), much less support the development of new ones. There is also significant variability in the proportion of preparedness funds that reaches the local level. As discussed in Chapter 3, an additional

---

[17] HUD monitors periodic program reports from grantees to verify that the required benefit to low-/moderate-income individuals and families is being met (generally required to be 70 percent of total expenditures unless a waiver is granted) (HUD, 2015).

[18] This section draws on a paper commissioned by the Committee on Post-Disaster Recovery of a Community's Public Health, Medical, and Social Services on "Disaster Recovery Funding: Achieving a Resilient Future?" by Gavin Smith (see Appendix B).

[19] In 2008, PHEP funds totaled just over $700 million, but in 2013, states and territories received only $584 million. Similarly, HPP funds decreased from nearly $400 million in 2008 to $331 million in 2013 (Pines et al., 2013).

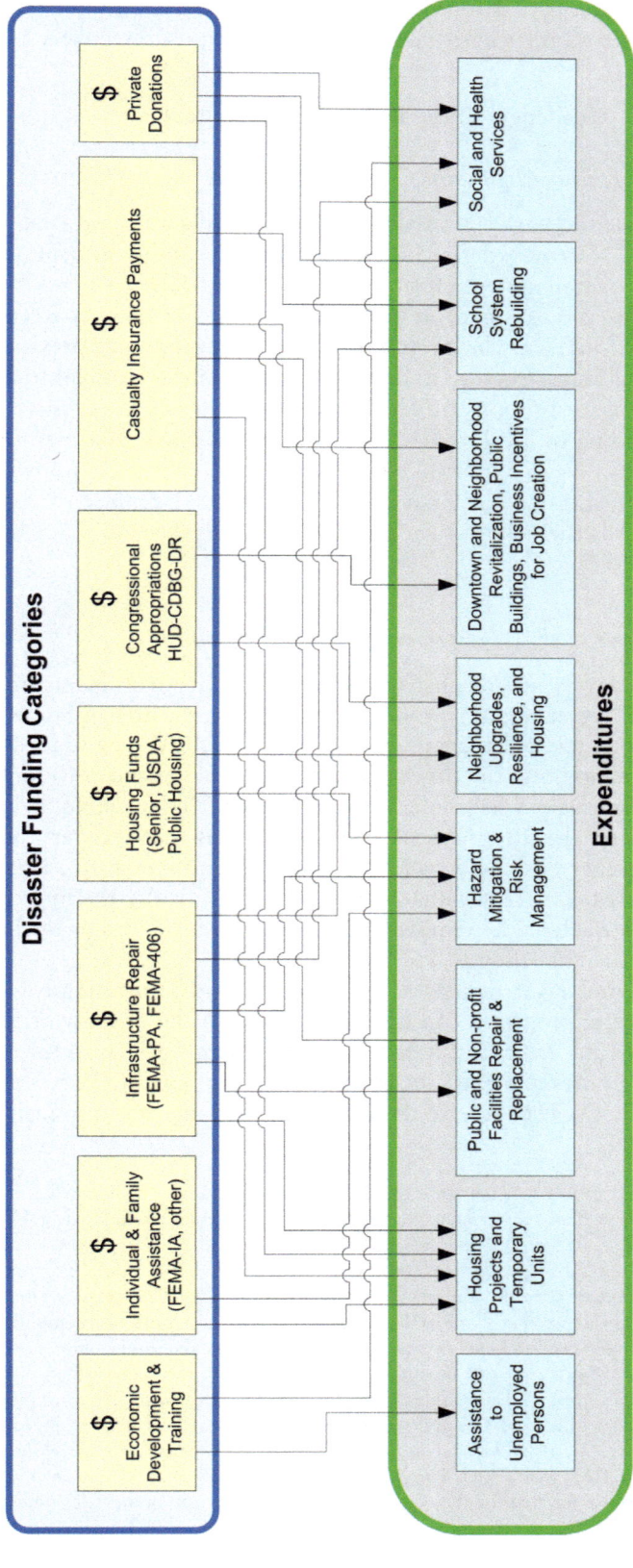

FIGURE 4-4 Funding pathways for disaster recovery.

NOTES: This schematic is not intended to comprehensively describe all disaster assistance categories but shows the complexity of the process by which funds from a multitude of sources are woven together to support comprehensive disaster recovery. This scenario assumes that there has been a presidential declaration of a major disaster and that Congress provided Community Development Block Grant Disaster Recovery funds through a supplemental appropriation.

SOURCE: B. Hokanson/PLN Associates.

challenge related to the use of preparedness funds for recovery planning is the paucity of specific guidance to aid state and local organizations, particularly with respect to long-term recovery.

Challenges in the Post-Disaster Context

Restrictive Requirements That Fail to Align with Community Needs

A common complaint alluded to earlier regarding federal and in some cases state funding programs is their restrictive requirements. Narrowly defined criteria impede the ability of communities to rebuild in ways that improve health and overall system effectiveness. As noted earlier in the discussion of FEMA's Public Assistance funds, this situation is changed somewhat by the 2013 Sandy Recovery Improvement Act, now Section 428 of the Stafford Act, which removed disincentives that may previously have prevented decision makers from rebuilding infrastructure to any state other than its original form and function.

States can implement further restrictions on federal funding that is passed on to local jurisdictions. When states lack an understanding of local needs, these restrictions may impose an undesirable burden. However, these strictures also can be an opportunity for forward-looking states to promote practices that support increased resilience and sustainability. For example, states may require receiving jurisdictions to adopt higher codes and standards than those currently in place or to develop plans before the release of federal funds[20] (Smith et al., 2013).

Coordination Challenges Related to the Timing and Flow of Funding

In the implementation of recovery and reconstruction efforts, local governments frequently face uncertainty regarding when they will receive grant program funding (Smith, 2011). Some programs, such as CDBG-DR and SSBG-DR, require a supplemental appropriation, so the timing of these funds will depend on the speed of congressional action and the time required for federal agencies to implement the legislation. The inability to determine easily when federal assistance will be available to carry out the many projects necessary for recovery in the aftermath of a disaster means that recovery outcomes are driven by such ambiguous timelines rather than by a more clear, logical, and integrative process (Smith, 2011). This ambiguity has widespread effects, especially on the ability to consider the interconnected nature of post-disaster recovery activities, such as the removal of debris, the repair of damaged infrastructure, and the reconstruction of damaged neighborhoods (see Box 4-2).

Each additional governmental layer increases the complexity and uncertainty of the post-disaster recovery process. Rules for federal programs can delay the timing of the delivery of funds. The administration of Hazard Mitigation Grant Program funds, for instance, can be delayed for extended periods of time (Smith, 2011). Individual grant recipients, such as homeowners slated to have their homes acquired, frequently must wait more than a year to receive these funds.[21] The agencies responsible for the adminis-

---

[20] In North Carolina following Hurricane Fran, the state required communities receiving Hazard Mitigation Grant Program funds to develop hazard mitigation plans. This requirement predated the similar stipulation adopted by FEMA under the Disaster Mitigation Act of 2000.

[21] Developing a pre-disaster hazard mitigation project can speed up the administration of federal program funds. Such a project, when linked to a disaster recovery plan that provides a method for post-disaster decision making, can improve the efficiency and efficacy of future post-disaster federal assistance. The value of the development of such a project is exemplified in the following case, which compares the post-disaster recovery process between two disasters that struck the same community: "Following Hurricane Fran, which struck North Carolina in 1996, it took one year to develop and approve the acquisition of approximately 360 flood-damaged homes using HMGP funds. After all of the available HMGP funds were expended, Kinston, North Carolina developed a HMGP application in anticipation of a future disaster and the release of additional funding. The grant was developed in close coordination with state and federal officials, all of whom had gained valuable knowledge in the development of an eligible grant application following Hurricane Fran. Three years later, Hurricane Floyd struck, devastating the town again. This time, it took approximately one week to have a grant approved for the acquisition of more than 300 homes and funds began to flow into the community shortly thereafter" (Smith, 2011).

BOX 4-2
Challenges in Merging Funding Streams for Disaster Recovery Projects

After a major disaster, many communities express a desire to "build back better" (e.g., in a way that improves quality of life and/or strengthens resilience). However, requirements attached to federal recovery funds and the staggered timing of different grant programs can pose significant challenges to making such improvements. For example, Federal Emergency Management Agency (FEMA) Public Assistance funds typically cover the cost (minimum of 75 percent) of restoring an eligible building to its original size or design capacity and function (FEMA, 2014b). Other federal funds (e.g., Community Development Block Grant for Disaster Recovery [CDBG-DR]) can be used to cover nonfederal cost shares and to finance improvements that are not covered by FEMA's Public Assistance program (duplication of benefits is prohibited). However, because CDBG-DR funds are dependent on a congressional appropriation, they may not be available as quickly as Public Assistance funds, necessitating delays in reconstruction. These kinds of delays can create a public outcry as community members seek a return to normalcy, thus deterring community betterment projects. Transparency and effective communication with the public are needed to ensure broad understanding that delays associated with betterment will ultimately yield positive change and improved quality of life in the community.

---

tration of such federal programs are located in a number of regional offices throughout the United States. The timeliness of funding is impacted by the capacity of these agencies to manage these programs, which varies dramatically depending on the staffing levels and post-disaster experience of each regional office. Variations in staffing capacity and post-disaster experience also characterize state and local agencies that administer federal grants, including the Hazard Mitigation Grant Program, Public Assistance, and the CDBGs. These variations, too, influence the speed with which federal funds reach the local governments and individuals carrying out the post-disaster recovery process (Smith, 2011; Smith et al., 2013).

As discussed earlier, coordination challenges can arise from the siloing of FEMA (specifically Hazard Mitigation Grant Program) and HUD CDBG-DR funding streams, both of which can be applied to hazard mitigation activities such as buyouts. In some cases, moreover, state grantees may choose to fund recovery activities directly rather than passing funds on to local governments. Should a city and the state in which it is located both receive CDBG-DR funding, the challenges for coordination are further increased. In such situations, proactive coordination among the administering agencies will be needed to merge the funds effectively. Public officials such as mayors and governors are key in ensuring such coordination occurs, but they may not always agree on spending approaches (Fossett, 2013).

OVERCOMING BARRIERS TO COORDINATION OF FUNDING TO SUPPORT A HEALTHY COMMUNITY APPROACH TO RECOVERY

There are two main mechanisms by which to drive use of disaster recovery funding to achieve a desired outcome—technical requirements and financial incentives. Both have been used successfully to advance other desired activities, such as hazard mitigation, and could likewise be used to overcome barriers that impede the post-disaster realization of healthier communities.

Technical Requirements

Technical requirements attached to funding programs are a powerful means of advancing a desired outcome and even best practices. This approach currently is being used by the federal government to foster resilience and sustainability in areas affected by a disaster. After Hurricane Sandy, for example, HUD required recipients of CDBG-DR funds to rebuild using green building standards, which, as discussed in more depth in Chapter 10, have been linked to improved health outcomes. Such requirements, however, should be considered carefully and ideally with input from stakeholders representing potential grantees because they increase the restrictiveness of funds, and this, as noted earlier, has been identified as a major impediment to the development of creative solutions that meet local needs.

In addition, funding agencies need to work to align the requirements for different grant programs around agreed-upon goals because diversity of requirements among funding sources creates a burden for applicants, and the requirements may even conflict, preventing the use of different funding streams in a cumulative manner to support large, multifaceted initiatives. Collaboration among funders is required to achieve the necessary coordination. The Partnership for Sustainable Communities, a joint effort of the U.S. Department of Transportation, the U.S. Environmental Protection Agency, and HUD, provides a model for how this coordination has been accomplished in a steady-state context (DOT et al., 2014). One mechanism that can aid such coordination efforts is establishment of a funding eligibility matrix tied to mutually agreed-upon goals.[22]

Financial Incentives

In recent years, financial incentives have been used to drive more progressive approaches to pre-disaster planning and resilience building. A similar approach may be warranted to catalyze the paradigm shift needed to facilitate a healthy community approach to recovery. The examples discussed below, while not exhaustive, could be examined for their applicability to incentivizing pre- and post-disaster investments in healthier communities.

Financial Incentives for Pre-Disaster Planning and Action

Several existing programs can serve as models for how pre-disaster planning can be supported through financial incentives:

- According to the Disaster Mitigation Act of 2000,[23] only communities with hazard mitigation plans in place prior to a disaster are eligible to receive Hazard Mitigation Grant Program funds for mitigation activities after a disaster.
- The Community Rating System provides a mechanism for incentivizing pre-disaster efforts to minimize flood damage for communities with flood insurance through the National Flood Insurance Program. The program is voluntary, but as communities undertake more extensive mitigation efforts, premiums are reduced. Policy holders in the Class 1 category have their premiums reduced by 45 percent.
- FEMA recently initiated a pilot program, authorized by the Sandy Recovery Improvement Act of 2013, to incentivize pre-disaster planning for timely debris clearance. Communities with FEMA-approved plans in place prior to a disaster receive a 2 percent increase in the federal cost share for debris removal using FEMA Public Assistance funds. FEMA provides a list of criteria that debris removal plans must meet to be accepted.

---

[22] This section draws on a paper commissioned by the Committee on Post-Disaster Recovery of a Community's Public Health, Medical, and Social Services on "Disaster Recovery Funding: Achieving a Resilient Future?" by Gavin Smith (see Appendix B).

[23] Disaster Mitigation Act of 2000, Public Law 106-390, 106th Cong., H.R.707 (October 30, 2000).

BOX 4-3
Rebuild by Design

Rebuild by Design is a competition sponsored by the U.S. Department of Housing and Urban Development (HUD) that is intended to spur redevelopment of resilient communities in Hurricane Sandy-impacted areas. The competition represents a collaboration among HUD, the Presidential Hurricane Sandy Rebuilding Task Force, and the Rockefeller Foundation, with financial contributions from other foundations. The competition's purpose is to protect communities that are most vulnerable to ever-more-intense weather events. The competition brings together the nation's most talented designers with the Sandy-affected area's active businesses, policy makers, and local groups to seek ways of redeveloping in an environmentally and economically healthier manner.

On April 3, 2014, HUD selected 6 winning designs from 10 finalists following 5 months of heightened analysis and public outreach to the populations living and working in Sandy-affected areas. Many of the proposals included measures that would increase not only the resilience of the area but also sustainability and ultimately health (Rebuild by Design, 2014b).

One of the winners was the "New Meadowlands Park and City," from a team of the Massachusetts Institute of Technology and several design firms. This $150 million project provides an integrated vision for protecting, connecting, and growing a land area—the Meadowlands basin—that is vital to both New Jersey and nearby metropolitan New York. The project weaves together transportation, ecology, and development to transform the Meadowlands basin into an area that can withstand a broad range of environmental risks, while also providing urban amenities, parks, and new opportunities for development. The project utilizes a series of intricate berms and marshes to protect against ocean surges, to collect rainfall, and to reduce sewer overflows in nearby towns. An aim of the project is to shift zoning from suburban to urban, with the expectation that doing so will enhance the identity of the basin, raise the value of the land, and provide for higher tax returns (Rebuild by Design, 2014a).

Competition-Based Incentives for Innovation and Resilience

In response to recommendations in the report of the Hurricane Sandy Rebuilding Task Force, HUD and its partners initiated a competition-based effort—Rebuild by Design (see Box 4-3)—to stimulate innovation in recovery approaches and promote multisector collaboration (notably public–private partnerships). According to HUD (2013b): "The goal of the competition is two-fold: to promote innovation by developing regionally-scalable but locally-contextual solutions that increase resilience in the region, and to implement selected proposals with both public and private funding dedicated to this effort. The competition also represents a policy innovation by committing to set aside HUD Community Development Block Grant Disaster Recovery funding specifically to incentivize implementation of winning projects and proposals." Rebuild by Design is considered so successful—it garnered recognition as one of CNN's Best Ideas for 2013—that it serves as a model for another new competition, the National Disaster Resilience Competition, announced by President Obama in summer 2014. That competition will be funded by $1 billion set aside from the CDBG-DR program. Communities that have been through natural disasters are invited to compete for funds to assist in rebuilding and increasing their resilience to future disasters. HUD is setting aside $181 million of that amount for applications from the states of New York and New Jersey and from New York City because of the catastrophic damage caused in those jurisdictions by Hurricane Sandy (HUD, 2014c). The competition is intended to spur creative resilience projects at the local level while also motivating communities to plan for the effects of extreme weather and climate change. While promising, however, this initiative does not address the need for support for pre-disaster planning since the competition is limited to communities that have recently been impacted by a natural disaster (HUD, 2014c).

SUMMARY OF FINDINGS AND RECOMMENDATION

The decisions made by those leading recovery efforts at the local level are inevitably based on the resources available to them. Through the Stafford Act, and in some cases supplemental appropriations from Congress, significant federal resources are made available to facilitate the rebuilding of communities, including many of the elements that contribute to healthy communities (e.g., housing, community centers). State and local governments, philanthropies, and the private sector also are key sources of recovery funding, particularly if there is no federal declaration of a major disaster. The amendments to the Stafford Act and other provisions of the Sandy Recovery Improvement Act represent a promising step forward in terms of removing impediments to rebuilding in ways that are forward thinking. However, the delivery of funding in isolation, which places the onus on communities to overcome barriers to coordinated use of the funds, remains a major challenge to achieving healthy community outcomes through recovery actions. Funding organizations need to better facilitate the coordinated expenditure of pre- and post-disaster funding. The first step to this end is broadening the understanding of resources that each stakeholder provides and the timing of assistance, as well as the various interests represented by funding organizations. Although a number of reports, websites, and other sources describe individual recovery programs,[24] funders need to seek opportunities to align around mutually compatible policies, which will have the dual benefit of coordinating the distribution of funds and reducing duplicative and counterproductive efforts.

Diverse resources are made available for rebuilding community features that impact health. Some federally funded rebuilding efforts focused on resilience and sustainability, such as those meeting HUD's requirement after Hurricane Sandy that communities applying for CDBG-DR funds rebuild green, may ultimately contribute to health. However, the various resources available to fund rebuilding generally are not mobilized with the explicit intent of improving community health status. The committee concludes that communities are missing opportunities in post-disaster recovery efforts to maximize resources devoted to health. Using mutually agreed-upon goals and policies to drive the coordinated use of resources, funders need to ensure that financial resources are mobilized more effectively by recovery decision makers to create healthy communities.

> **Recommendation 6:** *Leverage Recovery Resources in a Coordinated Manner to Achieve Healthier Post-Disaster Communities.*
>
> Federal agencies (the Federal Emergency Management Agency [FEMA], the U.S. Department of Housing and Urban Development [HUD], the U.S. Department of Health and Human Services [HHS], the U.S. Department of Transportation [DOT], and other federal partners) providing funding for recovery, including pre-event recovery planning, should lead and promote an integrated recovery approach by
>
> - aligning technical requirements and guidance for federal recovery funding opportunities within and across agencies around identified core needs;
> - including a requirement and financial incentives for grantees to demonstrate how health considerations will be incorporated into short- and long-term recovery planning conducted using those funds; and
> - identifying and removing disincentives that impede the coordination of efforts and the combining of different funding streams to support a healthy community approach to recovery.

Working with private and philanthropic organizations, elected and public officials should ensure that state and local funding regulations and guidelines are consistent with these federal integration efforts.

---

[24] For example, descriptions of disaster recovery programs can be found in FEMA disaster assistance guides (see http://www.fema.gov/pdf/rebuild/ltrc/recoveryprograms229.pdf and https://www.fema.gov/media-library/assets/documents/31850) and through the National Disaster Recovery Program Database at http://www.fema.gov/national-disaster-recovery-program-database (accessed March 4, 2015).

Annex 4-1

Funding for Disaster Recovery

TABLE 4-1 Funding for Disaster Recovery

Recovery Area	Source of Funds	Funding Pathway	Use of Funds (with notable restrictions)
Pre-disaster Funding			
Pre-disaster Mitigation	Federal Emergency Management Agency (FEMA)	Federal→state or local government	The Pre-Disaster Mitigation (PDM) program furnishes funds for hazard mitigation planning and projects on an annual basis. The PDM program was established to reduce overall risk to people and structures while reducing reliance on federal funding should an actual disaster occur. "Hazard mitigation is any sustained action taken to reduce or eliminate long-term risk to people and property from natural hazards and their effects" (FEMA, 2013a, p. 7-1).
Hospitals and Health Care Systems	Office of the Assistant Secretary for Preparedness and Response (ASPR)	Federal→state or local government	ASPR's Hospital Preparedness Program (HPP) provides cooperative agreements to state and local agencies for strengthening their capabilities in the areas of "health care system preparedness, health care system recovery, emergency operations coordination, fatality management, information sharing, medical surge, responder safety and health, and volunteer management" (ASPR, 2012, p. vii).

continued

TABLE 4-1 Continued

Recovery Area	Source of Funds	Funding Pathway	Use of Funds (with notable restrictions)
Public Health	Centers for Disease Control and Prevention (CDC)	Federal→state or local government	CDC's Public Health Emergency Preparedness (PHEP) cooperative agreements are provided to state and local health departments for developing the following capabilities needed to respond to a health emergency: community preparedness, community recovery, emergency operations coordination, emergency public information and warning, fatality management, information sharing, mass care, medical countermeasure dispensing, medical material management and distribution, medical surge, non-pharmaceutical interventions, public health laboratory testing, public health surveillance and epidemiological investigation, responder safety and health, and volunteer management (CDC, 2011).
Emergency Management	FEMA	Federal→state	The purpose of the Emergency Management Performance Grants (EMPG) Program is to assist state, local, territorial, and tribal governments in preparing for all hazards, as authorized by the Robert T. Stafford Disaster Relief and Emergency Assistance Act. The act authorizes FEMA to make grants for the purpose of "providing a system of emergency preparedness for the protection of life and property in the United States from hazards and to vest responsibility for emergency preparedness jointly in the federal government and the states and their political subdivisions" (FEMA, 2015b).
Homeland Security	FEMA	Federal→state	The Homeland Security Grant Program (HSGP) supports "the building, sustainment, and delivery of core capabilities" essential to achieving a secure and resilient nation. The funds support core capabilities across five mission areas: prevention, protection, mitigation, response, and recovery from acts of terrorism or other catastrophic events (FEMA, 2014c).

TABLE 4-1 Continued

Recovery Area	Source of Funds	Funding Pathway	Use of Funds (with notable restrictions)
Housing			
Private housing	FEMA	Federal→homeowner	FEMA's Individual Assistance grants are for homeowners to rebuild damaged properties. There is a $32,400 limit per homeowner.[a] The funds may be used for rental assistance; lodging expenses; home repairs; home replacement assistance; housing construction; personal property; moving and storage; transportation; and disaster-related medical, dental, and funeral expenses.
	Private homeowner's insurance	Private→homeowner	Homeowner's insurance payouts are made according to the contract between the insurance agency and the homeowner.
	Small Business Administration (SBA)	Federal→homeowner or renter	SBA provides low-interest disaster loans to homeowners or renters. SBA "disaster loans can be used to repair or replace the following items damaged or destroyed in a declared disaster: real estate and personal property" (SBA, 2015).
Public and private housing	U.S. Department of Housing and Urban Development (HUD)	Federal→state or local government (supplemental appropriation)	HUD's Community Development Block Grant-Disaster Recovery (CDBG-DR) can be used to rebuild homes and buildings, contingent on a presidential disaster declaration. Recipients must demonstrate a logical connection between the impacts of the covered disaster and the activity's contribution to community recovery (HUD, 2013a). Generally, at least 70 percent of the total grant must benefit persons of low and moderate income (HUD, 2015).
Public Infrastructure	FEMA	Federal state (local government or nonprofit organizations can be subgrantees)	"Through the Public Assistance program, FEMA provides supplemental federal disaster grant assistance for debris removal, emergency protective measures, and the repair, replacement, or restoration of disaster-damaged publicly owned facilities and the facilities of certain private nonprofit organizations" (FEMA, 2015c). Grants often are for rebuilding schools, municipal buildings, public hospitals, sewer systems, communication systems, and fire stations. Grantees generally are required to supply a 25 percent nonfederal cost share. The grants are contingent on a presidential disaster declaration (FEMA, 2015c).
	Municipal bonds	Bondholders→ municipalities	Cities borrow money from bondholders to finance municipal projects. Interest is usually tax free.

continued

TABLE 4-1 Continued

Recovery Area	Source of Funds	Funding Pathway	Use of Funds (with notable restrictions)
Hazard Mitigation	FEMA	Federal→state	FEMA's Hazard Mitigation Grant Program (HMGP) is intended to ensure that the opportunity to implement critical mitigation measures to reduce the risk of loss of life and property from future disasters is not lost during the reconstruction process following a disaster. Grants are provided only after a presidential disaster declaration. Grantees are required to supply a 25 percent nonfederal cost share. States are required to develop pre-disaster hazard mitigation plans to be eligible for funding (FEMA, 2007).
Business/ Economic Development	SBA	Federal→business	SBA provides low-interest disaster loans to businesses of all sizes and private nonprofit organizations. "SBA disaster loans can be used to repair or replace the following items damaged or destroyed in a declared disaster: real estate, machinery and equipment, and inventory and business assets" (SBA, 2015).
	HUD	Federal→state or local government (supplemental appropriation)	HUD's flexible CDBG-DR funding can be applied to economic development initiatives (e.g., workforce training) in a presidentially declared disaster area. Recipients must "demonstrate a logical connection between the impacts of the covered disaster and the activity's contribution to community recovery" (HUD, 2013a). Generally, at least 70 percent of the total grant must benefit persons of low and moderate income (HUD, 2015).
	Economic Development Administration	Federal→state, city, local government, university, or private nonprofit organization acting in cooperation with officials of a political subdivision of a state	Under the Public Works and Economic Development Act of 1965,[b] the Economic Development Administration (EDA) of the U.S. Department of Commerce provides recipients with flexible tools for developing and implementing regionally based long-term economic development strategies in response to presidentially declared major disasters. The EDA provides a wide range of technical, disaster recovery, economic recovery planning, and public works assistance. Applicants must demonstrate a clear relationship between the proposed scope of work and disaster recovery and resiliency efforts. The funding, which comes in the form of grants and cooperative agreements, is available only in presidentially declared disaster areas (EDA, 2013).

TABLE 4-1 Continued

Recovery Area	Source of Funds	Funding Pathway	Use of Funds (with notable restrictions)
Health	Red Cross, Salvation Army, and other private philanthropic organizations	Variable	These nongovernmental organizations fund the delivery of health care, rebuilding of health facilities, and health-related activities often not funded by public sources. The funds are for shelter, support, food, and supplies.
	HUD	Federal→state or local government (supplemental appropriation)	HUD's flexible CDBG-DR funding can be applied toward the rebuilding of hospitals and clinics as long as recipients "demonstrate a logical connection between the impacts of the covered disaster and the activity's contribution to community recovery" (HUD, 2013a). Its availability is contingent on presidential declaration of a disaster area. Generally, at least 70 percent of the total grant must benefit persons of low and moderate income (HUD, 2015).
Behavioral Health	FEMA	Federal→state	The Crisis Counseling Program (CCP) is a supplemental assistance program available to the states and territories in presidentially declared major disaster areas. The Substance Abuse and Mental Health Services Administration's (SAMHSA's) Center for Mental Health Services "works with FEMA through an interagency agreement to provide technical assistance, consultation, and training for state and local mental health personnel, grant administration, and program oversight" (FEMA, 2015a). Funds may not be used for "office-based" therapy or psychiatric treatment.
	Administration for Children and Families (ACF)	Federal→state	In the case of a special congressional appropriation, Social Services Block Grant (SSBG) funds can cover expenses for disaster mental health services for individuals, as well as repair, renovation, and rebuilding of mental hygiene facilities (ACF, 2014b).
	Substance Abuse and Mental Health Service Administration (SAMHSA)	Federal→state and local	SAMHSA's Emergency Response Grant (SERG), subject to availability of funds, can be used for behavioral health services during disaster recovery, including treatment for substance abuse and mental health disorders. A presidential disaster declaration is not required to request SERG funds.
	Red Cross and other private philanthropic organizations	Varied	These organizations provide psychological first aid, crisis counseling services, and other post-disaster behavioral health support.

continued

TABLE 4-1 Continued

Recovery Area	Source of Funds	Funding Pathway	Use of Funds (with notable restrictions)
	U.S. Department of Justice	Federal→Individual	Long-term mental health counseling is available to victims of crime.
Social Services	ACF	Federal→state	Through reprogramming of existing grant funds or in the case of a special congressional appropriation, Social Services Block Grant (SSBG) funds can cover unreimbursed expenses resulting from a disaster, including social, health, and mental health services for individuals, as well as repair, renovation, and rebuilding of health care facilities, mental hygiene facilities, child care facilities, and other social services facilities. Funds may go to daycare, foster care, case management, and housing, among other social services (ACF, 2014b).
Agriculture	U.S. Department of Agriculture (USDA)	Federal→eligible producers	USDA's Farm Service Agency provides assistance for natural disaster losses resulting from drought, flood, fire, freezes, tornadoes, pest infestation, and other calamities. The funding can be used for disaster-related losses to livestock, honeybees, farm-raised fish, forests, trees, bushes and vines, and noninsurable crops, as well as grazing losses due to drought or fire (FSA, 2015).
Transportation	Federal Highway Administration (FHWA)	Federal→state and local	Through its Federal-aid Highway Emergency Relief Program, FHWA within the U.S. Department of Transportation draws on the Highway Trust Fund for the repair or reconstruction of federal-aid highways and roads on federal lands that have suffered serious damage as a result of natural disasters or catastrophic failures from an external cause. A presidential declaration of a disaster is not required. Federal-aid highways include the more significant state, county, and city roads. There is a $100 million cap per state per disaster (FHWA, 2013).
	Federal Transit Administration (FTA)	Federal→state or local government or transit agency	FTA provides funding to transit agencies for emergency assistance when Congress has given supplemental appropriations to the agency for responding to a disaster (FTA, 2015).

[a] 78 F.R. 64523, Oct. 29, 2013.
[b] 42 U.S.C. § 3121 et seq.

REFERENCES

ACF (Administration for Children and Families). 2012. *SSBG grant awards allocations FY 2012.* http://www.acf.hhs.gov/programs/ocs/resource/allotments-for-states-2012 (accessed August 5, 2014).

ACF. 2013a. *SSBG fact sheet FY 2013.* http://www.acf.hhs.gov/programs/ocs/resource/social-services-block-grant-ssbg-fact-sheet (accessed August 5, 2014).

ACF. 2013b. *SSBG Q&As Hurricane Sandy supplemental FY 2013.* http://www.acf.hhs.gov/programs/ocs/resource/ssbg-qas-2013-sandy-supplemental (accessed August 5, 2014).

ACF. 2014a. *Hurricane Sandy supplemental round 2 Q&A.* http://www.acf.hhs.gov/sites/default/files/ocs/hurricanesandyround2.pdf (accessed August 5, 2014).

ACF. 2014b. *Social Services Block Grant Program (SSBG).* http://www.acf.hhs.gov/programs/ocs/programs/ssbg (accessed August 5, 2014).

ACF. 2014c. *SSBG contact info state officials & program contacts.* http://www.acf.hhs.gov/programs/ocs/resource/ssbg-state-officials-program-contacts (accessed August 5, 2014).

ASPR (Assistant Secretary for Preparedness and Response). 2012. *Healthcare preparedness capabilities: National guidance for healthcare system preparedness.* Washington, DC: ASPR.

CDC (Centers for Disease Control and Prevention). 2011. *Public health preparedness capabilities: National standards for state and local planning.* Atlanta, GA: CDC.

CPW (Community Planning Workshop). 2010. *Pre-disaster planning for post-disaster recovery: Case studies.* http://redevelopment.net/wp-content/uploads/2010/09/CRS-Case-Studies_Final.pdf (accessed April 4, 2015).

CRS (Congressional Research Service). 2011. *Community development block grant funds in disaster relief and recovery.* Washington, DC: CRS, Library of Congress.

CRS. 2012a. *Federal disaster recovery programs: Brief summaries.* Washington, DC: CRS, Library of Congress.

CRS. 2012b. *Social Services Block Grant: Background and funding.* Washington, DC: CRS, Library of Congress.

CRS. 2014a. *Congressional primer on major disasters and emergencies.* Washington, DC: CRS, Library of Congress.

CRS. 2014b. *FEMA's disaster relief fund: Overview and selected issues.* Washington, DC: CRS, Library of Congress.

DOT (U.S. Department of Transportation). 2012. *State & local funding resources.* http://www.dot.gov/highlights/disaster-recovery/funding/state-local (accessed October 14, 2014).

DOT, EPA (U.S. Environmental Protection Agency), and HUD (U.S. Department of Housing and Urban Development). 2014. *Partnership for sustainable communities: Five years of learning from communities and coordinating federal investments.* Washington, DC: DOT, EPA, and HUD.

Dunlop, A. L., K. M. Logue, and A. P. Isakov. 2014. The engagement of academic institutions in community disaster response: A comparative analysis. *Public Health Reports* 129(Suppl. 4):87-95.

EDA (Economic Development Administration). 2013. *Economic development administration overview.* http://www.eda.gov/annual-reports/fy2013/overview.htm (accessed March 31, 2015).

Erickson, D., and N. Andrews. 2011. Partnerships among community development, public health, and health care could improve the well-being of low-income people. *Health Affairs* 30(11):2056-2063.

FEMA (Federal Emergency Management Agency). 2007. *Selecting appropriate mitigation measures for floodprone structures.* Washington, DC: FEMA.

FEMA. 2009. *Emergency assistance for human influenza pandemic disaster assistance policy 9523.17.* Washington, DC: FEMA.

FEMA. 2011a. *National disaster recovery framework.* Washington, DC: FEMA.

FEMA. 2011b. *A whole community approach to emergency management: Principles, themes, and pathways for action.* Washington, DC: FEMA.

FEMA. 2013a. *Disaster Operations Legal Reference.* Washington, DC: FEMA.

FEMA. 2013b. *Public assistance alternative procedures pilot program guide for permanent work.* Washington, DC: FEMA.

FEMA. 2014a. *The declaration process.* http://www.fema.gov/declaration-process (accessed October 13, 2014).

FEMA. 2014b. *Public assistance: Local, state, tribal, and non-profit.* http://www.fema.gov/public-assistance-local-state-tribal-and-non-profit (accessed October 14, 2014).

FEMA. 2014c. *FY 2014 Homeland Security Grant Program.* https://www.fema.gov/fy-2014-homeland-security-grant-program-hsgp (accessed March 31, 2015).

FEMA. 2015a. *Additional Assistance.* https://www.fema.gov/additional-assistance (accessed March 31, 2015).

FEMA. 2015b. *Fiscal year 2014 emergency management performance grant program.* https://www.fema.gov/fiscal-year-2015-emergency-management-performance-grant-program (accessed March 31, 2015).

FEMA. 2015c. *Public Assistance: Local, state, tribal, and non-profit.* https://www.fema.gov/public-assistance-local-state-tribal-and-non-profit (accessed March 31, 2015).

FHWA (Federal Highway Administration). 2013. *Emergency relief manual (federal-aid highways).* http://www.fhwa.dot.gov/reports/erm/er.pdf (accessed March 5, 2015).

Fossett, J. W. 2013. *Let's stop improvising disaster recovery.* http://www.rockinst.org/observations/fossettj/2013-07-09-Improvising_Disaster_Recovery.aspx (accessed June 5, 2014).

FSA (Farm Service Agency). 2015. *Disaster assistance programs.* http://www.fsa.usda.gov/FSA/webapp?area=home&subject=diap&topic=landing (accessed April 1, 2015).

FTA (Federal Transit Administration). 2015. *Emergency Relief Program.* http://www.fta.dot.gov/map21_15025.html (accessed April 1, 2015).

GCHD (Galveston County Health District). 2007. *2007 Annual Report.* http://www.gchd.org/admin/07-annual-report/2007-Annual-%20Report.pdf (accessed March 26, 2015).

HUD. 2013a. *CDBG disaster recovery framework.* http://portal.hud.gov/hudportal/documents/huddoc?id=cdbg_training_2_2_13.pdf (accessed March 31, 2015).

HUD. 2013b. *Rebuild by design.* http://portal.hud.gov/hudportal/HUD?src=/sandyrebuilding/rebuildbydesign (accessed October 14, 2014).

HUD. 2014a. *CDBG-DR active disaster grants and grantee contact information.* https://www.hudexchange.info/cdbg-dr/cdbg-dr-grantee-contact-information (accessed March 31, 2015).

HUD. 2014b. *CDGB-DR eligibility requirements.* https://www.hudexchange.info/cdbg-dr/cdbg-dr-eligibility-requirements (accessed April 2, 2015).

HUD. 2014c. *National disaster resilience competition: FR-5800-N-29.* Washington, DC: HUD.

HUD. 2015. *Questions and answers about HUD.* http://portal.hud.gov/hudportal/HUD?src=/about/qaintro (accessed April 2, 2015).

Johnson, L. A., and R. B. Olshansky. 2013. The road to recovery: Governing post-disaster reconstruction. *Land Lines* 14-21. https://www.lincolninst.edu/pubs/2259_The-Road-to-Recovery--Governing-Post-Disaster-Reconstruction (accessed October 14, 2014).

Leydon, J. 2014. *Workforce development grants awarded.* http://www3.springfield-ma.gov/cos/1699.0.html (accessed March 5, 2015).

Lockwood, B. 2014. *Coordination among state and local government agencies.* Paper presented at IOM Committee on Post-Disaster Recovery of a Community's Public Health, Medical, and Social Services: Meeting Three, April 28-29, Washington, DC.

Meyers, D., C. E. Allien, III, D. Dunn, A. Wennerstrom, and B. F. Springgate. 2011. Community perspectives on post-Katrina mental health recovery in New Orleans. *Ethnicity and Disease* 21(3, Suppl. 1):S1-52-57.

Missouri SEMA. 2014. *State of Missouri COAD guidance manual.* http://sema.dps.mo.gov/programs/documents/mo-coad-manual.pdf (accessed November 5, 2014).

National VOAD (Voluntary Organizations Active in Disaster). 2014. *Who we are.* http://www.nvoad.org/about-us (accessed November 5, 2014).

Niquette, M. 2013. Joplin rebuilding after tornado saves on school bonds. *BloombergBusiness.* http://www.bloomberg.com/news/articles/2013-05-15/joplin-rebuilding-after-tornado-saves-on-school-bonds (accessed March 5, 2015).

Nolen, A. 2014. *A Health in All Policies approach to disaster recovery: Lessons from Galveston.* Paper presented at IOM Committee on Post-Disaster Recovery of a Community's Public Health, Medical, and Social Services: Meeting Four, June 13, Washington, DC.

Novogradac & Company, LLP. 2011. *Updated comprehensive housing market analysis, Joplin, Jasper County, Missouri.* http://joplinmo.org/DocumentCenter/View/1265 (accessed April 12, 2015).

Open Architecture Network. 2014. *Renew schools: Toms River High School North.* http://openarchitecturenetwork.org/projects/toms_river_hs (accessed October 14, 2014).

Pereira, E. 2013. Panel discussion at IOM Committee on Post-Disaster Recovery of a Community's Public Health, Medical, and Social Services: Meeting One, November 25, Washington, DC.

Pines, J. M., W. F. Pilkington, and S. A. Seabury. 2013. *Value-based models for sustaining emergency preparedness capacity and capability in the United States.* Washington, DC: IOM Forum on Medical and Public Health Preparedness for Catastrophic Events.

Rebuild by Design. 2014a. *New Meadowlands: Productive city + regional park.* http://www.rebuildbydesign.org/project/mit-cau-zus-urbanisten-final-proposal (accessed February 26, 2015).

Rebuild by Design. 2014b. *What is Rebuild by Design?* http://www.rebuildbydesign.org/what-is-rebuild-by-design (accessed February 26, 2015).

Riverside County VOAD. 2011. *VOAD vs. COAD.* https://sites.google.com/site/voadriversidecounty/about/voad-vs-coad (accessed November 5, 2014).

SBA (Small Business Administration). 2015. *Disaster loans.* https://www.sba.gov/category/navigation-structure/loans-grants/small-business-loans/disaster-loans (accessed March 31, 2015).

SAMHSA (Substance Abuse and Mental Health Services Administration). 2009. *Crisis Counseling Assistance and Training Program (CCP).* http://www.samhsa.gov/sites/default/files/ccp.pdf (accessed March 10, 2015).

Smith, G. 2011. *Planning for post-disaster recovery: A review of the United States disaster assistance framework.* Fairfax, VA: Public Entity Risk Institute.

Smith, G., W. Lyles, and P. R. Berke. 2013. The role of the state in building local capacity and commitment for hazard mitigation planning. *International Journal of Mass Emergencies and Disasters* 31(2):178-203.

Smith Parker, T. 2014. *CDBG disaster recovery overview.* Paper presented at IOM Committee on Post-Disaster Recovery of a Community's Public Health, Medical, and Social Services: Meeting Two, February 3, Washington, DC.

Thomas, E. A., A. Jerolleman, T. L. Turner, D. Punchard, and S. K. Bowen. 2011. *Planning and building livable, safe & sustainable communities: The patchwork quilt approach.* Metairie, LA: Natural Hazard Mitigation Association.

VAUMC (Virginia United Methodist Conference). 2014. *National VOAD members resource directory.* http://vaumc.org/NCFileRepository/Disaster/Disaster%20Response/National%20VOAD%20Resource%20Directory.pdf (accessed November 5, 2014).

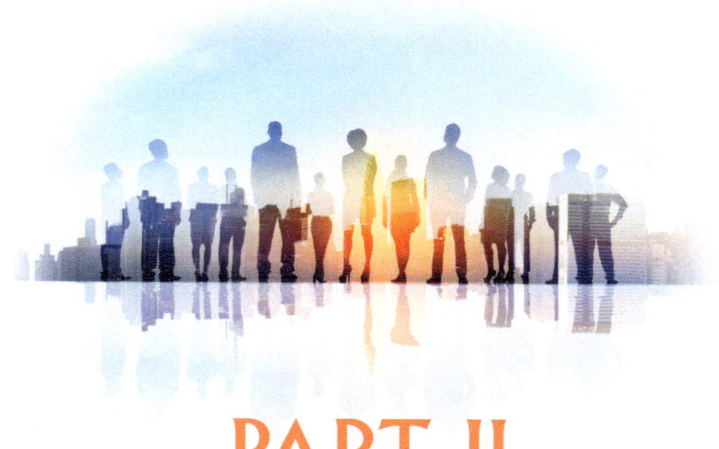

PART II

OPERATIONAL GUIDANCE TO SUPPORT A HEALTHY COMMUNITY APPROACH TO DISASTER RECOVERY

5

Public Health

Public health's mission is to ensure those conditions necessary for people to be healthy (IOM, 1988). The public health sector is unique in that its three core functions—assessment, policy development, and assurance (see Box 5-1)—are the foundation for a community's capability to address human needs, including those related to disasters. Because these functions cut across all other recovery domains (e.g., housing, transportation, health care delivery), successful recovery requires that the public health sector galvanize and lead an interdisciplinary, team-based approach to the continual assessment of health status and needs, the development and prioritization of plans and policies for addressing those needs, and the assurance of access to essential health services throughout the continuum of disaster response and recovery.

Given that components of the public health recovery mission cut across all other sectors, public health is integral to all of the committee's recommendations (as noted throughout this chapter) and is woven throughout this report. However, this chapter outlines specific tasks for the public health sector to support

---

BOX 5-1
Core Public Health Functions

Assessment—regularly and systematically collecting, assembling, analyzing, and making available information on the community's health, including health status, health needs, and causes of health problems.

Policy Development—facilitating evidence-based decision making in matters that impact public health and mobilizing the community in the development of public health policy that meets local needs.

Assurance—assurance that the full complement of services necessary to protect the public's health are accessible to all members of the community, either by providing such services directly, or encouraging other public or private entities to do so, using regulatory requirements when necessary.

SOURCE: IOM, 1988.

implementation of the committee's recommendations, and it describes the capabilities and resources that empower public health in the recovery process both pre- and post-disaster. In developing this guidance, the committee identified a number of key recovery strategies, which serve as cross-cutting themes throughout the chapter and apply to multiple pre- and post-disaster activities. Use of these strategies will facilitate the integration of health improvement into recovery planning before and after a disaster:

- Leverage existing relationships and networks (e.g., coalitions, collaboratives) to integrate public health and other community partners into recovery planning.
- Identify opportunities for alignment between ongoing public health improvement processes (e.g., accreditation prerequisites of community health assessments and community health improvement plans) and recovery planning.
- Educate nonhealth sectors and the community on why health is integral to recovery and how recovery activities impact health outcomes.
- Use and expand health technology infrastructure for data collection and analysis to facilitate data sharing, evidence-based decision making, and continual evaluation of progress toward an optimally healthy community.

The chapter concludes with a checklist of key activities that the public health sector needs to perform during pre-event planning, short-term recovery, and intermediate- to long-term recovery.

PUBLIC HEALTH IN THE CONTEXT OF A HEALTHY COMMUNITY

The public health sector has a central role to play in the realization of a healthy community. (Elements of a healthy community are detailed in Chapter 2, Box 2-2.) The process of creating healthier communities is not linear and has no end point; it is a continuous cycle (see Figure 5-1). Public health agencies and nongovernmental organizations protect and promote the health of individuals and communities through direct provision of health services, regulatory roles, education and advocacy efforts, sharing of health information to inform decision making, and creating and leveraging community partnerships. Through such measures (which are discussed in more detail throughout this chapter), the public health sector can spur within a community what the Robert Wood Johnson Foundation (RWJF) calls a culture of health. A culture of health encompasses a broader vision of what it means to be healthy, extending beyond health care to include work, family, and community life. According to RWJF, the characteristics of an American culture of health include

- "good health flourishes across geographic, demographic and social sectors;
- attaining the best health possible is valued by our entire society;
- individuals and families have the means and the opportunity to make choices that lead to the healthiest lives possible;
- business, government, individuals, and organizations work together to foster healthy communities and lifestyles;
- everyone has access to affordable, quality health care because it is essential to maintain, or reclaim, health;
- no one is excluded;
- health care is efficient and equitable;
- the economy is less burdened by excessive and unwarranted health care spending;
- the health of the population guides public and private decision-making; [and]
- Americans understand that we are all in this together" (RWJF, 2014, p. 5).

As discussed in Chapter 2, a healthy community is a prepared and resilient community. Planning for health improvement, recovery, and disaster response during steady-state periods should be concurrent,

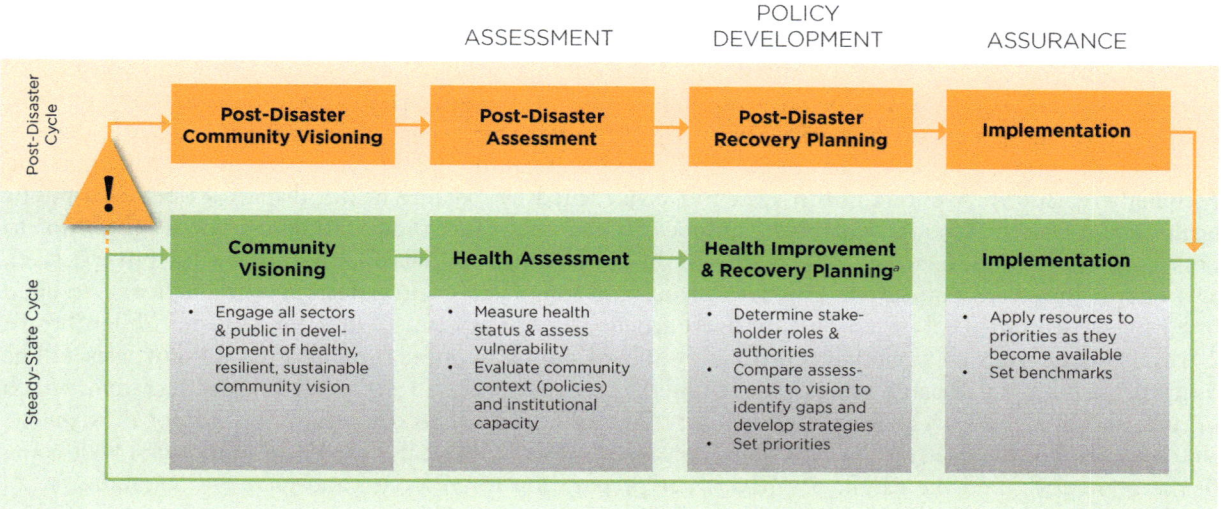

FIGURE 5-1 Linked community health improvement and disaster recovery cycles with associated core public health functions.

NOTE: This figure can assist public health agencies in articulating roles in and the cyclical nature of planning for health improvement and disaster recovery and encouraging pre-disaster recovery planning as a best practice.

[a] Disaster response planning also occurs during this phase and should be integrated with the recovery planning process to ensure integration across the emergency management phases and coordination of efforts and funding.

as illustrated in Figure 5-1. As discussed in Chapter 3, integration of health improvement and recovery planning ensures that a clear vision for a healthy, resilient, and sustainable community (and priorities for achieving that vision) is in place before a disaster to drive recovery activities. It should be noted that delineations between the phases in the cycle depicted in Figure 5-1 are not black and white, and various sectors engaged in these processes may be involved in different activities at any given time. Activities within sectors also may vary.

A disaster, which can occur in the community at any point in the steady-state health improvement cycle, initiates an event-specific cycle (detour) that mirrors the pre-disaster process, with cyclical phases of visioning, assessment, planning, and implementation. The diasater cycle persists until such time as the community transitions to a "new normal." This process can take years or even decades. The public health functions described in the following sections are a part of this phased approach to healthy community planning.

DISASTER-RELATED PUBLIC HEALTH CHALLENGES

As discussed in Chapter 2, a healthy community is contingent upon the optimal functioning and integration of the full spectrum of community and health services on which people depend to survive and thrive. A disaster can disrupt these systems directly through short-term impacts such as damage to health care facilities and indirectly through impacts such as destruction of other critical physical infrastructure (e.g., utilities, transportation, housing) and deterioration of the capacity of essential health and social services to meet a surge in post-disaster human needs. In the long term, a community's health may be impacted directly by an exodus of health care professionals (Berggren and Curiel, 2006; Rudowitz et al., 2006) or indirectly by unintended consequences of recovery decisions (e.g., unaddressed blight that deteriorates neighborhoods and is associated with increased crime).

After a disaster, the public health sector faces challenges well beyond the initial response phase because not only must it galvanize a multisectoral recovery effort to address long-term health needs, it must do so while also remaining focused on carrying out the core day-to-day functions of fostering good health, offering protection from unsafe or hazardous conditions, preventing disease, and disseminating credible health information. Lessons from the aftermath of the terrorist events of September 11, 2001, demonstrate the importance of balancing the crisis response and routine public health functions (Klitzman and Freudenberg, 2003). A public health system overburdened by existing health disparities before a public health emergency may be the least well equipped to maintain this balance (Runkle et al., 2012). Prior to Hurricane Katrina, for example, one quarter of the New Orleans population lived below the poverty level, and one in five were uninsured. The devastating and long-lasting aftereffects of the hurricane resulted in an overwhelming load on an already overburdened health system (Center for Disaster Philanthropy, 2012). A public health system that is just barely able to support a population on a day-to-day basis will be overwhelmed after a disaster strikes, weakening the recovery process for the overall health system, which in turn will hinder recovery for the community. The trajectory of recovery will depend not only on the characteristics of the disaster but also on the pre-event health (physical, behavioral) and social well-being of the population and the extent of pre-disaster preparation for response and recovery (Chandra et al., 2011). Thus, improving the health of communities is not just an ethical imperative; it must be viewed as a matter of national security and supported accordingly (HHS, 2009). Resilience to all manner of hazards depends not only on robust health systems but also on a robust population (Morton and Lurie, 2013).

The restoration of services and infrastructure, although critical and often regarded as full recovery, is not an end point in itself. The committee holds that within the tragedy of a disaster lies a unique opportunity for a community to reenvision itself through the lens of a healthy community. By leveraging new funding sources, partnerships, and technologies and redirecting existing funding streams, the process of recovery can be exploited to address previously identified gaps in a community, strengthen and expand existing programs and partnerships, and engage the community in a process of envisioning and building a better post-disaster future. Existing recovery guidance for the public health sector (discussed later in this chapter) focuses on the restoration of public health (as well as health care and behavioral health[1]) systems and mitigation of damage from future incidents. Greater recognition is needed of the broader public health responsibilities related to the building of healthier communities, including the social and physical environments, after disasters.

PUBLIC HEALTH SECTOR ORGANIZATION AND RESOURCES

The public health system comprises numerous governmental and nongovernmental organizations, working collectively to create conditions in which people can be healthy (IOM, 2003) (see Figure 5-2). In the disaster context, public health cuts across all other sectors because the ultimate goal for all preparedness, response, and recovery activities is the protection and betterment of the health and well-being of people (NBSB, 2014).

The Federal Public Health Enterprise[2]

The U.S. Department of Health and Human Services (HHS) is the main federal department tasked with protecting and improving the nation's health, and all agencies within it have roles in assuring public health through preparedness, response, and recovery activities. The Assistant Secretary for Preparedness and Response (ASPR) is responsible for coordinating, on behalf of the HHS Secretary, the HHS response activities under Emergency Support Function (ESF) #8 of the National Response Framework (Public Health

---

[1] For the purposes of this report, the term "behavioral health" encompasses "the interconnected psychological, emotional, cognitive, developmental, and social influences on behavior, mental health and substance abuse" (HHS, 2014a, p. 4).

[2] A broader synopsis of legislation and federal policy related to disaster recovery and health security can be found in Appendix A.

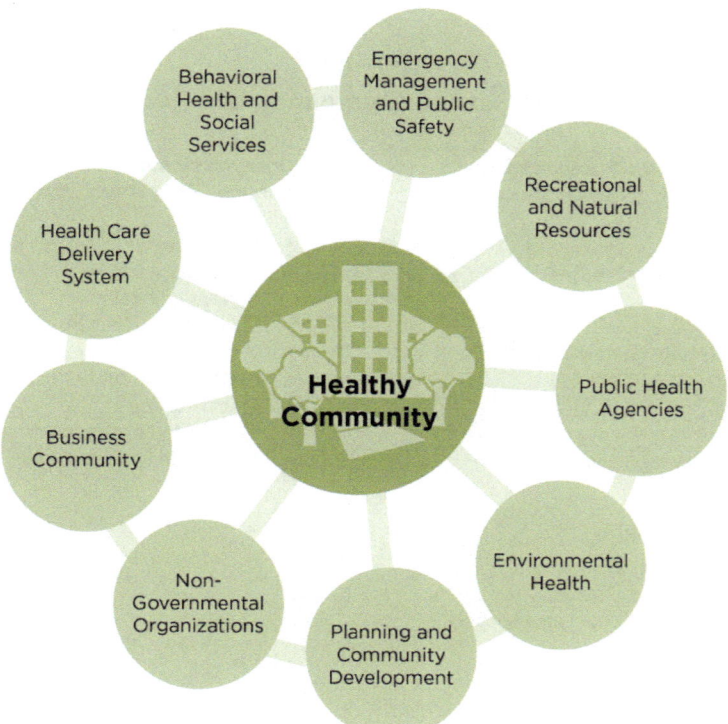

FIGURE 5-2 Key stakeholders in a healthy community.

and Medical Services), as well as recovery activities under the Health and Social Services Recovery Support Function (RSF) of the National Disaster Recovery Framework (NDRF), which is described in more detail in Chapter 3. Core mission areas for ESF #8 and the Health and Social Services RSF are listed in Box 5-2. Within these mission areas, public health activities include assessing the impact of the disaster; restoring the capacity of systems to meet post-disaster needs; ensuring the well-being of vulnerable populations, such as people with disabilities and the elderly; and providing the public with appropriate and accessible information. Although this report focuses primarily on recovery, it is important to recognize the need for integration across the two frameworks and the associated operational activities. Successful recovery will depend in part on the effectiveness of response activities.

In addition to its federal coordinating role for disaster response and recovery activities, HHS helps state, local, tribal, and territorial public health and health care organizations carry out strategic planning for preparedness, response, and recovery through grant funding (cooperative agreements). Public Health Emergency Preparedness (PHEP) cooperative agreement and Hospital Preparedness Program (HPP) funds are distributed on an annual basis by the Centers for Disease Control and Prevention (CDC) and ASPR, respectively, to all 50 states, 4 major metropolitan areas, and a handful of U.S. territories. These agencies have developed aligned sets of public health and health care preparedness capabilities (see Table 5-1) to guide the use of grant funds and prepare grantees to carry out the ESF and RSF functions described above (ASPR, 2012; CDC, 2011). This alignment of programs has enabled better coordination of the use of funds for preparedness activities at the state and local levels. The PHEP cooperative agreement funds preparedness activities aimed at cultivating emergency-ready, flexible, and adaptable public health departments. The Community Recovery capability is intended to help community partners "plan and advocate for the rebuilding of public health, medical, and mental/behavioral health systems to at least a level of functioning comparable to pre-incident levels, and improved levels where possible" (CDC, 2011, p. 10)

BOX 5-2
Core Mission Areas for Health-Related Emergency and Recovery Support Functions

Core mission areas under the Public Health and Medical Services Emergency Support Function (ESF #8)[a]

- Assessment of public health/medical needs
- Health surveillance
- Medical care personnel
- Health/medical/veterinary equipment and supplies
- Patient evacuation
- Patient care
- Safety and security of drugs, biologics, and medical devices
- Blood and blood products
- Food safety and security
- Agriculture safety and security
- All-hazard public health and medical consultation, technical assistance, and support
- Behavioral health care
- Public health and medical information
- Vector control
- Potable water/wastewater and solid waste disposal
- Mass fatality management, victim identification, and decontaminating remains
- Veterinary medical support

Core mission areas under the Health and Social Services Recovery Support Function[b]

- Public health
- Health care services
- Behavioral health
- Environmental health
- Food safety and medical products
- Responders' long-term health
- Social services
- Referral to case management
- Children in disasters

SOURCES:
[a] Excerpted from FEMA, 2008, p. 1-2.
[b] ASPR, 2015.

(see Box 5-3). Recovery involves identifying and monitoring recovery needs, coordinating recovery operations, and implementing corrective actions to mitigate damages from future incidents.

The CDC, whose mission is to protect America from health, safety, and security threats, is in a unique position to support a healthy community approach to disaster recovery. In addition to its support for preparedness activities through the PHEP cooperative agreement, the CDC has a number of programmatic activities and grants focused on advancing healthy and safe communities that could be leveraged after a disaster. As is the case for many other governmental and professional organizations involved in both preparedness and healthy community development, however, the two efforts are poorly connected. An important opportunity is being missed to expand and leverage the PHEP guidance on recovery capabilities to encourage grantees to incorporate a healthy community vision into recovery planning before and after disasters.

Although community health improvement is a key CDC programmatic area, it is important to note that many other departments across the federal government support the development of healthier communities. The Partnership for Sustainable Communities, for example, which promotes and coordinates improvements in transportation, housing, and land use, is a joint project of the U.S. Department of Housing and

TABLE 5-1 Lists of Public Health Emergency Preparedness (PHEP) and Hospital Preparedness Program (HPP) Capabilities, with Rows Showing Alignment

PHEP Capabilities[a]	HPP Capabilities[b]
Community preparedness	Health care system preparedness
Community recovery	Health care system recovery
Emergency operations coordination	Emergency operations coordination
Emergency public information and warning	
Fatality management	Fatality management
Information sharing	Information sharing
Mass care	
Medical countermeasure dispensing	
Medical material management and distribution	
Medical surge	Medical surge
Non-pharmaceutical interventions	
Public health laboratory testing	
Public health surveillance and epidemiological investigation	
Responder safety and health	Responder safety and health
Volunteer management	Volunteer management

[a] CDC, 2011.
[b] ASPR, 2012.

Urban Development (HUD), the U.S. Environmental Protection Agency (EPA), and the U.S. Department of Transportation (DOT). Through the Partnership, which was formalized in 2009, these departments are working together to align policies, funding opportunities, and technical assistance to "better serve American communities" (DOT et al., 2014, p. 2). As discussed in Chapter 2, health and sustainability are closely interconnected, and sustainability initiatives often yield co-benefits to health. Thus, many of the activities supported by the Partnership and its component departments individually (e.g., mixed-use development, affordable housing initiatives, and protection of open green space) are relevant to post-disaster efforts to build healthier communities. In fact, the committee noted that in the post-disaster context, EPA and the other members of the Partnership are leading these efforts under the banner of sustainability and smart growth, facilitated through a 2010 memorandum of agreement between the Federal Emergency Management Agency (FEMA) and EPA (DHS and EPA, 2010). The committee found little evidence of CDC involvement in post-disaster recovery sustainability initiatives led by Partnership agencies. Given the opportunities for the CDC noted above, the committee believes the agency's increased engagement in Partnership efforts to support post-disaster recovery could (1) help ensure that health considerations are explicitly included in recovery-related sustainability initiatives, (2) avoid separate and potentially duplicative activities across government agencies, and (3) encourage public health professionals at the state and local levels to expand recovery responsibilities beyond the restoration of public health services and participate in a more comprehensive discussion on building healthier post-disaster communities.

State and Local Health Departments

State, local, tribal, and territorial health departments are the backbone of the public health system (IOM, 2003). They are responsible for conducting epidemiology and surveillance activities to prevent

---

BOX 5-3
**Public Health Emergency Preparedness (PHEP) Cooperative Agreement
Guidance on Community Recovery**

Under the *Public Health Preparedness Capabilities: National Standards for State and Local Planning*, funding allocated for the Community Recovery capability should be focused on enabling the following three critical functions, each of which specifies several tasks and planning resource elements:

Function 1—Identify and monitor public health, medical, and mental/behavioral health system recovery needs.
Task 1: In collaboration with jurisdictional partners, document short-term and long-term health system delivery priorities and goals.
Task 2: Identify the services that can be provided by the public health agency and by community and faith-based partners that were identified prior to the incident as well as by new community partners that may arise during the incident response.
Task 3: Activate plans previously created with neighboring jurisdictions to provide identified services that the jurisdiction does not have the ability to provide during and after an incident.
Task 4: In conjunction with healthcare organizations (e.g., healthcare facilities and public and private community providers) and based upon recovery operations, determine the community's health service priorities and goals that are the responsibility of public health.

Function 2—Coordinate community public health, medical, and mental/behavioral health system recovery operations.
Task 1: Participate with the recovery lead jurisdictional agencies (e.g., emergency management and social services) to ensure that the jurisdiction can provide health services needed to recover from a physical or mental/behavioral injury, illness, or exposure sustained as a result of the incident, with particular attention to the functional needs of at-risk persons (e.g., those displaced from their usual residence).
Task 2: In conjunction with jurisdictional government and community partners, inform the community of the availability of mental/behavioral, psychological first aid, and medical services within the community, with par-

---

epidemics and the spread of disease, preventing injuries, providing laboratory services, protecting against environmental hazards, promoting healthy behavior, ensuring quality and accessible health services, and responding to disasters and assisting in community recovery. Although public health agencies are ubiquitous across the nation, health departments vary greatly from jurisdiction to jurisdiction in

- governance[3] and organizational structure;
- size relative to the population; and
- roles, responsibilities, and authorities (NACCHO, 2014a).

In addition to variation across jurisdictions, responsibilities and authorities at the state and local levels may vary as well. For example, state public health agencies may have more responsibility than their local-level counterparts related to ensuring access to health care. This variability in responsibilities and governance among state and local public health agencies must be taken into consideration in national-level planning efforts and policy development as it will translate to variable roles and authorities, as well as

---

[3] Some local health departments are local or regional units of the state health department (i.e., centralized), others are agencies of the local government, and still others are governed by both state and local authorities (called shared governance, accounting for 6 percent of states) (NACCHO, 2014a).

ticular attention to how these services affect the functional needs of at-risk persons (including but not limited to children, elderly, their caregivers, the disabled, or individuals with limited economic resources).

Task 3: Notify the community via community partners of the health agency's plans for restoration of impacted public health, medical, and mental/behavioral health services.

Task 4: Solicit community input via community partners regarding health service recovery needs during and after the acute phase of the incident.

Task 5: Partner with public health, medical, and mental/behavioral health professionals and other social networks (e.g., faith-based, volunteer organizations, support groups, and professional organizations) from within and outside the jurisdiction, as applicable to the incident, to educate their constituents regarding applicable health interventions being recommended by public health.

Task 6: In conjunction with jurisdictional government and community partners, inform the community of the availability of any disaster or community case management services being offered that provide assistance for community members impacted by the incident.

Function 3—Implement corrective actions to mitigate damages from future incidents.

Task 1: In conjunction with jurisdictional government and community partners, conduct post-incident assessment and planning as part of the after action report process that affects short- and long-term recovery for those corrective actions that are within the control and purview of jurisdictional public health, including the mitigation of damages from future incidents.

Task 2: Collaborate with sector leaders to facilitate collection of community feedback to determine corrective actions.

Task 3: Implement corrective actions for items that are within the scope or control of public health to affect short- and long-term recovery, including the mitigation of damages from future incidents.

Task 4: Facilitate and advocate for collaborations among government agencies and community partners so that these agencies can fulfill their respective roles in completing the corrective actions to protect the health of the public.

SOURCE: Excerpted from CDC, 2011.

access to resources, in disaster preparedness, response, and recovery. As a result, the committee's recommendations and guidance (like other national-level guidance materials) will have to be considered in the local context. In all cases, strong relationships with elected officials are critical to ensure funding and political support for health-related policies.

Although public health involvement in pre- and post-disaster community planning for recovery presents a new challenge for the sector, it should be recognized that many of the essential capabilities required for successful recovery are already in place in communities. These capabilities within different jurisdictions may vary, as well as the availability of resources needed for full implementation. Nevertheless, the committee has identified alignments among activities requisite for public health accreditation, performance of the ten essential public health services,[4] and the development of plans and procedures recommended under HHS preparedness guidance (PHEP and HPP) and FEMA recovery guidance (NDRF) that may be exploited to achieve recovery goals (see Table 5-2 for illustrative examples of potential alignments).

Unfortunately, the ability of state and local health agencies to carry out essential public health

---

[4] Following a 1988 report of the Institute of Medicine (IOM, 1988) that defined the 3 core public health functions (assessment, policy development, and assurance), the 10 essential public health services were developed as a framework for public health activities that all communities should undertake. These 10 essential services are generally accepted as minimum functions for health departments and serve as the foundation for the National Public Health Performance Standards (CDC, 2014b; NACCHO, 2011).

TABLE 5-2 Alignment of 10 Essential Public Health Services, Public Health Accreditation Board Standards, and Interrelated Preparedness and Recovery Functions

10 Essential Public Health Services[a]	Public Health Accreditation Board Standards[b]	Associated Disaster Preparedness and Recovery Functions[c]
1 Monitor health status to identify and solve community health problems	Conduct and disseminate assessments focused on population health status and public health issues facing the community	Pre-disaster community health assessment to inform recovery planning (vulnerabilities, unmet needs) • **Public Health Emergency Preparedness (PHEP) Community Preparedness capability:** Determine risks to the health of the jurisdiction • **PHEP Community Recovery capability:** Identify and monitor public health, medical, and mental/behavioral health system recovery needs
2 Diagnose and investigate health problems and health hazards in the community	Investigate health problems and environmental public health hazards to protect the community	Post-disaster assessment of disaster impact on health and medical needs (including environmental health hazards) • **PHEP Community Recovery capability:** Identify and monitor public health, medical, and mental/behavioral health system recovery needs • **PHEP Public Health Surveillance and Epidemiological Investigation capability:** Conduct public health surveillance and detection • **NDRF, Health and Social Services RSF activity:** Maintain situational awareness to identify and mitigate potential recovery obstacles • **NDRF, Health and Social Services RSF activity:** Provide technical assistance in the form of impact analyses and support recovery planning of public health, health care and human services infrastructure.
3 Inform, educate, and empower people about health issues	Inform and educate about public health issues and functions	Public messaging (health and safety risks, access to resources); health literacy as it relates to recovery; management of expectations • **PHEP Community Preparedness capability:** Coordinate training or guidance to ensure community engagement in preparedness efforts • **PHEP Emergency Public Information and Warning capability** • **NDRF, Health and Social Services RSF activity:** Establish communication and information-sharing forum(s) for Health and Social Services RSF stakeholders with the state and/or community
4 Mobilize community partnerships and action to identify and solve health problems	Engage with the community to identify and address health problems	Community partner engagement in health aspects of recovery • **PHEP Community Preparedness capability:** Engage with community organizations to foster public health, medical, and mental/behavioral health social networks • **PHEP Community Recovery capability:** Coordinate community public health, medical, and mental/behavioral health system recovery operations • **NDRF, Health and Social Services RSF activity:** Identify and coordinate with other local, state, tribal and federal partners to assess food, animal, water and air conditions to ensure safety

TABLE 5-2 Continued

10 Essential Public Health Services[a]	Public Health Accreditation Board Standards[b]	Associated Disaster Preparedness and Recovery Functions[c]
5 Develop policies and plans that support individual and community health efforts	Develop public health policies and plans	Participation in recovery planning to ensure that short- and long-term population health needs are considered • **PHEP Community Recovery capability:** Implement corrective actions to mitigate damages from future incidents • **NDRF, Health and Social Services RSF activity:** Develop strategies to address recovery issues for health, behavioral health, and social services
6 Enforce laws and regulations that protect health and ensure safety	Enforce public health laws	Advocate for changes to codes that improve resiliency • **PHEP Community Recovery capability:** Implement corrective actions to mitigate damages from future incidents • **NDRF, Health and Social Services RSF activity:** Promote the principles of sustainability, resilience and mitigation into preparedness and operational plans
7 Link people to needed personal health services and assure the provision of health care when otherwise unavailable	Promote strategies to improve access to health care	Support for clinical care sector recovery to ensure population access to needed health care providers • **PHEP Mass Care capability:** Coordinate public health, medical, and mental/behavioral health services
8 Assure a competent public and personal health care workforce	Maintain a competent public health workforce	Expansion of workforce capacity as needed to meet community recovery needs • **PHEP Volunteer Management capability** • **NDRF, Health and Social Services RSF activity:** When activated, deploy in support of the Health and Social Services RSF mission, as appropriate
9 Evaluate effectiveness, accessibility, and quality of personal and population-based health services	Evaluate and continuously improve processes, programs, and interventions	Continual assessment of health status and progress toward recovery goals to inform planning and develop and share lessons learned • **PHEP Community Recovery capability:** Identify and monitor public health, medical, and mental/behavioral health system recovery needs • **PHEP Community Recovery capability:** Implement corrective actions to mitigate damages from future incidents • **NDRF, Health and Social Services RSF activity:** Evaluate the effectiveness of federal health and social services recovery efforts
10 Research for new insights and innovative solutions to health problems	Contribute to and apply the evidence base of public health	

NOTE: This table can assist public health agencies in identifying existing departmental assets for recovery.
[a] CDC, 2014b.
[b] PHAB, 2013.
[c] CDC, 2011; FEMA, 2011.

functions—including ensuring the health of communities and preparing for disasters and other hazards—is compromised by continuing budget cuts and the resultant loss of workforce capacity. Local health departments have lost 44,000 jobs since 2008. In 2012, almost half of all local health departments cut health services, and emergency preparedness was among the areas most affected (NACCHO, 2013). These cuts in staff, programming, and funding mean that local health departments are less able to provide essential services, whether in steady-state times or during and after a disaster. During a large-scale disaster, public health departments need to be able to leverage the entire agency workforce to meet surge needs. During Hurricane Katrina, for example, personnel as varied as mosquito control sprayers, restaurant inspectors, and staff of the Special Supplemental Nutrition Program for Women, Infants, and Children (WIC) were tapped for the disaster response efforts (Shah, 2014). When health departments lose staff—from any part of the department—it affects their ability to effectively respond to disasters.

Public Health Partners for Healthier Post-Disaster Communities

As depicted in Figure 5-2, a number of organizations are included in broad descriptions of the public health system because of their demonstrated influence on population health outcomes, although some, such as planning and community development organizations, would not traditionally consider themselves part of the public health sector. Both in normal times and after a disaster, public health agencies can act as integrators, leveraging partnerships with health and traditionally nonhealth sectors to drive improvements in health at the individual and community levels. However, the success of the public health sector in disaster recovery depends heavily on pre-planning, knowledge of pre-disaster community demographics and health status, and knowledge of and partnerships with other governmental and nongovernmental sectors to ensure alignment of priorities and activities. Public health needs to have effective relationships in place with other governmental and nongovernmental stakeholders across sectors (e.g., housing, behavioral health, transportation, education) before a disaster to ensure that the actions that each sector takes during recovery not only will accomplish that sector's primary function but also will advance improved health outcomes and a healthier post-disaster community. As described in Chapter 2, this type of approach has been termed Health in All Policies (HiAP), which is described as "a collaborative approach to improving the health of all people by incorporating health considerations into decision-making across sectors and policy areas" (Rudolph et al., 2013, p. 5). The development of cross-sector collaborations to support HiAP will depend on an understanding among other sectors of the assets public health can bring to the table (see Box 5-4).

Health Care Providers

The interface between public health agencies and health care providers at the state and local levels is variable. Governmental public health agencies can act in a direct health care delivery role, sometimes running various care delivery systems such as public hospitals, nursing homes, psychiatric and substance abuse centers, rehabilitation hospitals, provider networks, and community health centers. More often, public health agencies with care delivery roles are gap fillers in the community, assisting those in need in accessing services. For example, the public health department may run clinics for the homeless or uninsured. The state or local public health agency may also be the regulatory entity in a given jurisdiction, with authority extending to facilities, health care provider licensing, and other responsibilities.

This close connection between public health and health care delivery systems has myriad implications for pre- and post-disaster public health activities. Disasters place heightened demands on health care services, demands that can also strain public health agencies with health care responsibilities (the role of the health care delivery system in disaster recovery is discussed in depth in Chapter 6). Working to facilitate the restoration of the health care delivery system should be one of the primary responsibilities of public health after a disaster (ASTHO, 2007). Public health agencies may collaborate with health care delivery partners through

---

BOX 5-4
Public Health Sector Assets to Leverage in Disaster
Recovery Planning for Optimal Health Outcomes

In building cross-sector collaboratives for health improvement planning before and after disasters, stakeholders need to be aware of the assets that the public health sector brings to the table. Relevant public health areas of expertise identified by the committee include

- early childhood development;
- data analysis, including use of geographic information systems;
- social network analysis;
- public health and health care economics;
- clinical—chronic and acute disease states;
- epidemiology;
- policy and legislative actions;
- health education;
- preventive medicine;
- public health– and health care–related legal issues;
- ethical issues;
- lead poisoning;
- continuous quality improvement;
- oral health;
- vital statistics;
- immunizations; and
- special-needs populations.

- risk and threat assessments, both community-wide and for specific facilities;
- evaluation of overall community health status;
- evaluation and identification of at-risk/vulnerable populations;
- evaluation of services needed and identification of mechanisms for filling gaps;
- assessment of local capabilities to fulfill ESF #8 responsibilities;
- engagement of the health care system, ideally through local health care coalitions[5] (discussed further in Chapter 6), in healthy community planning, disaster response, and optimal healthy community recovery; and
- collaboration with behavioral health/substance abuse service providers and social services providers.

The federal government has taken steps to promote alignment between preparedness planning conducted by public health and health care systems by jointly awarding PHEP and HPP grants. The goals of this alignment are to promote cross-sector planning, training, and exercising as well as to reduce the administrative burden for grant recipients. This cooperation between sectors can make disaster planning more efficient and the health system more robust and resilient in the face of a disaster. The Patient Protection and Affordable Care Act[6] (ACA) is facilitating increased alignment between the two sectors,

---

[5] Health care coalitions consist of a collaborative network of health care organizations and their respective public and private sector response partners within a defined region. They serve as a multi-agency coordinating group that assists emergency management and Emergency Support Function (ESF) #8 with preparedness, response, recovery, and mitigation activities related to health care organization disaster operations (ASPR, 2012).

[6] The Patient Protection and Affordable Care Act, Public Law 111-148, 111th Cong., H.R.3590 (March 23, 2010).

particularly with regard to the use of population-level data from health information systems to improve surveillance and service delivery (IOM, 2014). Moreover, the ACA requirement that nonprofit hospitals conduct community health needs assessments motivates collaborative efforts with public health agencies that are also conducting such assessments.

Behavioral Health and Social Services Providers

Disasters can cause or exacerbate behavioral health issues, and social services providers can become overwhelmed by the increased need for their services after a disaster. Public health is a natural partner to these sectors because the client populations served by behavioral health and social services correspond closely to the key populations at risk for adverse health outcomes after a disaster (White, 2014). Consequently, collaboration between public health and these sectors can vastly improve the health and well-being of affected individuals and communities after a disaster. In Galveston, Texas, for example, a preexisting and ongoing coalition of the Galveston County Health District, the Gulf Coast Center (the regional mental health authority), and local social services providers proved invaluable when Hurricane Ike struck. After the hurricane, the coalition sprang into action using already-proven methods such as telepsychiatry and mobile crisis response teams to reconnect clients with services, meet mental health needs, and simultaneously help clients apply for needed federal assistance (UTMB, 2011). By collaborating before a disaster strikes, public health, behavioral health, and social services providers can improve the care provided to individuals, share resources, and reduce the burden on individual sectors and organizations.

The following committee recommendations are applicable to this public health priority area:

- **Recommendation 8:** *Develop a National Disaster Behavioral Health Policy.* (see Chapter 7)
- **Recommendation 9:** *Develop an Integrated Social Services Recovery Framework.* (see Chapter 8)

Emergency Management and Public Safety Entities

Emergency managers and emergency medical services/fire departments have key roles in pre-disaster planning and post-disaster coordination (e.g., evacuation, distribution of medical countermeasures). In recent years, homeland security grant programs such as the Metropolitan Medical Response System and Urban Area Security Initiative programs have been integral in promoting better integration of local emergency management, public health, and medical systems (e.g., health care coalitions). In addition to their responsibilities for ensuring the safety of people and property, law enforcement agencies are also increasingly involved in health care response and recovery planning groups and are often employed in specific roles supporting the public health and health care sectors after a disaster, such as distribution of cached supplies and security for the receipt and movement of medical materials from federal stockpiles. As a critical early component of the community planning process, emergency managers and public safety agencies may partner with public health and health care stakeholders to develop hazard or threat vulnerability analyses.[7] These assessments are integral in identifying and prioritizing issues for planners.

During the early recovery period, public safety personnel are key partners in outreach efforts to inform the public on such issues as avoiding health and safety threats and scams. The relationships forged between public health officials and emergency management/public safety entities during preparedness activities related to response planning can be leveraged to ensure that public health is also engaged in recovery planning.

---

[7] Hazard or threat vulnerability analysis is a "systematic approach to identifying all hazards [and threats] that may affect an organization, assessing the risk (probability of hazard or threat occurrence and the consequence for the organization) associated with each hazard [or threat] and analyzing findings to create a prioritized comparison of hazard [and threat] vulnerabilities. The consequence, or vulnerability, is related to both the impact on organizational function and the likely service demands created by hazard [or threat] impact" (HHS, 2007, p. D-6).

Recreational and Natural Resources Organizations

Public health and recreational/natural resources organizations have cross-cutting areas of interest and can be partners in the creation of healthier communities through the development and maintenance of community features that promote active living, such as bike and walking paths, as well as green spaces community members can use to congregate. These kinds of projects (e.g., trails) may fall within the Natural and Cultural Resources RSF of the NDRF, but public health organizations can support their implementation through advocacy efforts and active partnerships between public health and recreational professionals and by providing data to support the strategic placement of resources so as decrease health disparities.

Environmental Health Agencies

Governmental environmental health agencies can be housed within the state or local public health department or may be separate entities. In either case, the two must work in partnership to assess the interrelationships between people and their environment and to foster a safe and healthy environment. Cross-cutting functions include monitoring to identify and mitigate health threats from adulterated food and poor water and air quality, disease vectors, and pests. In partnership with the housing sector, public health and environmental health agencies may also play a role in mitigating health risks (e.g., mold, debris) for recovery workers and homeowners involved in cleaning and reconstruction of housing (see Chapter 10) and other indoor environments. Given the potential negative impacts of disasters on environmental quality (both indoor and outdoor), respective roles and responsibilities of these two sectors, as well as mechanisms for their collaboration, should be discussed as part of pre-disaster planning. A process for joint operations, such as health assessments and risk identification and enforcement, during the response and recovery phases should be in place.

Planning and Community Development Entities

Health concerns are increasingly falling within the purview of urban and regional planning departments (e.g., climate change-related issues) and the public health field has discovered the power of comprehensive plans and other planning tools for altering the physical and social environments that impact health. Partnerships with urban and regional planning agencies are critical to ensuring that a healthy community vision and health improvement priorities are incorporated into the community's strategic (comprehensive) plan (see Recommendation 1 in Chapter 3). These partnerships can then be leveraged during recovery to ensure that the health implications of planning decisions are considered through such mechanisms as health impact assessments (discussed in Chapter 3).

Partnerships with community development organizations also represent important opportunities to create physical and social environments that better support health and, in particular, to address health equity issues. The community development enterprise is a network of governmental, nongovernmental, and private organizations (e.g., banks, real estate investors) working together to transform impoverished, blighted neighborhoods and improve quality of life and economic security for low- and middle-income individuals by investing in affordable housing and access to community services and amenities (e.g., child care centers, health clinics, grocery stores, charter schools). As with other sectors, public health can offer data to inform these investments and can help promote initiatives that benefit low- and middle-income populations by making explicit links to potential health impacts. Community development agencies often have a key role in disaster recovery as HUD Community Development Block Grants have become a more common vehicle for providing funding for recovery assistance.

According to a RWJF report, collaboration between the health sector and community development organizations is already fairly widespread (Mattessich and Rausch, 2013). In a survey of 661 professionals in health and community development fields, nearly half of the respondents reported successful cross-sector initiatives on such issues as physical activity, access to health care, and promotion of a culture of health and wellness. However, barriers to the development of these relationships remain. Two-thirds of respondents said that "inadequate funding and resources" was a major barrier, while more than half stated that a "lack of shared vision and common goals" prevented successful cross-sector collaboration (Mattessich and Rausch, 2013). Eighty-six percent of respondents cited an absence of pre-existing relationships and communication with potential partners as a barrier (Mattessich and Rausch, 2013)—perhaps pointing to an opportunity for conveners to promote these collaborations by bringing the health and community development sectors together for recovery planning.

Nongovernmental Organizations and the Business Community

A number of nongovernmental organizations, including community-based nonprofits and academic institutions, play important roles in the public health system, providing health services, training and education, and research capacity, among others. During and after a disaster, nongovernmental organizations and businesses provide invaluable assistance to the community. In the immediate aftermath of a disaster, community organizations that are already integrated into the community can step in to meet immediate needs such as shelter and food (The Alliance for a Just Rebuilding et al., 2014). This local mobilization of resources is particularly important when government is slow to respond or when outside help has not yet arrived. Private businesses assist by ensuring that individuals have access to medications and supplies. CVS Caremark, for example, assisted communities during Hurricane Sandy by setting up mobile pharmacies and delivering prescriptions to stranded customers (CVS Caremark, 2014). Public–private partnerships have enabled Wi-Fi access in shelters and recovery centers to help survivors seek help and connect with their social networks (Morton and Lurie, 2013). This type of collaboration among public health, nongovernmental organizations, and the business community can help reduce disparities in health outcomes following a disaster by accessing difficult-to-reach populations and providing services and supplies to all in need.

Building these partnerships in the pre-disaster phase is critical to ensuring that they are utilized to the fullest extent possible should a disaster occur. In Iowa, for example, the Safeguard Iowa Partnership was created in response to a concern that private-sector businesses wanted to assist during disasters but lacked an organized means for doing so (Beardsley, 2014). The Safeguard Iowa Partnership is an ongoing collaboration between private- and public-sector organizations that leverages community resources by facilitating the donation of private-sector resources and expertise to disaster response and recovery efforts (Beardsley, 2014; FEMA, n.d.). The Safeguard Iowa Partnership played a key role in promoting the sharing of both information and resources following flooding in Iowa in 2008 and again in 2013 (Safeguard Iowa Partnership, 2013).

PRE-DISASTER PUBLIC HEALTH SECTOR PRIORITIES

The best opportunity for improving community health beyond pre-disaster levels following a disaster arises when key elements are in place before a disaster to inform recovery efforts. As indicated during testimony to the committee by one state public health official, "to bring those types of issues up to a community that's still reeling from a disaster, it would not be well received" (Clements, 2014). Thus, as discussed in Chapter 3, community health improvement goals need to be incorporated into recovery planning prior to a disaster. The key elements that need to be in place for recovery planning include community health assessments, community health improvement plans, and health department strategic plans. These elements are also prerequisites for national accreditation of health departments (PHAB, 2012); however, few communities have linked these existing processes with preparedness activities, even though they can help identify opportunities to build resiliency and improve community health in recovery. Siloing of public health roles and responsibilities, particularly for public health preparedness (Duncan et al., 2007), has impeded integration of community health improvement and recovery planning, resulting in less than optimal health outcomes after disasters.

There are several reasons why it is challenging for communities to make pre-disaster plans that include opportunities to improve health in the recovery process. First, from a community standpoint, the focus is generally on immediate disaster response and on recovery as a means of returning to normalcy. Recovery as a means of creating a healthier community is a years-long process that for some communities is too far down the road to be a focus (Shah, 2014). Second, federal funding for disaster preparedness does not make long-term community health improvement a priority. The PHEP guidance on the Community Recovery capability, for example, has three foci: identify the recovery needs of health systems, coordinate recovery of these systems, and mitigate damages from future incidents. As James Blumenstock, the chief program officer for public health practice at the Association of State and Territorial Health Officials (ASTHO), pointed out, what is missing is an emphasis on making the community better and healthier in the recovery process (Blumenstock, 2014). Finally, public health professionals may not be engaged in pre-disaster recovery planning; thus, their perspective on long-term recovery is not reflected in the recovery plans.

The committee identified four key pre-disaster priorities in which the public health sector should be engaged to support implementation of the recommendations in this report and to ensure better short- and long-term health outcomes after a disaster:

- Conduct community health assessments.
- Engage community stakeholders in pre-disaster community health improvement and recovery planning.
- Ensure that public health community programs and services are integrated into healthy community and disaster recovery planning processes.
- Leverage pre-disaster preparedness activities in recovery planning.

The following discussion of the operational aspects of these activities, along with some best practices and other examples, is not exhaustive but is intended to be generalizable across a multitude of environments. In each case, there are opportunities to capitalize on traditional, preexisting public health programs, relationships, and resources.

Conduct Community Health Assessments

As discussed in earlier chapters, to optimally leverage disaster recovery-related opportunities to build healthier communities, health improvement goals must be integrated into pre-disaster recovery plans. The health improvement planning process should be informed by an assessment of community health status and needs. Monitoring of population health status is an essential public health function (see Table 5-2); public health departments continually collect, analyze, interpret, and report on community health needs and indicators. Commonly collected surveillance data include disease prevalence as well as individual and community risk factors and gaps in health care delivery (Salinsky, 2010). This type of information is incorporated into the community health assessment (sometimes called a community health needs assessment)— "a systematic examination of the health status indicators for a given population that is used to identify key problems and assets in a community" (PHAB, 2011, p. 8) (see also the discussion of community health assessments in Chapter 3). Assessment data can be used to prioritize interventions and provide a baseline against which change can be measured (Barnett, 2012).

Conducting community health assessments is one of the Public Health Accreditation Board's prerequisites for accreditation (PHAB, 2013). Nonprofit hospitals, under provisions of the ACA, are now required by the Internal Revenue Service to perform these assessments as well (IRS, 2013). A collaboration between these hospitals and their state and local health departments is desirable in completing these assessments so as to identify the most comprehensive data sets and the elements necessary to improve the health of the community (NACCHO, 2012). Community health assessments have traditionally been separate from assessments related to disaster planning, which have historically focused on ensuring that ESF #8 functions are in place. This separation is due in part to compartmentalization of public health services.

A number of tools are available to guide a community health assessment (and the subsequent community health improvement planning process). Examples include Mobilizing for Action through Planning and Partnerships (MAPP) and the Community Commons Community Health Needs Assessment Toolkit. MAPP, a framework designed by the National Association of City and County Health Officials (NACCHO), uses a six-phase process (organizing, visioning, assessments, strategic issues, goals/strategies, and action cycle) that focuses on community engagement and participation throughout (NACCHO, 2014b). For each phase, MAPP resources available on the NACCHO website[8] suggest recommended participants and describe each step in that phase. The Community Health Needs Assessment Toolkit is an online tool that brings publicly available data together in one place so users can find and compare data on health indicators within and across communities (Community Commons, 2014a). Users can create printable maps or reports on the indicators and communities they have chosen, or they can run a report on their community that includes preselected indicators (Community Commons, 2014b). The toolkit pulls data from numerous sources, including the CDC, *Healthy People 2020*, and the Health Resources and Services Administration (Community Commons, 2014a).

Disaster recovery necessitates a process of decision making regarding the use of scarce resources. In the competition for resources, entities that can present a strong position using convincing data and arguments stand to benefit (Smith, 2011). Health assessment data that public health officials are already collecting and analyzing can inform decision making during pre- and post-disaster recovery planning by providing pre-disaster baseline information on health status and identifying gaps in services, communities at risk, and strengths and resources in the community. Public health can use these data to help focus recovery efforts on at-risk populations and "winnable battles" that have a large impact on health and known, effective solutions (CDC, 2014c). Public health professionals have skills in data collection and analysis that can be valuable assets during recovery planning efforts. One of public health's core capabilities is data collection from multiple sources, including but not limited to health care providers, statistics on chronic disease, vital statistics (births, deaths, causes of death), information on utilization of programs such as Medicaid and WIC, community surveys, and geographic information systems. Public health professionals have experience in analyzing these data and creating reports, or in providing data to various organizations and agencies for purposes of research, grant making, and community and state decision making.

Interdisciplinary relationships established during broad stakeholder engagement in community health assessments or through data sharing arrangements (e.g., between public health and community-based organizations that require data for grant applications) also are valuable assets that can be leveraged during recovery planning. In many jurisdictions, however, public health's data collection and relationship building currently are not being carried out with disaster recovery in mind. As a result, opportunities to use these data and relationships to make a strong case for investing in healthier communities are being missed.

Engage Community Stakeholders in Pre-Disaster Community Health Improvement and Recovery Planning

Based on the pre-disaster community health assessment, a community health improvement plan should be developed. A community health improvement plan is a "long-term, systematic effort to address public health problems on the basis of the results of community health assessment activities and the community health improvement process" (PHAB, 2011, p. 8). Through a broad-based community stakeholder consensus-building process, agreement should be reached on the elements of a healthy community and the strategies for achieving this goal. Integrating these strategies into the community health improvement plan creates a road map for closing the gap between the current health assessment and the optimal healthy community. The development of a community health improvement plan utilizes many of the essential capabilities of the public health sector: mobilizing community partnerships; developing plans and policies that aid health improvement efforts; and educating and empowering the community with respect to health issues.

---

[8] Information on the MAPP process is available at http://www.naccho.org/topics/infrastructure/mapp/framework/index.cfm (accessed April 10, 2015).

To be successful, health improvement planning needs to move beyond the health sector. Public health stakeholders should participate in broader strategic community planning for healthy places to live, work, learn, and play. As discussed in Chapter 2, integration of health improvement plans with a community's comprehensive plan and recovery plan can better ensure uptake and resourcing of public health goals before and after a disaster (see Recommendation 1 in Chapter 3). Table 5-3 shows steps public health stakeholders can take to ensure that health considerations are incorporated into the comprehensive planning process (APA, 2006).

At the same time, the development of cross-sector partnerships, including public-private partnerships and partnerships with local planning, transportation, and housing departments and others, is critical since the public health sector typically does not design or build a community's physical environment. Thus, a Health in All Policies approach is well suited to steady-state community planning and disaster recovery planning alike. In fact, recovery can accelerate the adoption of HiAP (Stevenson et al., 2014). A case study on how the disaster recovery process has enabled public health leadership in Canterbury, New Zealand, to "leapfrog" to an enduring HiAP approach is presented in Chapter 2 (see Box 2-10). However, as noted in the testimony of James Blumenstock, although current ASTHO educational materials and position statements on HiAP are relevant to post-disaster recovery, "there is absolutely no reference to post-disaster recovery as an opportunity or an issue or a circumstance where Health in All Policies needs to apply. No examples, no case studies, no verbiage basically linking the two" (Blumenstock, 2014). This is a gap that professional public health organizations (governmental and nongovernmental) need to address in the near term. Doing so will require a significant continued effort to educate health sector and nonhealth sector stakeholders, including the general public, on the value of HiAP and such tools as health impact assessments. This upfront investment can pay off in the event of a disaster. As discussed in the Galveston Health in All Policies case study in Chapter 2 (see Box 2-11), the time required to conduct such health literacy efforts after a disaster can significantly delay progress toward the building of healthier and more resilient and sustainable communities (Nolen, 2014).

The incorporation of health improvement goals from the health improvement plan into the recovery plan should be guided by an advisory committee for the Health and Social Services RSF (see Box 5-5). This advisory committee should have clear roles within the overarching organizational structure for recovery decision making, consistent with the principles of the NDRF. Public health officials should be heavily involved in the process, and individuals familiar with local community health programs and activities should be represented on the committee. The advisory committee may or may not have the same composition as the group leading a community health improvement planning process but should, in collaboration with emergency management and urban and regional planning agency officials, identify opportunities to advance toward a healthier and more resilient community should a disaster strike.

The following committee recommendations are applicable to this public health priority area:

- Recommendation 1: *Develop a Healthy Community Vision for Disaster Recovery.* (see Chapter 3)
- Recommendation 2: *Integrate Health Considerations into Recovery Decision Making Through the National Disaster Recovery Framework.* (see Chapter 3)
- Recommendation 3: *Facilitate the Engagement of the Whole Community in Disaster Recovery Through Simplified and Accessible Information and Training.* (see Chapter 3)

Ensure That Public Health Community Programs and Services Are Integrated into Healthy Community and Disaster Recovery Planning Processes

The programs and services that are the foundational care functions of public health—for example, creation of programs for prevention and education, disease control measures for outbreaks, immunizations, and direct health care provision and referrals to services—all are critical tools for health protection and promotion during post-disaster recovery. After disasters, demand for public health organizations to carry out these routine health functions surges concurrently with new responsibilities related to emergency

TABLE 5-3 Public Health Roles in the Comprehensive Planning Process

Comprehensive Plan Action	Public Health Agency Role
Step 1: Visioning and Goal Setting	
• Engage the public and stakeholders; discuss community goals and values • Refine and articulate a vision for the future • Set goals and priorities • Establish plan scope	• Attend, initiate, or facilitate visioning sessions • Familiarize public health staff with planning process and potential roles for health • Educate planners on role of public health in planning • Recommend inclusion of a Health Element and/or health goals in the plan • Chair or participate in plan committees, work groups
Step 2: Data Collection and Needs Assessment	
• Collect data, track trends, conduct capacity studies, etc. • Survey the public, hold forums and hearings • Use GIS to map needs • Analyze needs and address how to meet them	• Provide health data and statistics to planners, stakeholders, and decision makers • Attend planning and zoning meetings • Disseminate information to the public, including "real-life" stories • Introduce Health Impact Assessment (HIA) options (e.g., walkability audit)
Step 3: Drafting the Plan	
• Use technical data and community input to form plan policies that meet established goals • Develop alternative growth scenarios • Develop implementation strategies reflecting costs and potential funding sources • Make plan available for public comment • Hold hearings on final draft plan, formal adoption by governing body	• Continue participation in the plan preparation process; comment on health concerns • Provide decision makers with model or sample functional plans (i.e., pedestrian plan, housing plan) that address health • Encourage citizens to use comment time to address health concerns • Attend planning and zoning meetings • Appoint or elect public health officials to decision-making boards
Step 4: Adoption and Implementation	
• Plan goes to legislative body for adoption • Plan serves as a guide to future land use decisions • Additional functional plans are prepared (i.e., pedestrian plans) • Plan is implemented through schedule set forth in the plan	• Be an advocate for adoption of the plan if it meets health goals • Take responsibility for implementation of health goals, or work to keep them as a priority • Review development proposals for health aspects • Attend public planning and zoning meetings
Step 5: Revise Development Regulations and Evaluate Plan Performance	
• Revise zoning and subdivision regulations to be consistent with the new plan • Support rezoning initiatives when applicable • Schedule public investments (e.g., streetscape improvements, housing upgrades) • Monitor plan implementation using benchmarks and indicators	• Provide decision makers with model zoning codes, comprehensive plans, and land use ordinances that relate to public health • Support rezoning initiatives when applicable • Attend planning and zoning meetings

SOURCE: Copyright 2006 by the American Planning Association. Reprinted by permission.

BOX 5-5
Promising Practice: Recovery Support Function Advisory Committees

Recovery Support Functions under the National Disaster Recovery Framework are designed to support and supplement local disaster recovery efforts. These local efforts can be strengthened by the creation of local advisory committees. The Health and Social Services advisory committee should be charged with collaborating with emergency management and planning agency officials on the integration of the community health improvement plan into disaster recovery planning. The advisory committee should identify opportunities to improve the overall health status of the community after a disaster. It should exercise flexibility and responsiveness to input from an ongoing assessment process, adjust the recovery plan accordingly, and continuously gauge movement toward implementation of the elements essential for improved community health. The opportunities identified by the advisory committee need to be integrated into the recovery plan framework for the community to advance toward a healthier and more resilient community should a disaster strike.

These types of advisory committees are already in development in some communities. Florida's Hillsborough County has created a Post-Disaster Redevelopment Plan (PDRP) to guide long-term recovery. Eight voluntary Technical Advisory Committees (TACs) on such topics as environmental restoration, housing recovery, and health and social services form the backbone of the PDRP. The TACs coordinate on issues that overlap. The Health and Social Services TAC focuses on meeting the health, social services, and public safety needs of the population after a disaster, and ensuring a smooth transition from short-term recovery to long-term redevelopment. Examples of organizations that may serve on the Health and Social Services TAC include the health department, the school district, health care providers, the Red Cross, and advocates for homeless or disabled residents (Hillsborough County Government, 2010). Similarly, in Fairfax County, Virginia, the Pre-Disaster Recovery Plan includes a provision for the establishment of subcommittees that would advise on areas of subject-matter expertise, such as housing or community services, should a disaster occur. These subcommittees might meet on an ongoing or ad hoc basis, and could coordinate regional issues or provide a venue for public input on recovery. They might include residents of the county as well as outside experts from academia, government, or nongovernmental organizations (Fairfax County, 2012).

---

operations (Klitzman and Freudenberg, 2003). Inability to meet this increased demand for ongoing public health services will have adverse effects on population-level health outcomes; therefore, strengthening these programs before a disaster will pay dividends should such an event occur.

As discussed earlier in this chapter, the community-based programs and services of the public health sector (e.g., health care delivery clinics, immunizations, nutrition and food services, wellness programs, home care, education programs) vary greatly by community depending on needs, authorities, and resources. These existing programs and services provide an interface to the community and can be leveraged to identify gaps and populations at risk and to educate and mobilize the community to develop a vision for health. Relationships with community partners involved in public health programs (e.g., social services, behavioral health) can be used to integrate these groups into disaster recovery planning.

The following committee recommendation is applicable to this public health priority area:

- **Recommendation 4:** *Enhance and Leverage Social Networks in Community Health Improvement and Recovery Planning.* (see Chapter 3)

Leverage Pre-Disaster Preparedness Activities in Recovery Planning

Much public health pre-disaster planning takes place under the guidance of the PHEP cooperative agreement, administered by the CDC. PHEP funding is provided to state public health departments (with a few exceptions) to help communities become more resilient and better prepared to respond to disasters. The CDC releases guidance on how PHEP awardees should use the funding (CDC, 2011). The 15 public health preparedness capabilities are split into two tiers. Tier 1, the highest-priority activities, includes Community Preparedness, Public Health Surveillance and Epidemiological Investigation, and Public Health Laboratory Testing. Tier 2 includes Medical Surge, Fatality Management, and Community Recovery (CDC, 2011). This prioritization—with Community Recovery in the bottom tier—demonstrates the lack of emphasis on disaster recovery during preparedness planning. Further, not only is Community Recovery a low priority, it is also currently defined in terms of systems recovery rather than overall community health: "the ability to collaborate with community partners ... for the rebuilding of public health, medical, and mental/behavioral health systems to at least a level of functioning comparable to pre-incident levels, and improved levels where possible" (CDC, 2011, p.10).

The lack of emphasis on recovery is further demonstrated in data on actual preparedness activities carried out by PHEP awardees. More than one-third of grantees (37 percent) reported that they had not undertaken any kind of activities related to the Community Recovery capability. Fewer than half (45 percent) had begun the process of recovery planning but were in early stages of identifying community partners or holding training meetings.[9] Recovery—particularly long-term recovery—is simply not a priority for many public health officials during disaster preparedness planning. As the President of the International Association of Emergency Managers, Bruce Lockwood, emphasized, "We were allowed to bullet vote at the public health advisory meeting as to which capabilities were our priorities. Where do you think recovery ended up? It is at the bottom of the list" (Lockwood, 2014).

PHEP funding offers an opportunity to support integration of health into recovery planning both horizontally (across sectors) and vertically. Despite the lack of emphasis on recovery in PHEP grant-related activities, myriad other preparedness efforts are directly linked to the recovery process and can be leveraged for that purpose. Some examples are described below.

Community preparedness (PHEP Capability 1) encompasses cross-disciplinary processes that include the development of plans, training exercises, and participation in coalitions. These activities are where relationships are built and agencies are exposed to each other's capabilities and challenges. Under the Community Recovery function, PHEP guidance encourages the development of community partnerships in order to identify the health system needs after a disaster and to coordinate the provision of services and health systems recovery. However, partnerships developed for community preparedness purposes can and should be utilized in recovery planning as well (see the example in Box 5-6).

Enhancement of the information-sharing environment (PHEP Capabilities 3 and 6) includes public information and warning as well as information sharing among agencies. Exploiting preexisting channels of communication can accelerate recovery planning at any stage. Having technology and data systems in place that allow for patient monitoring at a time when basic infrastructure may be compromised may prove critical, especially for vulnerable populations (Zucker, 2014). Based on experiences during Hurricane Sandy, for example, New York State accelerated development of its eFINDS system, a patient tracking system that had been initiated before the disaster and uses barcodes on wristbands to track patients evacuated from state-regulated and state-run medical and adult care facilities (Zucker, 2014). Electronic health records also may be lifesaving, providing up-to-date information on medications, such as those for older adults and people with psychiatric disorders, as well as information on individuals who may have mobility issues or may be homebound. Systems that allow for quick and systemic identification of those requiring medical devices and specialized equipment and treatment may also be critical. Although there may be concerns regarding Health Insurance Portability and Accountability Act (HIPAA) protections, a

---

[9] E-mail communication, C. Singleton, Centers for Disease Control and Prevention, to A. Downey, Institute of Medicine, regarding a request for information on PHEP recovery capability, October 6, 2014.

BOX 5-6
Los Angeles County Community Disaster Resilience Project

The Los Angeles County Community Disaster Resilience (LACCDR) project is intended to promote community resilience in the event of a disaster. The project defines community resilience as "the capacity of the community as a whole to prepare for, respond to, and recover from adverse events and unanticipated crises that threaten the health of all" (LACCDR, 2014; Plough et al., 2013). To foster community resilience, public and private community-based organizations work together in preparedness, response, and recovery planning activities, seeking to focus disaster planning not solely on individual preparedness but more broadly on community preparedness and social connections. The project's message is that community resilience is about "transforming disaster planning and response from just 'me' to include 'we'" (LACCDR, 2014). The project is a collaborative venture supported by the Centers for Disease Control and Prevention (CDC), the National Institute of Mental Health, and the Robert Wood Johnson Foundation. The project is an outgrowth of awareness that the absence of sustainable engagement with community organizations hampered recovery from Hurricane Katrina, the H1N1 pandemic of 2009, and Hurricane Sandy and explained the disparities between communities that recovered successfully and those that did not (Plough et al., 2013).

One of the LACCDR project's first activities was to survey health department staff and community organizations to identify barriers to and facilitators of resilience building. The survey revealed that minimal time was devoted to community resilience and emergency preparedness, even though many populations in the community stood to benefit from such efforts (Chandra et al., 2013). Building upon the results of this survey, the project is undertaking the following five activities: (1) improving the community engagement skills of Los Angeles County health department staff to enable them to build sustainable multisector community partnerships; (2) developing a best practices and resilience curriculum for engagement of county health department staff with community organizations; (3) creating a resilience toolkit for use by community organizations in building coalitions that increase community preparedness; (4) developing a countywide media campaign around the theme of "Just Be Ready" in order to encourage social connectivity (i.e., "Know your neighbors. Plan together. Be ready."); and (5) identifying metrics for gauging whether the LACCDR project has successfully achieved community resilience, including a social network analysis tool called "PARTNER" that measures and monitors collaboration among people and organizations (Plough et al., 2013).

2014 bulletin from HHS's Office for Civil Rights, *HIPAA Privacy in Emergency Situations*, notes that "the HIPAA Privacy Rule protects the privacy of patients' health information (protected health information) but is balanced to ensure that appropriate uses and disclosures of the information still may be made when necessary to treat a patient, to protect the nation's public health, and for other critical purposes" (HHS, 2014b, p. 1). According to the bulletin, the Privacy Rule allows for disclosure of protected health information to a public health authority (federal, state, or local) as necessary to carry out its public health mission. For example, Medicare claims data recently were used in an emergency preparedness drill to identify locations of individuals who rely on electricity-dependent medical equipment, a key vulnerable population. The data were securely transmitted to the local health department. The success of this model depends on having appropriate protocols and privacy protections in place in advance of a disaster, as well as on local capabilities to receive and manage the data for preparedness purposes (DeSalvo et al., 2014).

Emergency operations center operations and surge (medical, fatality, mass care, volunteers) management (PHEP Capabilities 3, 5, 7, 9, 10) require evaluation and coordination of resources (including human resources) both vertically and horizontally. The knowledge and relationships built in developing these capabilities form the basis for initiating recovery planning discussions. An example of pre-disaster surge preparedness is the development of local and regional Medical Reserve Corps (MRCs), disaster medical assistance teams (DMATs), and other medical teams to be deployed in the immediate aftermath of a disaster. In many cases, a disaster prompts a generous outpouring of volunteerism from the medical community across the country. The MRC and DMAT models give volunteer health professionals access to specific disaster-related training and provide pre-event credentialing, both of which are equally important to response and recovery efforts.

Additional activities pivotal to public health pre-disaster planning take place under the guidance of the HPP, which, as noted earlier, is administered by ASPR within HHS. These activities, detailed in Chapter 6, require engagement of state and local public health agencies in planning, training, and exercise events with partners from the health care delivery sector, often in the context of health care coalitions.

THE CONTINUUM OF POST-DISASTER PUBLIC HEALTH RESPONSE AND RECOVERY PRIORITIES

Early recovery and response operations need to begin concurrently (ASTHO, 2007), and in fact, the effectiveness of the response to a disaster can significantly impact the trajectory of recovery. The most pressing issues typically facing a community during and immediately following a disaster are ensuring the immediate safety and security of those present and the continuity of essential services. Coordination among stakeholders during this period should occur through ongoing operation of an incident command system that allows for active participation in public health recovery activities by social services agencies, behavioral health agencies, volunteer organizations, the medical examiner/coroner, mass sheltering organizations, and businesses and organizations regulated by the public health department. Steps necessary to ensure safety and continuity of services are discussed in the following sections. As circumstances change during response and then throughout recovery, however, opportunities to invest in changes that will strengthen resiliency and add those elements of a healthy community that may previously have been absent ought to be actively pursued.

Some jurisdictions may require an emergency declaration to assist with various aspects of response and recovery. In some cases, the use of certain stockpiles or procedures or even funding may be tied to the issuance of an emergency declaration. Such declarations may be made at various levels of government, making available resources held at that level for emergency use. A presidential declaration is necessary to activate federal reimbursement funding for specific emergencies covered under the Stafford Act (see Chapter 4).

Post-disaster response and early recovery priorities for public health include

- participating in a shared communication effort;
- conducting impact assessments of the community's health and medical needs;
- reestablishing critical public health infrastructure;
- delivering public health services to meet post-disaster needs of the community; and
- providing support to impacted health care delivery systems.

There are also a number of priorities for which efforts may be initiated in the short-term post-disaster period but will extend into long-term recovery. These include

- facilitating health-informed recovery decision making through data;
- engaging in health-informed community rebuilding and redevelopment planning; and
- sharing lessons learned with other communities to improve disaster recovery planning.

EARLY POST-DISASTER PUBLIC HEALTH RECOVERY PRIORITIES

Participating in a Shared Communication Effort

During disaster response and recovery, clear and bidirectional communication within and across sectors and with the public is critical to providing needed health-related information and preventing further illness or injury. Coordination of communication efforts across sectors should be conducted within the structure of a joint information system. Emergency management officials often lead shared communication efforts, but the joint information system should include spokespersons from all major agencies to make it possible to develop, maintain, and disseminate a coordinated message; manage media inquiries and press conferences; and ensure that early and accurate information is provided to the public. The joint information system may or may not have a formal physical location but must provide capabilities for message review, conference calls, and secure communications between agencies. As the event unfolds and the transition from response to recovery begins, the communication methods used must be sustainable throughout.

When communicating with the public, the health sector (including public health, health care, behavioral health) and social services providers should focus on messaging, education, and outreach. Communication about the health risks of a disaster and how to prevent further injury and illness can be accomplished through such channels as press releases, interviews with experts, and news conferences. Disaster-related communications should be written and designed to ensure that the general public can comprehend the basic health information necessary to make appropriate health-related decisions.

The use and monitoring of social media during disaster response and recovery are increasingly important functions for public health agencies. The use of preestablished social media outlets to provide messaging to followers (e.g., Facebook and Twitter) is now a common vehicle for communication. Monitoring social media is critical to identify trends and discredit false rumors that can be detrimental to successful response and recovery activities or even pose a danger to the public and responders (Knearl, 2014).

In addition to social media and more traditional media venues, public health officials should consider using community partners to help reach the public, especially vulnerable populations. A best practice is to identify in advance of a disaster those community partners that serve vulnerable populations, faith-based groups, and other culturally unique populations. These partners can serve as agents of the public health entity, providing a trusted source of information and visible leaders who can translate public health messaging in linguistically and culturally appropriate ways using their unique access to their constituents. In King County, Washington, for example, public health officials learned to use community partners to reach out to immigrant populations after a storm-related power outage in 2006 resulted in eight carbon monoxide poisoning fatalities and scores of hospital admissions when people used grills indoors for heat. In a similar outage in 2012, when public health officials used communication channels suggested by their community partners—including flyers in multiple languages and robo-calls from a mosque—carbon monoxide poisoning was reduced by 90 percent and caused no fatalities (NRC, 2012).

Within the health sector, a well-designed health information technology recovery plan can help ensure continued access to health information such as vital records, immunization records, and medical histories. Information-sharing systems can help health care systems share resources and manage capacity; the Hospital Available Beds for Emergencies and Disasters (HAvBED) system, for example, tracks available hospital beds in real time to facilitate management of a surge in patients during a large-scale disaster (AHRQ, 2005). Likewise, the CDC's Health Alert Network can keep public health practitioners and clinicians up to date on ongoing or emerging threats to public health (CDC, 2014a).

Conducting Impact Assessments on the Community's Health and Medical Needs

A critical post-disaster task for the public health sector is to conduct an assessment of the immediate health and medical needs of the impacted community. This process needs to be rapid, flexible, and data driven, with a focus on actively seeking opportunities to strengthen community resiliency and health.

The information gathered, along with any relevant pre-disaster assessment data (e.g., from a community health assessment), is then used to inform planning efforts and forms the basis for resource and funding requests. As indicated in Figure 5-1 presented earlier, assessment is part of a continuous feedback loop. A multidisciplinary task force (such as the advisory committee discussed previously in Box 5-5) should be responsible for recommending course corrections based on the most recent data gathered through the ongoing assessment process throughout recovery.

The following committee recommendation is applicable to this public health priority:

- **Recommendation 5:** *Establish Pathways by Which Health Information Can Inform Recovery Decision Making.* (see Chapter 3)

Reestablishing Critical Public Health Infrastructure

In the aftermath of a disaster that compromises public health capabilities, it is critical for services to be restored as soon as possible, even in a degraded mode (e.g., paper rather than computerized forms). To this end, it is important to have a robust continuity of operations plan and/or continuity of government plan with pre-identified mission-essential functions, alternative work sites, vendors and suppliers, and backup systems. Such a plan should, when possible, identify primary, secondary, and tertiary alternative locations that include at a minimum sanitation facilities, parking, adequate work and rest spaces, and backup electricity/phones/computers. Emergency procurement procedures should be identified to enable the agency to obtain the necessary goods and services. The agency succession process should be activated if needed to ensure that key leadership roles are filled. Access to vital records is imperative during the immediate response to a disaster and during recovery. Methods of operation for a vital records agency may be severely degraded in a disaster, requiring the development of plans for keeping records intact and secure and for distributing and collecting information in a degraded mode when necessary.

Once an agency has identified its emergency needs related to reconstitution and recovery, numerous sources of human capital can be called upon to increase workforce capacity. These sources include federal or state assistance (such as the Emergency Management Assistance Compact), temporary employees, volunteers, the Medical Reserve Corps, and contracted employees or agencies. Recent legislative changes under the reauthorization of the Pandemic and All Hazards Preparedness Act (PAHPA)[10] have mitigated some of the legal and logistical barriers that previously impeded deployment of local public health personnel funded through federal grants for alternative functions during a disaster. If licensed personnel, certified personnel, or those with special skills are used to augment public health recovery resources, care should be taken to verify their credentials and skills before deployment. Disaster response plans should include provisions for the licensing and certification of incoming volunteer resources in two categories: those that are planned and those that are spontaneous.

Delivering Public Health Services to Meet Post-Disaster Needs of the Community

In addition to the essential services provided during steady-state times, a number of services must be ensured by the public health sector in the aftermath of a disaster. These services are described below.

Environmental Services

In a post-disaster community, ensuring the safety of food and water is a critical function of public health. If a disaster involves flooding or power outages, there is the risk that food and water supplies will be contaminated or spoiled. Mass feeding operations, such as at shelters, must be inspected for proper

---

[10] Pandemic and All-Hazards Preparedness Reauthorization Act of 2013, Public Law 113-5, 113th Cong., H.R.307 (March 13, 2013).

food handling and storage to prevent the spread of foodborne illness. To monitor the safety of food and water, public health laboratories must have the capacity to test samples and obtain results reasonably quickly. Public health agencies should take appropriate actions to protect the public when contamination is suspected, and they should coordinate their food and water safety efforts with media outreach to ensure the confidence of the public. Disaster impact assessments should address potential releases of toxins, radiation, or other hazards into the environment (both indoors and outdoors). Public health agencies should work with municipal and private water and sewer systems and environmental protection agencies to ensure environmental health.

Fatality Management

Public health involvement in fatality management will vary by jurisdiction. Typical public health support for fatality management may include providing or coordinating the receipt of supplies, as well as facilitating federal efforts such as the disaster mortuary operational response team (DMORT). Public health agencies may also be involved in the coordination of assets and processes for identification, storage, embalming, and interment of remains. Public health laboratories may be needed for these efforts. Usually, public health coordinates with the local medical examiner or coroner and the local emergency management agency on mass fatality issues. Agencies should be well versed in their roles as assigned by their local fatality management plan.

Access and Functional Needs Populations

In all post-disaster efforts, public health should consider individuals with access and functional needs and the community-based agencies that serve them. Individuals with access and functional needs include but are not limited to people with disabilities that affect their ability to function independently without assistance, women in late stages of pregnancy, children and the elderly, non-English speakers, and people needing special medical equipment (FEMA, 2010). All planning for recovery operations should take into account these populations, and public health should consider taking a lead role in coordinating volunteer and advocacy groups to ensure that recovery efforts are meeting their needs. For example, public health should be part of a multisector task force on interim and temporary housing to ensure that access needs are addressed.

Providing Support to Impacted Health Care Delivery Systems

Working with other community stakeholders (e.g., emergency management), public health agencies can facilitate the recovery of a jurisdiction's health care system through a variety of activities. Most jurisdictions have mutual aid plans that can be implemented automatically to ensure emergency medical coverage. Depending on the nature of the event, these plans may be disrupted or hindered. When the resources needed outweigh those available, a public health agency may be asked to assist in augmenting those resources. Volunteers in the local Medical Reserve Corps or registered through the Emergency System for Advance Registration of Volunteer Health Professionals (ESAR-VHP; discussed further in Chapter 6) can be mobilized to support these efforts. Interstate and federal assistance can also be requested, such as implementation of the National Disaster Medical System to facilitate patient transport to other areas; deployment of DMAT, DMORT, and federal medical station teams; and other critical resources. Advance planning, combined with training and exercising of plans on a regular basis, is essential. An adequate health operations center should be identified and equipped for long-term continuous operations in support of health care system recovery, and health care coalition leadership should be integrated into the public health incident command system. Past disaster experience has demonstrated that health care coalitions are critical to bridging the gap between public health and the medical community (Clements, 2014).

Public health agencies may also be asked to coordinate transitions to and from contingency or crisis standards of health care delivery to ensure the most comprehensive care for the greatest number of people. Such measures may be required in inpatient and outpatient settings and other environments, such as coordination of additional health care personnel to establish a shelter-based clinic and pharmacy. The effects of a disaster on the community may create a need to change EMS or dispatch protocols temporarily to facilitate care or to require a modification of transportation patterns for health responders.

Changes to licensing or certification requirements and suspension or modification of protocols, rules, or even certain laws may be necessary to coordinate the restoration of a health care system. For example, communities may decide to recognize medical credentials of out-of-state volunteer providers to meet a surge in care delivery needs. Ideally, systems for verifying credentials (e.g., ESAR-VHP) should be developed in advance of a disaster. Some changes also may need to be made in nonmedical areas (such as spending and personnel rules). Public health agencies should anticipate in advance and plan for situations that may require this type of response and determine the best way to obtain the necessary legal permissions.

Public health should work with appropriate authorities to assess damaged health care facilities in accordance with priorities based on the community's needs. Rapid mobilization of public health department staff to conduct reviews of medical facility plans and surveys of facilities can expedite the process of reopening facilities to the public. Some normal facility requirements may be temporarily waived to facilitate bringing a given building back to operational status.

INTERMEDIATE- TO LONG-TERM RECOVERY: OPPORTUNITIES TO ADVANCE HEALTHIER AND MORE RESILIENT AND SUSTAINABLE COMMUNITIES

After a disaster, the emphasis is on immediate response and short-term recovery—getting things back to normal. While these restoration efforts are critical to meeting the most immediate needs of the community, they may well fall short of moving the community closer to a consensus-derived vision of a health community. During its efforts to engage the public health sector in discussions about recovery, the committee noted a lack of focus on long-term recovery concerns. Public health officials agreed that long-term health improvement opportunities were of interest to them but not a priority because of their strong mission focus on disaster response and early recovery and the scarcity of resources and funding for existing public health programs. As described by one public health director: "As soon as the waters recede or there's no more disease going around or we've administered all the vaccine, it's really [about getting] back to business as usual. We really don't have a plan or a thought about what are we going to do now long term in assessing the community" (Beardsley, 2014). Yet despite the challenges involved in long-term recovery, previous events have shown that long-term disaster recovery presents an opportunity for public health officials to facilitate the development of healthier and more resilient and sustainable communities. The sections below describe how the public health sector can engage in long-term recovery efforts and help inform decision makers and the community at large about how they can exploit this opportunity.

Facilitating Health-Informed Recovery Decision Making Through Data

Long-term recovery requires a commitment on the part of the community to continually assess itself and identify the best uses for recovery resources and funding. Public health agencies are positioned to be among the main providers of data and analysis on health-related issues. Through preexisting community health assessments and public health-related data sets, new disaster needs assessments, disaster-related research projects, and health impact assessments targeting community rebuilding projects, public health stakeholders can promote a HiAP approach to long-term recovery. (See Chapter 2 for a discussion of this approach.) Continual outreach to and education of decision makers and the community at large must occur during this process to ensure buy-in. A cyclical process of continual assessment, analysis, planning, and evaluation of early outcomes, such as that depicted earlier in Figure 5-1, is a best practice.

The following committee recommendations are applicable to this public health priority area:

- Recommendation 5: *Establish Pathways by Which Health Information Can Inform Recovery Decision Making.* (see Chapter 3)
- Recommendation 7: *Ensure a Ready Health Information Technology Infrastructure.* (see Chapter 6)

Engaging in Health-Informed Community Rebuilding and Redevelopment Planning

Based on impact and damage assessments, public health leadership should work with elected and public officials, as well as leaders from relevant nonhealth sectors (e.g., housing, transportation), to identify opportunities for integrating some or all of the goals and objectives of the community health improvement plan with long-term community recovery efforts. Familiarity with and support for these goals and objectives prior to a disaster will greatly facilitate their implementation. Success can still be achieved even when this integration has not been done in advance (see Box 5-7 for an example from New Orleans in the wake of Hurricane Katrina), although the task will most likely be more challenging and take significantly longer. Public health can assist community decision makers in the use of a HiAP approach—for example,

---

BOX 5-7
New Orleans After Hurricane Katrina: A New Approach to Public Health

New Orleans has been honored with the inaugural 2013 Robert Wood Johnson Foundation Culture of Health Prize for its progress in transforming community health. The award honors New Orleans' exemplary community partnerships, which are encouraging its citizens to live healthier lives (RWJF, 2013).

In the aftermath of Hurricane Katrina, New Orleans made public health and prevention a priority as a critical part of the continuing recovery effort. To advance community health, a cross-sector partnership was developed among New Orleans' Health Department, businesses, nonprofit organizations, and schools (RWJF, 2013). Prior to Katrina, New Orleans' approach to health emphasized clinical care over prevention and public health, a common emphasis throughout the nation. New Orleans Health Commissioner Dr. Karen DeSalvo attributes the public health department's rapid transformation from "broken and outmoded" to a modern public health agency to the city's use of the Public Health Accreditation Board's accreditation blueprint (RWJF, 2013). According to DeSalvo, "That is how we're getting from a place where we were treating the consequences of poor health decisions and the impacts of social determinants of health, and actually move into a place where we're upstream and we can prevent it, but then work with other sectors" (RWJF, 2013).

DeSalvo stresses that a single department alone cannot solve all the health challenges a community faces. The development of a cross-sector partnership that reflects the various social determinants of health plays a crucial role in advancing community health further and ensuring that health remains an important consideration in every new policy (RWJF, 2013).

Key steps in New Orleans' transformation included

- reinvesting in the local health system,
- ensuring access to healthy food and opportunities to be physically active, and
- implementing new education models.

While New Orleans has made impressive strides in advancing community health, its new approach to public health and emphasis on prevention remains a "work in progress" (RWJF, 2013). The ongoing nature of this transformation will ensure that New Orleans continues to make progress toward resolving the health challenges caused and brought to light by Hurricane Katrina.

SOURCE: RWJF, 2013.

by conducting health impact assessments—to help them seek opportunities for improved health within their areas of jurisdiction and responsibility. These opportunities may include

- promoting more resilient design of new construction;
- promoting consideration of quality of life in planning for community redesign (e.g., bicycle lines, walking/jogging trails, parks and green spaces, locations of community amenities);
- identifying priority areas for redevelopment based on data showing health disparities;
- implementing strategies designed to retain the health services workforce; and
- promoting access to care as part of action plans.

To facilitate post-disaster health improvement planning, community leaders can activate a health-related advisory committee or subcommittee of the jurisdictional long-term recovery effort (discussed earlier in Box 5-5). Based on the pre-disaster community health assessment and the community health improvement plan, the advisory committee can identify opportunities to implement strategies designed to improve the overall health status of the community. Flexibility and responsiveness will be important to integrate input from the ongoing assessment process, adjust the recovery plan accordingly, and continuously gauge movement toward implementation of the elements essential for improved community health (see Chapter 3 for discussion of measurement tools). This process will help close the gap between the community's current health status and its agreed-upon criteria for an optimally healthy community, which will likewise be continuously monitored and evaluated for effectiveness (see Figure 5-1).

When opportunities to improve quality of life and public safety are identified, local and state public health agencies should promote efforts to seize these opportunities at the system, policy, and legislative levels. These efforts should cut across nonhealth areas such as housing, land use, and the business community to incorporate health considerations into all governmental decision-making processes. This HiAP approach will enable sustainable strategies to improve community health in the long term. Support from such key partners as local planners, city managers, and school districts will be essential to the success of such efforts. In communities that have established a HiAP approach to decision making prior to a disaster, the event will strengthen the practice and perhaps galvanize support from additional stakeholders. In communities without such an approach, a disaster may open doors for collaboration that have previously been closed and provide a forum for educating the community on the value of considering health in developing community projects.

The following committee recommendations are applicable to this public health priority area:

- **Recommendation 6:** *Leverage Recovery Resources in a Coordinated Manner to Achieve Healthier Post-Disaster Communities.* (see Chapter 4)
- **Recommendation 10:** *Design for Healthy Post-Disaster Communities.* (see Chapter 9)
- **Recommendation 11:** *Mitigate Against Future Health Hazards.* (see Chapter 9)
- **Recommendation 12:** *Ensure Healthy and Affordable Post-Disaster Housing.* (see Chapter 10)

Sharing Lessons Learned with Other Communities to Improve Disaster Recovery Planning

After a disaster, a communication strategy should be developed to share lessons learned and opportunities for improvement so other jurisdictions can benefit from experiences with recovery. Local, tribal, territorial, and state health officials should utilize state, regional, and national conferences, workshops, and discipline-specific professional meetings for this purpose and reach out to professional organizations representing traditionally nonhealth sectors to discuss opportunities for improved public health. Increased opportunities to share lessons learned both with other health departments and with other sectors—such as cross-training, mentorships, cross-disciplinary articles, and urban planning webinars—should be pursued. Examples of mechanisms for sharing lessons learned include but are not limited to

- after-action reports in FEMA's Lessons Learned Information Sharing System;
- presentations at state and national public health association meetings, including the Public Health Preparedness Summit, the National Healthcare Coalition Conference, and other applicable national emergency management conferences;
- engagement with professional organizations representing traditionally nonhealth sectors, such as the United States Council of Mayors, the National Governors Association, the International City/County Management Association, the American Planning Association, the International Association of Emergency Managers, and the Council of State Community Development Agencies;
- presentations at conferences of state hospital associations, mental health associations, and other applicable professional associations;
- engagement with philanthropic organizations and foundations regarding the rationale for building resiliency in the face of disasters;
- discussions with intra- and interstate medical system coalitions;
- presentations to emergency management partners at state conferences and meetings;
- leveraging of NACCHO and ASTHO to share lessons learned with other local and state health departments; and
- discussions during PHEP and HPP conference calls and reporting opportunities.

RESEARCH NEEDS

In the process of developing its guidance specific to the public health sector, the committee noted that further research is needed to address the following questions:

- For those with chronic health problems exacerbated by the effects of disasters, what are the stages of exacerbation?
- How can identifying persons that are at highest risk for most rapid deterioration assist in prioritization of limited resources during recovery?

SUMMARY OF FINDINGS AND CONCLUSIONS

Although a disaster causes significant disruption to the status quo, the subsequent recovery period presents a unique opportunity to shift existing funding streams, leverage one-time funding opportunities, and coalesce community stakeholders to build the resiliency of a community intentionally and strategically and to close the gap between the pre-disaster state of health and what the community envisions as an optimally healthy community.

The development of a healthy community requires a solid public health system foundation. The public health enterprise incorporates many activities focused on improving the health of a community. These activities include conduct of a community health assessment and development of community health improvement plan, as required by the national Public Health Accreditation Board. Although communities nationwide are currently engaged in improving their health, their progress to that end is often steady but slow. Disasters can catalyze bold change over a shorter period of time than would otherwise have been possible. However, successful movement toward optimal health—especially in the face of a disaster, which understandably demands attention to the immediate needs of the community—requires strategic use of a comprehensive community health assessment and a community health improvement plan that is fully integrated into the disaster recovery decision-making process. This integration will not occur without the integration of public health into pre- and post-disaster planning for long-term recovery.

PUBLIC HEALTH SECTOR RECOVERY CHECKLIST

The committee has identified four pre-event and eight post-disaster critical recovery priorities for the public health sector that are inextricably linked to strengthening the health, resilience, and sustainability of a community. Action steps for each of these priorities are provided in the following checklist. Although public health leaders will need to adapt these actions to the local context, this guidance provides an indicative set of concerns to be considered during recovery. The checklist illustrates how the following four key recovery strategies, identified as recurring themes at the beginning of this chapter, apply to individual priority areas:

- Leverage existing relationships and networks (e.g., coalitions, collaboratives) to integrate public health and other community partners into recovery planning.
- Identify opportunities for alignment between ongoing public health improvement processes (e.g., accreditation prerequisites of community health assessments and community health improvement plans) and recovery planning.
- Educate nonhealth sectors and the community on why health is integral to recovery and how recovery activities impact health outcomes.
- Use and expand health technology infrastructure for data collection and analysis to facilitate data sharing, evidence-based decision making, and continual evaluation of progress toward an optimally healthy community.

Pre-Event

Priority: Conduct Community Health Assessments

Primary Actors[1]: State/Local Health Departments[2]
Key Partners: Social Services Agencies, Health and Medical System Partners, Urban and Regional Planning Agencies, Emergency Management Agencies

Key Recovery Strategies:

- Leverage existing relationships and networks (e.g., coalitions, collaboratives) to integrate public health and other community partners into recovery planning.
- Use and expand health technology infrastructure for data collection and analysis to facilitate data sharing, evidence-based decision making, and continual evaluation of progress toward an optimally healthy community.

Activities include but are not limited to:

☐ Examine all existing public health data sources and relationships and crosswalk with disaster recovery data needs.
☐ Develop disaster data needs in the pre-disaster environment.
☐ Define how current analyses and reports can support recovery planning; develop new reports for recovery if needed.
☐ Create innovative methods for sharing data with disaster recovery planners, political leaders, and the community.
☐ Link data to economic opportunities and challenges.
☐ Utilize existing adjunct technologies such as geographic information systems (GIS) and spatial analysis to articulate findings to broader audiences.
☐ Utilize newer vehicles such as social media to share findings with broader audiences and obtain feedback.
☐ Examine opportunities for public health access to electronic medical records from inpatient, outpatient, and prehospital services.
☐ Proactively engage in health information technology infrastructure planning to connect relevant data sets and develop sharing policies across agencies.

- -

Priority: Engage Community Stakeholders in Pre-Disaster Community Health Improvement and Recovery Planning

Primary Actors: State/Local Health Departments
Key Partners: Elected Officials and Community Leaders, Urban and Regional Planning Agencies, Emergency Management Agencies, Community- and Faith-Based Organizations

---

[1] See Appendix F for further description of terms used to describe Primary Actors and Key Partners in this checklist.
[2] Throughout this checklist, "State/Local" is used for the purposes of brevity but should be inferred to include tribal and territorial as well.

Pre-Event

Key Recovery Strategies:
- Identify opportunities for alignment between ongoing public health improvement processes (e.g., accreditation prerequisites of community health assessments and community health improvement plans) and recovery planning.
- Leverage existing relationships and networks (e.g., coalitions, collaboratives) to integrate public health and other community partners into recovery planning.
- Educate nonhealth sectors and the community on why health is integral to recovery and how recovery activities impact health outcomes.

Activities include but are not limited to:
- ☐ Reach out to community, government, and private-sector leaders and create a list of all stakeholder groups, including existing coalitions. Consider maintaining this list within one program for continuity. Existing coalitions may include
  - HIV/Ryan White;
  - those that focus on the elderly, children, and special populations;
  - school/education groups;
  - faith-based groups;
  - health care coalitions;
  - public safety/homeland security; and
  - groups that focus on specific diseases or conditions (e.g., homelessness, poverty, domestic violence).
- ☐ Assess each group/meeting for the potential to integrate in recovery planning, by either using group time for parallel meetings or soliciting participation in a newly formed recovery coalition.
- ☐ Evaluate for potential funding streams to facilitate and support groups.
- ☐ Ensure that public health is engaged in recovery planning.
- ☐ Engage urban and regional planners and city/county managers in the development of the community health improvement and recovery plans.
- ☐ Create materials to educate nonhealth partners on health impacts that should be included in disaster recovery planning and impacts to their sector, as well as the value of a Health in All Policies approach and the cost of failure.
- ☐ Educate on recovery-related funding and strategies for its future use.
- ☐ Educate emergency managers and community planners on integrating health improvement into disaster recovery and the importance of engaging those with community health knowledge in pre-disaster recovery planning.

- -

Priority: Ensure That Public Health Community Programs and Services Are Integrated into Healthy Community and Disaster Recovery Planning Processes

Primary Actors: State/Local Health Departments
Key Partners: Elected Officials and Community Leaders, Urban and Regional Planning Agencies, Community- and Faith-Based Organizations, Emergency Management Agencies

Pre-Event

Key Recovery Strategies:

- Leverage existing relationships and networks (e.g., coalitions, collaboratives) to integrate public health and other community partners into recovery planning.
- Identify opportunities for alignment between ongoing public health improvement processes (e.g., accreditation prerequisites of community health assessments and community health improvement plans) and recovery planning.

Activities include but are not limited to:

For external programs and services:

☐ Work with partner agencies to identify gaps and prioritize recovery resources.
☐ Identify community-based organizations with capacities that can be used in recovery (e.g., food services, shelters, counseling).
☐ Use face-to-face contact with community members to educate on disaster preparedness to improve individual and community resiliency.
☐ Develop post-disaster communications strategies with partner agencies.

For internal programs and services:

☐ Pre-identify essential services to be priorities during recovery and areas in which recovery resources can be used to develop new programs to improve health.
☐ Identify program areas within public health departments in which alignment exists.
☐ Exploit cross-cutting activities for accreditation and public health emergency planning.
☐ Connect program leads with the goal of information and resource sharing and the creation of synergy among programs.
☐ Establish strategic plans to leverage activities/resources/contacts.
☐ Exploit the opportunity to cross-train public health staff and volunteers and partners.
☐ Document overlapping areas to show progress toward strategic goals.
☐ Exercise and train for recovery activities.

- -

Priority: Leverage Pre-Disaster Preparedness Activities in Recovery Planning

Primary Actors: State/Local Health Departments
Key Partners: Emergency Management Agencies, Health and Medical System Partners, Community- and Faith-Based Organizations

Key Recovery Strategy:

- Identify opportunities for alignment between ongoing public health improvement processes (e.g., accreditation prerequisites of community health assessments and community health improvement plans) and recovery planning.

Pre-Event

Activities include but are not limited to:
- ☐ Enhance regulatory and accreditation requirements to support more intensive pre-event recovery planning by local and state public health agencies, health care organizations, behavioral health agencies, social services agencies, and local and state emergency management agencies using standard criteria.
- ☐ Develop health department continuity of operations plans that enable impacted jurisdictions to rapidly overcome damage and engage in recovery efforts by utilizing either local health department staff or public health staff from other jurisdictions.
- ☐ Promote and develop public health rapid assessment teams familiar with local and state emergency response and recovery plans and trained to conduct post-disaster community assessments.
- ☐ Educate and train medical system and emergency management partners regarding the roles and responsibilities of the public health assessment team during recovery efforts.
- ☐ Routinely train and engage personnel assigned assessment responsibilities in local, regional, state, and national disaster exercises.
- ☐ Build in the capacity to identify gaps to be closed to achieve an optimally healthy community.

Short-Term Recovery

Priority: Participate in a Shared Communication Effort

Primary Actors: State/Local Health Departments, Emergency Management Agencies
Key Partners: Elected Officials and Community Leaders, Health and Medical System Partners, Behavioral Health Authorities

Activities include but are not limited to:
- ☐ Establish and operate a recovery joint information system staffed with representatives from all engaged sectors.
- ☐ Assign health department public information officer(s) to the public health incident command system.
- ☐ Engage both internal and external subject matter experts as necessary.
- ☐ Ensure that public health agency information officers participate actively in the jurisdictional joint information center or joint information system.
- ☐ Identify outreach methods and key messages.
- ☐ Integrate health messages with general emergency management messages related to ongoing recovery efforts, focusing on safety and injury prevention and other event-specific public health messages.
- ☐ Ensure that communication plans address appropriate risk communication strategies.
- ☐ Engage leaders of community-based organizations in communications to vulnerable or nonmainstream audiences.
- ☐ Develop a plan for outreach through and monitoring of social media.

- -

Priority: Conduct Impact Assessments on the Health and Medical Needs of the Community

Primary Actors: State/Local Health Departments
Key Partners: Health and Medical System Partners, Social Services Agencies, Emergency Management Agencies

Key Recovery Strategy:
- Use and expand health technology infrastructure for data collection and analysis to facilitate data sharing, evidence-based decision making, and continual evaluation of progress toward an optimally healthy community.

Activities include but are not limited to:
- ☐ Deploy public health rapid assessment teams familiar with local and state emergency response and recovery plans and trained to conduct pre- and post-disaster community assessments.
- ☐ Work with health system leaders to assess impacts on health care facilities, emergency medical services, long-term care facilities, and specialty facilities (e.g., dialysis centers).
- ☐ Work with emergency management agencies and applicable volunteer agencies to assess the need and potential duration for mass shelters, including special needs shelters and needs within existing shelter operations.

Short-Term Recovery

- ☐ Work with emergency management agencies to assess the need for a public health emergency declaration and provide data to support requests for assistance.
- ☐ Collect and compile service restoration timelines from key public health and medical system partners.
- ☐ Evaluate data, create reports, and communicate findings to responding agencies, stakeholders, and the community at large.

- -

Priority: Reestablish Critical Public Health Infrastructure

Primary Actors: State/Local Health Departments
Key Partners: Elected Officials and Community Leaders

Activities include but are not limited to:
- ☐ Reestablish public health department programs based on preestablished (as identified in continuity of operations/continuity of government) departmental service priorities, using temporary service sites if needed.
- ☐ Develop strategies for increasing workforce capacity to meet surge in needs.
- ☐ Restore access to vital records.
- ☐ As reestablishment takes place, identify opportunities and organize activities in a manner that may close the gap between existing conditions, or even the pre-disaster state, and an optimal healthy community.

- -

Priority: Deliver Public Health Services to Meet Post-Disaster Needs of the Community

Primary Actors: State/Local Health Departments
Key Partners: Social Services Agencies, Community- and Faith-Based Organizations

Activities include but are not limited to:
- ☐ Conduct licensed and unlicensed food vendor inspections (including mass shelters with feeding operations).
- ☐ Focus immunization efforts on responders, victims, and volunteers.
- ☐ Provide behavioral health support.
- ☐ Ensure the availability of services related to functional needs/at-risk populations.
- ☐ Provide mass shelter support as needed.
- ☐ Provide fatality management support.
- ☐ If necessary, issue a public health emergency declaration to assist with debris removal and cleanup.

Short-Term Recovery

Priority: Provide Support to Impacted Health Care Delivery Systems

Primary Actors: State/Local Health Departments, Health and Medical System Partners
Key Partners: Social Services Agencies, Emergency Management Agencies, Behavioral Health Authorities

Activities include but are not limited to:
- Engage health and medical system partners and/or health care coalition members early in the Emergency Support Function (ESF) #8 response and recovery efforts.
- Integrate health care coalition leadership within the public health incident command system.
- Establish needed emergency medical treatment capabilities within impacted area.
- Mobilize and deploy Medical Reserve Corps or Emergency System for Advance Registration of Volunteer Health Professionals (ESAR-VHP) volunteers to support efforts.
- Implement strategies designed to retain the health and medical services workforce.
- Coordinate necessary patient transport out of impacted areas.
- Engage in a process for wellness checks.
- Ensure access to and availability of pharmaceuticals, including psychotropics.
- Coordinate health care (including behavioral health) resources and volunteers responding to the area.
- Rapidly mobilize health department staff to expedite reviews of medical facility plans and surveys of facilities to determine readiness to be reopened to the public; reopen minimally damaged facilities.
- Identify opportunities to improve care and the configuration and location of services to best meet the needs of the community.

Intermediate- to Long-Term Recovery

Priority: Facilitate Health-Informed Recovery Decision Making Through Data

Primary Actors: State/Local Health Departments
Key Partners: Health and Medical System Partners, Social Services Agencies, Urban and Regional Planning Agencies

Key Recovery Strategies:
- Leverage existing relationships and networks (e.g., coalitions, collaboratives) to integrate public health and other community partners into recovery planning.
- Educate nonhealth sectors and the community on why health is integral to recovery and how recovery activities impact health outcomes.
- Use and expand health technology infrastructure for data collection and analysis to facilitate data sharing, evidence-based decision making, and continual evaluation of progress toward an optimally healthy community.

Activities include but are not limited to:
- ☐ Ensure ongoing operation of an incident command system that provides for routine assessment of health and medical needs by public health staff working jointly with health, social services, and medical community partners.
- ☐ Assess access to mental/behavioral health services, health care services, public health services, and social services.

- -

Priority: Engage in Community Rebuilding and Redevelopment Planning to Identify Opportunities to Enhance Population Health

Primary Actors: State/Local Health Departments
Key Partners: Emergency Management Agencies, Urban and Regional Planning Agencies, Education System, Transportation Agencies, Housing Agencies

Key Recovery Strategies:
- Leverage existing relationships and networks (e.g., coalitions, collaboratives) to integrate public health and other community partners into recovery planning.
- Educate nonhealth sectors and the community on why health is integral to recovery and how recovery activities impact health outcomes.

Activities include but are not limited to:
- ☐ Engage community leaders early in the process to encourage their interest in participating in broader community redevelopment processes.
- ☐ Educate community leaders, in conjunction with urban and regional planners, on the elements of a resilient and healthy community, the important opportunity to utilize recovery efforts to achieve that goal, and the applicability of such tools as health impact assessments to inform decision making.
- ☐ Assist with identifying sources of capital and financing for rebuilding in ways that promote health.

Intermediate- to Long-Term Recovery

- ☐ Continuously measure progress toward healthy community goals and adapt recovery and health improvement plans accordingly.
- ☐ Organize and implement a health-related advisory committee or subcommittee of the jurisdictional long-term recovery effort.
- ☐ Inform and advocate for infrastructure investments that strengthen safety and resilience, such as improved construction standards, safe rooms and storm shelters (where appropriate), underground utilities, and energy-efficient standards/construction.
- ☐ Educate local and state leaders on lessons learned as a result of the disaster and ways to build stronger, more resilient communities.

- -

Priority: Share Lessons Learned with Other Communities to Improve Post-Disaster Recovery Planning

Primary Actors: State/Local Health Departments, Health and Medical System Partners, Emergency Management Agencies

Key Partners: Community- and Faith-Based Organizations, Elected Officials and Community Leaders

Activities include but are not limited to:
- ☐ Participate in after-action processes, including analysis of lessons learned and identification of opportunities for improvement.
- ☐ Utilize state, regional, and national conferences, workshops, and discipline-specific professional meetings to share lessons learned and opportunities for improvement so that other jurisdictions can benefit from recovery experiences.
- ☐ Disseminate information regarding opportunities for improved public health to health sector and nonhealth groups, such as the council of mayors, city managers, city councilors, emergency management agencies, and urban and regional planners.

REFERENCES

AHRQ (Agency for Healthcare Research and Quality). 2005. *National Hospital Available Beds for Emergencies and Disasters (HAvBED) system: Final report.* AHRQ Publication No. 05-0103. Rockville, MD: AHRQ.

The Alliance for a Just Rebuilding, ALIGN, Community Development Project at the Urban Justice Center, Community Voices Heard, Faith in New York, Families United for Racial and Economic Equality, Good Old Lower East Side, Red Hook Initiative, and New York Communities for Change. 2014. *Weathering the storm: Rebuilding a more resilient New York City Housing Authority post-Sandy.* http://www.rebuildajustny.org/wp-content/uploads/2014/03/Weathering_The_Storm.pdf (accessed October 20, 2014).

APA (American Planning Association). 2006. *Integrating planning and public health (PAS 539/540).* APA Planning Advisory Service. Washington, DC: APA.

ASPR (Office of the Assistant Secretary for Preparedness and Response). 2012. *Healthcare preparedness capabilities: National guidance for healthcare system preparedness.* Washington, DC: HHS.

ASPR. 2015. *Core mission areas.* http://www.phe.gov/about/oem/recovery/Pages/rsf-core.aspx (accessed February 26, 2015).

ASTHO (Association of State and Territorial Health Officials). 2007. *Disaster recovery for public health.* http://www.astho.org/programs/preparedness/disaster-recovery-for-public-health (accessed November 18, 2014).

Barnett, K. 2012. Best practices for community health needs assessment and implementation strategy development: A review of scientific methods, current practices, and future potential. In *Report of proceedings from a public forum and interviews of experts.* http://www.phi.org/uploads/application/files/dz9vh55o3bb2x56lcrzyel83 fwfu3mvu24oqqvn5z6qaeiw2u4.pdf (accessed August 25, 2014).

Beardsley, D. 2014. *Session I: Public health, panel discussion.* Paper presented at IOM Committee on Post-Disaster Recovery of a Community's Public Health, Medical, and Social Services: Meeting Two, February 3, Washington, DC.

Berggren, R. E., and T. J. Curiel. 2006. After the storm—health care infrastructure in post-Katrina New Orleans. *New England Journal of Medicine* 354(15):1549-1552.

Blumenstock, J. 2014. *Coordination among state and local government agencies.* Paper presented at IOM Committee on Post-Disaster Recovery of a Community's Public Health, Medical, and Social Services: Meeting Three, April 28-29, Washington, DC.

CDC (Centers for Disease Control and Prevention). 2011. *Public health preparedness capabilities: National standards for state and local planning.* Washington, DC: HHS.

CDC. 2014a. *Health Alert Network (HAN).* http://www.bt.cdc.gov/han (accessed November 18, 2014).

CDC. 2014b. *The public health system and the 10 essential public health services.* http://www.cdc.gov/nphpsp/essential services.html (accessed February 6, 2014).

CDC. 2014c. *Winnable battles.* http://www.cdc.gov/winnablebattles (accessed November 18, 2014).

Center for Disaster Philanthropy. 2012. *The impact of disasters on public health.* http://disasterphilanthropy.org/the-impact-of-disasters-on-public-health (accessed November 26, 2014).

Chandra, A., J. Acosta, S. Howard, L. Uscher-Pines, M. Williams, D. Yeung, J. Garnett, and L. S. Meredith. 2011. *Building community resilience to disasters: A way forward to enhance national health security.* http://www.sciencedirect.com/science/article/pii/S0277953612005953 (accessed November 18, 2014).

Chandra, A., M. Williams, A. Plough, A. Stayton, K. B. Wells, M. Horta, and J. Tang. 2013. Getting actionable about community resilience: The Los Angeles County Community Disaster Resilience Project. *American Journal of Public Health* 103(7):1181-1189.

Clements, B. 2014. *Public health and community recovery: Texas' experience.* Paper presented at IOM Committee on Post-Disaster Recovery of a Community's Public Health, Medical, and Social Services: Meeting Two, February 3, Washington, DC.

Community Commons. 2014a. *Community Health Needs Assessment (CHNA).* http://assessment.communitycommons.org/chna/About.aspx (accessed November 18, 2014).

Community Commons. 2014b. *Indicator data list.* http://assessment.communitycommons.org/CHNA/Datalist.aspx (accessed November 18, 2014).

CVS Caremark. 2014. *CVS disaster relief.* http://info.cvscaremark.com/newsroom/featured-topics/disaster-relief (accessed November 18, 2014).

DeSalvo, K., N. Lurie, K. Finne, C. Worrall, A. Bogdanov, A. Dinkler, S. Babcock, and J. Kelman. 2014. Using Medicare data to identify individuals who are electricity dependent to improve disaster preparedness and response. *American Journal of Public Health* 104(7):1160-1164.

DHS (U.S. Department of Homeland Security) and EPA (U.S. Environmental Protection Agency). 2010. *Memorandum of agreement between the Department of Homeland Security (DHS), Federal Emergency Management Agency (FEMA) and the Environmental Protection Agency (EPA)*. http://www.epa.gov/dced/pdf/2011_0114_fema-epa-moa.pdf (accessed November 18, 2014).

DOT (U.S. Department of Transportation), EPA (U.S. Environmental Protection Agency), and HUD (U.S. Department of Housing and Urban Development). 2014. *Partnership for sustainable communities: Five years of learning from communities and coordinating federal investments*. Washington, DC: DOT, EPA, and HUD.

Duncan, W. J., P. M. Ginter, A. C. Rucks, M. S. Wingate, and L. C. McCormick. 2007. Organizing emergency preparedness within United States public health departments. *Public Health* 121(4):241-250.

Fairfax County. 2012. *Fairfax County pre-disaster recovery plan*. http://www.fairfaxcounty.gov/oem/pdrp/pdrp-complete-doc-march2012.pdf (accessed November 18, 2014).

FEMA (Federal Emergency Management Agency). 2008. *Emergency support function #8—public health and medical services annex*. http://www.fema.gov/media-library-data/20130726-1825-25045-8027/emergency_support_function_8_public_health__medical_services_annex_2008.pdf (accessed February 26, 2015).

FEMA. 2010. *Guidance on planning for integration of functional needs support services in general population shelters*. Washington, DC: DHS.

FEMA. 2011. *National disaster recovery framework*. Washington, DC: FEMA.

FEMA. n.d. *State partnership—Safeguard Iowa Partnership*. http://www.fema.gov/pdf/privatesector/ia_ppp.pdf (accessed November 18, 2014).

HHS (U.S. Department of Health and Human Services). 2007. *Medical surge capacity and capability: A management system for integrating medical and health resources during large-scale emergencies*. http://www.phe.gov/preparedness/planning/mscc/handbook/documents/mscc080626.pdf (accessed March 24, 2015).

HHS. 2009. *National health security strategy of the United States of America*. Washington, DC: HHS.

HHS. 2014a. *HHS disaster behavioral health concept of operations*. http://www.phe.gov/Preparedness/planning/abc/Documents/dbh-conops-2014.pdf (accessed October 21, 2014).

HHS. 2014b. *HIPAA privacy in emergency situations*. Washington, DC: HHS.

Hillsborough County Government. 2010. *Post-disaster redevelopment plan*. http://www.hillsboroughcounty.org/index.aspx?nid=1795 (accessed November 18, 2014).

IOM (Institute of Medicine). 1988. *The future of public health*. Washington, DC: National Academy Press.

IOM. 2003. *The future of the public's health in the 21st century*. Washington, DC: The National Academies Press.

IOM. 2014. *The impacts of the Affordable Care Act on preparedness resources and programs: Workshop summary*. Washington, DC: The National Academies Press.

IRS (Internal Revenue Service). 2013. *IRB 2013-21*. http://www.irs.gov/irb/2013-21_IRB/ar09.html (accessed December 1, 2014).

Klitzman, S., and N. Freudenberg. 2003. Implications of the World Trade Center attack for the public health and health care infrastructures. *American Journal of Public Health* 93(3):400-406.

Knearl, E. 2014. *Role of public information in health systems recovery*. Paper presented at IOM Committee on Post-Disaster Recovery of a Community's Public Health, Medical, and Social Services: Meeting Three, April 28-29, Washington, DC.

LACCDR (Los Angeles County Community Disaster Resilience). 2014. *What is community resilience?* http://www.laresilience.org (accessed August 26, 2014).

Lockwood, B. 2014. *Coordination among state and local government agencies*. Paper presented at IOM Committee on Post-Disaster Recovery of a Community's Public Health, Medical, and Social Services: Meeting Three, April 28-29, Washington, DC.

Mattessich, P. W., and E. J. Rausch. 2013. *Collaboration to build healthier communities: A report for the Robert Wood Johnson Foundation Commission to Build a Healthier America*. http://www.rwjf.org/content/dam/farm/reports/surveys_and_polls/2013/rwjf406479 (accessed November 18, 2014).

Morton, M. J., and N. Lurie. 2013. Community resilience and public health practice. *American Journal of Public Health* 103(7):1158-1160.

NACCHO (National Association of County and City Health Officials). 2011. *National public health performance standards: Local implementation guide version 3.0*. http://www.naccho.org/topics/infrastructure/NPHPSP/loader.cfm?csModule=security/getfile&pageid=256555 (accessed March 2, 2015).

NACCHO. 2012. *Role of local health departments in community health needs assessments*. http://naccho.org/advocacy/positions/upload/12-05-Role-of-LHDs-in-CHNA.pdf (accessed November 18, 2014).

NACCHO. 2013. *Local health department job losses and program cuts: Findings from the 2013 profile study.* http:// www.naccho.org/topics/infrastructure/lhdbudget/upload/Survey-Findings-Brief-8-13-13-3.pdf (accessed November 18, 2014).

NACCHO. 2014a. *2013 national profile of local health departments.* http://www.naccho.org/topics/infrastructure/ profile/upload/2013-National-Profile-of-Local-Health-Departments-report.pdf (accessed November 5, 2014).

NACCHO. 2014b. *MAPP framework.* http://www.naccho.org/topics/infrastructure/mapp/framework/index.cfm (accessed November 18, 2014).

NBSB (National Biodefense Science Board). 2014. *Community health resilience report.* Washington, DC: NBSB.

Nolen, A. 2014. *A health in all policies approach to disaster recovery: Lessons from Galveston.* Paper presented at IOM Committee on Post-Disaster Recovery of a Community's Public Health, Medical, and Social Services: Meeting Four, June 13, Washington, DC.

NRC (National Research Council). 2012. *Disaster resilience: A national imperative.* Washington, DC: The National Academies Press.

PHAB (Public Health Accreditation Board). 2011. *Acronyms and glossary of terms.* http://www.phaboard.org/wp-content/uploads/PHAB-Acronyms-and-Glossary-of-Terms-Version-1.0.pdf (accessed November 18, 2014).

PHAB. 2012. *National public health department accreditation prerequisites.* http://www.phaboard.org/wp-content/ uploads/PrerequisitesJuly-2012.pdf (accessed November 18, 2014).

PHAB. 2013. *Standards & measures.* http://www.phaboard.org/wp-content/uploads/SM-Version-1.5-Board-adopted-FINAL-01-24-2014.docx.pdf (accessed November 18, 2014).

Plough, A., J. E. Fielding, A. Chandra, M. Williams, D. Eisenman, K. B. Wells, G. Y. Law, S. Fogleman, and A. Magaña. 2013. Building community disaster resilience: Perspectives from a large urban county department of public health. *American Journal of Public Health* 103(7):1190-1197.

Rudolph, L., J. Caplan, K. Ben-Moshe, and L. Dillon. 2013. *Health in all policies: A guide for state and local governments.* http://www.phi.org/uploads/files/Health_in_All_Policies-A_Guide_for_State_and_Local_Governments. pdf (accessed November 18, 2014).

Rudowitz, R., D. Rowland, and A. Shartzer. 2006. Health care in New Orleans before and after Hurricane Katrina. *Health Affairs* 25(5):w393-w406.

Runkle, J. D., A. Brock-Martin, W. Karmaus, and E. R. Svendsen. 2012. Secondary surge capacity: A framework for understanding long-term access to primary care for medically vulnerable populations in disaster recovery. *American Journal of Public Health* 102(12):e24-e32.

RWJF (Robert Wood Johnson Foundation). 2013. *New Orleans, Louisiana: 2013 RWJF culture of health prize.* http:// www.rwjf.org/en/about-rwjf/newsroom/newsroom-content/2013/02/new-orleans--louisiana--2013-roadmaps-to-health-prize.html (accessed November 18, 2014).

RWJF. 2014. *Building a culture of health: 2014 President's message.* http://www.rwjf.org/content/dam/files/rwjf-web-files/Annual_Message/2014_RWJF_AnnualMessage_final.pdf (accessed April 5, 2014).

Safeguard Iowa Partnership. 2013. *2013 annual report.* https://safeguardiowa.wildapricot.org/Resources/Documents/ Annual%20Meeting/2013/2013%20SIP%20ANNUAL%20REPORT.pdf (accessed November 18, 2014).

Salinsky, E. 2010. *Governmental public health: An overview of state and local public health agencies.* National Health Policy Forum, background paper no. 77. http://www.nhpf.org/library/background-papers/BP77_GovPublicHealth_08-18-2010.pdf (accessed March 2, 2015).

Shah, U. 2014. *Coordination among state and local government agencies.* Paper presented at IOM Committee on Post-Disaster Recovery of a Community's Public Health, Medical, and Social Services: Meeting Three, April 28-29, Washington, DC.

Smith, G. 2011. *Planning for post-disaster recovery: A review of the United States disaster assistance framework.* Fairfax, VA: Public Entity Risk Institute.

Stevenson, A., A. Humphrey, and S. Brinsdon. 2014. A health in all policies response to disaster recovery. *Perspectives in Public Health* 134(3):125-126.

UTMB (University of Texas Medical Branch at Galveston). 2011. *Mental health continuum of care program.* http:// www.utmbhpla.org/doc/Page.asp?PageID=DOC000725 (accessed November 18, 2014).

White, J. 2014. *Post-disaster social services and health outcomes in recovery.* Paper presented at IOM Committee on Post-Disaster Recovery of a Community's Public Health, Medical, and Social Services: Meeting Two, February 3, Washington, DC.

Zucker, H. 2014. *Post-disaster recovery: New York State Department of Health experience with Superstorm Sandy.* Paper presented at IOM Committee on Post-Disaster Recovery of a Community's Public Health, Medical, and Social Services: Meeting Two, February 3, Washington, DC.

Health Care

Recovery planning and post-event recovery activities for the health care sector—which includes pre-hospital resources, hospital-based care, and out-of-hospital care delivery systems—are ideally focused on a continuum of community needs, ranging from short-term early recovery needs to decisions about long-term healthy community goals. If developed properly, these latter goals can help communities not only recover from a disaster but also address chronic community health concerns such as access to health care services. In the early recovery period, health care recovery planning should be initiated with assessment of residual health care sector capacities and challenges and, for long-term planning, acknowledgment of current and planned changes in health care delivery and financing systems. For example, as of the writing of this report, planning for long-term community health needs might include consideration of possible expanded access to preventive services stemming from the Patient Protection and Affordable Care Act[1] (ACA). The committee urges local health systems to continue or initiate proactive recovery-focused planning to build health care sector resilience. This planning will facilitate actions that (1) stabilize, strengthen, and integrate existing resources; (2) identify resources that should be rebuilt or replaced; and (3) identify de novo preventive and health care delivery approaches that are sustainable and affordable and will lead to improved health and public health outcomes in the community.

To accelerate the recovery of the health care sector in the event of a disaster, the community must assess the health care services currently in place and develop an agreed-upon comprehensive community disaster response and recovery plan prior to a disaster. This planning process should leverage data derived from health information systems and solicit input and feedback from a variety of stakeholders and sectors invested in building and sustaining a strong and robust health care infrastructure within the community. During short- and intermediate-term recovery, the health care sector should identify both patient and system gaps that occurred during the response that could be improved upon should another disaster occur. During long-term recovery, identified patient and system gaps should be addressed and goals set for an improved healthy community.

Disasters often cause health systems to adjust the way health care services are delivered, moving care delivery out of hospitals and into the community and using team-based strategies to meet multifaceted needs of survivors (DeSalvo, 2013). In many ways, these adjustments better meet patient needs and are

---

[1] Patient Protection and Affordable Care Act, 42 U.S.C. § 18001. Aug. 25, 2010.

consistent with contemporary policies such as those of the ACA. As a community addresses disaster-related impacts during recovery, it needs to think about opportunities to leverage disaster experiences, relationships, and recovery resources to shift to these new models of care.

This chapter presents the committee's assessment of major health care sector resources and operational processes that are mobilized along the continuum from pre-disaster planning to post-disaster recovery, and its guidance for enhancing and supporting the optimal use of these assets to create healthier communities after disasters. The chapter addresses four key strategies that drive the success of recovery for the health care sector and ultimately the building of a healthier community:

- Use multidisciplinary team-based care strategies to meet multifaceted health care needs.
- Ensure continuity of access to health care services.
- Use health information technology to drive decision making for individual and community health, and to inform future planning.
- Leverage health care coalitions and other relationships with local care providers for health services strategic decision making and alignment of clinical resources.

The chapter concludes with a checklist of key activities that the health care sector needs to perform during each of the three phases of recovery: pre-event, short-term recovery, and intermediate- to long-term recovery.

HEALTH CARE IN THE CONTEXT OF A HEALTHY COMMUNITY

The degree of integration of health care services with each other and across the continuum of public health, behavioral health, and social services contributes significantly to overall community health and, relatedly, the community's resilience to withstand the impacts of a disaster. This comprehensive and integrated vision of health has been incorporated into major influential initiatives that continuously assess the health of the nation, including America's Health Rankings, the Commonwealth Fund's Scorecard, and the Robert Wood Johnson Foundation's County Health Rankings (County Health Rankings, 2014; Radley et al., 2014; United Health Foundation, 2013).

Unfortunately, given the importance of the health care system to realizing maximally healthy and resilient communities, it has long been known that America as a whole, and most of its communities in particular, experiences suboptimal quality in health care delivery (IOM, 2000, 2001, 2013a). As discussed in Chapter 1, the United States has the highest per capita health care costs but poorer health relative to its peer nations. In an effort to address this disparity, the Institute for Healthcare Improvement developed the Triple Aim—better experience of care at lower cost and improved population health—which serves as the foundation for organizations and communities to transition from a focus on health care to a focus on optimizing health for individuals and populations (IHI, 2007). Key strategies for the Triple Aim include

- "Innovative financing approaches;
- New models of primary care, such as patient-centered medical homes" to meet comprehensive needs of individuals (see Box 6-1 for characteristics of optimal coordinated care systems);
- "Sanctions for avoidable events, such as hospital readmissions or infections; and
- Integration of information technology"—advancing data and knowledge sharing (IHI, 2007).

As communities conduct planning to enhance the resiliency and sustainability of their health care infrastructure, prepare for rapid response to crises, and engage in the activities necessary to recover from a disaster, the logic of the Triple Aim and its underlying conceptual foundations outlined above provide a useful and aligned strategic model to focus the efforts of the multiple stakeholders with a voice in health care activities relevant to disaster planning. At the same time, the disaster management cycle, along the continuum from pre-disaster planning to immediate- and long-term recovery, provides currently under-

---

BOX 6-1
Optimal Coordinated Care Systems

Characteristics of an optimal coordinated care system include

- the right person delivering the right care at the right time;
- interdisciplinary teams and multiple levels of care that address various aspects and steps of the treatment process; and
- a decentralized referral structure, such that the system can "capture" clients in a wide variety of settings, including nonclinical ones.

Examples include accountable care organizations and patient-centered medical homes.[a]

---

[a] A patient-centered medical home, as defined by the Agency for Healthcare Research and Quality (AHRQ), is "a model of the organization of primary care that delivers the core functions of primary health care," including comprehensive, patient-centered, and coordinated care; accessible services; and quality and safety (AHRQ, 2015). An example of this model includes CMS-sponsored "health homes" for Medicaid beneficiaries.
SOURCE: HHS, 2011.

---

leveraged opportunities for the infusion of new resources that can facilitate the reorganization of health care infrastructures to support the broader goal of realizing maximally healthy communities.

In addition, as communities engage in the spectrum of health care activities related to disaster preparedness, response, and recovery, they should take advantage of prevailing shifts in the delivery and funding of medical care. Two relevant and related movements are occurring synergistically. First, the recommendations contained in the landmark Institute of Medicine (IOM) report *Crossing the Quality Chasm: A New Health System for the 21st Century* (IOM, 2001) introduced new concepts in "comprehensive patient-centered care" that continue to guide the care delivery system toward reorganization that meets the needs of patients more effectively through enhanced cooperation and continuity of healing relationships across clinical disciplines and settings of care. Advances in data and knowledge sharing via new health information technology and data infrastructures are essential to implementing this vision. Second, the concept of "population health"—proposed by Kindig and Stoddart (2003, p. 380) as "the health outcomes of a group of individuals, including the distribution of such outcomes within the group"—that focuses on the patterns of health determinants and the policies and interventions that result in health outcomes has now migrated from the public health community to become an emphasis of the health care delivery system, driven by pressures for greater value being exerted by the purchasers of care. "Value," generally defined as the relationship between outcomes of care and the cost of providing that care, entails a focus not only on the care of individual patients but also on the total population of patients treated by care delivery systems. The evolution of reimbursement away from a fee-for-service model toward models based on value provides financial fuel for a shift in focus favoring prevention (e.g., preventing hospital admissions and re-admissions). Of particular interest in the present context, this population-based approach for the health care system now begins to mirror the traditional population perspective typically associated with public health and provides a useful bridge for integrating health care delivery more effectively into the comprehensive effort of creating or rebuilding healthier communities. It also provides incentives for developing collaborative relationships among local care delivery organizations, which are key to building resilience.

Two related efforts provide guidance and opportunities relevant to the ongoing task of strengthening and integrating communities' clinical care and prevention systems. First, the IOM produced a report in 2012 entitled *Primary Care and Public Health: Exploring Integration to Improve Population Health* (IOM,

2012b). That report observes that, although both of these fields "share a common goal, historically they have operated independently of each other. However, new opportunities are emerging that could bring the two sectors together in ways that will yield substantial and lasting improvements in the health of individuals, communities, and populations" (IOM, 2013c). The report describes the interactions between the two sectors as so varied that no single specific model or template for integration can be prescribed for all communities. However, it does identify the following set of principles reflecting the components essential to successful integration efforts, which the committee endorses as key to integrating health into broader disaster recovery efforts:

- having a shared goal of improving population health;
- involving the community in defining and addressing its needs;
- strong leadership that bridges programs, disciplines, and jurisdictions;
- sustainability; and
- the collaborative use of data and analysis (IOM, 2012b).

The second effort, convened by the Association of State and Territorial Health Officials (ASTHO)—the ASTHO-Supported Primary Care and Public Health Collaborative[2]—arose from the above IOM report and aims to "inform, align, and support the implementation of integrated efforts that improve population health and lower healthcare costs" (ASTHO, 2014). Given the need to maximally leverage existing resources, the committee urges ASTHO and its partners in this effort to include disaster planning and preparedness as an explicit activity.

DISASTER-RELATED HEALTH CARE CHALLENGES

Disasters are often accompanied by significant threats to the immediate- and long-term physical health of individuals living in affected communities and by disruptions of the health care delivery infrastructure. Health status can be affected by injury associated with the disaster; exposure to toxins and environmental contaminants; and exacerbation of preexisting risk factors and clinical conditions due to stress, lack of access to health care and social support resources, and disruption of continuity of care. Health care delivery infrastructure can be compromised by loss of facilities; migration of health professionals away from the impacted area; and disruption of critical supports such as information and data technology, medical supplies and pharmaceuticals, transportation, and medically necessary social services (a more detailed description of disaster impacts on health is presented in Box 1-1 in Chapter 1). The obvious paradox is that at a time when medical care is urgently needed, its capacity is often diminished. These effects are especially pronounced among already vulnerable populations and individuals who have little ability to withstand health insults or further erosion in previously overburdened care delivery systems. For medically vulnerable individuals, disaster-related disruption in primary care can create a secondary surge of increased demand for medical services during recovery due to a rise in chronic health issues exacerbated by the disaster (Runkle et al., 2012). In the long term, the disaster's impact on the social vulnerability of the population can have a ripple effect that further strains the health care delivery system. Shifts in patient demographics featuring disaster-related increases in numbers of indigent patients can create significant burdens for weakened health systems (Colias, 2005). Such effects are felt not just by hospitals but also by the entire spectrum of care delivery providers (public, private, and nonprofit). A healthy community

---

[2] More than 50 organizations participated within this collaborative including, but not limited to, "ASTHO, the National Association of County and City Health Officials, Trust for America's Health, Association of Public Health Nurses, and Association of Schools and Programs of Public Health. Primary care is represented by lead medical societies including the American Medical Association, American Academy of Family Physicians, American Academy of Pediatrics, and American College of Preventive Medicine. Health insurer partners include the National Association of Medicaid Directors, America's Health Insurance Plans, and Alliance of Community Health Plans. Federal partners include HRSA, CDC, CMS, CMMI, and AHRQ" (ASTHO, 2014).

BOX 6-2
Capability Targets for the Health and Social Services Recovery Support Function

Core Capability: Restore and improve health and social services networks to promote the resilience, independence, health (including behavioral health), and well-being of the whole community.

Capability Targets:

1. Restore basic health and social services functions. Identify critical areas of need for health and social services, as well as key partners and individuals with disabilities and others with access and functional needs and populations with limited English proficiency (LEP) in short-term, intermediate, and long-term recovery.
2. Complete an assessment of community health and social service needs and develop a comprehensive recovery timeline.
3. Restore and improve the resilience and sustainability of the health and social services networks to meet the needs of and promote the independence and well-being of community members in accordance with the specified recovery timeline.

SOURCE: Excerpted from FEMA, 2014a, p. 42.

---

approach to recovery focused on reducing post-disaster social vulnerabilities by addressing the social determinants of health may ameliorate these detrimental impacts.

HEALTH CARE SECTOR ORGANIZATION AND RESOURCES

A 2012 IOM report emphasizes that preparedness, crisis standards of care, response, and recovery require a systems approach to planning "to integrate all of the values and response capabilities necessary to achieve the best outcomes for the community as a whole" (IOM, 2012a, p. 3). The report states further that

> Successful disaster response depends on coordination and integration across the full system of the key stakeholder groups: state and local governments, EMS, public health, emergency management, hospital facilities, and the outpatient sector. Vertical integration among agencies at the federal, state, and local levels also is crucial. At the cornerstone of this coordination and integration is a foundation of ethical obligations—the values that do not change even when resources are scarce—and the legal authorities and regulatory environment that allow for shifts in expectations of the best possible care based on the context of the disaster in which that care is being provided. (IOM, 2012a, p. 3)

A complex mosaic of federal, state, and local resources is available for health care–related pre-disaster planning and disaster response and recovery. The roles of stakeholders at each of these different levels, along with resources available to support them in their activities, are discussed briefly below.

Federal Level[3]

Under the structure of the National Disaster Recovery Framework (NDRF; described in more detail in Chapter 3), health care falls within the Health and Social Services Recovery Support Function (RSF) (see Box 6-2), which is coordinated by the Assistant Secretary for Preparedness and Response (ASPR) within

---

[3] A broader synopsis of legislation and federal policy related to disaster recovery and health security can be found in Appendix A.

BOX 6-3
Health Care Coalitions

Healthcare Coalitions consist of a collaborative network of health care organizations and their respective public- and private-sector response partners within a defined region. Healthcare Coalitions serve as a multi-agency coordinating group that assists Emergency Management and Emergency Support Function (ESF) #8 with preparedness, response, recovery, and mitigation activities related to health care organization disaster operations. The primary function of the Healthcare Coalition includes sub-state regional health care system emergency preparedness activities involving the member organizations. Healthcare Coalitions also may provide multi-agency coordination to interface with the appropriate level of emergency operations in order to assist with the provision of situational awareness and the coordination of resources for healthcare organizations during a response.

SOURCE: Excerpted from ASPR, 2012, p. 1.

---

the U.S. Department of Health and Human Services (HHS) on behalf of the HHS Secretary. The NDRF supports a "whole-community" approach to recovery planning and operations. Thus, the audience for its guidance is specifically intended to include a broad range of stakeholders, including the health care delivery system.

The primary source of federal funding to support health care system preparedness, including pre-event planning for health care system recovery, is the Hospital Preparedness Program (HPP), established in 2002 and administered by ASPR. The original goal of the HPP was to enhance the ability of hospitals to prepare for and respond to bioterrorism attacks on the United States, as well as other public health emergencies, such as influenza pandemics and natural disasters. Today, the HPP is a crucial element of community resilience and enhances the response and recovery capabilities of the nation's health care system. Recognizing that a resilient health care system requires the engagement of all the system's components, ASPR has shifted the focus of the program from hospitals to health care coalitions (health care coalitions are described in Box 6-3). This shift reflects the recognition that, as demonstrated by such events as Hurricanes Katrina and Sandy and the H1N1 influenza pandemic, hospitals cannot be successful in response and recovery without the support and cooperation of a variety of critical community partners (ASPR, 2012). State HPP grantees, who are responsible for disseminating HPP funds to health care coalitions, are expected to encourage representation from the full spectrum of health care services in the building and sustaining of these regional coalitions—a goal the committee suggests warrants continued emphasis by federal and state leadership.

Currently, all 50 states, as well as the District of Columbia, eight U.S. territories and freely associated states, and the nation's three largest municipalities (Chicago, Los Angeles, and New York City), receive HPP funding. A core element of the contemporary version of the HPP is the capabilities-based framework developed in January 2012 titled *Healthcare Preparedness Capabilities: National Guidance for Healthcare System Preparedness* (ASPR, 2012). This guidance document lays out the eight health care system preparedness capabilities, one of which is Healthcare System Recovery. Importantly, these eight capabilities align with the Public Health Emergency Preparedness (PHEP) capabilities outlined in the Centers for Disease Control and Prevention's (CDC's) *Public Health Preparedness Capabilities: National Standards for State and Local Planning* (CDC, 2011), supporting the coordinated use of preparedness grant funds (see Table 5-1 in Chapter 5). Although only one of the HPP capabilities focuses specifically on recovery, the premise is that building and sustaining these eight core capabilities will provide the requisite infrastructure for short- and long-term disaster response and recovery.

According to the HPP guidance, "healthcare system recovery involves the collaboration with Emer-

---

BOX 6-4
Hospital Preparedness Program (HPP) Guidance on Health Care System Recovery

Under *Healthcare Preparedness Capabilities: National Guidance for Health System Preparedness*, funding allocated for the Healthcare System Recovery capability should be focused on enabling the following two critical functions.

Function 1   Develop recovery processes for the healthcare delivery system. Identify healthcare organization recovery needs and develop priority recovery processes to support a return to normalcy of operations or a new standard of normalcy for the provision of healthcare delivery to the community.
Function Alignment: [Public Health Emergency Preparedness] (PHEP) Capability 2, Community Recovery; Function 1: Identify and monitor public health, medical, and mental/behavioral health system recovery needs
Task 1 Assess the impact of an incident on the healthcare system's ability to deliver essential services to the community and prioritize healthcare recovery needs
Task 2 Promote healthcare organization participation in state and/or local pre-and post-disaster recovery planning activities as described in the National Disaster Recovery Framework (NDRF) in order to leverage recovery resources, programs, projects, and activities

Function 2   Assist healthcare organizations to implement Continuity of Operations (COOP). Maintain continuity of the healthcare delivery by coordinating recovery across functional healthcare organizations and encouraging business continuity planning
Function Alignment: [Public Health Emergency Preparedness] (PHEP) Capability 2, Community Recovery; Function 1, Resource P3: Continuity of Operations Plans
Task 1 Identify the healthcare essential services that must be continued to maintain healthcare delivery following a disaster.
Task 2 Encourage healthcare organizations to identify the components of a fully functional COOP and develop corresponding plans for implementation.
Task 3 If a disaster notice can be provided, alert healthcare organizations within communities threatened by disaster and if requested and feasible, assist them with the activation of COOP such that healthcare delivery to the community is minimally impacted.
Task 4 Develop coordinated health care strategies to assist healthcare organizations transition from COOP operations to normalcy or the new norm for healthcare operations

SOURCE: Excerpted from ASPR, 2012, pp. 12-14.

---

gency Management and other community partners (e.g., public health, business, and education) to develop efficient processes and advocate for the rebuilding of public health, medical, and mental/behavioral health systems to at least a level of functioning comparable to pre-incident levels and improved levels where possible. The focus is an effective and efficient return to normalcy or a new standard of normalcy for the provision of healthcare delivery to the community" (ASPR, 2012, p. 12). HPP staff report to the committee that 36 of the 50 state public health department HPP awardees have allocated funds for the Healthcare System Recovery capability and its two functions (see Box 6-4). The majority have focused on establishing a designated lead for recovery work, performing health care risk assessments, and engaging in the development of a recovery plan and process for hospitals and other facilities. Additional funded recovery activities include conducting trainings and workshops on building recovery and continuity of operations (COOP) processes.[4]

---

[4] E-mail communication, R. Dugas, HPP, to A. Downey, Institute of Medicine, regarding HPP funds, August 26, 2014.

The committee notes that the HPP cooperative agreement guidance document includes limited discussion of recovery planning beyond the early recovery phase. It is the committee's view that planning aimed only at achieving a preexisting and likely suboptimal state fails to exploit an opportunity to achieve more desirable longer-term goals of maximally healthy communities through improvements in care delivery and health care access. Thus, the committee strongly urges ASPR to take leadership in working with its fellow agency partners to expand the vision that informs its efforts. The HPP guidance would then be updated to articulate that the goal of health care sector recovery should not be simply to return to the pre-disaster state but to strengthen the sector so that the community will emerge from recovery healthier, more resilient, and sustainable. The checklist at the end of this chapter can be used to review and update this guidance accordingly. Further, the recovery functions identified in the updated HPP cooperative agreement should be aligned with similar changes to other federal grant programs, including the CDC's PHEP cooperative agreement and the preparedness grants of the Federal Emergency Management Agency (FEMA) (see Recommendation 1 in Chapter 3).

Although health care system recovery is a key ASPR programmatic area, it is important to note that many other departments within HHS and across the federal government (e.g., the U.S. Department of Veterans Affairs [VA]) have important roles in defining and expanding the role of health care in a healthy community. The Centers for Medicare & Medicaid Services (CMS), for example, has great influence as a result of its authority to determine the services that can be covered by Medicare and Medicaid. For instance, effective January 1, 2014, a change in the federal rule on essential health benefits allows Medicaid reimbursement for preventive services delivered by nonlicensed providers as long as those services have been recommended by a physician or another licensed provider (ASTHO, 2015). This rule change has important implications in terms of transitioning to community-based models of care (e.g., utilization of community health workers), as described later in this chapter. Other agencies whose efforts need to be integrated into the recovery planning process include the Health Resources and Services Administration, which provides support for federally qualified health centers, and the Agency for Healthcare Research and Quality.

Federal Legislation Relevant to Health Care Sector Preparedness and Recovery

Waivers and Authorizations   Waivers of certain federal regulatory requirements are available following presidentially declared disasters and emergency declarations to ensure that health care systems and providers have the flexibility necessary to provide care when their infrastructure has been impacted by the disaster. Often these waivers are issued during the initial stages of disaster response, but they may be extended during the short-term recovery period as warranted. Waivers and their justification are subject to congressional notification.

Under Section 1135 of the Social Security Act, the Secretary of HHS may waive requirements under Medicare and Medicaid upon declaring a public health emergency.[5] Such waivers allow, for example, bed capacity increases, cessation of all but emergency survey activities, relaxed length-of-stay requirements in skilled nursing facilities, and relaxed supervision requirements for staff in home health and hospice agencies. The waiver authority may also be used to enable health care professionals who hold out-of-state licenses to operate legally and obtain reimbursement in the state experiencing the emergency. Waivers may be retroactive to the beginning of the emergency. Also under Section 1135 of the Social Security Act, the Secretary of HHS may waive sanctions for hospitals engaging in inappropriate transfer or relocation of patients for medical evaluation under federally declared disaster conditions. Under normal conditions, the Emergency Medical Treatment and Active Labor Act (EMTALA) of 1986 requires hospitals to offer emergency screening and stabilization to all comers irrespective of citizenship, legal status, or ability to pay.[6] They may not transfer or discharge individuals with an emergency medical condition unless the

---

[5] Social Security Act § 1135, Aug. 14, 1935.

[6] Examination and Treatment for Emergency Medical Conditions and Women in Labor. 42 U.S.C. § 1395dd. 2005.

patient has stabilized or given informed consent, or if their condition necessitates transfer to a hospital better equipped to provide needed care. The Secretary's waiver applies only to relief from sanctions under EMTALA; it does not apply to actions brought by individuals or hospitals alleging harms owing to violations of EMTALA. Those individuals or hospitals may still sue for damages. Waivers from EMTALA sanctions were utilized during Hurricanes Katrina, Rita, Gustav, and Ike, among others.

Should the President declare an emergency or disaster and the Secretary of HHS also declare a public health emergency, the Secretary has the authority to waive sanctions against hospitals that fail to comply with specific provisions requirements of the Health Insurance Portability and Accountability Act (HIPAA) Privacy Rule (ASPR, 2013):

- the requirement to obtain a patient's consent to disclose protected health information to a family member or close personal friend involved in the patient's care (45 CFR 164.510(b));
- the requirement to honor an objection to being included in the facility directory (45 CFR 164.510(a));
- an individual's right to a notice of privacy practices for protected health information (45 CFR 164.520);
- an individual's right to request privacy restrictions (45 CFR 164.522(a)); and
- an individual's right to request confidential communications (45 CFR 164.522(b)).

When a waiver is issued, it pertains only to the region and timeframe described in the public health emergency declaration. Moreover, it pertains only to hospitals that have instituted a disaster protocol, and it lasts only up to 72 hours from the time the hospital begins to invoke its disaster protocol. When the presidential or secretarial declaration ends, a hospital must resume compliance with all HIPAA requirements for all patients under its care, irrespective of whether 72 hours has elapsed since its disaster protocol was invoked. In the absence of an emergency waiver, HIPAA rules still allow certain disclosures to disaster relief organizations and for treatment purposes (ASPR, 2013). For example, HIPAA regulations allow hospitals to disclose protected health information to the American Red Cross so it can inform family members of a patient's whereabouts (45 CFR 164.510(b)(4)).

CMS Proposed Rule   On December 27, 2013, CMS filed a Federal Register notice regarding the Proposed Rule for Emergency Preparedness Requirements for Medicare and Medicaid Participating Providers and Suppliers (still pending as of publication of this report). The rationale for this rule is that "disasters can disrupt the environment of health care and change the demand for health care services. This makes it essential that health care providers and suppliers ensure that emergency management is integrated into their daily functions and values."[7] CMS believes that the fragmented collection of current federal, state, and local laws and guidelines and accrediting organization emergency preparedness standards is inadequate for ensuring that health care providers and suppliers are prepared for a disaster. This assertion is based on extensive analysis of the literature and ongoing dialogue with various stakeholders and representatives of local, state, and federal entities.[8] Consistent with the point made earlier in this chapter that building a comprehensive and integrated care delivery system is fundamental to creating maximally healthy and resilient communities, the committee was pleased to note that this proposed rule is aligned with and in fact cites the program guidance for emergency preparedness grants from HHS.

The proposed rule addresses what most experts cite as the key elements of preparedness necessary to ensure that health care is available during response to and recovery from an emergency: "safeguarding

---

[7] 78 F.R. 79084, Dec. 27, 2013.

[8] The proposed rule reflects the guidance and input of key stakeholders in health care delivery infrastructure, including other federal agencies; the American College of Healthcare Executives (policy guidance); the American Osteopathic Association (standards for disaster preparedness); The Joint Commission (standards for emergency preparedness); the National Fire Protection Association (disaster and emergency management standards); and certain states, including California and Maryland, with salient state-level requirements.

human resources, ensuring business continuity, and protecting physical resources."[9] To these ends, the proposed rule focuses on four key functions for different categories of care providers and suppliers:

- risk assessment and planning utilizing an "all-hazards" approach, which means evaluating the full range of potential hazards and vulnerabilities;
- "develop[ing] and implement[ing] policies and procedures based on the emergency plan and risk assessment";
- developing and maintaining an emergency preparedness communication plan to facilitate well-coordinated patient care "within the facility, across health care providers, and with state and local public health departments and emergency systems"; and
- "develop[ing] and maintain[ing] an emergency preparedness training and testing program."[10]

The Patient Protection and Affordable Care Act In 2013, the Institute of Medicine (IOM) organized a workshop that examined the impacts of the ACA on preparedness (IOM, 2014a). While the ACA does not include many specific provisions that directly address preparedness, response, or recovery, a number of the provisions will have an impact on strengthening the resilience and health of a community and should be taken into consideration during disaster recovery. Examples include

- the impact of coverage expansion, changing reimbursement systems and new incentives on preparedness activities;
- the use of health information technology to strengthen preparedness, response, and recovery;
- the use of existing resources for improving daily operations and emergency response;
- workforce training needs;
- opportunities for building relationships and coalitions among health care delivery systems that may not previously have been involved in preparedness activities; and
- an emerging model for care delivery referred to as community paramedicine or mobile integrated health care practice (see Box 6-5) (IOM, 2014a, p. 37).

Many of the ACA provisions with more immediate impacts on improving community resilience and health are highlighted in Table 6-1.

Regional, State, and Local Levels

The highly decentralized health care delivery system encompasses a wide range of for-profit, nonprofit, and governmental (regional, state, and local) entities. Community health care is delivered through the interaction of hospitals, networks of outpatient providers, long-term care facilities, home health care and hospice, emergency medical services, behavioral health services, community and large chain pharmacies, and walk-in health services. A complex, sophisticated support system of financial, diagnostics, and logistics (e.g., supply chain, transportation) providers are less well understood facilitators of care. Technology, in particular health information technology, has an ever-increasing role in connecting patients to providers and structuring that connection in powerful ways. Planning, coordination, and financial support by regional, state, and local public health entities also are important elements of a community's health care system. Health care coalitions, described earlier, are key mechanisms for supporting a coordinated approach to planning at the regional level.

The goal of incident management in events entailing mass casualties or the catastrophic failure of crucial infrastructure is "to get the right resources to the right place at the right time." These same goals should also help guide recovery. As noted by the IOM,

---

[9] 78 F.R. 79085, Dec. 27, 2013.
[10] 78 F.R. 79085, Dec. 27, 2013.

This may involve anticipating shortfalls, adapting responses, partnering with other stakeholder agencies to provide alternate care sites for patient volumes that cannot be accommodated within the usual medical facilities, and other strategies. Therefore, a regionally coordinated response is imperative to facilitate consistent standards of care within all affected communities after a disaster. Regional coordination enables the optimal use of available resources; facilitates obtaining and distributing resources; and provides a mechanism for policy development and situational awareness that is critical to avoiding crisis situations and, when a crisis does occur, ensuring fair and consistent use of resources to provide a uniform level of care across the region. (IOM, 2012a, p. 10)

Health care systems and hospitals are well recognized as crucial partners in community health planning because of their organizational capacity, specialized workforce, health analytic capabilities, and significant stakeholder status in their communities. Often undervalued and overlooked as healthy community partners, however, are local outpatient providers and clinics, group homes, long-term care facilities, and home health providers, which can play key roles in surge response and recovery efforts (IOM, 2012a). The vast majority (approximately 89 percent) of health care encounters occur in these outpatient settings (Hall et al., 2010; Schappert and Rechtsteiner, 2011), and the increasing focus on preventive care is leading to an even greater role for outpatient care facilities and providers. Therefore, it is imperative that outpatient care assets be integrated as the systems framework for disaster prepared-

---

BOX 6-5
Community Paramedicine

Community paramedicine is an emerging model of collaborative, community-based health care in which emergency medical technicians and paramedics operate in expanded roles, beyond emergency response and transport. Community paramedicine utilizes the skills of emergency management personnel in addressing care gaps in the community to encourage more appropriate and efficient use of emergency care resources and to improve access to primary care, especially for underserved populations. As concerns regarding rising health care costs and the need to better connect underserved populations to the delivery of care persist, interest in and implementation of the community paramedicine model have grown, given its potential to improve the quality of and access to care while also reducing costs (Kizer et al., 2013).

While community paramedicine programs vary from place to place, most

- "begin with a community-specific health care needs assessment,
- community paramedics are specially trained to provide services to meet those local needs, and
- community paramedics provide services under clear medical control (i.e., under a physician's direction and supervision)" (Kizer et al., 2013, p. 7).

Specific examples of the benefits of community paramedicine programs include getting individuals who have accessed emergency services yet are not suffering from medical emergencies to more appropriate sources of care than a hospital emergency department. As part of the effort to increase access to primary care for underserved populations, some community paramedicine programs offer short-term follow-up visits for newly discharged patients, a practice that may help prevent emergency department or hospital readmissions (Kizer et al., 2013). The community paramedicine model has particular potential for rural communities. In these low-call-volume areas, the integration of emergency medical technicians and paramedics into the local or regional health care system allows these personnel to maintain their skills and expand their clinical experience (HRSA, 2012; Kizer et al., 2013).

TABLE 6-1 ACA Provisions That Could Potentially Affect Medical and Public Health Preparedness Activities[a]

Title/Subtitle (Section)	Topic Area	Summary of Provision[b]	Potential Impact on Preparedness as Presented by Individual Speakers
Title 3. A. I (3001)	Hospital Value-Based Purchasing	A percentage of hospital payment would be tied to hospital performance on quality measures related to common and high-cost conditions, such as cardiac, surgical, and pneumonia care.	Greater emphasis on overall health of patient, prevention and wellness; greater need to demonstrate value; ensuring patient needs are met before and after hospital visit.[1]
Title 3. F (3504-3505)	Regional Trauma Care	Provides funding to the Assistant Secretary for Preparedness and Response (ASPR) to support pilot projects that design, implement, and evaluate innovative models of regionalized, comprehensive, and accountable emergency care and trauma systems (3504); Reauthorizes and improves the trauma care program, providing grants administered by the Health and Human Services (HHS) Secretary to states and trauma centers to strengthen the nation's trauma system (3505).	Improved everyday care and emergency response at a regional level can improve response in a disaster;[2,5] housing under ASPR also can allow for better coordination between preparedness and daily emergency programs.[3]
Title 3. G (2551); Title 3. B (3133)	Disproportionate Share Hospital Allotments	Reduction in federal Medicaid Disproportionate Share Hospital Allotments at the state level, based on the assumption of increased coverage and reduced uncompensated care costs. While the statute sets forth reductions through fiscal year 2020, the final rule applies only to reductions in fiscal year 2014 and 2015.	For those states that do not expand their Medicaid program, the coverage increase will not occur. But their safety-net hospitals will still lose this allotment, and correspondingly, they may have fewer resources to bring to bear in a disaster.[1,16,17]
Title 4. D (4304)	Epidemiology-Laboratory Capacity Grants	Grant program to award funding to states and local and tribal jurisdictions to improve surveillance and threat detection and build laboratory capacity.	Increased funding and capacity at the state and local levels for threat detection and biosurveillance.[4]
Title 5. C (5210)	Ready Reserve Corps	Ready Reserve Corps members may be called to active duty to respond to national emergencies and public health crises and to fill critical public health positions left vacant by members of the Regular Corps who have been called to duty elsewhere.	Building a network of trained professionals ready to respond in disasters who can be deployed to assist in any public health emergency and augment response.[6]
Title 5. D (5314-5315)	U.S. Public Health Sciences Track	Increased emphasis on team-based service and merging of clinical and public health training. Public health recruitment and retention programs are also being expanded.	Potential for increased and better-educated workforce within the public health field.[6]

TABLE 6-1 Continued

Title/Subtitle (Section)	Topic Area	Summary of Provision[b]	Potential Impact on Preparedness as Presented by Individual Speakers
Title 5. F (5502)	Federally Qualified Health Center (FQHC) Improvements	Expansion of Medicare-Covered Preventive Services at FQHCs; Increased spending for FQHCs.	Could remove the burden of surge from community hospitals (and Disproportionate Share Hospital payments) if patients shift routine care visits throughout the FQHC network.[7]
Title 5. G (5601)	FQHC Improvements		
Title 6. D (6301)	Patient-Centered Outcomes Research Institute	Establishes private, nonprofit institute to identify priorities for and provide for the conduct of comparative outcomes research.	Increased data infrastructure and dissemination of research findings focused on improved patient outcomes could contribute to more standardized sharing of best practices.[8]
Title 9. A (9007, 6033(b), 4959)	Community Health Needs Assessment (CHNA)	Imposes new requirements on 501(c)(3) organizations that operate one or more hospital facilities to conduct a CHNA and adopt an implementation strategy at least once every 3 years (9007); Also added a tax penalty for failing to meet and report this requirement (6033(b), 4959).	Better awareness of community needs in an emergency and a more accurate population picture; opportunity for hospitals to partner more with public health departments to meet these requirements.[7,9]
Title 3. A. II (3015) Title 4. D (4302)	Data Collection, Public Reporting; Understanding Disparities, Data Collection and Analysis	Development of data collection standards for five different demographic factors and calls for them to be collected in all national population health surveys (4302); Requires the Secretary to collect and aggregate consistent data on quality and resource use measures from information systems used to support health care delivery to implement the public reporting of performance information (3015).	More data and information will be available for improved awareness of community needs and resources; more information will be available for surveillance and predictive modeling.[4,10,11,12]
Title 1. D. I (1302, 1311)	Mental Health	(1) By including mental health and substance use disorder benefits in the Essential Health Benefits; (2) by applying federal parity protections to mental health and substance use disorder benefits in the individual and small group markets; and (3) by providing more Americans with access to quality health care that includes coverage for mental health and substance use disorder services.	Individuals can have better coverage for daily mental health and substance abuse issues and after a disaster may have better access to services because they are already familiar with care and providers.[9]

continued

TABLE 6-1 Continued

Title/Subtitle (Section)	Topic Area	Summary of Provision[b]	Potential Impact on Preparedness as Presented by Individual Speakers
Title 1. G (1561); Title IV. D (4304)	Health Information Technology, Interoperability, and Standards	Requires the development of standards and protocols to promote the interoperability of systems for enrollment of individuals in federal and state health and human services programs (1561); Requires the Director of the Centers for Disease Control and Prevention (CDC) to issue national standards on information exchange systems to public health entities for the reporting of infectious diseases and other conditions of public health importance in consultation with the National Coordinator for Health Information Technology (4304).	While everyone is collecting data, the data may not reach their potential utility unless they can be shared across county, state, and agency lines; standards and interoperability are key to building on Health Information Technology for Economic and Clinical Health Act and Meaningful Use standards.[8,13,14]
Title 3. F (3510); Title 3. D (3306); Title 4. A (4003); Title 4. C (4201, 4202)	Community Resilience	Patient navigator program (3510); Funding outreach and assistance for low-income programs (3306); Clinical and Community Preventive Services (4003); Community Transformation Grants (4201); Healthy Aging, Living Well: evaluation of community-based prevention and wellness programs for Medicaid beneficiaries (4202).	Patient navigator program can assist patients in continuity of care and in staying healthy in steady-state times. Opportunity for improved care and overall health at the community level through transformation grants and preventive services; evaluation of community-based programs could allow for improvements and ability to share lessons across cities and states.[15]

[a] The information presented in this table was compiled by the rapporteurs of a 2014 IOM workshop (IOM, 2014a) based on presentations made by workshop speakers. Each potential impact has been referenced to the workshop speaker(s) who discussed the relevant topic as follows: [1]Lisa Tofil, [2]Norman Miller, [3]Gregg Margolis, [4]Georges Benjamin, [5]Charles Cairns, [6]Ellen Embrey, [7]Karen DeSalvo, [8]Justin Barnes, [9]Nicole Lurie, [10]Gus Birkhead, [11]Nathaniel Hupert, [12]Brandon Dean, [13]Kevin Larsen, [14]Roland Gamache, [15]Connie Chan, [16]Xiaoyi Huang, and [17]Jack Ebeler.

[b] Summary items garnered from https://www.govtrack.us/congress/bills/111/hr3590/text# (accessed June 8, 2014).
SOURCE: IOM, 2014a, p. 4-7.

ness, response, and recovery is developed. However, the committee recognizes that health care providers based outside of hospitals, particularly private providers, have limited and sometimes no funding for participating in a comprehensive disaster planning effort. Greater attention to incentivizing the participation of the full spectrum of health care providers is needed to actualize a systems approach to disaster preparedness and recovery.

PRE-DISASTER HEALTH CARE SECTOR PRIORITIES

The speed and success of the health care system's post-disaster recovery depend to a large extent on pre-disaster planning both within the health care sector and across sectors. A robust pre-disaster planning process also is key to capitalizing on the opportunities presented by a disaster to improve the health care system during the recovery process because it prepares the community to make the needed improvements.

In the pre-disaster preparedness stage, specific attention is devoted to planning for the transitions from response to recovery and then back to steady state. The planning includes

- identifying and developing relationships with key local and regional partners;
- identifying [and strengthening] programs and systems that could be leveraged after a disaster; and
- building an understanding of current program and system resources, capabilities, and needs (FEMA, 2014a.

This section identifies several key activities that should be undertaken prior to a disaster to increase the capacity of the health care sector to respond to the surge in health needs that may occur in the early recovery phase as well as to the long-term community health care needs that may arise later during the recovery period. These activities include

- assessing the capacity and vulnerability of the health care system,
- establishing, sustaining, and exercising health care coalitions and other coordinating groups,
- developing continuity of operations (COOP) and recovery plans, and
- establishing a resilient health information technology system.

As indicated earlier in this chapter, a variety of federal, state, and local funding resources may be available to aid in these activities.

Assessing the Capacity and Vulnerability of the Health Care System

The success of the recovery of any community's health care sector is informed by an assessment of the community's health status and the strengths and weaknesses of its health and social service systems and resources prior to disaster. It is imperative that recovery planning for the health care sector be informed by an assessment of the community's overall risks, threats, and vulnerabilities, such as those that could impact community infrastructure (buildings), transportation (roadways, bridges, tunnels), utility services (water/sewage treatment, electricity), and its vulnerable populations. Such assessments also should include a vision of what post-disaster recovery should look like for that community from the health care and health systems perspectives.

Community Health Needs Assessment

Under the provisions of the ACA, nonprofit hospitals are now required to conduct a community health needs assessment.[11] A community health needs assessment (CHNA)[12] is:

> a process that uses quantitative and qualitative methods to systematically collect and analyze data to understand health within a specific community. An ideal assessment includes information on risk factors, quality of life, mortality, morbidity, community assets, forces of change, social determinants of health and health inequity, and information on how well the public health system provides essential services. Community health assessment data inform community decision-making, the prioritization of health problems, and the development, implementation, and evaluation of community health improvement plans. (NACCHO, 2014)

To avoid a tax penalty, nonprofit hospitals conducting CHNAs must demonstrate a community benefit. One such benefit that could stem from CHNAs and associated implementation plans is community health resilience. By providing information on vulnerable populations in the community, preparing to meet the

---

[11] 26 U.S.C. § 501(r).

[12] The term "community health needs assessment" is often used interchangeably with the term "community health assessment."

needs of those populations, and increasing public awareness regarding the threat of social vulnerability, nonprofit hospitals can help build a more prepared community (IOM, 2014a). To this end, Internal Revenue Service (IRS)-required CHNAs should be conducted in collaboration with the regional, state, or local department of health (NACCHO, 2012) and, where possible, utilize data from existing health information technology systems, which are discussed later in this chapter.

Hazard Vulnerability Analysis

Recovery planning for the health care sector should also be informed by a health care facility assessment that includes a hazard vulnerability analysis (HVA). HVA is defined as "a systematic approach to identifying all hazards that may affect an organization, assessing the risk (probability of hazard occurrence and the consequence for the organization) associated with each hazard and analyzing findings to create a prioritized comparison of hazard vulnerabilities. The consequence, or vulnerability, is related to both the impact on organizational function and the likely service demands created by hazard impact" (HHS, 2007).

An HVA examines physical infrastructure risks based on environmental (e.g., wind, fire, storm, flood) and other vulnerabilities (e.g., insufficient quantities of medical equipment and pharmaceuticals, food, water, limitations of insurance coverage). This assessment helps identify facilities or systems for which more robust advance planning is necessary to ensure continuity of operations after a disaster (Knowlton and Rotkin-Ellman, 2014). Typically, an HVA is required as part of the Joint Commission's accreditation process, and it is a requirement under CMS's proposed emergency preparedness rule discussed above.

As mentioned earlier, a facility's HVA should also be informed by overall community risks and vulnerabilities. Most local emergency management planners routinely conduct a threat and hazard identification and risk assessment (THIRA)[13] based on their jurisdiction and region; health care facility planners should collaborate with their local emergency management agency in the development of their facility/health system HVA.

In addition to collaboration with local public health and emergency management agencies, both a pre-disaster CHNA and an HVA must be informed by a broad range of public- and private-sector perspectives that encompasses citizens, community- and faith-based organizations, health care providers and other nearby health care systems, government and elected officials, insurers, and representatives of the business community. Representation of these groups in recovery planning for the health care sector is critical to identifying what capabilities the health care system and its partners may need to bring to bear during the response to and recovery from a disaster.

Establishing, Sustaining, and Exercising Health Care Coalitions and Other Coordinating Groups

ASPR's HPP emphasizes the importance of communities building and sustaining health care coalitions, as discussed previously in this chapter. To aid in these efforts, ASPR's HPP cooperative agreement supports the establishment of these coalitions and provides guidance on how they can strengthen a jurisdiction's medical surge and other health care preparedness capabilities. As highlighted in the 2012 IOM report *Crisis Standards of Care: A Systems Framework for Catastrophic Disaster Response*, health care coalitions have two key functions:

- "Develop strategies and tactics to support emergency preparedness, response, and recovery activities of substate regional health care systems involving member organizations; and
- Provide multiagency coordination for the interface with the appropriate level of emergency

---

[13] A THIRA is a four-step process that assists the entire community, including individuals, businesses, faith-based organizations, nonprofit groups, schools, and governments, in determining and comprehending its risks and estimating capability requirements (FEMA, 2014b).

operations to assist with the provision of situational awareness and the coordination of resources for health care organizations during a response" (p. 45).

The multistakeholder composition of health care coalitions is important not only in preparedness planning and response but also in bringing together the relevant multisector expertise during short- and long-term recovery (see Box 6-6). The coalition can serve as a primary mechanism for local and regional coordination (for planning and operations) among care providers, as well as in public health and emergency management. If coalitions are to serve these functions, however, they must participate in state and local recovery planning and be integrated into the organizational structures of the RSFs specified in the NDRF. Relationships with the public health and emergency management sectors can facilitate this integration.

Historically, many health care coalitions have limited their membership to representatives of hospitals, public health, and emergency management. Given the complex health care needs of a community during recovery from a disaster, however, coalition membership needs to expand beyond those sectors (see Table 6-2).

Efforts to expand representation on health care coalitions to reflect the full complement of stakeholders presented in Table 6-2 may face considerable challenges. For example, private outpatient providers care for the majority of the population (including most patients on Medicaid [O'Shea, 2007; Paradise, 2015]) but generally have little incentive to participate in recovery planning or health care coalitions. Outpatient providers (including behavioral health care providers) are decentralized, mainly privately owned businesses that have increasingly limited regular contact with hospitals (because of an increase in hospital-based providers who handle inpatient duties) and may see little value in participating in such organizations and planning efforts. Professional organizations (particularly those specific to specialties such as pediatrics) may be helpful in facilitating efforts to engage nonhospital providers in the recovery planning process.[14]

Task forces and workgroups may be formed before and after disasters to address specific needs related to health care recovery and may require the participation of health care providers. For example, pediatricians should participate in children and youth task forces, as discussed in Chapter 8. Other examples include behavioral health workgroups and workgroups formed to meet the needs of frail elderly persons (e.g., those in nursing homes) (Hillsborough County Government, 2010).

Developing Continuity of Operations and Recovery Plans

COOP is "an effort within individual organizations to ensure they can continue to perform their essential functions during a wide range of emergencies, including localized acts of nature, accidents, and technological or attack-related emergencies" (DHS, 2012, p. P-3). Because health care systems provide a critical array of services after a disaster, they must develop a COOP plan as part of their overall disaster recovery plan (DHS, 2012). ASPR's *Healthcare Preparedness Capabilities: National Guidance for Healthcare System Preparedness* emphasizes that health care facilities must develop a COOP plan as part of achieving the Healthcare System Recovery capability (ASPR, 2012). This guidance document identifies four important tasks associated with the implementation of COOP:

- "Identify the healthcare essential services that must be continued to maintain healthcare delivery following a disaster;
- Encourage healthcare organizations to identify the components of a fully functional COOP and develop corresponding plans for implementation;
- If a disaster notice can be provided, alert healthcare organizations within communities threatened by disaster and if requested and feasible, assist them with the activation of COOP such that healthcare delivery to the community is minimally impacted; [and]

---

[14] E-mail communication, S. Needle, Healthcare Network of Southwest Florida, to A. Downey, Institute of Medicine, regarding experience with disaster recovery, August 23, 2014.

HEALTHY, RESILIENT, AND SUSTAINABLE COMMUNITIES AFTER DISASTERS

BOX 6-6
Key Features of Hospital and Health Care Coalitions

Over the past decade, robust regional hospital and health care coalitions have developed that often started as mutual-aid agreements or simply meetings as part of hospital preparedness grant programs. Some are led by an executive director, with hospital administrators serving as the board of directors (Northern Virginia Hospital Alliance); others are led by a public health agency (e.g., King County, Washington) or a consortium of state public health and health departments (Southeastern Regional Pediatric Disaster Surge Network); and still others are led by elected members of the emergency preparedness group (e.g., Minneapolis/St. Paul). These coalitions have been extremely successful in planning and exercising for disasters, as well as demonstrated operational response functions during actual incidents. Key features of strong coalitions are

- collaborative and invested leadership;
- written agreements specifying how and when the coalition is to be activated and its delegated responsibilities;
- a trusted agency or entity to represent the facilities to the emergency management and public health communities;
- collaborative work in concrete response areas (e.g., regional HAZMAT training and planning);
- linkages to cooperative agreements, grants, and programs such as the Hospital Preparedness Program, Metropolitan Medical Response System, Urban Area Security Initiative, and the Centers for Disease Control and Prevention's (CDC's) Public Health Emergency Preparedness (PHEP) cooperative agreements (notably, the PHEP cooperative agreement has adopted the conventional/contingency/crisis framework for health care surge capacity);
- operational experience in representing or coordinating policy and resources during exercises and incidents; and
- multiagency collaboration and integration with other response partners, ensuring recognition of the coalition as a defined entity within the emergency response framework of the community.

SOURCE: Excerpted from IOM, 2012a, p. 230.

- Develop coordinated healthcare strategies to assist healthcare organizations transition from COOP operations to normalcy or the new norm for healthcare operations" (ASPR, 2012, p. 14).

In addition, the Joint Commission identifies four elements of performance related to recovery that it uses to accredit and certify hospitals:

- "EM 02.01.01 EP4—The hospital develops and maintains a written Emergency Operations Plan that describes the recovery strategies and actions designed to help restore the systems that are critical to providing care, treatment, and services after an emergency;
- EM 02.01.01 EP5—The Emergency Operations Plan describes the processes for initiating and terminating the hospital's response and recovery phases of the emergency, including under what circumstances these phases are activated;
- EM 02.02.03 EP2—[EOP describes the following] How the hospital will obtain and replenish medical supplies that will be required throughout the response and recovery phases of an emergency, including personal protective equipment where required; and

TABLE 6-2 Potential Members of Health Care Coalitions to Address Recovery Considerations

Essential Partners	Additional Health Care Coalition Partners/Members
Emergency Medical Services, hospitals, and other health care administrators	Local and state law enforcement and fire services
Emergency management/public safety	Public works
Long-term care providers	Private organizations
Mental/behavioral health care providers	Nongovernmental organizations
Private entities associated with health care (e.g., hospital associations)	Nonprofit organizations
Specialty service providers (e.g., dialysis, pediatrics, women's health, stand-alone surgery, urgent care)	Volunteer Organizations Active in Disaster (VOAD)
Support service providers (e.g., laboratories, pharmacies, blood banks, poison control)	Faith-based organizations
Primary care providers	Community-based organizations
Community health centers	Volunteer medical organizations (e.g., American Red Cross)
Public health	
Tribal health care	
Federal entities (e.g., National Disaster Medical System, U.S. Department of Veterans Affairs [VA] hospitals, Indian Health Service facilities, U.S. Department of Defense facilities)	

SOURCE: ASPR, 2012, p. 2.

- EM 02.02.03 EP3—[EOP describes the following] How the hospital will obtain and replenish non-medical supplies that will be required throughout the response and recovery phases of an emergency." (The Joint Commission, 2013)

COOP plans should also guide a health care facility or system on "how key resources from governmental, nongovernmental, and private sector agencies can be used to support the sustainment and reestablishment of essential services for healthcare organizations. This coordination assists healthcare organizations to maintain their functional capabilities during and after an all hazards incident and enables a rapid and more effective recovery" (ASPR, 2012, p. 13).

In developing COOP and recovery plans, health care sector planners need to extend beyond surge scenarios to include major infrastructure loss contingencies. Planning for infrastructure loss requires the identification of potential temporary sites and facilities, as well as measures to ensure continuity of supply chain operations. The following considerations apply to supply chain continuity planning[15]:

- Administrators should have a plan in place for sourcing post-disaster supplies, including a supply list (e.g., based on a disaster formulary or records of past orders) with anticipated quantities, binding contracts with suppliers and pre-authorization for placing orders. Special consideration should be given to assessing whether a supplier is providing products or services to other facilities and determining the prioritization of those products/services.

---

[15] Personal communication, G. Kirtser, ROi, to A. Downey, Institute of Medicine, regarding lessons learned from Mercy Health Joplin Experience, July 16, 2014.

- Disaster recovery plans, operating procedures, and supply lists need to be documented and available in digital and paper forms, and multiple staff members need to be aware of them.
- Large distribution companies (which most health facilities use) have planned extensively for disaster scenarios and can be a good resource. Distributors may not share disaster plans as a matter of course, but facility administrators can request this information to help with their own plans.

Just as important as establishing a COOP plan is establishing a plan for the transition from continuity of operations to normal operations following disaster recovery (ASPR, 2012).

Finally, much of the emphasis in disaster drills and exercises focuses on preparing for disaster response, with little attention given to testing a facility's COOP and recovery plans. Failure to conduct such testing could impact the availability essential services of a health care facility or system following a disaster.

Establishing a Resilient Health Information Technology System

The nation is advancing toward the widespread adoption of personal health records and electronic health records, which facilitate the collection of patient-specific medical information that can be shared among providers to help maintain continuity of care. Federal legislation—most notably the ACA and the Health Information Technology for Economic and Clinical Health Act,[16] included in the American Recovery and Reinvestment Act of 2009—encourages the use and spread of health information technology. These two acts include specific provisions aimed at increasing the use of electronic health records throughout the health care sector, as well as the implementation of meaningful use guidelines with which to monitor and reward health care providers and organizations using the technology (ONC, 2012). Additionally, efforts at the state and local levels to create health information exchanges are facilitating the flow of clinical information across centers of care.

The emergence of information technology in health care has presented both opportunities and challenges for its use in disaster scenarios. Concerns remain about privacy and information and data sharing, as well as costs associated with new technology. Nonetheless, experience from past disasters has shown that health information technology tools (e.g., electronic medical records, health information exchanges) are valuable assets in addressing many of the challenges associated with the interruption of health care relationships that occurs as patients relocate temporarily or permanently away from their regular providers, thereby losing the benefit of their providers' records (see Box 6-7). Because access to health information and other vital records is imperative during recovery, health systems need to be more proactive in planning for continuing access to these resources following a disaster (Horahan et al., 2014). Electronic records that can be accessed from cloud-based storage, for example, ensure access to critical health information if physical records are destroyed. Health systems also should consider storing copies of electronic health records on a local physical server to ensure access in the event of a disruption in Internet service. In addition, personal health records are increasingly available through consumer-mediated exchange initiatives, such as the Blue Button initiative (Health IT, 2014), and mobile personal health apps such as Microsoft's HealthVault (HealthVault, 2015). These technologies can empower individuals and families to be prepared for all kinds of emergencies, increase health literacy, and reduce some of the post-disaster challenges related to lack of access to critical health information. Differences in the responses to Hurricanes Katrina and Sandy demonstrate the benefits of health information technology for preparedness, planning, response, and recovery (IOM, 2014a).

In addition to facilitating individual care, health data also can be used to develop a better understanding of the community (e.g., through baseline data) and to evaluate program effectiveness as health protection and promotion measures are implemented. The expansion of coverage through the ACA has increased participation in the health care system. As a result, more people are now visible to the system and more data are available with which to understand a community's potential vulnerabilities, to plan for

---

[16] 42 U.S.C. § 300jj et seq.; § 17901 et seq.

BOX 6-7
Health Information Technology as a Critical Resource for
Health Care System Recovery:
Lessons from the U.S. Department of Veterans Affairs (VA) After Hurricane Katrina

In August 2005, catastrophic flooding in New Orleans after Hurricane Katrina forced approximately 80 percent of the city's population to evacuate, including most of the nearly 40,000 veterans who received care at the New Orleans VA Medical Center before the storm hit (Brown et al., 2007). Because of the population dispersal, veterans were frequently treated at locations outside their normal health system. VA's electronic health records became a critical tool for maintaining continuity of care for displaced veterans (Claver et al., 2012; Hogan et al., 2011), a benefit that largely was not present in the health system at the time. Between August 29 and September 30, 2005, data requests for 14,941 New Orleans VA patients were processed, totaling 38 percent of the pre-Katrina patient group. The requests came from 125 sites across 48 states and Washington, DC (Brown et al., 2007). While VA's use of electronic health records to provide continued care following Katrina is generally considered a success, Brown and colleagues (2007) suggest several steps to improve the use of these systems in a post-disaster setting. These include improved integration among multiple electronic health record operating systems to further enhance coordination, as well as improved availability of health data beyond prescriptions and lab results, which were the most commonly available data in electronic record systems (Brown et al., 2007).

---

individuals with specific or complex health needs, and to foster resiliency. Likewise, data from electronic health records, syndromic surveillance, and other sources can facilitate modeling, predictive analytics, and real-time situational awareness that informs pre-disaster planning and provides decision support during and after an event (IOM, 2014a).

Health information technology also is expanding beyond health care to enable better integration of different kinds of care providers, a capability that could be of great value after a disaster when people need to reconnect with their entire care support network. For example, Parkland Center for Clinical Innovation (PCCI), a nonprofit organization in Dallas, Texas, has developed an information exchange portal that captures social health components important to public health preparedness and response (PCCI, 2014). The aim is to include more than 400 community organizations that provide a range of social services, including shelter, food and nutrition assistance, transportation assistance, housing assistance, and financial support (IOM, 2014a). A goal is to connect health care organizations and providers in the region, as well as behavioral health professionals and first responders, through the information portal. Thus, the portal can serve to provide coordination of care for patients whose care involves various health and social services providers, enabling the sharing of information about medications and medical history and facilitating the identification of patients with mobility needs who may require additional assistance, especially during a disaster.

Many of the benefits of health information technology, including information exchange portals, are useful during daily operations but can provide extra benefit during and after disasters or emergencies (see Table 6-3). For example, health information technology makes it possible to develop a unified patient, victim, materiel, and fatality tracking system. Having a single unified tracking system that conforms to a consistent set of standards reduces unnecessary redundancy and improves interoperability, facilitating efforts to address the challenges encountered during all facets of disaster response and recovery as well as throughout the provision of care, from prehospital settings through rehabilitation facilities.

TABLE 6-3 Potential Applications of an Information Exchange Portal in a Disaster

Before	• Builds collaborative relationships to strengthen community resilience • Builds redundancy into technology systems • Collects baseline data on community health • Clinical and social providers document needs in case of a disaster • Provides data to inform disaster resource planning
During	• Identifies individuals or populations at highest risk to target and receive delivery of scarce resources • Assists with on-the-ground workforce and resource management, coordination, and communication • Enables real-time surveillance of emergent health issues and community trends • Mitigates impact of any loss of public health infrastructure • Mobilizes tools that support response efforts in the field • Documents needs for first responders or response coordinators • Marshalls the primary care network to support hospitals, Red Cross • Prevents exacerbation of disaster effects
After	• Enables communicating back to primary care providers after a disaster • Helps relocated individuals thrive in new settings • Enhances community recovery efforts, particularly for vulnerable populations • Provides data to improve disaster response planning for future disaster events • Enables long-term surveillance of populations affected by a disaster

SOURCE: Chan, 2013.

EARLY POST-DISASTER HEALTH CARE RECOVERY PRIORITIES

As noted by FEMA (2014a, C-6), "Disaster response and recovery operations are interdependent, overlapping, and often conducted concurrently." The assessment of community health and social service needs and of the recovery resources available to meet those needs may occur while response operations are ongoing. Further, health system recovery happens in phases, entailing a gradual/staged reintroduction of services. As the community progresses to intermediate- and long-term recovery, ongoing evaluation of resources and the changing needs of individuals is essential. In the post-disaster environment, for example, the number of people who are newly homebound and in need of home care may increase.

Conducting Post-Disaster Assessments

Immediately following a disaster and throughout the recovery period, assets must be aligned with the identified on-the-ground requirements of the community. To ensure that the needs of the impacted population are being met, not only infrastructure assessments but also community health assessments and assessments of supplies are required. However, a standardized tool for rapid, simplified needs and impact assessment is currently unavailable. ASPR, working with other relevant agencies from within HHS and other federal departments—including FEMA, the U.S. Department of Transportation (DOT), and the National Institutes of Health (NIH) (National Library of Medicine)—is well positioned to establish a standardized assessment tool that can be used by state and local officials to assess the impact of a disaster on the health system both immediately following the event and during recovery. Any such tool should be based on the common principles outlined in the Post-Disaster Needs Assessment developed by the European Commission, the United Nations Development Group, and the World Bank (GFDRR, 2013).

Restoring Care Delivery Infrastructure and Services

In the short term following a disaster, recovery of the health care system should be focused first on ensuring that the immediate medical needs of the population are being met. Meeting those needs requires ensuring the accessibility of urgent care centers and shelters with appropriate supports for at-risk individuals, as well as functioning supply chains for acquiring medicines and needed medical supplies. As short-term recovery continues, the focus should shift to restoring not only emergency health care services (inpatient and outpatient) but also the health care delivery infrastructure necessary for reestablishing primary care (Runkle et al., 2012). This is especially critical for medically vulnerable populations, such as those requiring ongoing care for chronic diseases. If primary care is not restored in a timely manner, a secondary surge in disaster casualties could result from exacerbation of preexisting conditions.

Consistent with the principles laid out in the IOM reports on crisis standards of care, it may not be feasible immediately to provide the same level of care as that previously available; however, providing some level of care is a moral and legal imperative (IOM, 2009, 2012a, 2013b). To this end, it may be necessary to allocate scarce resources or conserve, adapt, and/or substitute some supplies to ensure that functionally equivalent or crisis care is provided, depending on the situation. In the event of significant damage to health care infrastructure, it may be necessary to adapt facilities or to use temporary facilities to ensure continuity of care. Such strategies may include the following:

- Tent facilities may be used to meet immediate emergent care needs in the impacted community. Such facilities and guidance on operating within them may need to be sought from external parties such as the disaster medical assistance team (DMAT), the National Guard, or other military units.
- Mobile clinics may be operated both by governmental (see Box 6-8) and by nongovernmental (including faith-based) organizations, but coordination between these two sectors is needed.
- If permanent reconstruction of hospitals and other medical facilities will require an extended period of time, temporary modular buildings can be used in the interim. Such facilities must be able to accommodate auxiliary services to support staff. Important partners include state emergency management to help with permits and regulations, as well as utility companies to set up water, power, and communications infrastructure (e.g., to support access to electronic health records).
- Rented office spaces may serve as temporary physician offices, but attention to accessibility is necessary for those with limited transportation options.

Given that much of the health care delivery system is privately owned (and often runs on thin margins), funding support for restoring infrastructure can be a significant challenge, particularly when organizations are underinsured (ASTHO, 2007). Lost revenue due to disruption of services adds to this challenge. In many communities, the private health care industry is a major part of the economy, so that delays in recovery of the health care sector translate into delays in recovery for the community as a whole. Consequently, special attention should be paid during pre- and post-event planning to mechanisms that can expedite financial aid for these critical services. The private sector is not eligible for FEMA Public Assistance funds that are provided for nonprofit health care systems and facilities after a major disaster to fund the reconstruction of damaged infrastructure (see Chapter 4). In the event of a supplemental appropriation, funds from a Community Development Block Grant for Disaster Recovery (CDBG-DR) can be applied to reconstruction of privately owned facilities but will not be available immediately, and there will be many competing priorities for these funds. Low-interest loans from the Small Business Administration and Federal Housing Administration (FHA)-insured loans for health care facilities may be important mechanisms for handling costs not covered by insurance.

BOX 6-8
Continuity of Care for Veterans

Following a disaster, all health care providers have a moral obligation to ensure (to the extent possible) continuity of care for the impacted members of their community. In the case of the U.S. Department of Veterans Affairs (VA), this responsibility is also statutory. VA is required by law to provide timely and quality care to the nation's veterans. This is particularly important for those with conditions (e.g., chronic diseases) that require ongoing care, but may be a challenge when facilities are damaged by a disaster, particularly in the case of a regional-scale disaster that disrupts multiple VA medical facilities (such as Hurricanes Katrina and Sandy).

In past disasters, VA has met the health care needs of veterans by establishing mobile clinics and by providing transportation services to nearby facilities (Eagan, 2013). In the case of mobile clinics, veterans benefited from being able to access care within their own communities, which may have encouraged help-seeking behavior (Lafuente et al., 2007). Additionally, the collaborative, team-based approach used in these mobile clinics provided opportunities for health care providers to encourage veterans' adherence to treatment regimens. VA also has the ability to reimburse non-VA providers for care given to veterans, and in the past has contracted with federally qualified health centers for this purpose. This strategy has been proposed as a mechanism for ensuring veterans' access to care in rural areas lacking nearby VA facilities (CRS, 2013) and may have potential as an approach for ensuring post-disaster continuity of care for veterans as well.

Ensuring Availability of the Required Medical Workforce

Retaining a damaged health care facility's workforce following a disaster is critical to ensure that skilled workers will be available when the facility is again fully operational (see Box 6-9 for one health system's approach to workforce retention after a disaster). Guaranteeing pay and jobs provides employees with needed financial security, the opportunity to maintain their clinical skills, and enhanced psychological recovery through a sense of being useful to the community. Additionally, other local health care facilities that remain operational will likely experience a surge in people seeking care as a result of the community's reduced capacity. Temporary transfer of displaced medical staff to such facilities can help alleviate this burden.

As part of COOP plans, specific consideration should be given to ensuring that the needs of the health care workforce are met. Otherwise, the permanent migration of providers away from the impacted community, as occurred following Hurricane Katrina, will have a direct impact on the quality of care provided to a population in the short and long term (Berggren and Curiel, 2006; Rudowitz et al., 2006). Following a disaster, however, the needs of a community may change. Therefore, accurate assessments are critical to ensuring that the appropriate workforce is available to meet post-disaster needs. Determination of how many and what types of providers will be required during recovery requires assessment of the disaster's impact on local populations, and these needs may change as the recovery progresses. Strategies that may be used to help retain the health care workforce include the following:

- In the immediate post-disaster period, health system employers can assist staff and their families with personal recovery priorities (e.g., housing, child care, rental cars, cash advances to meet basic needs).
- Health systems and governments can help offset the costs of or provide temporary offices for physicians.
- Temporary care facilities can be provided, with flexibility to use them either within or outside of the employing health system.

Although retention of existing providers is critical after a disaster, needs assessments may reveal the need to recruit personnel with additional skills and expertise. Following Hurricane Katrina, for example, loan forgiveness programs and other incentives were used for this purpose (DeSalvo, 2011). Local medical education institutions also can help recruit medical professionals. In recruiting efforts, consideration should be given to long-term needs that may be associated with contemporary changes in health care policy. For example, increased numbers of insured patients as a result of the ACA may create a need for more primary care physicians.

Coordinating Volunteers and Other Medical Professionals from Outside the Community

Depending on the nature and scope of a disaster, local health care organizations may be bolstered by additional personnel with medical expertise (e.g., through the Emergency Management Assistance Compact and other mutual aid agreements). Acute care facilities typically serve as hubs for disaster-related

---

BOX 6-9
Retaining the Medical Workforce Through a Talent-Sharing Program:
St. John's Regional Medical Center in Joplin, Missouri

When St. John's Regional Medical Center was destroyed in the 2011 tornado that struck Joplin, Missouri, the leadership of Mercy Health System, the hospital's parent company, created a talent-sharing program. St. John's coworkers were assured from the first day of the disaster that their salaries and benefits would be continued as the health system sought opportunities to put them back to work. Displaced employees were matched to other facilities based on experience, facility need, and geographic availability. Lessons from this experience include the following:

- Competitors in a medical care market, as well as sister facilities in other communities within the same health system, may temporarily absorb staff from temporarily and permanently closed facilities to meet their increased demand for services. Agreements must be carefully structured to cover payment of salary (including any difference in salary between the employee's previous and interim positions), benefits, noncompete agreements, and conditions and duration of employment.
- Information regarding such a program should be disseminated quickly and widely to employees. Mercy distributed a detailed Q&A document to communicate the details of the talent-sharing program.
- In implementing a talent-sharing program, it is helpful for the human resources organization to have comprehensive information regarding the employees' backgrounds (e.g., education, licenses, certifications, additional skills) to better match them with positions. This can be a strong case for employers to invest in a performance management system.
- Maintaining staff on payroll represents a significant financial commitment. For practical reasons, it may be necessary to consider different job categories separately when making commitments to the continuation of salaries and positions.
- If the talent-sharing program would result in employees practicing in a different state, licensure laws must be considered. Many, but not all, states have reciprocity provisions for health professionals from other states.

SOURCE: Personal communication, C. Mercer, Mercy Health System, to A. Downey, Institute of Medicine, regarding lessons learned from the Joplin experience, July 14, 2014.

medical care, but additional staff and interim facilities may be required to supplement local capacity or replace it if it has been destroyed. U.S. Department of Defense personnel, Medical Reserve Corps (MRC) personnel, disaster relief organizations, emergency management agencies, and/or staff and resources from other localities may be involved, depending on the disaster's scope. While the MRC is a national program administered by ASPR, these units comprise local volunteers positioned to meet the disaster-related needs of the communities in which they live and serve. Each local unit is required to uphold minimal national standards to be officially recognized by ASPR, but the mission and training of MRC personnel are determined largely by the local unit leadership and the organization in which they are housed. There are currently around 1,000 local MRC units across the country and in U.S. territories (MRC, 2015).

The influx of providers that may occur primarily during the response phase may extend into the recovery period to address ongoing critical gaps; therefore, both preparedness and recovery plans need to take into account the challenges associated with the use of volunteer providers. Increasing the number of available paid and volunteer personnel alone does not constitute a successful response if these human resources lack the skills, training, and expertise necessary to meet the needs of a community struck by a disaster. After-action reports following some of the nation's largest and even smallest disasters have suggested that identifying, mobilizing, and integrating health care and other workers into a disaster response is one of the most significant challenges.

Mechanisms for addressing the legal issues surrounding licensing and credentialing of out-of-state medical providers include both state-enacted legislation and federally sponsored registries. The Emergency System for Advance Registration of Volunteer Health Professionals (ESAR-VHP), a federal program administered by ASPR, was created to establish a standardized volunteer registration process for disasters and public health and medical emergencies. The program is managed at the state or territorial level in collaboration with local agencies and organizations; however, ASPR's national ESAR-VHP program staff provide guidance and technical assistance in the development of these registration systems. The ESAR-VHP program provides an efficient and coordinated process for verifying the identities, licenses, credentials, accreditations, and hospital privileges of health care volunteers, a process which saves vital time during emergencies (ASPR, 2015). The Uniform Emergency Volunteer Health Practitioners Act is a model bill that, if enacted by a state, recognizes the licensure of health care providers in other states during an emergency or disaster if those providers are registered with a public or private registration system, including ESAR-VHP. More than a dozen states have enacted this legislation (ACS, 2015).

In addition to the issues surrounding volunteer credentialing and liability, free services provided by volunteers can have unintended consequences if allowed to operate for too long. Free clinics may be critical sources of care during the early days or even weeks after a disaster; during the recovery period, however, these facilities can place further financial strain on private providers who would otherwise be receiving payment to care for those patients (IOM, 2014b). Thus, it is important that decisions on both deploying and demobilizing volunteer services be based on continual assessment of the capacity of the local health care infrastructure, including private providers, to deliver care to the community after a disaster.

INTERMEDIATE- TO LONG-TERM RECOVERY: OPPORTUNITIES TO ADVANCE HEALTHIER AND MORE RESILIENT AND SUSTAINABLE COMMUNITIES

Rebuilding Health Care Facilities After Disasters for Increased Resilience and Sustainability

Health systems and services must be able to ensure continuous operation in disaster situations, particularly in light of the expected increase in the number and severity of disasters as a result of climate change. However, health systems themselves may contribute to climate change through high energy usage, carbon emissions, and use of chemical materials. Thus, the health sector must become resilient to the impacts of climate change *and* be environmentally friendly. The health sector can help ameliorate climate change by reducing its carbon footprint through efficient energy use and by reducing water consumption and contamination. Two recent demonstration projects carried out by the Pan American Health Organization demonstrate that it is feasible and economically beneficial to implement interventions that are both safe and green in health facilities (PAHO, 2014).

During the long-term recovery period, the rebuilding of health care facilities gives a community the opportunity to establish environmentally friendly permanent facilities in which previous vulnerabilities have been addressed, making the facility—and thus, the community—more resilient and sustainable. The American Meteorological Society has identified three approaches—a combination of structural, nonstructural, and functional interventions—to addressing vulnerabilities while bolstering resilience and sustainability:

- Structural hardening—the use of construction elements (e.g., impact-resistant glass; waterproofing measures; backup systems for critical utilities such as electricity, heating, ventilation, and air-conditioning [HVAC], plumbing) that maximize resiliency.
- Incremental adaptation—an approach to addressing operational vulnerabilities that could cause loss of function. For example, critical systems (HVAC, electricity) can be moved out of basement/lower-level floors in flood-prone areas, and some hospitals are locating emergency departments on the second floor and parking and/or administrative offices on the ground floor. In addition, critical systems can be made redundant (e.g., multiple emergency power generators).
- Innovative practice—means of increasing resilience by transforming the role of health care in communities. For example, facilities can be relocated to improve community access, and health services can be expanded beyond acute care to encompass health and wellness. A network of providers outside of hospitals can be leveraged to fill this latter role, allowing hospitals to focus on acute care. This type of systemic change benefits communities during day-to-day operations as well as during disaster recovery. Improving access and quality of care is discussed further in the next section (American Meteorological Society, 2014).

Further, as part of the President's 2013 Climate Action Plan for preparing communities for the impacts of climate change, HHS established a Sustainable and Climate Resilient Health Care Facilities Initiative to help health care facilities increase their resilience (White House Office of the Press Secretary, 2014). To assist in this effort, a best practices toolkit was created to help all stakeholders enable continuity of care in the face of extreme weather events and other disasters. This toolkit identifies the current status of the resilience of health care infrastructure to extreme weather risks and best practices that health care organizations can adopt to improve their climate readiness (White House Office of the Press Secretary, 2014).[17]

These resilience and sustainability principles have been applied in both large metropolitan and smaller suburban and rural facilities. Rebuilding and renovation also provide an opportunity to improve facility design features that can impact patient care and experiences (e.g., locating the emergency room, operating rooms, and radiology in proximity to one another). Newer, more effective technologies that would otherwise have been too costly to install may also be integrated into facilities. This process should involve input from the community, which can help identify current and future needs. Additionally, assessments should be conducted to ensure that renovations and upgrades are based on a full understanding of the current health care system, community populations, their chronic health issues, and the behaviors that influence medical care (Hillsborough County Government, 2010). The examples described in Box 6-10 highlight these opportunities.

Improving Health Care System Access and Quality of Care

Reducing the social and economic costs of health care services through actions taken during recovery can contribute to a healthier and more resilient and sustainable community. Viewed through the lens of

---

[17] The Best Practices Toolkit for Sustainable and Climate Resilient Health Care Facilities can be found at http://toolkit.climate.gov/sites/default/files/SCRHCFI%20Best%20Practices%20Report%20final2%202014%20Web.pdf (accessed April 8, 2015).

BOX 6-10
Rebuilding Health Care Infrastructure for Increased Resilience and Sustainability

Mercy Hospital Joplin, Joplin, Missouri: After the 2011 tornado destroyed St. John's Regional Medical Center, construction began on a new hospital, Mercy Hospital Joplin. The new facility's design is based on extensive community input and is intended not only to provide resilience against disasters but also to apply green sustainability principles. Hardening features include impact resistant windows, concrete roof decks, and a reinforced core. Of particular interest given this chapter's premise that rebuilding should comport with modern trends in reorganization of care delivery and financing, the design reflects a modular approach that promotes flexible patient-centric care and the incorporation of telehealth capabilities to link the new facility with other care settings in the region (HHS, 2014a).

Memorial Sloan Kettering, New York, New York: Memorial Sloan Kettering is investing $1 billion in the construction of a new ambulatory care center along the East River in New York City (NYS DOH, 2013). Having recently experienced hurricanes Irene and Sandy, the hospital is instituting a variety of measures to ensure the resiliency of the new facility to future extreme weather events. For example, the only component below grade in the building is the parking area. The entire footing and foundation system were designed to be completely waterproof. Flood barriers were installed along the property line. All mission-critical infrastructure systems are in elevated floors, and emergency generators provide backup energy for the heating, ventilation, and air-conditioning systems and mechanical, electrical, and plumbing systems (MSKCC, 2013).

Kiowa County Memorial Hospital, Greensburg, Kansas: Having been destroyed by a tornado in 2007, this small community chose to rebuild its hospital so that it would be Leadership in Energy & Environmental Design (LEED) Platinum certified, with features that include but are not limited to

- day-lighting in 75 percent of interior space;
- high performance, low-energy, double-glazed windows and well-insulated buildings (R-25 polyurethane foam insulation);

---

creating optimally healthy post-disaster communities, maximizing the accessibility, quality, and effectiveness of medical care should be an obvious and defining requirement. Nonhospital settings—including ambulatory clinics, medical and dental offices, nursing homes, rehabilitative and assisted living centers, hospices, pharmacies, urgent and emergency services, and home health care services—are essential to realizing maximally health communities. As noted earlier, moreover, the degree of integration of these services with each other and across the continuum of public health, prevention, behavioral health, and social services significantly determines overall community health and, relatedly, the resilience of the community.

After a disaster, communities have an opportunity to evolve their health systems beyond the typical high-cost, low-quality care that is prevalent throughout the country today. The cost of avoidable health care utilization is high. For example, the top 5 percent of health care utilizers generate half of all health care spending (Cohen and Uberoi, 2013), and one county found that the cost of poverty in its jurisdiction was an annual $2.5 billion, consisting largely of costs for emergency room visits ($663.5 million) and hospitalizations ($1.5 billion) (Pinellas County, 2013). During the long-term recovery of health systems, communities can address unsustainable costs by improving health care infrastructure and resources to prevent emergency room visits and hospital admissions (see Box 6-11).

As highlighted in Box 6-12, following hurricanes Katrina and Rita, HHS supported the establishment of the Louisiana Health Care Redesign Collaborative, which developed and oversaw the implementation of a practical guide for an evidence-based, quality-driven health care system for New Orleans (HHS, 2006).

- a rainwater collection system that stores water in underground cisterns that can be used for irrigation and flushing toilets;
- on-site wind turbines; and
- low-flow toilets to conserve water (DOE, 2010).

In addition, the facility added a Federal Emergency Management Agency (FEMA)-approved storm shelter, with its own power generation and air system; moved the records department to the interior of the building where there are no windows; and built a second community emergency operations center in the storm shelter (DOE, 2010; HHS, 2014a).

Spaulding Rehabilitation Hospital, Boston, Massachusetts: Highlighted in the Department of Health and Human Services' Best Practices Toolkit for Sustainable and Climate Resistant Health Care Facilities is Spaulding Rehabilitation Hospital, which employed dual-use approaches to both build resilience into its new facility and reduce its impact on the environment. Leveraging the experiences of hospitals during hurricane Katrina in 2005, the hospital was elevated much higher than required by code during recent renovations—its first floor is 30 inches above the 500-year flood elevation, a step that should keep water out even in the event of a catastrophic flood (Wilson, 2015). Some additional important hazard mitigation measures that were undertaken include the following:

- Plantings and retaining walls act as protective barriers against storm surge.
- Critical patient programs are located above the ground floor.
- Operable windows are keyed open in the event of systems failure.
- Mechanical, electrical, and emergency services are located in the penthouse to avoid flooding issues.

A spokesperson for the project, David Burson, senior project manager at Partners Healthcare, estimated that $700,000—or ½ of 1 percent—of the project funds was spent on resilience-building features (Wilson, 2015). As a result of multiple sustainability measures, the energy use intensity of the 262,000-square foot, 132-bed hospital is 150 Btu per square foot per year, which is approximately 50 percent less than the energy used by the average American hospital (Wilson, 2015). Rain gardens and green roofs absorb rainfall, which helps reduce runoff and also provides a therapeutic environment for resident patients (Wilson, 2015).

Four key principles guided the long-term recovery of the health care sector, and the committee supports these as guiding principles for any community:

- Delivery redesign—All stakeholders—including health care organizations, professional groups, public and private purchasers, and other health system participants—focused on reducing the burden of disease and improving health through primary care and prevention. They exploited opportunities to leverage the work of other sectors—for example, by working with community development organizations that fund community health centers.
- Improved quality—The plan established a team-based care and medical home model, and incorporated an all-hazards approach for effective emergency preparedness.
- Tools—The system emphasized the creation and use of provider tools, such as standardized and interoperable health information technology to improve safety and effectiveness.
- Realignment of incentives—Coverage was expanded through realignment of incentives, including the use of innovative payment models to support team-based care and the integration of behavioral health into primary care (HHS, 2006).

Importantly, many of the approaches used by a community to address entrenched health disparities and high health care costs (such as those described in Box 6-11) are similar to those used to meet post-

---

BOX 6-11
Transforming Health, Social Welfare, and Economic
Stability in Pinellas County, Florida

As part of a larger effort to address the cost of poverty, Pinellas County, Florida, is redesigning its health care system. Its Plan for a Quality Pinellas Community began with a data-driven report on the economic impact of poverty. The report found that 45 percent of impoverished people in the county reside in five at-risk zones and that in these zones, seven interrelated factors contributed to the cycle of poverty: "insufficient transportation, limited access to food, lower educational attainment, limited access to health care, increased crime rates, high unemployment, and inadequate and insufficient housing" (Pinellas County, 2013, p. 4). The report found further that the cost of poverty to the county was an annual $2.5 billion, consisting largely of costs for emergency room visits ($663.5 million) and hospitalizations ($1.5 billion).

With the report in hand, the county sought to address some of the factors that contribute to poverty by focusing on healthy, safe, and sustainable communities in a manner that would increase transparency, accountability, and accessibility. Under the health care system redesign, the goal is to develop an integrated, family-focused care delivery system consisting of a one-stop health campus in each of the county's five at-risk zones. The campus integrates medical and social services by providing wraparound care for low-income residents and linkage to support services. Some of the costs of the new system are absorbed by the federal government through an expansion of the county's federally qualified health center (FQHC) designation. Additional sources of revenue come from the expansion of Medicaid coverage under the Patient Protection and Affordable Care Act of 2010. The centerpiece of the new system is the patient-centered medical home, which offers team-based health care led by a primary care physician who provides comprehensive care by coordinating with specialty care; behavioral health services, prescription drugs services, dental services, and wellness and health education also are incorporated. In addition, the county provides health care for the homeless through a mobile medical unit and it created and expanded a network of school-based clinics; community paramedicine; hospital clinics; and other community partners, including community free clinics and substance abuse treatment facilities.

Pinellas County's system redesign addresses many of the elements needed to improve human recovery after a disaster. In the event of a disaster, increased collaboration across partners, access to quality data, service integration, and a focus on the most vulnerable are all strategies that can dramatically enhance recovery efforts.

SOURCE: Pinellas County, 2013.

---

disaster health care needs. Sustaining these approaches beyond the response and early recovery phases of a disaster is one way to improve long-term access to care. Examples of such complementary approaches include but are not limited to the following:

- Community-based care, such as mobile clinics and the emerging community paramedicine model described earlier in this chapter (see Box 6-5).
- Employment of community health workers to better link community members to needed health services. Community health workers can facilitate the integration of health and human services partners (including health care, public health, social services, and housing) and have been shown to improve patient compliance with chronic disease management (see Box 6-13).
- Collocation and integration of clinical services with other types of services (e.g., social services) using a team-based care approach. These integrated care models follow naturally from the care that is provided immediately following a disaster, when case managers and health professionals work in a collaborative and coordinated manner to meet the comprehensive needs of survivors (see Box 6-14).

RESEARCH NEEDS

In the process of developing its guidance and recommendation specific to the health care sector, the committee noted that further research is needed to address the following questions:

- How can team-based and community-based care approaches that emerge after a disaster be sustained?
- What is the effect of the Affordable Care Act on health care system recovery approaches?
- How can health care coalitions be optimally leveraged to better integrate health care leadership into recovery planning and operations?
- What are the long-term impacts on health when access to care is disrupted?

BOX 6-12
Redesigning Health Care for Increased Access in the Wake of Hurricane Katrina

Before Hurricane Katrina struck, the health and health care system of New Orleans were less than ideal. A high percentage of the population was uninsured; the prevalence of heart disease, stroke, and diabetes exceeded the national averages; and there were wide disparities in health status (New Orleans Health Department, 2013). For Medicare patients, the quality of care in Louisiana ranked the lowest in the nation at the highest cost (Baicker and Chandra, 2004). Some of the proposed reasons for this poor performance were limited access to primary and preventive care, low density of primary care physicians and high density of specialty care physicians, high use of emergency departments, and minimal use of health technology (DeSalvo, 2011). Care for the poor and uninsured was supplied largely by a state-run safety-net system of public hospitals, the largest and most prominent of which was Charity Hospital, responsible for 83 percent of all inpatient care and 88 percent of outpatient uncompensated care delivered in the city (Rudowitz et al., 2006). After Hurricane Katrina, the damage to the health care system—an 80 percent reduction in hospital capacity, over 75 percent of safety-net clinics closed, and permanent closure of Charity Hospital (Bascetta and Siggerud, 2006)—left hundreds of thousands of people without access to care. Nevertheless, the destruction of the health care infrastructure afforded "an unprecedented opportunity to redesign a major American health care sector from the ground up," according to Karen DeSalvo, former health commissioner of the city of New Orleans (DeSalvo, 2011, p. 45).

System Redesign

The U.S. Public Health Service convened a broad group of stakeholders to formulate a vision of change for the New Orleans health care system. Buoyed by grassroots efforts that had resulted in the opening of makeshift primary care clinics throughout the city, the group envisioned a move away from the hospital-centered system to a distributed safety-net primary care system. This vision was undergirded by evidence that primary care leads to fewer unnecessary emergency department visits, better preventive care, better management of chronic conditions, reduced disparities, lower cost, and lower mortality (Shi et al., 2003; Starfield et al., 2005). The Louisiana Health Care Redesign Collaborative was developed, with the aim of transforming health care along the following four dimensions: (1) focus on primary care and prevention delivered in community health centers that ideally are collocated with other community programs, such as day care and job training; (2) improve quality of care by creating the Louisiana Health Care Quality Forum; (3) expand the use of health information technology; and (4) expand insurance coverage through increased public and private funding (DeSalvo, 2011). These guidelines informed the effort to implement an evidence-based and quality-driven health care system (DeSalvo, 2011).

The Louisiana Health Care Redesign Collaborative was awarded a 3-year, $100 million grant from the U.S. Department of Health and Human Services (HHS) known as the Primary Care Access and Stabilization Grant (DeSalvo, 2011). The state of Louisiana partnered with the Louisiana Public Health Institute to

continued

BOX 6-12 Continued

administer the federal funds and to provide technical assistance, and identified 68 public and nonprofit clinics eligible to receive the funds. Local leaders set minimum quality standards, such as the establishment of a quality assurance program, 24-hour phone response in urgent cases, same-day appointments, and the use of evidence-based clinical guidelines (Rittenhouse et al., 2012). HHS awarded an additional $35 million for expanding and retaining the workforce to support the primary care sites, which enabled the state to provide financial incentives that attracted hundreds of primary care and mental health clinicians. This infusion of medical expertise was badly needed since many medical professionals had left the area after the hurricane, further degrading an already inadequate health care infrastructure (DeSalvo, 2011).

Evaluation of the System Redesign

From September 2007 through September 2010, more than 329,320 patients were seen in the new network of primary care clinics (DeSalvo, 2011). A survey of clinic users found that in 2010, 73 percent had a usual source of care other than the emergency department, compared with 66 percent in 2006 (DeSalvo, 2011). Another survey found that 74 percent of New Orleans patients had confidence in their quality of care, compared with 39 percent of adults nationwide (DeSalvo, 2011).

The most ambitious evaluation of the New Orleans system redesign was performed by researchers from the University of California, San Francisco. In a survey of New Orleans clinics receiving federal grant funding, researchers assigned points for three global domains: enhanced access (e.g., open on weekends; responds to urgent phone calls after hours); quality and safety (e.g., alerts providers to abnormal test results; sends patients reminders about care for chronic illnesses); and care coordination and integration (e.g., uses care managers for chronic diseases; uses electronic health records) (Rittenhouse et al., 2012). These are the same domains used to garner recognition by the National Committee on Quality Assurance as a patient-centered medical home (PCMH), defined as a primary care clinic that delivers an array of evidence-based comprehensive services and coordinated care. Through the federal grant funds, clinics in New Orleans became eligible for bonus payments for achieving recognition as a PCMH. Over the study period, 2008-2010, investigators found increased numbers of PCMHs, patient encounters, and patients served. Using the point system, the investigators found substantial progress in improving access, quality and safety, and care coordination and integration. However, they observed declines in these three domains toward the end of the study period, when clinics were no longer eligible for bonus payments from the federal grant, and they cautioned that, with the loss of federal grant funding, clinics could be losing ground in sustaining change (Rittenhouse et al., 2012).

SUMMARY OF FINDINGS AND RECOMMENDATION

While emergency responses that provide essential life-sustaining interventions in the immediate aftermath of a disaster take obvious priority at such times, preparing the health care delivery system for resilience before a disaster, restoring and preferably enhancing the health care infrastructure after a disaster, and engaging this rebuilt infrastructure more successfully in realizing healthier communities overall warrant increased attention and priority. The ultimate goal of planning and rebuilding toward a comprehensively defined healthy community often is not a vision or priority for recovery efforts. In fact, much of the language in disaster recovery guidance focuses on restoring the community to a "normal or new normal" status. Active participation by the health sector is essential in defining a community's "new normal" and using the tragedy of the disaster experience as an opportunity to rebuild to achieve optimal health, resilience, and sustainability—in short, a healthy community capable of withstanding such events in the future.

BOX 6-13
Community Health Workers

Many studies have shown benefit from the use of community health workers (CHWs) in chronic disease management, although more research is needed on this issue (AHRQ, 2007). CHWs have been found more effective than standard care in the areas of patient knowledge and treatment compliance for chronic diseases such as hypertension, mental health, diabetes, and asthma (AHRQ, 2007). For example, a review of the evidence on the care of diabetes patients showed that the use of CHWs resulted in improvements in knowledge and self-management practices (Norris et al., 2006), while studies on managing hypertension among urban African American men showed that the use of CHWs resulted in significant improvements in keeping appointments and adhering to medication (Brownstein et al., 2007). Involvement of CHWs also can lead to more appropriate health care utilization. One study of African American Medicaid patients with diabetes and hypertension, for example, showed that weekly home visits and phone calls by CHWs resulted in declines in emergency room visits, hospital admissions, and Medicaid reimbursements (Fedder et al., 2003). Evidence is mixed, however, on whether use of CHWs can improve health outcomes. One review of eight randomized controlled trials on the use of CHWs in managing hypertension found that in seven of the trials, CHW involvement was correlated with a significant improvement in controlling blood pressure (Brownstein et al., 2007). Another review, however, which excluded studies of poor quality, found that the majority of CHW interventions for management of chronic diseases, with the exception of asthma, "failed to show consistently greater improvement in health outcomes" (AHRQ, 2007, p. 6). Two of four diabetes studies showed improvement in blood sugar levels among the CHW groups, while none of the four hypertension studies showed any difference in blood pressure between the CHW and control groups (AHRQ, 2007). More research is needed to determine whether the use of CHWs in managing chronic conditions can result in better health outcomes.

Few studies have examined the use of CHWs in a disaster context. Yet despite the lack of hard evidence, the public health community recognizes the role of CHWs in disasters and has called for a scaling up of the CHW workforce for emergencies. A joint statement of global health organizations outlines the important roles played by CHWs in all phases of emergency management, from planning and preparedness to response and recovery. For example, CHWs can prepare by identifying high-risk groups in the community and educating them about preparedness, and they can respond to a disaster by assessing community needs, providing psychosocial support, and referring individuals to appropriate health professionals (WHO et al., 2011).

CHWs have been vital to recovery efforts in disasters around the world. For example, Barangay health workers in the Philippines come from the neighborhoods they serve and have good relationships with and knowledge of the community (Emergency Physicians International, 2014). After Typhoon Haiyan, these health workers were trained in psychosocial support for survivors, managed communicable disease outbreaks with a vaccination campaign, and assisted with management of chronic diseases (Emergency Physicians International, 2014). In New Orleans, a pilot program trained CHWs to help with post-disaster mental health services after Hurricane Katrina (Springgate et al., 2011). The CHWs reported high satisfaction with the program and a desire for further training, and noted that they were still providing mental health services to clients up to 5 years after the hurricane (Springgate et al., 2011). The results of this pilot program suggest that training CHWs can help build community capacity to respond to disasters (Springgate et al., 2011).

BOX 6-14
A Continuum of Care Model: Gulf Coast Center

The Gulf Coast Center serves as the regional mental health authority for Galveston and Brazoria Counties in southeast Texas. In 2005, the Gulf Coast Center created a continuum of care model to improve communication among the mental health authority, the community, and local hospitals so as to provide better access for mental health services while minimizing costs (Tiernan et al., 2010). This model identified sites around the community where it was critical for Gulf Coast Center staff to work and provide mental health care services, including the regional hospital, free clinics, a social services organization, and county jails. Through the use of telepsychiatry and mobile response teams, the center was able to provide access to services for community members living in rural areas. In addition, the mobile response teams proved particularly valuable in providing follow-up care and crisis intervention, as well as dealing with complaints and missed evaluations, lab tests, and appointments (Tiernan et al., 2010). The successful management and provision of these services was made possible by cross-sector collaboration between Gulf Coast Center case managers and local medical professionals.

Under this continuum of care model, the Gulf Coast Center was able to provide continuous and easily accessible mental health services to the local community, improving social and health outcomes for its clients. Furthermore, the center used this model to avoid unnecessary emergency room visits and the use of hospital resources, resulting in impressive savings of approximately $2.3 million (UTMB, 2011). The development and use of a continuum of care model thus offer communities the potential for significant cost savings.

The Gulf Coast Center model further proved its value and resilience in 2008, when Hurricane Ike struck southeast Texas. During the course of this disaster, center staff effectively "adapted to the crisis using their mobile tools and experience with integrated community-based crisis management" (Tiernan et al., 2010). This continuum of care model thus played an essential role in allowing the Galveston and Brazoria Counties community to mobilize and respond quickly in the aftermath of the hurricane, providing relief and mental health services even as the regional emergency room and psychiatric hospital remained closed.

The Gulf Coast Center offers an example of a community utilizing integrated health services to bring about cost savings while at the same time improving and expanding access to health services overall. The success and adaptability of this continuum of care model when tested by a crisis such as Hurricane Ike that displaced most social services demonstrate how "by planning and practicing integrated services, many community mental health agencies will be better prepared" in the event of a disaster (Tiernan et al., 2010).

Through its research and testimony provided for this study, the committee learned how important, and how difficult, it is for health care leaders to understand the many sources of available support and to participate in decision-making forums with local, state, and federal leaders at every stage in the process. The complexity of the various bureaucratic processes and the jargon that is often used can be daunting to anyone who is not an emergency manager or other disaster management specialist. A community's health care leaders and executives are especially likely to be unfamiliar with their roles and responsibilities during a disaster. As a result, disaster planning and operations leaders at the federal, state, and local levels need to reach out to clinical leaders as they conduct their activities, with the specific intent of engaging them in the collaborative work necessary to envision and strive toward a maximally healthy community and to build a more resilient health care system. At the same time, however, the responsibility for ensuring that health care is integrated into a multisector effort does not lie solely with governmental planners. Health care leaders themselves need to be sensitized to the importance of engaging proactively in community preparedness efforts that extend to planning not only for response but also for recovery. Health care coalitions provide an important mechanism for this multistakeholder, multisector approach and should be supported in expanding this role. Guidance and training for health care sector grantees under the HPP (see Recommendation 4 in Chapter 3) should bring greater awareness of this responsibility.

"Organized information is key to resiliency" (Coastal Recovery Commission of Alabama, 2010, p. 6.06). The ability of the health care sector to meet the medical needs of a disaster-impacted population and monitor health outcomes as the community progresses through the recovery process toward a healthier and more resilient and sustainable future will depend on a robust health information technology infrastructure. According to the Office of the National Coordinator for Health Information Technology, "The best way to ensure that health information can be accessed during an emergency is to ensure that it can be accessed during routine care" (ONC, 2012, p. ES-1). Despite the clear advantages noted earlier in this chapter of advancing the nation's clinical and health data and related analytic competencies, progress has been suboptimal for many reasons. Common barriers to the adoption of electronic health records by physicians include cost (initial purchase and maintenance), training requirements, and concerns regarding lost productivity (HHS, 2014b). The threat of disaster provides one more motivating factor for overcoming these barriers and establishing a robust health information technology infrastructure. In the event that such systems are not in place before a disaster, however, the recovery process should be leveraged as an opportunity to advance both this infrastructure and plans for utilizing it to ensure continuity of care and to facilitate a learning system approach to recovery in the context of health.

Recommendation 7: *Ensure a Ready Health Information Technology Infrastructure.*

State and local governmental officials should ensure the necessary leadership and accountability to support establishment of the interconnected data systems and analytic capacity that are essential to the continuity of health care and social services delivery across the continuum of disaster response and recovery. To this end, coordination of efforts will be required among local and regional public health, health care, health insurance plans, private-sector information technology innovators and vendors, and regulatory and governmental stakeholders at all levels.

At the federal level, the Office of the National Coordinator for Health Information Technology should build on its current efforts and develop a 3-year implementation plan for health information technology integration. This plan should be designed to facilitate data sharing and portability of individual health records across health care settings in support of pre- and post-disaster recovery health planning and optimal recovery of essential infrastructure for medical and behavioral health care, public health, and social services.

Concrete steps that can be taken to implement this recommendation at the state and local levels include the following recommendations from a recent report by the Office of the National Coordinator for Health Information Technology (ONC, 2012), written for public and private organizations interested in sharing health information during and after a disaster:

- "Understand the State's disaster response policies and align with the State agency designated for Emergency Support Function #8 (Public Health and Medical Services) before a disaster occurs.
- Develop standard procedures approved by relevant public and private stakeholders to share electronic health information across State lines before a disaster occurs.
- Consider enacting the Mutual Aid Memorandum of Understanding to establish a waiver of liability for the release of records when an emergency is declared and to default state privacy and security laws to existing Health Insurance Portability and Accountability Act (HIPAA) rules in a disaster. States should also consider using the Data Use and Reciprocal Support Agreement in order to address and/or expedite patient privacy, security, and health data-sharing concerns.

- Assess the State's availability of public and private health information sources and the ability to electronically share the data using HIE(s) [health information exchanges] and other health data-sharing entities.
- Consider a phased approach to establishing interstate electronic health information-sharing capabilities" (ONC, 2012, p. ES-3).

In addition, emergency management and health sectors (including public health and health care) should work together to undertake public education/outreach efforts that promote the use of mobile applications for transporting personal health records to increase individual readiness.

HEALTH CARE SECTOR RECOVERY CHECKLIST

The committee has identified four pre-event and nine post-disaster critical recovery priorities for the health care sector that are inextricably linked to strengthening the health, resilience, and sustainability of a community. Action steps for each of these priorities are provided in the following checklist. Health care sector leaders will need to adapt these actions to local context, but this guidance provides an indicative set of concerns to be taken into consideration during recovery. The checklist illustrates how the following 4 key recovery strategies, identified as recurring themes at the beginning of this chapter, apply to individual priority areas:

- Use multidisciplinary team-based care strategies to meet multifaceted health care needs;
- Ensure continuity of access to health care services;
- Use health information technology to drive decision making for individual and community health, and to inform future planning;
- Leverage health care coalitions and other relationships with local care providers for health services strategic decision making and alignment of clinical resources.

Pre-Event

Priority: Assess Capacity and Vulnerability of the Health Care System

Primary Actors[1]: Health and Medical System Partners, State/Local Health Departments[2]
Key Partners: Emergency Management Agencies, Social Services Agencies, Community- and Faith-Based Organizations

Key Recovery Strategies:
- Use health information technology to drive decision making for individual and community health and to inform future planning.
- Leverage health care coalitions and other relationships with local care providers for health services strategic decision making and alignment of clinical resources.

Activities include but are not limited to:
- ☐ Conduct a community health needs assessment (CHNA), ensuring hospital-conducted assessments are coordinated with public health agencies.
  - Use CHNA data to derive information on vulnerable populations that will need to be considered in recovery planning at facility and community levels.
- ☐ Conduct a health system hazard vulnerability assessment.
  - Develop scenario-based vulnerability assessments to determine potential vulnerabilities to the health sector infrastructure (inpatient and outpatient facilities).
  - Coordinate vulnerability assessments with state and/or local emergency management and, when possible, incorporate information from the community Threat and Hazard Identification and Risk Assessment (THIRA).
- ☐ Plan to meet recovery needs of at-risk populations, including those with special medical needs.
  - Develop a registry of community members with special medical needs.
  - Use data from health information technology, CMS, and other relevant sources to help pre-identify individual and community health vulnerabilities and to inform potential recovery plans.

- -

Priority: Establish, Sustain, and Exercise Health Care Coalitions and Other Coordinating Groups

Primary Actors: Health and Medical System Partners, State/Local Health Departments
Key Partners: Emergency Management Agencies

Key Recovery Strategy:
- Leverage health care coalitions and other multisector partnerships among local care providers for health services strategic decision making, alignment of clinical resources, and coordination with public health and emergency management sectors.

---

[1] See Appendix F for further description of terms used to describe Primary Actors and Key Partners in this checklist.
[2] Throughout this checklist, "State/Local" is used for the purposes of brevity but should be inferred to include tribal and territorial as well.

Pre-Event

Activities include but are not limited to:
- ☐ If not already established, form health care coalition with clear governance structure and responsibilities to serve as a regional (substate) planning and coordination group for disaster preparedness, response, and recovery.
- ☐ Ensure health care coalition membership encompasses, to the degree possible, all essential partners specified in ASPR's *Healthcare Preparedness Capabilities: National Guidance for Healthcare System Preparedness.*
- ☐ Identify and seek alignment with other area health coalitions and collaboratives.
- ☐ Ensure that health care coalition plans and exercises address recovery activities.
- ☐ Consider the need for task forces/workgroups to address specific health care issues (e.g., behavioral health) or the needs of special populations (e.g., children and youth).
- ☐ Establish pathways for integrating the health care coalition into state, regional, or local coordinating structures under the NDRF.

- -

Priority: Develop Continuity of Operations (COOP) and Recovery Plans

Primary Actors: Health and Medical System Partners, State/Local Health Departments
Key Partners: Emergency Management Agencies, Private Sector Suppliers and Distributors

Key Recovery Strategies:
- Ensure continuity of access to clinical care services.
- Use health information technology to drive decision making for individual and community health and to inform future iterations of planning.
- Leverage health care coalitions and other relationships among local care providers for health services strategic decision making, alignment of clinical resources, and coordination with public health and emergency management sectors.

Activities include but are not limited to:
- ☐ Proactively engage in discussions with emergency management with regards to disaster recovery planning and community organizational structures aligned with the NDRF, including recovery coordinators and local recovery managers.
- ☐ Ensure alignment of planning occurring through all relevant federal grants and cooperative agreements (public health and emergency management).
- ☐ Identify essential health care services and develop contingency plans for continuity of operations based on health care facility vulnerability assessments.
- ☐ Pre-identify shelters and facilities where specialized care will be provided.
- ☐ Include major medical infrastructure loss and supply chain interruptions in scenario-based planning and continuity of operations plan.
  - – Ensure that contracts with supply vendors and pre-authorization are in place.
- ☐ Understand array of resources for recovery assistance and requirements and processes for reimbursement.
- ☐ Exercise and drill continuity of operations and recovery plans on a regular basis.

Priority: Establish a Resilient Health Information Technology System

Primary Actors: Health and Medical System Partners, State/Local Health Departments
Key Partners: Health Insurers, Private-Sector Information Technology (IT) Innovators and Vendors

Key Recovery Strategies:
- Ensure continuity of access to clinical care services.
- Use health information technology to drive decision making for individual and community health and to inform future planning.

Activities include but are not limited to:
- ☐ Support the establishment of a health IT infrastructure (interconnected data systems and analytic capacity) that is essential to the continuity of health care and social services delivery across the continuum of disaster response and recovery.
  - – Promote and support the adoption of electronic health records.
  - – Include social vulnerability risk factors as standard data elements.
  - – Establish data sharing agreements to support intra- and interstate electronic health information sharing capabilities.
  - – Ensure capacity to protect privacy while transferring personal health information.
  - – Employ system redundancies to improve resilience of health IT infrastructure.
- ☐ Promote the use of personal health records as a critical aspect of individual/family preparedness.

Short-Term Recovery

Priority: Conduct Post-Disaster Assessment

Primary Actors: Health and Medical System Partners, State/Local Health Departments
Key Partners: Emergency Management Agencies

Key Recovery Strategies:
- Leverage health care coalitions and other relationships among local care providers for health services strategic decision making, alignment of clinical resources, and coordination with public health and emergency management sectors.
- Use health information technology (IT) to drive decision making for individual and community health and to inform future iterations of planning.

Activities include but are not limited to:
- ☐ Integrate health care coalition leadership within the public health incident command system.
- ☐ Establish capacity of local hospitals, outpatient facilities, emergency physician networks, etc. to deliver care.
  - – Determine disaster impact on health system infrastructure (facilities, supply chain, and health IT systems), medical workforce capacity, and critical services.
  - – Estimate magnitude of surge.
- ☐ Assess damages and estimate reconstruction costs.
- ☐ Identify urgent disaster-related risks to community health.
- ☐ Identify the most vulnerable populations that will require assistance/consideration.

- -

Priority: Restore Care Delivery Infrastructure and Services

Primary Actors: Health and Medical System Partners, State/Local Health Departments
Key Partners: Behavioral Health Authorities, Social Services Agencies

Key Recovery Strategies:
- Leverage health care coalitions and other relationships among local care providers for health services strategic decision making, alignment of clinical resources, and coordination with public health and emergency management sectors.
- Use multidisciplinary team-based care strategies to meet multifaceted health care needs.
- Ensure continuity of access to clinical care services.

Activities include but are not limited to:
- ☐ Utilize local staff to establish fusion ambulatory and urgent care site.
- ☐ Ensure accessible community-based emergency department with follow-up and hospital transfer relations.
- ☐ Reestablish essential primary care clinics and ensure coordination with other components of the health system.
- ☐ Secure damaged facilities to prevent access and subsequent injury/exposure and salvage working equipment if possible. Store damaged equipment for FEMA/insurance claims.
- ☐ Track activity and cost for FEMA/insurance reimbursement.

Short-Term Recovery

- □ Request expedited medical facility plan reviews and surveys of facilities ready to reopen to the public. Reopen minimally damaged facilities.
- □ Identify community resources available for intermediate facility arrangements until health facilities are recovered.
- □ Restore access to vital records.

- -

Priority: Ensure Availability of the Required Medical Workforce

Primary Actors: Health and Medical System Partners, State/Local Health Departments
Key Partners: Federal Agencies (including ASPR), Behavioral Health Authorities

Key Recovery Strategies:
- Leverage health care coalitions and other relationships among local care providers for health services strategic decision making, alignment of clinical resources, and coordination with public health and emergency management sectors.
- Ensure continuity of access to clinical care services.

Activities include but are not limited to:
- □ If needed, implement strategies (e.g., incentives) designed to retain a health and medical services workforce in the affected area.
- □ Mobilize and deploy Medical Reserve Corps or ESAR-VHP volunteers to support efforts.
- □ Engage in a process for wellness checks and monitor behavioral health needs of medical workforce.
- □ Coordinate health (including behavioral health), medical resources, and volunteers responding to the area.
- □ Ensure transition of medical system partners and/or health care coalition members from ESF-8 response efforts to health and social services RSF recovery efforts.

- -

Priority: Locate and Meet Needs of At-Risk Community Members with Special Medical Needs

Primary Actors: State/Local Health Departments
Key Partners: Health and Medical System Partners, Emergency Management Agencies, Community- and Faith-based Organizations

Key Recovery Strategies:
- Use team-based care strategies to meet multifaceted clinical care needs.
- Use health information technology to drive decision making for individual and community health and to inform future iterations of planning.
- Ensure continuity of access to clinical care services.

Short-Term Recovery

Activities include but are not limited to:
- ☐ Utilize registries if available or other electronic health information to locate at-risk community members.
- ☐ Track vulnerable patients transferred from long-term care facilities and other institutions.
- ☐ Ensure access to and availability of pharmaceuticals, including psychotropics, and critical medical equipment for those with special medical needs.
- ☐ Utilize mobile services to meet needs of community members without access to transportation.

- -

Priority: Coordinate Provision of Clinical Services

Primary Actors: Health and Medical System Partners
Key Partners: State/Local Health Departments, Social Services Agencies, Behavioral Health Authorities, Emergency Management Agencies

Key Recovery Strategies:
- Leverage health care coalitions and other relationships among local care providers for health services strategic decision making, alignment of clinical resources, and coordination with public health and emergency management sectors.
- Use team-based care strategies to meet multifaceted clinical care needs.

Activities include but are not limited to:
- ☐ Engage social services and community health workers to ensure comprehensive care needs of survivors are met.
- ☐ Identify opportunities for collocating health care services with behavioral health and social services.

Intermediate- to Long-Term Recovery

Priority: Monitor Ongoing Health and Medical Needs of Post-Disaster Population

Primary Actors: State/Local Health Departments
Key Partners: Social Services Agencies, Health and Medical System Partners

Key Recovery Strategy:
- Use health assessments and health information technology to drive decision making for individual and community health and to inform future iterations of planning.

Activities include but are not limited to:
- ☐ Conduct community health needs assessments.
- ☐ Utilize aggregate data from health IT systems to evaluate ongoing clinical care needs and changes to patient demographics.

- -

Priority: Rebuild Health Care Facilities After Disasters for Increased Resilience and Sustainability

Primary Actors: Health and Medical System Partners, State/Local Health Departments
Key Partners: Emergency Management Agencies

Key Recovery Strategies:
- Leverage health care coalitions and other relationships among local care providers for health services strategic decision making, alignment of clinical resources, and coordination with public health and emergency management sectors.
- Ensure continuity of access to clinical care services.

Activities include but are not limited to:
- ☐ Adopt construction standards and practices that ensure safety and continued functionality in the event of a disaster.
- ☐ Rebuild and strengthen health care infrastructure through such methods as:
  - Structural hardening—use of construction elements (impact-resistant glass, waterproofing measures, backup systems for critical utilities like electricity, HVAC, plumbing) that maximize resiliency.
  - Incremental adaptation—address operational vulnerabilities that could cause loss of function. Ex. Relocating critical systems (HVAC, electricity) out of basement/lower level floors or redundancy for critical systems (multiple emergency power generators).
  - Innovative practice—increase resilience by transforming role of health care in communities and functionality. Ex. Relocating facilities to improve community access and expanding health services beyond acute care to health and wellness. Leverage network of providers outside hospitals for this role to allow hospitals to focus on acute care. Benefits communities during blue sky times and after disasters. Improving access and quality of care is discussed further in section below.
- ☐ When necessary and feasible, rebuild significantly damaged medical facilities outside of known hazard areas.

Intermediate- to Long-Term Recovery

☐ Consider opportunities to improve sustainability of health care facilities (e.g., reduced carbon footprint, reduced water waste).

- -

Priority: Improve Health Care System Access and Quality of Care

Primary Actors: Health and Medical System Partners, State/Local Health Departments
Key Partners: Emergency Management Agencies, Urban and Regional Planning Agencies, Community Development Organizations

Key Recovery Strategies:
- Leverage health care coalitions and other relationships among local care providers for health services strategic decision making, alignment of clinical resources, and coordination with public health and emergency management sectors.
- Use team-based care strategies to meet multifaceted clinical care needs.

Activities include but are not limited to:
☐ Ensure that all stakeholders—health care organizations, professional groups, public and private purchasers, and other health system participants—are focused on reducing the burden of disease and improving health through primary care and prevention.
☐ Engage community leaders early in the process to express interest in participating in broader community redevelopment processes.
☐ Improve quality by identifying opportunities to improve type of care, configuration and location of services to best meet the needs of the community.
  – Consider opportunities and benefits to adopting team-based and community-based care models (patient-centered medical homes, community paramedicine).
  – Identify opportunities to integrate health services with other assistance for vulnerable populations (e.g., public housing, senior housing).
  – Incorporate an all-hazards approach for effective emergency preparedness into the health care system.
☐ Expand coverage in part through realignment of incentives.
☐ Evaluate opportunities to fill preexisting gaps in health care capacity (e.g., primary care, behavioral health capacity).

- -

Priority: Update Planning Documents and Share Lessons Learned with Other Communities to Improve Post-Disaster Recovery Planning

Primary Actors: Health and Medical System Partners
Key Partners: Emergency Management Agencies, State/Local Health Departments

Intermediate- to Long-Term Recovery

Key Recovery Strategies:
- Leverage health care coalitions and other relationships among local care providers for health services strategic decision making, alignment of clinical resources, and coordination with public health and emergency management sectors.
- Use health assessments and health information technology to drive decision making for individual and community health and to inform future iterations of planning.

Activities include but are not limited to:
- ☐ Update COOP plans based on lessons learned.
- ☐ Participate in after-action process, including analysis of lessons learned and identification of opportunities for improvement.
- ☐ Utilize state, regional, and national conferences, workshops, and discipline-specific professional meetings to share lessons learned and opportunities for improvement so that other jurisdictions can benefit from their recovery experiences.

REFERENCES

ACS (American College of Surgeons). 2015. *Uniform Emergency Volunteer Health Practitioners Act.* https://www. facs.org/advocacy/state/uevhpa (accessed March 14, 2015).

AHRQ (Agency for Healthcare Research and Quality). 2007. *Outcomes of community health worker interventions.* http://www.ahrq.gov/research/findings/evidence-based-reports/comhwork-evidence-report.pdf (accessed December 3, 2014).

AHRQ. 2015. *Defining the PCMH.* http://pcmh.ahrq.gov/page/defining-pcmh (accessed March 3, 2015).

American Meteorological Society. 2014. *A prescription for the 21st century: Improving resilience to high-impact weather for healthcare facilities and services.* http://www2.ametsoc.org/ams/assets/File/health_workshop_report. pdf (accessed December 3, 2014).

ASPR (Office of the Assistant Secretary for Preparedness and Response). 2012. *Healthcare preparedness capabilities: National guidance for healthcare system preparedness.* Washington, DC: HHS.

ASPR. 2013. *Public health emergency declaration Q&As.* http://www.phe.gov/Preparedness/legal/Pages/phe-qa. aspx#q5 (access April 6, 2015).

ASPR. 2015. *About ESAR-VHP.* http://www.phe.gov/esarvhp/Pages/about.aspx (accessed February 12, 2015).

ASTHO (Association of State and Territorial Health Officials). 2007. *Disaster recovery for public health.* http://www. astho.org/programs/preparedness/disaster-recovery-for-public-health (accessed January 2, 2014).

ASTHO. 2014. *ASTHO supported primary care and public health collaborative.* http://www.astho.org/PCPH Collaborative/Overview (accessed December 2, 2014).

ASTHO. 2015. *Community health workers.* http://www.astho.org/community-health-workers (accessed April 6, 2015).

Baicker, K., and A. Chandra. 2004. Medicare spending, the physician workforce, and beneficiaries' quality of care. *Health Affairs (Millwood)* Suppl Web Exclusives W4-184-197.

Bascetta, C., and K. Siggerud. 2006. *Status of the health care system in New Orleans.* Washington, DC: U.S. Government Accountability Office.

Berggren, R. E., and T. J. Curiel. 2006. After the storm—health care infrastructure in post-Katrina New Orleans. *New England Journal of Medicine* 354(15):1549-1552.

Brown, S. H., L. F. Fischetti, G. Graham, J. Bates, A. E. Lancaster, D. McDaniel, J. Gillon, M. Darbe, and R. M. Kolodner. 2007. Use of electronic health records in disaster response: The experience of Department of Veterans Affairs after Hurricane Katrina. *American Journal of Public Health* 97(Suppl. 1):S136-S141.

Brownstein, J. N., F. M. Chowdhury, S. L. Norris, T. Horsley, L. Jack, Jr., X. Zhang, and D. Satterfield. 2007. Effectiveness of community health workers in the care of people with hypertension. *American Journal of Preventive Medicine* 32(5):435-447.

CDC (Centers for Disease Control and Prevention). 2011. *Public health preparedness capabilities: National standards for state and local planning.* Washington, DC: HHS.

Chan, C. 2013. *The Dallas Information Exchange Portal: New technologies for public health preparedness.* Paper presented at IOM Forum on Medical and Public Preparedness for Catastrophic Events: The Impact of the Affordable Care Act on U.S. Preparedness Resources and Programs: An IOM Workshop, November 18-19, Washington, DC.

Claver, M., D. Friedman, A. Dobalian, K. Ricci, and M. Horn Mallers. 2012. The role of Veterans Affairs in emergency management: A systematic literature review. *PLoS Currents* 4:e198d344bc140a175f927c199bc5024279815.

Coastal Recovery Commission of Alabama. 2010. *A roadmap to resilience: Towards a healthier environment, society and economy for south Alabama.* http://crcalabama.org/wp-content/uploads/2011/02/CRC-Report-02-2011.pdf (accessed March 31, 2015).

Cohen, S., and N. Uberoi. 2013. Differentials in the concentration in the level of health expenditures across population subgroups in the US, 2010. *Medical Expenditure Panel Survey* 1-9.

Colias, M. 2005. Hurricane Katrina. The disaster after the disaster. *Hospitals and Health Networks* 79(10):36-38, 40, 42.

County Health Rankings. 2014. *County health rankings & roadmaps.* http://www.countyhealthrankings.org (accessed December 2, 2014).

CRS (Congressional Research Service). 2013. *CRS report for Congress prepared for members and committees of Congress health care for rural veterans: The example of federally qualified health centers.* Washington, DC: CRS, Library of Congress.

DeSalvo, K. 2011. Delivering high-quality, accessible health care: The rise of community centers. In *Resilience and opportunity: Lessons from the U.S. Gulf Coast after Katrina and Rita,* edited by A. Liu, R. V. Anglin, R. Mizelle, and A. Plyer. Washington, DC: Brookings Institution Press. Pp. 45-63.

DeSalvo, K. B. 2013. *The Katrina experience: Considerations for health system recovery.* Paper presented at IOM Committee on Post-disaster Recovery of a Community's Public Health, Medical, and Social Services: Meeting One, November 25, Washington, DC.

DHS (U.S. Department of Homeland Security). 2012. *Federal continuity directive 1: Federal executive branch national continuity program and requirements.* http://www.gpo.gov/pdfs/about/fcd_1_october_2012.pdf (accessed December 3, 2014).

DOE (U.S. Department of Energy). 2010. *Rebuilding it better: Greensburg, Kansas.* http://www1.eere.energy.gov/office_eere/pdfs/47461.pdf (accessed April 8, 2015).

Eagan, A. 2013. Panel Discussion at IOM Committee on Post-disaster Recovery of a Community's Public Health, Medical and Social Services: Meeting One, November 25, Washington, DC.

Emergency Physicians International. 2014. *Community health workers prove the key to Philippines relief efforts.* http://www.epijournal.com/articles/122/community-health-workers-prove-the-key-to-philippines-relief-efforts (accessed December 3, 2014).

Fedder, D. O., R. J. Chang, S. Curry, and G. Nichols. 2003. The effectiveness of a community health worker outreach program on healthcare utilization of west Baltimore City Medicaid patients with diabetes, with or without hypertension. *Ethnicity & Disease* 13(1):22-27.

FEMA (Federal Emergency Management Agency). 2014a. *Recovery federal interagency operational plan.* http://www.fema.gov/media-library-data/1406719669673-6081c9249705bc59153d724abcb2e7ca/Recovery_FIOP_FINAL_20140729.pdf (accessed December 2, 2014).

FEMA. 2014b. *Threat and hazard identification and risk assessment.* https://www.fema.gov/threat-and-hazard-identification-and-risk-assessment (accessed December 2, 2014).

GFDRR (Global Facility for Disaster Reduction and Recovery). 2013. *Post-disaster needs assessment guidelines, Volume A.* http://www.recoveryplatform.org/assets/publication/PDNA/PDNA%20Volume%20A%20FINAL%20for%20Web.pdf (accessed April 4, 2015).

Hall, M. J., C. J. DeFrances, S. N. Williams, A. Golosinskiy, and A. Schwartzman. 2010. National hospital discharge survey: 2007 summary. *National Health Statistics Reports* (29):1-20, 24.

Health IT. 2014. *About blue button.* http://www.healthit.gov/patients-families/blue-button/about-blue-button (accessed December 3, 2014).

HealthVault. 2015. *What is HealthVault?* https://www.healthvault.com/us/en (accessed April 7, 2015).

HHS (U.S. Department of Health and Human Services). 2006. *Louisiana healthcare redesign collaborative charter.* http://archive.hhs.gov/louisianahealth/collaborative/Charter/charter.html (accessed March 14, 2015).

HHS. 2007. *Medical surge capacity and capability: A management system for integrating medical and health resources during large-scale emergencies.* http://www.phe.gov/Preparedness/planning/mscc/healthcarecoalition/Pages/glossary.aspx (accessed December 2, 2014).

HHS. 2011. *National strategy for quality improvement in health care.* Washington, DC: HHS.

HHS. 2014a. *Primary protection: Enhancing health care resilience for a changing climate.* Washington, DC: HHS.

HHS. 2014b. *Update on the adoption of health information technology and related efforts to facilitate the electronic use and exchange of health information.* Washington, DC: HHS.

Hillsborough County Government. 2010. *Post-disaster redevelopment plan.* http://www.hillsboroughcounty.org/index.aspx?nid=1795 (accessed November 3, 2014).

Hogan, T. P., S. A. Holmes, L. M. Rapacki, C. T. Evans, L. Lindblom, H. Hoenig, B. Goldstein, B. Hahm, and F. M. Weaver. 2011. Disaster preparedness and response practices among providers from the Veterans Health Administration and veterans with spinal cord injuries and/or disorders. *Journal of Spinal Cord Medicine* 34(4):353-361.

Horahan, K., H. Morchel, M. Raheem, and L. Stevens. 2014. Electronic health records access during a disaster. *Online Journal of Public Health Informatics* 5(3).

HRSA (Health Resources and Services Administration). 2012. *Community paramedicine: Evaluation tool.* Washington, DC: HHS.

IHI (Institute for Healthcare Improvement). 2007. *The IHI Triple Aim.* http://www.ihi.org/engage/initiatives/tripleaim/pages/default.aspx (accessed March 24, 2015).

IOM (Institute of Medicine). 2000. *To err is human: Building a safer health system.* Washington, DC: National Academies Press.

IOM. 2001. *Crossing the quality chasm: A new health system for the 21st century.* Washington, DC: The National Academy Press.

IOM. 2009. *Guidance for establishing crisis standards of care for use in disaster situations: A letter report.* Washington, DC: The National Academies Press.

IOM. 2012a. *Crisis standards of care: A systems framework for catastrophic disaster response.* Washington, DC: The National Academies Press.

IOM. 2012b. *Primary care and public health: Exploring integration to improve population health.* Washington, DC: The National Academies Press.

IOM. 2013a. *Best care at lower cost: The path to continuously learning health care in America.* Washington, DC: The National Academies Press.

IOM. 2013b. *Crisis standards of care: A toolkit for indicators and triggers.* Washington, DC: The National Academies Press.

IOM. 2013c. *Primary care and public health: Exploring integration to improve population health.* http://www.iom.edu/Reports/2012/Primary-Care-and-Public-Health.aspx (accessed April 6, 2015).

IOM. 2014a. *The impacts of the Affordable Care Act on preparedness resources and programs: Workshop summary.* Washington, DC: The National Academies Press.

IOM. 2014b. *Preparedness, response, and recovery considerations for children and families: Workshop summary.* Washington, DC: The National Academies Press.

The Joint Commission. 2013. *2013 CAMH: Comprehensive Accreditation Manual for Hospitals.* Oakbrook Terrace, IL: The Joint Commission.

Kindig, D., and G. Stoddart. 2003. What is population health? *American Journal of Public Health* 93(3):380-383.

Kizer, K. W., K. Shore, and A. Moulin. 2013. *Community paramedicine: A promising model for integrating emergency and primary care.* Sacramento, CA: UC Davis Institute for Population Health Improvement.

Knowlton, K., and M. Rotkin-Ellman. 2014. *Preparing for climate change: Lessons for coastal cities from Hurricane Sandy.* New York: Natural Resources Defense Council.

Lafuente, C. R., V. Eichaker, V. E. Chee, and E. Chapital. 2007. Post-Katrina provision of health care to veterans in a mobile clinic: Providers' perspectives. *Journal of the American Academy of Nurse Practitioners* 19(8):383-391.

MRC (Medical Reserve Corps). 2015. *About the Medical Reserve Corps.* https://www.medicalreservecorps.gov/pageViewFldr/About (accessed April 2, 2015).

MSKCC (Memorial Sloan Kettering Cancer Center). 2013. *74th Street Project Report for Public Health and Health Planning Council Ad HOC Advisory Committee on Environmental and Construction Standards Regarding Storm Mitigation Design.* https://www.health.ny.gov/facilities/public_health_and_health_planning_council/meetings/2013-06-27/docs/gillson_storm_mitigation_exec_summary.pdf (accessed April 12, 2015).

NACCHO (National Association of County and City Health Officials). 2012. *Role of local health departments in community health needs assessments.* http://naccho.org/advocacy/positions/upload/12-05-Role-of-LHDs-in-CHNA.pdf (accessed November 18, 2014).

NACCHO. 2014. *Definitions of community health assessments (CHA) and community health improvement plans (CHIPS).* http://naccho.org/topics/infrastructure/community-health-assessment-and-improvement-planning/upload/Definitions.pdf (accessed December 2, 2014).

New Orleans Health Department. 2013. *New Orleans community health improvement report: Community health profile and community health improvement plan.* http://www.naccho.org/topics/infrastructure/CHAIP/upload/UPDATED-NOLA-Community-Health-Improvement-Final-Report.pdf (accessed April 4, 2015).

Norris, S. L., F. M. Chowdhury, K. Van Le, T. Horsley, J. N. Brownstein, X. Zhang, L. Jack, Jr., and D. W. Satterfield. 2006. Effectiveness of community health workers in the care of persons with diabetes. *Diabetic Medicine* 23(5):544-556.

NYS DOH (New York State Department of Health). 2013. *New York State Department of Health Public Health and Health Planning Council Ad Hoc Advisory Committee on Environmental and Construction Standards Final Report and Recommendations.* https://www.health.ny.gov/facilities/public_health_and_health_planning_council/meetings/2013-10-03/docs/e_and_cs_committee_final_report.pdf (accessed April 12, 2015).

ONC (Office of the National Coordinator for Health Information Technology). 2012. *Southeast Regional HIT-HIE Collaboration (SERCH): Final report: ONC State Health Policy Consortium Project.* http://disasterlit.nlm.nih.gov/record/5904 (accessed December 3, 2014).

O'Shea, J. S. 2007. *More Medicaid means less quality health care.* http://www.heritage.org/research/reports/2007/03/more-medicaid-means-less-quality-health-care (accessed March 14, 2015).

PAHO (Pan American Health Organization). 2014. *Smart hospitals toolkit.* http://www.paho.org/disasters/index.php?option=com_content&view=article&id=1742%3Asmart-hospitals-toolkit&catid=1026%3Ageneral-information&Itemid=911&lang=en (accessed March 14, 2015).

Paradise, J. 2015. *Medicaid moving forward.* http://kff.org/health-reform/issue-brief/medicaid-moving-forward (accessed March 14, 2015).

PCCI (Parkland Center for Clinical Innovation). 2014. *The Dallas Information Exchange Portal.* http://iep.pccipieces.info (accessed December 3, 2014).

Pinellas County. 2013. *Update on the economic impact of poverty report for the Pinellas County Board of County Commissioners.* Pinellas County, FL: Pinellas County.

Radley, D. C., D. McCarthy, J. A. Lippa, S. L. Hayes, and C. Schoen. 2014. *Aiming higher: Results from a scorecard on state health system performance, 2014.* New York: The Commonwealth Fund.

Rittenhouse, D. R., L. A. Schmidt, K. J. Wu, and J. Wiley. 2012. The post-Katrina conversion of clinics in New Orleans to medical homes shows change is possible, but hard to sustain. *Health Affairs (Millwood)* 31(8):1729-1738.

Rudowitz, R., D. Rowland, and A. Shartzer. 2006. Health care in New Orleans before and after Hurricane Katrina. *Health Affairs* 25(5):w393-w406.

Runkle, J. D., A. Brock-Martin, W. Karmaus, and E. R. Svendsen. 2012. Seconday surge capacity: A framework for understanding long-term access to primary care for medically vulnerable populations in disaster recovery. *American Journal of Public Health* 102(12):e24-e32.

Schappert, S. M., and E. A. Rechtsteiner. 2011. Ambulatory medical care utilization estimates for 2007. *Vital and Health Statistics* 13(169):1-38.

Shi, L., J. Macinko, B. Starfield, J. Wulu, J. Regan, and R. Politzer. 2003. The relationship between primary care, income inequality, and mortality in US states, 1980-1995. *Journal of the American Board of Family Medicine* 16(5):412-422.

Springgate, B., A. Wennerstrom, and C. Carriere. 2011. Capacity building for post-disaster mental health since Katrina: The role of community health workers. *The Review of Black Political Economy* 38(4):363-368.

Starfield, B., L. Shi, and J. Macinko. 2005. Contribution of primary care to health systems and health. *Milbank Quarterly* 83(3):457-502.

Tiernan, K. M., G. M. Winburn, and B. G. Raimer. 2010. Coalition weathers a storm. *Behavioral Healthcare* 30(9):16-18.

United Health Foundation. 2013. *America's health rankings: A call to action for individuals & their communities.* http://www.unitedhealthfoundation.org/Publications/AHR.aspx (accessed December 2, 2014).

UTMB (University of Texas Medical Branch at Galveston). 2011. *Mental health continuum of care program.* http://www.utmbhpla.org/doc/Page.asp?PageID=DOC000725 (accessed November 18, 2014).

White House Office of the Press Secretary. 2014. *Fact sheet: Strengthening the climate resilience of the health care sector.* https://www.whitehouse.gov/administration/eop/ceq/Press_Releases/December_15_2014 (accessed March 5, 2015).

WHO (World Health Organization), UNICEF, Global Health Workforce Alliance, UNHCR (United Nations High Commissioner for Refugees), and International Federation of Red Cross and Red Cresent Societies. 2011. *Scaling-up the community-based health workforce for emergencies.* http://www.who.int/workforcealliance/knowledge/publications/alliance/jointstatement_chwemergency_en.pdf?ua=1 (accessed December 3, 2014).

Wilson, A. 2015. *How to make a hospital resilient: A tour of Spaulding Rehab.* http://www.resilientdesign.org/how-to-make-a-hospital-resilient-a-tour-of-spaulding-rehabilitation-center (accessed March 3, 2015).

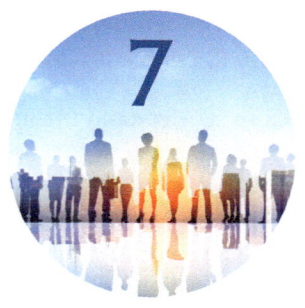

Behavioral Health

Behavioral health[1] problems and disorders are among the most frequent adverse health effects after exposure to a disaster—this despite chronic underreporting due to the stigma often associated with these conditions, the lack of visible or physical wounds, the separation of mental health services from medical services, and the lag time between exposure and the onset of disorder. Almost everyone in a community struck by a disaster will feel some type of emotional effect. For most, the acute reactions will be transient, and functional recovery will occur without intervention. For some, however, the impacts of a disaster on behavioral health can be severe and long-lasting, and if not addressed, can impede the recovery of individuals, families, and communities, resulting in significant long-term health burdens. Consequently, it is critically important to identify those individuals at risk for more severe and persistent psychopathology after a disaster and link them with the appropriate preventive and/or rehabilitative services. To this end, however, significant pre-disaster planning is required to establish clear roles and responsibilities for the myriad stakeholders at all levels, an agile and resilient system for delivery of behavioral health services, and a process for evaluating the needs for those services and ensuring that those in need are receiving timely and effective treatment. Where such conditions do not exist in advance, the disaster recovery process can represent an opportunity for advancing toward that more optimal state.

This chapter examines the linkages among behavioral health, resilience, and healthy communities; activities that mitigate adverse behavioral health effects in survivors; the gaps in the current system for addressing disaster-related behavioral health needs; and the opportunities for strengthening the behavioral health sector and integrating it with other sectors by leveraging disaster-related resources and experiences. Based on documented expert consensus on the important elements of behavioral health interventions (Watson et al., 2011, p. 485), the committee proposes the following key recovery strategies for the behavioral health sector that should cut across all phases of the disaster cycle and that represent recurring themes throughout this chapter:

---

[1] For the purposes of this report, the term "behavioral health" encompasses "the interconnected psychological, emotional, cognitive, developmental, and social influences on behavior, mental health and substance abuse" (HHS, 2014, p. 4).

- Integrate behavioral health activities and programming into other sectors (e.g., education, health care, social services) to reduce stand-alone services, reach more people, foster resilience and sustainability, and reduce stigma.
- Provide a spectrum of behavioral health services and use an approach based on stepped care (from supportive intervention to long-term treatment).
- Maximize the participation of the local affected population in recovery planning with respect to behavioral health, and identify and build on available resources and local capacities and networks (community, families, schools, and friends) in developing recovery strategies.
- Promote a sense of safety, connectedness, calming, hope, and efficacy at the individual, family, and community levels.

BEHAVIORAL HEALTH IN THE CONTEXT OF A HEALTHY COMMUNITY

Behavioral health and its integration with health promotion, health care, education, and social services are increasingly appreciated as essential to the realization of healthy communities and healthy individuals (SAMHSA, 2003). The U.S. surgeon general's landmark 1999 report on mental health significantly advanced the nation's understanding of these conditions and their importance to the overall health of the American population:

> "(M)ental health" and "mental illness" … may be thought of as points on a continuum. Mental health is a state of successful performance of mental function, resulting in productive activities, fulfilling relationships with other people, and the ability to adapt to change and to cope with adversity. Mental health is indispensable to personal well-being, family and interpersonal relationships, and contribution to community or society. (HHS, 1999, p. 4)

In the context of this report, the observation that good behavioral health is key to the ability to adapt to change and cope with adversity (i.e., resilience) is of particular importance. Additionally, the surgeon general's report emphasizes the importance of viewing mental health through a public health lens. It asserts that public health has a critical role in identifying risk factors for mental illnesses and in undertaking interventions to prevent their emergence and promote overall mental health. These concepts are reinforced by the recent *Healthy People 2020* report (Secretary's Advisory Committee, 2010). Despite the increased attention to mental health conditions resulting from these reports, however, these conditions remain among the most frequent causes of disability. The Substance Abuse and Mental Health Services Administration (SAMHSA) reports that an estimated 9.6 million American adults are afflicted by a serious mental illness on an annual basis (SAMHSA, 2013b). In the United States, mental health disorders are the leading cause of disability, and these conditions account for a quarter of all years of life lost to disability and premature mortality (NIH, 2014). Moreover, approximately 40,000 Americans take their own lives each year; suicide ranks as the tenth leading cause of death in the United States (CDC, 2014, 2015).

Unfortunately, the consensus among experts is that behavioral health still does not receive the attention it deserves. Specific to the committee's focus on the interrelationship between healthy communities and disaster experiences, the committee was concerned to hear testimony that long-term behavioral health planning and programming are not adequately considered by federal, state, and local disaster and health officials in post-disaster recovery planning (Herrmann, 2014; NBSB, 2010; North and Pfefferbaum, 2013). And although the committee does note growing awareness of the importance of improving the delivery of mental health care, as evidenced by vigorous legislative and other efforts under way to ensure parity in reimbursement[2] for treatment of mental health disorders and medical clinical care, as well as greater coordination between the two (AHA, 2012; Goodell, 2014), much more effort in this regard is required.

Pertinent to the goals of this report, it is important to gain a better understanding of how to optimize

---

[2] Mental Health Parity and Addiction Equity Act of 2008, Public Law 110-343, Title V, Subtitle B, 110th Cong. (October 3, 2008).

the integration of behavioral health planning components into overall healthy community planning; how to incorporate the consultation of behavioral health professionals (e.g., leadership and policy consultation, assistance with behavioral health needs assessments, advice on risk and crisis communications, program evaluation) into pre-disaster planning; and how to use the opportunities and resources available along the disaster recovery continuum appropriately to advance toward the realization of more mentally healthy communities and, ultimately, healthier communities overall.

DISASTER-RELATED BEHAVIORAL HEALTH CHALLENGES

Disasters affect the biological-physical, psychological, and sociocultural well-being of survivors in a number of ways, including

- the acute psychological trauma of the disaster itself (including the bereavement associated with the loss of loved ones), whose effects can be immediate or delayed;
- the stress and upheaval associated with the cascade of adversities experienced in the post-disaster environment, such as displacement from homes, challenges in accessing disaster relief benefits, loss of business revenue, uncertainty related to employment, and the increased need to care for others (e.g., children and the frail elderly);
- disruption of health protective medical services, social services, and behavioral health support services;
- disruption of social networks that can leave people feeling isolated and without support (social effects); and
- an increased propensity for risky and destructive behavior, such as cigarette smoking (Vlahov et al., 2002), alcohol abuse and binge drinking (Adams et al., 2006), and domestic violence (Phua, 2008; Weisler et al., 2006).

Patterns of mental illness after a disaster are variable depending upon preexisting local factors and disaster specifics, such as the individual's direct proximity to the disaster, the number of lives lost, the number of injured (which will impact rehabilitation issues), the extent of damages (which determines the level of disruption of normal activities such as economic and family functioning), the type of disaster (e.g., naturally occurring versus human-caused, novelty of the event); the degree of disruption of behavioral health services/infrastructure; the demographics of the affected population; the resilience of the residents; and the ability of community systems/services to support those in need. As a result, some people within a community may experience more severe adverse behavioral health effects than others. For example, one study conducted after the Oklahoma City bombing in 1995 found that women were more at risk and developed new-onset psychiatric disorders at a rate nearly double that of men (North et al., 2005) (see Table 7-1). Individuals with previous psychiatric disorders may also be at heightened risk following a disaster. The pattern after exposure to Hurricane Katrina was notably characterized by exacerbation of preexisting diagnoses, primarily depression and substance use disorders (North, 2010). The prevalence of posttraumatic stress disorder (PTSD) in a sample of residents affected by Katrina increased from a baseline rate of nearly 15 percent, measured 5-8 months after the Hurricane, to nearly 21 percent when measured again one year later (Kessler et al., 2008). Although rates of mental illness of this order of magnitude will present significant challenges to a community's recovery from a disaster, these data show that even after the most horrific disasters, the majority of the exposed population will not develop diagnosable behavioral health disorders. However, the distress of the event and the recovery process still can generate a wide range of responses—including stress, anxiety, grief, sleeplessness, fatigue, irritability, gastrointestinal distress, and poor concentration (Freedy and Simpson, 2007)—that can interfere with community members' roles within the family, community, workplace, or school (NBSB, 2010). Beyond the impacts on quality of life for individuals, these long-term behavioral health sequelae have a cumulative negative effect on the functioning of society.

TABLE 7-1 Incidence of Psychiatric Diagnoses After Oklahoma City Bombing

New-Onset Psychiatric Diagnoses	Men (%)	Women (%)
Posttraumatic stress disorder	19.8	35.1
Major depression	8.0	17.0
Panic disorder	5.8	3.2
Generalized anxiety disorder	0.0	5.3
Alcohol use disorder	0.0	0.0
Any diagnosis	20.5	40.4

SOURCE: North et al., 2005.

Moreover, while most will be resilient in the face of disaster and experience only mild, transient stress reactions, certain populations are especially vulnerable to behavioral health disorders and require targeted outreach and intervention. These populations warrant special consideration and proactive planning to meet their unique disaster recovery needs:

- **Children and youth**—Children and youth are more likely than adults to be severely impaired after a disaster, most commonly with PTSD or its symptoms (Norris et al., 2002). They also experience anxiety disorders, depression, grief, bereavement, and behavioral and academic difficulties (Pfefferbaum et al., 2014). Children's vulnerability is dependent upon their age, cognitive level, and degree of exposure to the event, as well as how their parents/caregivers are doing after the event (Pfefferbaum et al., 2014). Parent/caregiver status is of particular importance because children are dependent on adults to identify their needs and to access behavioral health and other support services for them. Problems can arise when caregivers themselves are experiencing symptoms of behavioral health disorders or emotional disturbances. Disasters threaten children's perception that the world is safe and predictable; thus, recovery for children requires that parents, caregivers, and the community reestablish a protective shield for them (Pynoos et al., 2007). Media portrayals of disasters also can adversely impact children. A number of studies have explored the direct relationship between media coverage and behavioral health problems following disasters. A study conducted after the Oklahoma City bombing found an association between the amount of disaster-related television viewing and PTSD and depression in children (Pfefferbaum et al., 2002). This association has been documented in numerous other studies examining children's responses to traumatic events, prompting recommendations from researchers (Fairbrother et al., 2003), federal agencies such as the Federal Emergency Management Agency (FEMA), and organizations such as the American Red Cross (FEMA and ARC, 2004) to limit children's disaster-related television viewing.
- **Individuals with a preexisting behavioral health disorder (mental illness or substance abuse disorder) and those having experienced prior trauma**—Pre-disaster functioning is an important predictor of post-disaster functioning (Dirkzwager et al., 2006). For example, among directly exposed survivors of the Oklahoma City bombing with a mental health disorder, 63 percent had some form of mental illness prior to the bombing (North et al., 1999). Meeting the needs of individuals with preexisting behavioral health disorders requires special consideration to ensure continuity of care throughout response and recovery.
- **Responders and recovery workers**—First responders and other recovery workers also are at increased risk for developing mental or substance use disorders (Ehring et al., 2011; Flannelly et al., 2005; Mitani et al., 2006; Rosser, 2008). One key study of 27,449 police officers, firefighters, construction

workers, and municipal workers who responded to the September 11 terrorist attacks in New York City found that among police officers, 7.0 percent developed depression, 9.3 percent developed PTSD, and 8.4 percent developed panic disorder (Wisnivesky et al., 2011). Among other rescue and recovery workers, cumulative incidence of depression was 27.5 percent, PTSD 31.9 percent, and panic disorder 21.2 percent. Before the attacks, only 1 percent of these workers had a history of physician-diagnosed PTSD and 3 percent a history of depression (Wisnivesky et al., 2011). Another study, which looked at psychiatric disorders in rescue workers following the Oklahoma City bombing, found that 13.0 percent of firefighters who served as rescue workers developed PTSD (North et al., 2002). Behavioral health impacts in this population can seriously compromise response and recovery efforts by interfering with workers' abilities to carry out essential job functions.

Other disaster response personnel—including health care professionals and those providing social support and counseling to victims (e.g., social workers, mental health professionals)—are susceptible to burnout and compassion fatigue (reduced capacity to be empathic), which can result from secondary trauma (hearing about the traumas experienced by patients/clients) (Adams et al., 2008). Burnout—"a state of physical, emotional, and mental exhaustion caused by long term involvement in emotionally demanding situations" (Pines and Aronson, 1988, p. 9)—can develop when responders attempt to tackle too much. Compassion fatigue similarly involves the depletion of one's physical, mental, or spiritual resources. Workers with compassion fatigue frequently suffer from a sense of isolation and may be unable to offer emotional support to their patients (Mendenhall, 2006).

The U.S. Department of Health and Human Services' (HHS's) definition of at-risk individuals[3] identifies a number of other population groups that may also be at increased risk for adverse behavioral health outcomes after a disaster. They include senior citizens (e.g., frail elderly displaced from damaged nursing homes), pregnant women, individuals who have disabilities or live in institutionalized settings, people who have limited English proficiency or are non-English-speaking, the transportation disadvantaged, and those with chronic medical disorders (ASPR and ABC, 2012). Vulnerability in many of these populations stems from barriers to their access to behavioral health services such as inadequate finances, lack of health care coverage, language impediments, and difficulties arranging for transportation or daycare. Bridging the language and cultural barriers of different minority groups is a special challenge for successful response and recovery efforts.

BEHAVIORAL HEALTH SECTOR ORGANIZATION AND RESOURCES

The behavioral health sector consists of a fragmented collection of federal, national, state, and local (public and private) resources that "aims to provide a continuum of services and activities—including communication, education, basic support, as well as access to clinical behavioral health services when needed—in order to mitigate the progression of adverse reactions into more serious physical and behavioral health conditions" (HHS, 2014, p. 5). The sector's roles and responsibilities and the associated challenges related to integrating behavioral health effectively at each level are described in the sections below. Although much of the focus is on those agencies and organizations directly supporting behavioral health services, it is important to remember that the trauma of the event itself is only one contributor to psychosocial sequelae after a disaster. The cascade of challenges experienced by disaster survivors after the immediate threat has passed is a key factor as well; thus, behavioral health interventions can in the broadest sense include all actions that reduce the adversities and associated stress of the short-term response and

---

[3] "Before, during, and after an incident, members of at-risk populations may have additional needs in one or more of the following functional areas: communication, medical care, maintaining independence, supervision, and transportation. In addition to those individuals specifically recognized as at-risk in the All Hazards Preparedness Act (i.e., children, senior citizens, and pregnant women), individuals who may need additional response assistance include those who have disabilities, live in institutionalized settings, are from diverse cultures, have limited English proficiency or are non-English speaking, are transportation disadvantaged, have chronic medical disorders and have pharmocological dependency" (HHS, 2013, p. 1).

long-term recovery periods. By providing accessible small business loans and loans for repair of homes, for example, the Small Business Administration can be viewed as a key federal agency providing a form of behavioral health support, removing one stressor from individuals and families. The same may be said when efforts are made to reopen schools as quickly as possible and to train teachers in how to support students in facing the myriad issues they encounter after a disaster. Such initiatives may be just as beneficial as more traditional behavioral health interventions in reducing individual, family, and community stress.

Federal Level[4]

At the federal level, several government agencies carry out an array of behavioral health activities across the disaster continuum (see Figure 7-1). HHS and its subcomponents—including the Office of the Assistant Secretary for Preparedness and Response (ASPR), SAMHSA, the Administration for Children and Families (ACF), the Administration for Community Living (ACL), and the Centers for Disease Control and Prevention (CDC)—play key roles specifically in the integration of behavioral health into disaster preparedness, response, and recovery activities (HHS, 2014). Other key federal partners, such as FEMA, the U.S. Department of Housing and Urban Development (HUD), the U.S. Department of Education, the U.S. Department of Veterans Affairs (VA), and the U.S. Department of Defense (DoD), also have important roles in supporting the behavioral health needs of individuals both before and after a disaster.

Although the federal agencies cited above offer an array of resources, both financial and technical, their primary role is to support state and local assets based on locally defined behavioral health needs (HHS, 2014). The availability of many federal resources after a disaster, including behavioral health assets, depends on a presidential disaster declaration even though those that do not receive such a declaration may generate significant mental health needs in the impacted population (Hyde, 2014). Even in the absence of a presidential disaster declaration, however, federal agencies can offer technical assistance and support to current grantees of existing (steady-state) federal programs. It should be noted that mass violence events—which are relevant to this report because, like natural and technological disasters, they can exceed a community's capacity to recover without outside assistance—result in the activation of different federal services and funding streams in the absence of a presidential disaster declaration.[5]

As noted above and depicted in Figure 7-1, HHS and its subcomponents, especially ASPR, play a significant role in the preparation for, response to, and recovery from disasters as well as public health emergencies. This role includes providing financial resources in the form of grant funding (cooperative agreements), as well as technical assistance and tools to augment state and local planning and preparedness efforts, including addressing behavioral health. ASPR's national Hospital Preparedness Program (HPP) grant, discussed in more detail in Chapter 6, is intended to prepare health care systems, both public and private, for the surge in services that typically occurs after a disaster. The program focuses on, among other things, building health care coalitions at the state and local levels to enhance the coordination and integration of disaster planning and response activities (see Boxes 6-3 and 6-6 in Chapter 6 for discussion of health care coalitions). Public and private behavioral health organizations are highly encouraged by ASPR to join and participate actively in these coalitions.

The federal government workforce is also a vital resource, especially during disaster response and early recovery. It encompasses a variety of health care professionals, including behavioral health specialists serving under ASPR's National Disaster Medical System as well as public health and health care personnel serving as part of the U.S. Commissioned Corps, a program managed nationally by the Office of the Surgeon General within HHS. The ASPR-based Medical Reserve Corps (MRC) program, a network of approximately 1,000 local units comprising volunteers from a variety of health- and nonhealth-related

---

[4] A broader synopsis of legislation and federal policies related to disaster recovery and health security can be found in Appendix A.
[5] Examples of federal programs specific to mass violence events include Victims of Crime funding, the U.S. Department of Justice's Antiterrorism and Emergency Assistance Program for Crime Victims, and the U.S. Department of Education's School Emergency Response to Violence Program.

PREPAREDNESS

Action	Leads
☐ Convene *Disaster Behavioral Health Preparedness Forum* and *Federal Community Health Resilience Coalition* to facilitate interagency collaboration and planning	ASPR
☐ Participate in the development of *National disaster and emergency plans and exercises* to ensure behavioral health is appropriately included	ASPR / Federal Agencies
☐ Engage in *behavioral health promotion* to enhance day-to-day mental and behavioral functioning and promote resilience following emergencies or disasters	SAMHSA
☐ Develop and disseminate *behavioral health educational, messaging, and guidance materials*	SAMHSA / ASPR
☐ Engage in *Scientific Preparedness* activities to coordinate and catalyze the research agenda for disaster behavioral health issues	ASPR / NIH / CDC

RESPONSE

Action	Leads
☐ Upon imminent threat or occurrence of major disaster or public health emergency, the *health and medical services function* of the National Response Framework and the National Disaster Medical System activate	ASPR
☐ HHS's *Incident Response Coordination Team*, which includes a behavioral health liaison officer, stands up to coordinate and support the response	ASPR
☐ *HHS agencies and response partners activate*; depending on the activation level, agency liaison officers may report to the Secretary Operations Center	ASPR / Federal Agencies
☐ *SAMHSA contacts behavioral health agencies*, state disaster behavioral health coordinators, and behavioral health grantees in the impacted region to offer technical assistance and support	SAMHSA
☐ *SAMHSA engages their disaster-related programs* to provide support, such as Crisis Counseling Program, Disaster Technical Assistance Center, and Disaster Distress Helpline	SAMHSA
☐ *Federal Disaster Behavioral Health Group*, comprised of federal agencies with behavioral health expertise, convenes and establishes communication and information gathering channels	ASPR
☐ If indicated, *behavioral health mission assignments* are developed and enacted to provide federal behavioral health responders to the disaster impacted region	ASPR / NDMS / DCCPR (PHS)
☐ *Behavioral health force protection* is carried out to safeguard deployed HHS responders	ASPR / NDMS
☐ *Behavioral health educational and messaging materials* specific to the needs of the event are disseminated through multiple mechanisms	ASPR / SAMHSA
☐ *Surveillance/assessment* mechanisms are queried to gather behavioral health data to inform response and recovery	CDC / ASPR / SAMHSA

RECOVERY

Action	Leads
☐ When National Disaster Recovery Framework activation is imminent, Health & Social Services **Recovery Support Function Primary & Supporting agencies are activated**	ASPR
☐ The Federal Disaster Behavioral Health Group transitions to recovery and continues to meet in support of health and social services recovery efforts	ASPR
☐ **Agencies maintain bi-directional communication through relevant agency programs** and grant programs to assess and address recovery needs and gaps and share information	ASRP / Federal Agencies
☐ **Agencies identify behavioral health informational resources** related to disaster recovery/resilience and mobilize access to this information through information channels	ASPR / Federal Agencies
☐ Agencies plan for and implement the transition from recovery operations to steady-state activity within their agency's programs	ASPR / Federal Agencies
☐ **Longer term responder health monitoring** post-event is carried out	CDC / ASPR

FIGURE 7-1 Federal roles in behavioral health preparedness, response, and recovery.
SOURCE: HHS, 2014, p. 7.

professional backgrounds, can be another valuable resource for expanding the nation's public health and medical response capability (MRC, 2015). The vast majority of MRC units are collocated in public health departments; others are housed in emergency management or law enforcement agencies or are independent, not-for-profit organizations.

Other HHS components play key roles across the disaster continuum. SAMHSA supports "states, territories, tribes, and local entities to deliver an effective mental health and substance abuse (behavioral health) response to disasters" (SAMHSA, 2014b). It develops and disseminates behavioral health educational, messaging, and guidance materials, in addition to providing technical assistance and training manuals for state and local governments to ensure the adoption of behavioral health practices that are evidence-informed. Many of these behavioral health resources (e.g., tip sheets, guidance documents, training resources) are available from SAMHSA's Disaster Technical Assistance Center[6] (SAMHSA, 2014b). Some of the agency's grant-funded initiatives (e.g., the National Child Traumatic Stress Network) also provide technical assistance, training, and services in the preparedness and recovery phases of a disaster. SAMHSA's national Disaster Distress Helpline provides a virtual connection with trained professionals offering tips for coping and referral to local crisis call centers (Hyde, 2014). To address post-disaster domestic violence issues, the HHS Administration for Children and Families provides emergency sheltering, statewide services coordination, and the National Domestic Violence Hotline (HHS, 2014).

The Crisis Counseling Assistance and Training Program (CCP), which is funded by FEMA and administered through an interagency agreement with SAMHSA, is the largest federal program supporting short-term disaster-related mental health services. Authorized under the Stafford Act, CCP grants are available only after a presidential disaster declaration and are of two types: the Immediate Services Program, which lasts 60 days, and the Regular Services Program, which lasts 9 months (SAMSHA, 2014a). The main goals of the CCP are to contact a large number of people through face-to-face outreach, to provide basic crisis counseling and connection to community support systems, and to make referrals to traditional mental health or substance abuse treatment services when necessary. CCP-funded services include individual crisis counseling; supportive educational contact; group crisis counseling; assessment, referral, and resource linkage; and media and public service announcements. These services are typically provided by behavioral health staff from organizations under contract to the state or territory mental health authority. CCP funds can be used to train and educate these staff. CCP crisis counselors, consisting of both mental health professionals and paraprofessionals, do not diagnose or treat people with behavioral health disorders, nor are they allowed to create a record of the type of services provided to an individual (FEMA, 2015; HHS, 2014).

Although the CCP is a critical resource for increasing workforce capacity after a major disaster, the committee learned of multiple challenges with the program as currently designed and administered. A number of problems are highlighted in a 2008 report of the U.S. Government Accountability Office (GAO, 2008). For example, the administrative aspects of applying for CCP services are time-consuming and cumbersome for states, particularly in the midst of a crisis. According to testimony provided to the committee by SAMHSA (Hyde, 2014), 6 years after release of the GAO report, many of these problems had not yet been resolved. Specific concerns include the following:

- Those seeking the two types of available CCP funds must apply for them separately (funding is not automatic after a presidential disaster declaration), and applicants must demonstrate that no other funding sources are available.
- The application for the Immediate Services Program is due within 14 days of a disaster declaration (FEMA, 2013), when states (and localities) may still be in the midst of the emergency response phase. The time required for review of an Immediate Services Program application, receipt of an award, and contracting and training of service providers means that the time for service provision is significantly less than 60 days—in some cases, less than 30 days—unless an extension request is

[6] Resources from SAMHSA's Disaster Technical Assistance Center can be found at http://www.samhsa.gov/dtac/dtac-resources (accessed November 2, 2014).

granted (GAO, 2008). States have suggested extending the length of the Immediate Services Program to 90 days to help alleviate these timing challenges.[7]

- Applications for the Regular Services Program are due about 6 weeks later (by day 60) and duplicate information from the Immediate Services Program application (FEMA, 2013). Some states have recommended that funding through the Immediate Services Program be made available automatically after a presidential disaster declaration.[8] The review process for the Regular Services Program also is lengthy, sometimes necessitating multiple extensions of the Immediate Services Program, which is disruptive to counseling and can delay training of Crisis Counseling Assistance and Training Program staff (FEMA, 2013; Walker, 2014).
- The lack of an electronic system for data collection and reporting to SAMHSA on encounters, assessments, and referrals by crisis counselors creates a large administrative burden by necessitating the compilation of individual paper forms to transfer to the state and, ultimately, SAMHSA.
- Neither CCP grant covers indirect costs, thereby preventing some states from seeking the funds because the local provider agencies often cannot afford to cover those costs.
- Neither mental health treatment (short- or long-term) nor financial coverage for such services is available under the CCP.

Mechanisms for streamlining CCP processes are urgently needed. The committee noted that SAMHSA and FEMA have already initiated a collaborative process to relieve some of the burden of the application process,[9] and it applauds these efforts. However, some needed changes (automatic availability of Immediate Services funds after a presidential declaration, support for electronic data collection and reporting systems, and coverage of indirect costs) require congressional action.

It should be noted that although HHS programs, such as those offered through ASPR and SAMHSA, support behavioral health preparedness and immediate response efforts,[10] little in the way of post-disaster federal resources and funding to support behavioral health activities during long-term recovery is available from HHS unless there is a supplemental appropriation, such as through the Social Services Block Grant (discussed in Chapter 4). SAMHSA also has a relatively small amount of discretionary funds available through the SAMHSA Emergency Response Grant (SERG) program that can be used for behavioral health services during long-term recovery. For example, these funds were used after Hurricane Katrina to continue methadone treatment for displaced individuals (SAMHSA, 2013a). The annual amount of available funds under this program is modest ($750,000-$1,000,000) (Hyde, 2014), and there is no specific congressional appropriation for SERG funds. Instead, SAMHSA must estimate annually the amount of appropriated discretionary funds that needs to be set aside for this purpose. Consequently, during periods of budgetary constraint, no SERG funds may be available to support disaster-stricken communities (Hyde, 2014). While funding limitations for recovery activities are a particular challenge, the administrative burdens associated with demonstrating need within the allotted time window for applications presents further challenges to states. For example, the committee heard that one state withdrew its request for funding "because providing such information took their time and energy away from directly responding to the people, community and state in crisis."[11]

---

[7] Letter, P. Hyde, SAMHSA, to A. Downey, Institute of Medicine, regarding questions posed at Committee on Post-Disaster Recovery of a Community's Public Health, Medical, and Social Services: Meeting Five, October 7, 2014.

[8] Letter, P. Hyde, SAMHSA, to A. Downey, Institute of Medicine, regarding questions posed at Committee on Post-Disaster Recovery of a Community's Public Health, Medical, and Social Services: Meeting Five, October 7, 2014.

[9] Letter, R. Glover, Executive Director, NASMHPD (National Association of State Mental Health Program Directors), to Desk Officer, FEMA, regarding NASMHPD comments on FEMA's Crisis Counseling Assistance and Training Program (CCP), September 25, 2014.

[10] It should also be noted that HHS preparedness funds do not always flow to mental health agencies, which are frequently separate from state public health agency grantees.

[11] Letter, P. Hyde, SAMHSA, to A. Downey, Institute of Medicine, regarding questions posed at Committee on Post-Disaster Recovery of a Community's Public Health, Medical, and Social Services: Meeting Five, October 7, 2014.

National-Level Nongovernmental Resources

A variety of nongovernmental resources and programs are available to assist states, territories, and localities in behavioral health preparedness, response, and recovery. Nongovernmental organizations, including Voluntary Organizations Active in Disasters (VOAD) such as the American Red Cross, play a key role in providing psychosocial support and spiritual care after disasters. Under its congressional charter, the Red Cross provides an array of services and offers substantial behavioral health capacity for disasters through its corps of trained mental health volunteers that respond to such events across the country. "Red Cross has well-defined procedures to provide disaster behavioral health support, identify behavioral health needs through triage and assessment, promote resilience and coping, and target interventions—including crisis interventions, secondary assessments, referrals, and psychoeducation" (HHS, 2014, p. 12). Other National VOAD members such as the Salvation Army, Catholic Charities USA, and Save the Children, as well as private organizations such as Doctors without Borders, provide essential services, including psychosocial support, in the immediate aftermath of disaster.

To take advantage of the support offered by these organizations, they and the services they provide must be coordinated and integrated into the overall disaster response. Still, many of these national organizations provide only short-term response and recovery services, leaving the states and localities to address their long-term recovery needs. Thus, expanding the capacity of first responders and other disaster workers is critical, especially for large-scale events in which such state and local resources are limited. The Emergency Management Assistance Compact (EMAC), a program established in 1996 and administered by the National Emergency Management Association, meets this need during states of emergency declared by governors and in presidentially declared disasters. EMAC is a mutual-aid agreement among all 50 states; the District of Columbia; and the U.S. territories of Puerto Rico, Guam, and the U.S. Virgin Islands. It allows for the sharing of personnel, equipment, and commodities across jurisdictions during disasters and is a vehicle through which behavioral health assets can be requested from other member states (EMAC, 2015).

State Level

The behavioral health system at the state level varies from state to state, with behavioral health services being offered through a complex web of government, nonprofit, and private-sector agencies. Since the enactment of the Stafford Act, state mental health authorities have been required to have plans addressing the mental health aspects of disasters. In some instances, inadequate planning has delayed federal funding (SAMHSA, 2003). Two years after the events of September 11, 2001, SAMHSA provided preparedness grants to mental health and substance abuse agencies in many states to enhance behavioral health disaster planning. This grant funding augmented that provided at the time by other federal agencies (i.e., the CDC and the U.S. Department of Homeland Security) to build state and local capability for responding to future terrorist events and other emergencies (GAO, 2008). Many of the state grant awardees used the funding to support a designated disaster behavioral health coordinator. This individual was assigned the responsibility of coordinating behavioral health disaster planning and response activities, often working with state emergency management and public health agencies to ensure integration with broader response and recovery operations. Today, all states have such a position (ASPR, 2014). However, with the decline and subsequent elimination of this SAMHSA-specific preparedness funding stream, and despite the advances made in preparedness planning since 2001, the committee found that mental health and substance abuse issues are not adequately integrated into recovery efforts at the state level, and the capacity to do so is widely lacking. A 2013 report from the Council of State and Territorial Epidemiologists indicates that fewer than 20 percent of states reported having systems for monitoring the efficacy of mental health services delivered following a disaster and only 15 percent said they had the ability to monitor the population to identify mental health needs arising in the later post-disaster stages (CSTE, 2013). These assessments are critical to targeting behavioral health services where they are most needed and need to be integrated into existing public health and comprehensive state emergency management planning processes.

Some state mental health authorities and public health agencies have made a concerted effort to prepare for the surge in behavioral health care needs typically seen after a disaster by providing disaster-related mental health education and training to health and mental health clinicians and other providers (Cross et al., 2010). While generally viewed as a local resource, these trained professionals can be activated as a team to respond to incidents within their region or state. Additional efforts are needed at the state level to ensure that local behavioral health teams are integrated into the statewide disaster plan and that adequate training is provided to these professionals to ensure a consistent and coordinated response in the acute aftermath of a disaster. More important, it is essential to ensure that this expanded capacity also is available to meet a community's long-term behavioral health recovery needs, when more severe and complex behavioral health disorders are more likely to arise.

State financial resources to aid in behavioral health preparedness, response, and recovery are limited. Typically, states rely on federal funding to support behavioral health planning. Federal funding mechanisms previously mentioned in this report, such as the CDC's Public Health Emergency Preparedness (PHEP) cooperative agreements and ASPR's HPP grants, offer support to states, territories, and selected metropolitan cities for building and strengthening their behavioral health preparedness and response capabilities. Following a disaster, states also may be eligible for SAMHSA CCP funding, discussed above, which in turn can be used to establish local contracts to train service providers and offer relevant post-disaster crisis services (e.g., crisis counseling).

Local Level

At the local level, the behavioral health sector consists of a fragmented collection of local mental health agencies, public and private community mental health centers, psychiatric hospitals, general hospitals with psychiatric beds, nursing homes, addiction services, and local networks of behavioral health and other medical providers (primary care physicians, pediatricians).[12] Behavioral health services are integrated into other community service systems and institutional settings, including corrections, education, and child welfare. As discussed in Chapter 8, a variety of human services are available at the county/city level that provide support to individuals and families on a day-to-day basis, assisting them with housing, food, and child care services. Having ready access to these agencies and their services after a disaster can greatly mitigate stress due to a disaster and enhance the recovery process.

As mentioned earlier in this chapter, access to behavioral health services can be challenging even in the absence of a disaster. Stigma, diminished capacity to provide such services, and cost contribute to the inadequate availability and utilization of such services. Even if access to such services were improved in the steady-state period, communities might still be faced with a lack of clinicians trained and skilled in disaster-related behavioral health treatments and interventions. Most behavioral health professionals receive no specific training and education in this area during their normal course of study. Greater effort is needed to provide these professionals with the knowledge and skills needed to respond to the myriad behavioral health issues that can be expected to emerge after a disaster among both their existing patients and new patients they will encounter.

To accommodate the surge in behavioral health needs that typically occurs after a disaster, local mental health and emergency management authorities may look to nonprofit and private-sector partners to assist in the community's behavioral health response. Many local Red Cross chapters provide mental health services following community emergencies such as a fire or motor vehicle accident resulting in fatalities, as well as larger disasters such as floods or tornadoes. As noted above, these services typically

---

[12] Behavioral health service providers receive information and other forms of support from professional organizations such as the American Academy of Child and Adolescent Psychiatry, the American Psychiatric Association, and the American Psychological Association.

BOX 7-1
The Red River Resilience Project

One example of a community-led coalition that emerged to support coordinated behavioral health care following a disaster is the Red River Resilience Project, initiated in Fargo, North Dakota, in the aftermath of a flood. Partners in the coalition, which is led by the local Red Cross chapter, include the county mental health department, health insurers, a university, Catholic Charities, and local mental health centers. The Red River Resilience Project strives to educate the public on simple steps that can be taken toward resilience, such as fostering hope, engaging in active coping, acting with purpose, connecting with others, taking care of oneself, and searching for meaning (Red River Resilience, 2010).

---

are short-term in nature and, when warranted, often result in referral to other community-based mental health organizations, although on some occasions, the Red Cross has coordinated longer-term support for survivors by organizing community-based coalitions (see Box 7-1). Local Medical Reserve Corps units, alluded to earlier in this chapter, provide an array of medical and nonmedical services, including behavioral health care, at the local level following a disaster.

Disaster behavioral health services also may be delivered through private-sector for-profit organizations under contract to state and local governments or private employers. Examples of these private providers include Crisis Care Network, Kenyon International, and the KonTerra Group. These organizations offer a range of mental health services, including crisis intervention, individual counseling, health promotion, stress management, and psychoeducation. Some states establish contracts with such behavioral health organizations prior to a disaster to ensure the availability of behavioral health workers should such an event occur. Such contracts may be of particular value in those areas in which disasters are recurring events, not only to ensure that their services will be available immediately following a disaster but also to reduce reliance on local providers, who may themselves be suffering the effects of the disaster (Clements, 2014).

Sometimes overlooked, but more recently gaining visibility, are local faith-based organizations, which often are well positioned to deliver spiritual and emotional care both in the immediate aftermath of disaster and during the recovery phase. Although disaster spiritual care has long existed, it only recently has been acknowledged as a critical part of holistic healing for individuals and communities.[13] Disaster spiritual care is "a process through which individuals, families, and communities affected by disaster draw upon their rich heritage of faith, hope, community, and meaning as a form of strength that bolsters the recovery process" (National VOAD, 2014, p. 5). A disaster can tear apart the fabric of a community; thus, a critical part of the recovery process is rebuilding a sense of community (e.g., through community gatherings). Disaster spiritual care providers can support this process and also offer individuals grief support for the many kinds of losses that accompany disasters. Disaster spiritual care providers often do not share the same faith as the individuals and families they care for (Massey, 2006); however, they find ways to connect spiritually with those in need of their services in a manner that is supportive and comforting. Bonding of local faith-based groups into an alliance may reinforce the message that spiritual care is appropriate for all people and may diminish concerns about the focus on any one religious group (Paget, 2014).

Other key recovery partners include national (e.g., the Robert Wood Johnson Foundation) and local

---

[13] No government agency has authority over spiritual care, so until recently there were no standards or guidelines for such care. To fill this gap, National Voluntary Organizations Active in Disaster (VOAD), through its Emotional and Spiritual Care Committee, has used a consensus process to develop a number of resources to support the provision of appropriate and respectful disaster spiritual care, including the National VOAD Disaster Spiritual Care Guidelines, released in 2014. For more information, see http://www.nvoad.org/resource-center (accessed October 13, 2014).

foundations. During past disasters, these philanthropic organizations have been important contributors of funding to support behavioral health recovery. For example, the Missouri Foundation for Health provided funding to the Ozark Center, the behavioral health division of Freeman Health System, for behavioral health recovery efforts in Joplin, Missouri, following the May 2011 tornado. These efforts included employment of community crisis workers; telepsychiatry services; and a text/online messaging service that could be used by students to discuss such issues as depression, suicidal thoughts, and family problems (Freeman Health System, 2012).

Finally, the media, including companies representing print, radio, and television communications, can be instrumental local partners in the aftermath of disaster and throughout the recovery process. Early on, effective crisis and emergency risk communication can help alleviate fear among individuals and communities and aid in obtaining compliance with emergency management directions or other response activities. As recovery proceeds, the media can be an important resource for conveying strategies developed by the public and private sectors for improving emotional well-being and resilience, including coping skills and community prosocial activities (i.e., volunteering to help others). At the same time, however, as stated earlier in this chapter, it is necessary to be aware of the potentially negative influences of the media on behavioral health. Media hype following disasters or other traumatic events and repetitive television coverage (e.g., the replaying of footage of the aircrafts crashing into the World Trade Center towers) can amplify feelings of risk and uncertainty (Vasterman et al., 2005) and contribute to behavioral health problems and disorders, especially in children. For adults who have previously experienced traumatic events, such as veterans, media coverage also can exacerbate symptoms of PTSD (Kinzie et al., 2002).

Challenges to Coordination and Integrated Planning

As discussed earlier in this chapter, the number of stakeholders, both public and private, with key roles in supporting behavioral health grows significantly when behavioral health interventions are viewed broadly to include the many activities that reduce adversity and stress during recovery. This multiplicity of individuals and organizations involved in disaster behavioral health requires effective leadership and coordination at all levels. Coordination is required horizontally among the public, nonprofit, faith-based, and private organizations that make up the local behavioral health sector, and it must also extend across other sectors, including local social services (e.g., case management, homeless programs), education, housing, and emergency management. Coordination also is required vertically to encompass state and federal agencies responsible for mental health and overall disaster response and recovery. Information and data sharing (e.g., sharing of electronic health records) and the development of partnerships and coalitions are critical to the coordination function. Unfortunately, coordination remains a challenge for many communities: data and information systems are inadequate; issues related to the Health Insurance Portability and Accountability Act (HIPAA) and confidentiality must be addressed; and behavioral health representatives are not routinely included at the table during planning discussions or in emergency operation centers (CSTE, 2013).

States and localities impacted by disasters have reported frustration associated with the lack of coordination within and across federal agencies, including HHS, HUD, and the U.S. Department of Homeland Security (NBSB, 2010). This lack of coordination results in overlap and duplication, as well as inconsistent guidance. A recent GAO report cites HHS and seven other federal agencies for failing to fully coordinate behavioral health programs targeting those with serious mental illness (GAO, 2015). The report also indicates that federal agencies failed to formally evaluate many of these mental health programs and thus were unable to ensure that the program activities were meeting the needs of those they were intended to serve. This report and its findings have important implications for disaster recovery in that some of the programs cited are those on which vulnerable populations, such as the severely mentally ill, rely to support them both before and after a disaster. The report also emphasizes the importance of establishing a robust evaluation component for programs that receive federal funding to ensure that they are reaching their targeted audiences and that the services they provide are effective.

By virtue of its coordinating role for both Emergency Support Function (ESF) #8 (Public Health and Medical Services) and the Health and Social Services Recovery Support Function (RSF), ASPR has a lead role in coordinating internal and external federal agencies for the purpose of ensuring that behavioral health issues are integrated into public health and emergency preparedness, response, and recovery. In 2014, HHS released the latest version of its Disaster Behavioral Health Concept of Operations (CONOPS), which provides a framework for ASPR's coordination of federal disaster behavioral health activities (HHS, 2014). Interagency coordination is further promoted by two ASPR-led interagency groups—the Disaster Behavioral Health Preparedness Forum (to support preparedness activities) and the Federal Disaster Behavioral Health Group—both of which can be utilized during a disaster response as well as during the recovery period, as needed (HHS, 2014).

The committee finds HHS's Disaster Behavioral Health CONOPS to be a welcome improvement in policy making and coordination of the department's behavioral health response to disasters. Nonetheless, there remains a need for a "clear and directive national policy" to establish behavioral health as an integral component of the response to and recovery from disasters and to delineate the governmental role in this area across all federal agencies (Pfefferbaum et al., 2012). Such a policy is particularly needed for events that do not result in a presidential disaster declaration; in such cases, further guidance is needed regarding the incident command structure, including delineation of the lead federal agency and the mechanisms for coordination among agencies.[14] In a 2010 report, the Disaster Mental Health Subcommittee of the National Biodefense Science Board concludes that "the most pressing and significant problem that hinders integration of disaster mental health and behavioral health is the lack of appropriate policy at the highest Federal level. Compounding that problem is the lack of any clear statement as to where the authority to devise, formulate, and implement such policy should reside" (NBSB, 2010, p. 3). Based on a review of the literature, the findings of the Disaster Mental Health Subcommittee's report, and testimony from key subcommittee members, the committee believes many of these issues and challenges remain salient today.

At the state and local levels, the structural organization of mental health agencies varies widely, which affects both vertical and horizontal coordination and integration of mental health into broader preparedness, response, and recovery efforts (NBSB, 2010). Mental health agencies often are separate from public health agencies, and siloing of these two sectors has been cited as a significant barrier to post-disaster mental health surveillance (CSTE, 2013). Because of the variation in structural organization, states, territories, and localities need to work proactively to overcome barriers to coordination and integration. Moreover, federal policies designed to promote integration need to account for this variation. States have reported that a lack of understanding of state and local structures and capabilities at the federal level has resulted in confusion in guidance materials (NBSB, 2010). Thus, it is important to engage state and local authorities, as well as nongovernmental, professional, and voluntary organizations that provide behavioral health services, in federal efforts to further integrate behavioral health into disaster preparedness, response, and recovery.

Testimony provided to the committee by experts in disaster behavioral health supported conclusions drawn from the literature that there is virtually no emphasis on integrating behavioral health into intermediate- and long-term recovery planning at the state and local levels (Herrmann, 2014). The committee heard that existing behavioral health programs are tailored primarily to meet short-term, immediate needs during the response phase. Although preparedness funds can be used to improve planning for behavioral health during later recovery stages, cutbacks in critical federal funding support from the HPP and the PHEP cooperative agreements pose significant challenges to making such improvements. Indeed, in the face of reduced funding, advances made in the last few years are being eroded as training opportunities are reduced or eliminated (Herrmann, 2014).

---

[14] M. Brymer, National Center for Child Traumatic Stress at University of California at Los Angeles, to A. Downey, Institute of Medicine, comments provided regarding draft Behavioral Health chapter October 30, 2014.

PRE-DISASTER BEHAVIORAL HEALTH SECTOR PRIORITIES

Not only is mental health essential to the realization of a healthy community; it is also a key component of community resilience (Chandra and Acosta, 2010). A resilient community is one that has fewer risk and resource inequities; engages residents in taking significant, resolute, and collaborative action to remedy a problem; creates linkages to various community resources; promotes and maintains healthy social connections; and successfully adapts to adversities in a flexible manner (Norris et al., 2008). The committee identified two key pre-disaster priorities in which the behavioral health sector should be engaged to support pre-disaster resilience building efforts:

- Strengthening the Existing System with Day-to-Day Responsibility for Promoting Behavioral Health and Delivering Behavioral Health Services
- Engaging in Disaster Preparedness and Recovery Planning Activities

Strengthening the Existing System with Day-to-Day Responsibility for Promoting Behavioral Health and Delivering Behavioral Health Services

To mitigate the behavioral health impacts of disasters (increase resilience) while also building healthier communities, pre-event activities need to focus on strengthening the existing systems with day-to-day responsibility for promoting behavioral health and delivering behavioral health services. Inadequate attention to individuals with prior trauma, for example, can result in a larger population at risk of developing more severe behavioral health disorders after a disaster (HHS, 2014). It is important to stress, however, that during steady-state times, as during recovery, a broad view of behavioral health interventions needs to be taken and the importance of behavioral health to individual and community health emphasized.

Strengthening existing systems is not just about treating those with disorders but also entails preventive measures such as integrating a curriculum for building emotional well-being, coping skills, and social competence into schools to foster healthy students. Another example is the development of programs to foster increased social connectedness[15] as part of preparedness activities (HHS, 2014; NBSB, 2014). An inverse relationship between individual-level social capital and mental health disorders has been observed (De Silva et al., 2005), suggesting that stronger social support may be a protective factor that can reduce the risk of post-disaster mental health disorders. An individual's social network is an important source of emotional support after a disaster (Chandra and Acosta, 2010), and cohesion among family members has been associated with reduced symptoms of PTSD following such events (Birmes et al., 2009). Investment in stronger systems for the delivery of behavioral health services, the integration of preventive behavioral health services into other community systems, and increased social connectedness can build resilience at the individual, family, and community levels, which in turn can reduce disaster-related effects on behavioral health and alter the trajectory of recovery. It is worth pointing out that some primary care practices and patient-centered medical homes are already integrating behavioral health with health care (NCQA, 2014). To encourage such integration, existing payment and reimbursement barriers need to be reduced or eliminated so that patient-centered medical homes can increase their everyday capacity and, as a result, their disaster-related capacity.

Engaging in Disaster Preparedness and Recovery Planning Activities

To ensure that behavioral health providers are prepared to function as part of a coordinated health system after a disaster, they need to be actively engaged in pre-disaster preparedness activities. One mechanism for integrating behavioral health into pre-disaster planning for response and recovery is through exist-

---

[15] An example of an emergency preparedness program focused on increasing social connectedness is SF72, which was developed by the San Francisco Department of Emergency Management. For more information, see http://www.sf72.org/home (accessed April 2, 2015).

ing or newly formed regional (substate) health care coalitions, which, as mentioned earlier in this chapter and discussed in greater detail in Chapter 6, serve as coordinating groups for the health system before and after disasters and provide an interface with the public health and emergency management sectors (ASPR, 2012). As noted earlier, the HPP supports the development of health care coalitions, and according to the National Guidance for Healthcare System Preparedness, behavioral health providers should be considered essential members of these groups. Included among program measures for state-level awardees of HPP funds is an indicator for whether the health care recovery plan, developed in collaboration with the health care coalition, addresses how the community's post-disaster behavioral health care needs will be met (ASPR, 2013). To ensure a specific focus on behavioral health challenges during planning activities, a behavioral health task force could be formed within the health care coalition. Another task for the health care coalition is to develop adequate continuity of operations plans for mental health agencies, organizations, and facilities providing behavioral health services. These plans should consider the surge in demand arising from the needs of individuals who were not utilizing these services before the disaster.

In addition to pre-event planning, providing disaster-specific training in advance of an event on behavioral health interventions can increase community resilience by enhancing self-sufficiency and enabling the community to better meet the surge in behavioral health needs. This type of training can be provided to community members, behavioral health professionals, and/or community partners. These trained individuals can then form a local disaster behavioral health response team that can be deployed after a disaster to offer supportive interventions that mitigate the acute and long-term behavioral health consequences of the disaster (University of Rochester et al., 2005). For example, one state invested PHEP cooperative agreement funds in a program used to teach community partners how to deliver psychological first aid (described in more detail in the section below), thus creating a cadre of individuals ready to provide behavioral health services when activated in subsequent disasters (Singleton, 2014). The American Red Cross offers a 4-hour training course, Coping in Today's World: Psychological First Aid and Resilience for Families, Friends and Neighbors, aimed at building community resilience by helping people learn to cope with stresses, including those related to a disaster, as well as to help their fellow community members (ARC, 2010).

To facilitate and expedite the deployment of behavioral health services after a disaster, behavioral health professionals who wish to assist can be encouraged to affiliate with a local or state-based disaster behavioral health team (e.g., American Red Cross, local MRC unit) and register in the Emergency System for Advance Registration of Volunteer Health Professionals (described in Chapter 6) or similar state registries so their credentials can be verified in advance of a disaster. Additionally, memorandums of understanding can be established with community partners who will offer behavioral health services after a disaster to articulate their roles and responsibilities. Participation in pre-disaster drills and exercises will further prepare community members, behavioral health professionals, and community partners to address disaster behavioral health needs.

THE CONTINUUM OF POST-DISASTER BEHAVIORAL HEALTH INTERVENTIONS

As discussed earlier in this chapter, most disaster survivors will not develop major psychological or psychiatric problems but short-term stress reactions that will resolve on their own or through minimal supportive care. Others, however, will go on to develop more significant behavioral health problems that will require more intensive, targeted intervention and treatment. According to Pfefferbaum and colleagues (2012, p. 60), "Timely mental and behavioral health interventions can improve response efficiency, prevent secondary adversities due to inappropriate or inadequate response, help affected populations recover and adjust to changed circumstances, improve adherence to future recommendations and directives, and increase confidence in government."

Behavioral health interventions help survivors adjust to the consequences of a disaster and its secondary adversities. However, three major challenges are encountered in efforts to deliver effective and adequate behavioral health services after a disaster. First, disasters generate an increased need for services in a system already strained by capacity limitations. Second, this disaster-related surge in mental and behavioral health

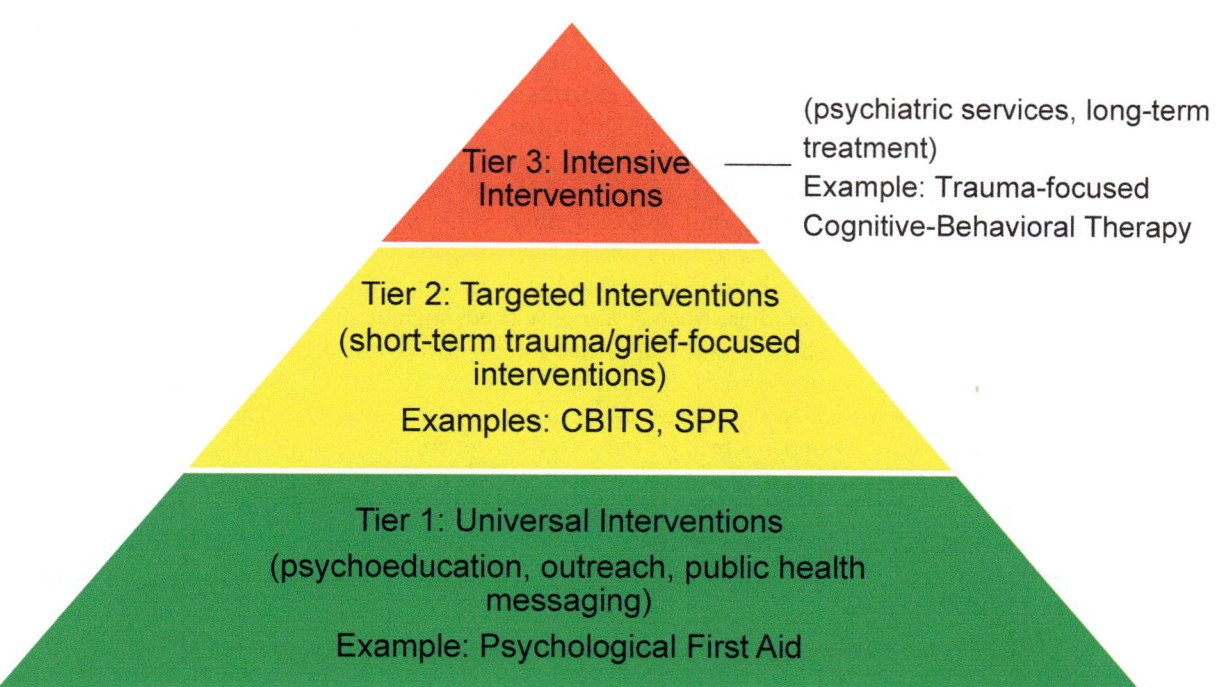

Tier 3: Intensive Interventions —— (psychiatric services, long-term treatment)
Example: Trauma-focused Cognitive-Behavioral Therapy

Tier 2: Targeted Interventions (short-term trauma/grief-focused interventions)
Examples: CBITS, SPR

Tier 1: Universal Interventions (psychoeducation, outreach, public health messaging)
Example: Psychological First Aid

FIGURE 7-2 A 3-tiered public health model for behavioral health interventions after disasters.
NOTE: CBITS = Cognitive-Behavioral Intervention for Trauma in Schools; SPR = Skills for Psychological Recovery.
SOURCE: Adapted from Pynoos et al., 1998.

needs occurs at the same time that the mental health infrastructure is weakened. And third, as discussed earlier, behavioral health systems often are fragmented so that it is difficult to coordinate the efforts of the many actors and sectors involved.

When post-disaster behavioral health needs are not adequately addressed, they can become chronic and subsequently lead to an increased demand for long-term behavioral health services. In the immediate post-disaster stage, interventions need to focus on alleviating the emotional suffering caused by the traumatic events, reinforce short- and longer-term adaptive functioning and coping, provide clear communication aimed at destigmatizing help seeking for those in distress, prevent the progression to mental illness or substance abuse, address the immediate mental health needs of those with preexisting behavioral health disorders, and refer those severely affected to appropriate therapeutic services. While each of these issues presents critical short-term needs, activities should be undertaken with the long-term goal of building a more socially supportive and cohesive environment and a resilient behavioral health infrastructure in which preventive and rehabilitative services are integrated with other community services.

Disasters affect different people in different ways as a result of factors specific to the disaster (e.g., exposure) and the individual (e.g., resilience).[16] Thus, different types of support will be required to meet the spectrum of needs within a community. A three-tiered public health approach that offers multiple intervention strategies at different post-disaster time points will ensure that survivors receive services based upon their disaster experience and current needs (see Figure 7-2). With a tiered approach, triage and assessment strategies are needed to determine the appropriate level of care in each case and to target

---

[16] A number of individual resilience factors have been identified and can inform the development and refinement of behavioral health interventions. These include personality traits, attributional style, social support, coping self-efficacy, and a variety of biological factors (Watson et al., 2011).

interventions to priority groups (Pynoos et al., 2007). For example, the Fast Mental Health Triage Tool (Brannen et al., 2013) and Psychological Simple Triage and Rapid Treatment (Schreiber et al., 2014) are examples of triage tools that can assist in identifying individuals who may be at risk of more serious mental health consequences and thus require further assessment from qualified behavioral health specialists. It is important that behavioral health responders and others using these triage tools be trained in their use and understand how to identify the most appropriate level of care based on the symptoms being assessed.

Although there is broad recognition of the value of population-level psychosocial support methods that provide comfort and promote resilience, and several such interventions are discussed in the sections below, the committee recognizes that studies are urgently needed to determine the effectiveness of these methods. Evaluation of other interventions that were once commonly used, such as psychological debriefing,[17] has demonstrated the importance of showing not only that interventions are beneficial but also that they cause no further harm. One challenge with evaluation studies, however, is that what constitutes meaningful change as opposed to statistically significant findings may not be clear. In the absence of adequate evidence from research studies, consensus methods are used to inform interventions. For example, a panel of experts on the study and treatment of survivors from disasters and mass violence events developed empirically supported consensus principles that can guide intervention and prevention efforts. Based on expert consensus, early and mid-term interventions should promote "1) a sense of safety; 2) calming; 3) a sense of self- and community efficacy; 4) connectedness; and 5) hope" (Hobfoll et al., 2007, p. 283).

Delivering Early Behavioral Health Interventions

The first priority after a disaster is to ensure that basic needs are met by addressing individuals' safety concerns; connecting them with their loved ones; providing practical assistance, information, and emotional support; and linking them with other community services (Tier 1 in Figure 7-2). The behavioral health needs of the community must be assessed if appropriate care is to be provided, and at-risk individuals or groups that may need further intervention should be identified during this assessment. If the disaster disrupted the usual provision of behavioral health services, it should be reestablished as soon as possible to assist survivors with preexisting mental health and substance abuse disorders (as well as a possible surge in demand due to the disaster). However, it is important to note that the steady state of behavioral health services often is inadequate for individuals with Medicaid or those lacking health or behavioral health insurance coverage. These are often, not coincidentally, the most vulnerable populations—impoverished children and adults, individuals for whom English is not the primary language spoken, and those who lack U.S. citizenship (ASPR and ABC, 2012). If necessary, mobile services, such as those provided by some community and faith-based organizations, can be used to reach patients when facilities are damaged or patients are displaced. Behavioral health response teams, such as those discussed in the previous section, can be activated after the disaster to begin assisting the community.

Psychological first aid (PFA) is a widely accepted technique used during the response phase by first responders and other disaster workers to address these initial priorities. In 2006, the National Center for Posttraumatic Stress Disorder and the National Child Traumatic Stress Network released the second edition of *Psychological First Aid Field Operations Guide,* a set of comprehensive guidelines on the definition and use of PFA (Brymer et al., 2006). This guide, produced after consultation with first responders and disaster mental health professionals, as well as disaster survivors, appears to represent the strongest attempt yet

---

[17] Psychological debriefing is "an intervention consisting of one or more individual or group sessions provided hours or days after a traumatic event." Its goals are to "normalize survivors' reactions, process their trauma experiences, address psychological distress, [and] enhance resilience." Its elements include "assist[ing] survivors in sharing their experiences and ventilating their emotional reactions, provid[ing] education about common reactions, [and] encourag[ing] further intervention if appropriate" (North and Pfefferbaum, 2013, p. 514). Psychological debriefing gained popularity internationally without evidence of efficacy. An influential review of numerous randomized controlled trials of single-session debriefing for individuals found that it lacked effectiveness for reducing distress or preventing PTSD and that it could worsen posttraumatic symptoms, but only in those at greatest risk for PTSD (Rose et al., 2002).

made to develop a consensus on guidelines for conducting PFA, which is defined as "a systematic set of helping actions aimed at reducing initial post-trauma distress and supporting short- and long-term adaptive functioning" (Ruzek et al., 2007, p. 17). The core actions for PFA are

- contact and engagement,
- safety and comfort (to enhance immediate and ongoing safety and provide physical and emotional comfort),
- stabilization to promote calm,
- information gathering to identify immediate needs and concerns,
- practical assistance to offer help in addressing immediate needs and concerns,
- connection with social supports,
- information on coping support, and
- linkage with collaborative services (Ruzek et al., 2007).

Psychological first aid can be performed by a wide variety of trained professionals and paraprofessionals in diverse settings, including general-population shelters, special-needs shelters, field hospitals and medical triage areas, schools, acute care facilities, staging or respite centers for first responders, and crisis hotlines or phone banks (Brymer et al., 2006). Training resources for PFA exist across the country and are offered through various organizations, including the American Red Cross (ARC, 2014), the World Health Organization (WHO) (2011), and the Bloomberg School of Public Health at Johns Hopkins University (Johns Hopkins Bloomberg School of Public Health, 2014). One Red Cross program—Coping in Today's World—can be offered throughout the recovery period to help community members better help themselves, their families, and their neighbors (CDMHC, 2011).

While PFA is a widely accepted and utilized technique within the mental health and disaster recovery communities and has received support from major stakeholders such as WHO, the National Institute of Mental Health, the American Red Cross, and several relief organizations (including The Sphere Project[18]), it has not been empirically evaluated for efficacy (Watson et al., 2011). Further scientific evaluation of this intervention is essential to determine its value and effectiveness.

Providing Ongoing Psychosocial Support

Following the acute post-disaster stage, one measure for judging the progress of recovery is how people feel they are coping with their lives. During the recovery period, therefore, it is critical to provide community members with the tools and resources they need to cope with the ongoing challenges they face (i.e., a self-help approach). According to Gluckman (2011, p. 2),

> A comprehensive and effective psychosocial recovery programme needs firstly to support the majority of the population who need some psychosocial support within the community (such as basic listening, information and community-led interventions) to allow their innate psychological resilience and coping mechanisms to come to the fore, and secondly to address the most severely affected minority by efficient referral systems and sufficient specialised care. Insufficient attention to the first group is likely [to] increase the number represented in the second group.

Although no single evidence-based psychosocial support program can be applied in all communities after a disaster, expert consensus documents highlight the important elements of a disaster behavioral health program (see Box 7-2), as well as evidence-informed and promising models. Ideally, programs should be

---

[18] The Sphere Project brings together humanitarian agencies around the common goal of improving the quality and accountability of humanitarian assistance and actors. The Sphere Project was established in 1997 and is "governed by a Board composed of representatives of global networks of humanitarian agencies." The Sphere Handbook, *Humanitarian Charter and Minimum Standards in Humanitarian Response*, offers a set of common guidelines and standards (The Sphere Project, 2015).

BOX 7-2
Expert Consensus on Disaster Behavioral Health Interventions

Commonalities across guidelines and recommendations from expert consensus on disaster behavioral health interventions include the following:

- Be proactive/prepared ahead of time, pragmatic, flexible, and plan on providing the appropriate services matched for phase across the recovery period.
- Promote a sense of safety, connectedness, calming, hope, and efficacy at every level.
- Do no harm, by:
  - participating in coordination of groups to learn from others and to minimize duplication and gaps in response;
  - designing interventions on the basis of need and available local resources;
  - committing to evaluation, openness to scrutiny, and external review;
  - considering human rights and cultural sensitivity; [and]
  - staying updated on the evidence base regarding effective practices.
- Maximize participation of local affected population, and identify and build on available resources and local capacities (family, community, school, and friends).
- Integrate activities and programming into existing larger systems to reduce stand-alone services, reach more people, be more sustainable, and reduce stigma.
- Use a stepped care approach: Early response includes practical help and pragmatic support, and specialized services are reserved for those who require more care.
- Provide multilayered supports (i.e., work with media or Internet to prepare the community at large; facilitate appropriate communal, cultural, memorial, spiritual, and religious healing practices).
- Provide a spectrum of services, including
  - provision of basic needs;
  - assessment at the individual level (triage, screening for high risk, monitoring, formal assessment) and the community level (needs assessment and ongoing monitoring, program evaluation);
  - psychological first aid/resilience-enhancing support;
  - outreach and information;
  - technical assistance, consultation, and training to local providers; [and]
  - treatment for individuals with continuing distress or decrements in functioning (preferably evidence-based treatments like trauma-focused cognitive-behavioral therapy).

SOURCE: Excerpted from Watson et al., 2011, p. 485.

---

tailored to the local community based on a continuous assessment of needs, preexisting assets that support community resilience, and the social environment. The behavioral health strategy should be incorporated into the larger social recovery strategy. Cultural barriers, including language, need to be considered in the development of broad-based psychosocial support programs so that subpopulations within the community are not excluded. Thus, programs should be informed by the community itself (e.g., using focus groups). Commonalities in effective programs include psychoeducation (i.e., helping people understand what kinds of emotional effects are common after a disaster and what signs may indicate that professional help is needed), skill building, and efforts to reconnect and strengthen social networks. These interventions may be universal (Tier 1 in Figure 7-2) or targeted to specific subgroups (Tier 2). A novel but promising example of a locally informed Tier 1 (universal) intervention designed to normalize emotional reactions to a disaster and reduce stigma is the "All Right?" social marketing campaign developed in the Canterbury region of New Zealand (see Box 7-3).

A crisis counseling program, which may begin in the early period after a disaster and extend into the recovery phase,[19] is a mechanism for delivering different kinds of psychosocial support interventions. Crisis counselors (trained crisis workers and paraprofessionals) conduct outreach and education in a full range of disaster settings, such as shelters, schools, workplaces, faith-based organizations, and homes (Norris and Bellamy, 2009). Counseling staff bring services to where residents spend most of their days. Visits usually last at least 15 minutes and usually are limited to one or two for an individual or a group. Crisis counseling can empower survivors by helping them understand and normalize their reactions, enhance coping, consider options, and be linked with other community resources. Its elements include door-to-door outreach, public education, supported individual and group counseling, and referral if necessary (FEMA, 2013).

Although crisis counseling is considered broadly helpful for dealing with post-disaster distress, its efficacy has not been evaluated in randomized controlled clinical trials. One survey of providers and patients found that participants' perceived benefits improved with increases in service intensity, service intimacy (in homes as opposed to shelters or on the street), and frequency of referrals, and with a decrease in provider job stress (Norris et al., 2009). As discussed earlier in this chapter, the Crisis Counseling Assistance and Training Program administered by SAMHSA is a common mechanism for delivering this type of psychosocial support within the first year following a disaster. However, the program's efficacy has not been evaluated in recent years, and as the committee learned through testimony, presents a significant administrative burden to jurisdictions seeking such support. A contemporary, independent review and evaluation of this program leveraging input from a variety of stakeholders, including behavioral health specialists, emergency managers, and others, is warranted. In the process, other models, such as an exposure-based model, should also be considered.

Skills for Psychological Recovery (SPR) is a skills-based, solution-focused intervention designed to assist children, adults, and families in recovery (Berkowitz et al., 2010). It is a flexible, modular approach developed by the National Center for Posttraumatic Stress Disorder and the National Child Traumatic Stress Network for use during the Crisis Counseling Regular Services Program. Unlike supportive counseling methods, Skills for Psychological Recovery is a skills-building approach aimed at empowering people to take control of their own recovery; skills emphasized include problem solving, managing reactions, promoting positive thinking and attitudes, and strengthening social connectedness. SPR can be delivered by non–behavioral health providers, although they should be supervised by a behavioral health provider. While each of the skills it supports stands on its own and can be taught in one session, multiple sessions are ideal to maximize the intervention's benefit. This intervention can be targeted to individuals or groups and delivered in various settings (Tier 2 in Figure 7-2) (Berkowitz et al., 2010). In Joplin, Missouri, for example, where a strong sense of community existed after the town was devastated by a tornado in 2011, health experts decided to leverage regular community potluck dinners as an opportunity for group outreach. The Mercy Community Connections program was built around those dinners, with case workers attending and teaching each SPR skill to thousands of community members (Walker, 2014).

Identifying and Treating Behavioral Health Disorders

Although early and ongoing population-level support interventions may have broad impact by reducing stress and potentially mitigating the later onset of behavioral health disorders, it is important as well to ensure that mechanisms are in place for assessing needs for clinical treatment of mental illness. These assessments should identify preexisting conditions and other vulnerabilities, as well as disaster-related psychopathology (Pfefferbaum et al., 2014). Care must be taken to differentiate psychopathology from normal emotional responses to the disaster. As noted earlier, most people experiencing distress after a disaster will rebound on their own, but as many as one-third of survivors with significant exposure to a traumatic event and/or loss may exhibit a behavioral health disorder (North and Pfefferbaum, 2013). For these individuals, mental health treatment services beyond broad-based interventions designed to address

---

[19] FEMA's Crisis Counseling Assistance and Training Program can last up to 9 months after an event (SAMHSA, 2014a).

BOX 7-3
Canterbury's "All Right?" Social Marketing Campaign

"All right?" is a social marketing campaign launched in February 2013 in the city of Christchurch and the wider Canterbury region of New Zealand to help residents heal and improve their mental well-being in the aftermath of a series of earthquakes that, between 2010 and 2012, left over 185 people dead, and damaged or destroyed homes, other buildings, and significant areas of the city (Rinard Hinga, 2015). The goals for the campaign were twofold: first, to address the psychosocial issues surrounding recovery from the earthquakes so as to prevent more acute mental health problems from developing; and second, to seize an opportunity offered by the recovery process to improve the region's well-being in general by increasing people's understanding and experience of good mental health (All Right?, 2014a).

To develop the "All Right?" campaign, research was carried out using a combination of focus groups and surveys to assess how the earthquakes impacted Cantabrians, how they were coping, and what specific issues they were dealing with (All Right?, 2013). The study also asked participants what they would want a well-being campaign to look like. Participants stressed that the recovery effort should focus on people rather than buildings, and suggested that a campaign should concentrate on four objectives (All Right?, 2013):

- Normalize concern about mental health.
- Give people the tools to improve their mental health.
- Provide credible examples of how others in similar circumstances have felt better.
- Help people feel empowered rather than focused on things that are beyond their control.

Key activities of the campaign. The campaign had three major phases. The first was designed to assure people that the range of emotions they were experiencing after the disaster were normal. Advertisements that declared a range of feelings to be "all right" were placed in public places (Healthy Christchurch, 2014b). The second phase encouraged Cantabrians to check in with themselves and each other and to take small steps to take care of their well-being. Posters encouraged people to have a "mate date," to "get your sweat on," or to

---

distress are indicated. In determining the appropriateness of treatment options (supportive versus intensive psychotherapy), the conditions of the treatment (e.g., voluntary or involuntary), and the background and training of the treatment providers (e.g., professional versus paraprofessional), it is important to be aware of potential ethical and legal implications. There also are other ethical and legal implications of disaster behavioral health that, while they need to be understood, are beyond the scope of this report (Flynn and Speier, 2014).

To enhance the recovery of behavioral health among people with diagnosable trauma-induced disorders, interventions include a combination of psychotherapy and pharmacotherapy—most typically, selective serotonin reuptake inhibitors or anxiolytics. Two commonly described psychotherapy interventions are trauma-focused cognitive-behavioral therapy and exposure-based therapy (North and Pfefferbaum, 2013). Trauma-focused cognitive-behavioral therapy is an evidence-based intervention that "uses behavioral and verbal techniques to identify and correct problematic thinking" and perceptual patterns that contribute to dysfunction (Nucifora et al., 2007). One example of discouraging negative appraisals is to replace thinking that the disaster is "the worst thing that has ever happened to me" with a more optimistic appraisal that the disaster, while harrowing, "has given me the courage and skills to survive and take charge of my life." Exposure-based therapy is an evidence-based intervention that helps the patient directly confront fearful situations, objects, memories, and images so as to desensitize their impact and modify emotional reactions.

Psychotherapy-based treatments can be short- or long-term and delivered to individuals or groups. An example of a Tier 2 (targeted, short-term) intervention is Cognitive-Behavioral Intervention for Trauma

have "a good boogie" (All Right?, 2014c). The third phase asked Cantabrians to share their own stories about what makes them feel happy, and started a community conversation by placing these stories on posters around town (All Right?, 2014c).

The "All Right?" campaign also initiated or supported such events as community fun days, a walking festival, and a body festival offering dance lessons (All Right?, 2014b). Another part of the campaign, "Outrageous Bursts of All Right," included flower bombing (handing out roses and coffee to some of the most affected communities), and surprise limousine rides for unsuspecting members of the public (All Right?, 2014b). These events were designed to "share a little love" and to remind people to take care of themselves and others (All Right?, 2014b). The campaign also disseminated a telephone helpline to provide free support to individuals struggling with mental health issues.

Evaluation of the campaign. To inform the continual development of the "All Right?" campaign, quantitative research was conducted in 2014 through phone interviews with a random sample of 800 individuals in the Christchurch area and compared to data collected in 2012 (All Right?, 2014d). Despite ongoing concerns and frustrations regarding the recovery process, more respondents in 2014 than in 2012 agreed that

- they had access to the support they needed to cope;
- they valued what they had more now than before the earthquakes;
- they connected with their neighbors more than before the earthquakes; and
- they were given the opportunity to contribute to the recovery effort (All Right?, 2014d).

"All Right?" as a model for other communities. The "All Right?" campaign has been connecting with international organizations that are interested in bringing the concept to other areas of the world (Healthy Christchurch, 2014a). Simplicity and flexibility are key attributes of the campaign that make it easily adaptable. "All Right?" works because it is informed by local research, local voices, and a consultative development process. Thus, it will be important for a community to develop its own culturally relevant messages and activities to help mitigate the mental health effects of disasters.

in Schools (CBITS), which incorporates cognitive-behavioral therapy skills. CBITS is delivered in school settings to groups of children who have been exposed to trauma, with the aim of relieving symptoms of behavioral health disorders such as PTSD, depression, and general anxiety (Jaycox et al., 2012). Like SPR, CBITS is a skills-based intervention and therefore helps children not only deal with a past trauma but also develop skills that can be used to handle future stress. Longer-term and more intensive interventions (delivered primarily to individuals) will be needed for those with persistent and severe reactions and impairments (Tier 3 in Figure 7-2).

A major challenge for communities that have experienced a disaster is that few resources have been allocated for the long-term planning or delivery of diagnostic and treatment services. Meager federal, state, and local funding is designated expressly for formal mental health services for people who have identified disorders and for whom personal recovery is the treatment goal. The little funding available often goes toward treating the chronic and persistently mentally ill. It is therefore not surprising that as few as 18.5 percent of people with new-onset psychiatric disorders after Hurricane Katrina received some treatment, primarily with pharmacotherapy (Wang et al., 2008). As discussed previously, formal treatment services may be funded with SAMHSA's SERG funds because they entail fewer restrictions than crisis counseling grants (a presidential disaster declaration is not required for states to request SERG funds); however, there is no guarantee that SERG funds will be available at the time of a disaster (Hyde, 2014). Existing federal block grants—the Substance Abuse Prevention and Treatment Block Grant and the Community Mental Health Services Block Grant, as well as the Social Services Block Grant—also can be used to fund formal treatment for disaster survivors not covered by health insurance, but there are multiple competing priorities for these funding streams, making them less likely to be a viable resource for states and localities (SAMHSA, 2015).

SPECIAL CONSIDERATIONS FOR VULNERABLE POPULATIONS

After the response phase, when many volunteers have left the area, there often remains significant unmet need related to mental health and emotional well-being that extends into the intermediate- and long-term post-disaster period, particularly among those most at risk of developing severe adverse reactions to the trauma. Many of the most vulnerable populations have difficulty accessing services or may refrain from doing so because of associated stigma. Programs that reach these vulnerable populations in community settings such as schools, community centers, and homeless shelters can help extend the reach of behavioral health and psychosocial support programs to those in greatest need. Integration of behavioral health into health care and other community services is critical to the success of such efforts.

Children and Youth

Children and youth spend most of their formative years in educational settings. Consequently, education systems are increasingly cognizant of the importance of creating environments that support physical well-being, social inclusiveness, and psychological resilience among children and youth (Layard and Hagell, 2014). Additionally, primary and secondary schools increasingly are seen as providers of health and mental health services. Therefore, getting schools operating as quickly as possible is critical in the aftermath of a disaster so that school-based programs can provide an opportunity to reach this at-risk population, promoting resiliency skills and identifying children in need of referral to more specialized treatment services (see the example in Box 7-4). While schools have increasingly been utilized to deliver psychosocial support services to children, further efforts are needed to reach younger children by working with preschools and Head Start programs (White, 2014). Mobile services also can help reach children, particularly in settings where they are concentrated after disasters, such as temporary housing sites. For example, the Children's Health Fund, in partnership with the Mailman School of Public Health at Columbia University, used mobile vans to provide medical services, including mental health services, to children living in FEMA villages after Hurricanes Katrina and Rita (Madrid et al., 2008). Additional resources on addressing behavioral health in children and youth after a disaster can be found in Appendix C.

As with interventions for the broader public, the evidence base for interventions used with children is inadequate. A review of the child disaster mental health intervention evidence base revealed nearly 50 different packaged interventions specifically for children in disaster situations. Most were found to be beneficial, but the interventions commonly included multiple components so it was unclear which components were responsible for the observed benefit, and few direct comparisons were made to determine comparative effectiveness (Pfefferbaum, 2014).

Community Members with Preexisting Behavioral Health Disorders

In addition to providing interventions for identified cases of new behavioral health disorders, it is essential to ensure the continuity of services for those with preexisting psychiatric illnesses or substance use disorders. For example, continuity of services for those in methadone treatment programs was identified as a problem after Hurricane Sandy.[20] SAMHSA's *Disaster Planning Handbook for Behavioral Health*

---

[20] Letter, P. Hyde, SAMHSA, to A. Downey, Institute of Medicine, regarding questions posed at Committee on Post-Disaster Recovery of a Community's Public Health, Medical, and Social Services: Meeting Five, October 7, 2014.

BOX 7-4
Project Fleur-de-lis™: A Tiered Intervention Approach for Children

Traumatic exposures during natural or man-made disasters put children at risk of posttraumatic stress disorder (PTSD) and depression (Pfefferbaum et al., 2006; Thienkrua et al., 2006), yet most children with these conditions go undetected and untreated during and after disasters (Madrid et al., 2008). Mercy Family Center created Project Fleur-de-lis™ in New Orleans in fall 2005 to address this deficiency. Its continuation for 3 years in 45 schools covering 20,000 students was made possible by piecing together funding from corporations, foundations, individual donors, and nonprofit agencies. The project's purpose was, in a school-based setting, to screen for, triage, and treat trauma-related disorders in children exhibiting traumatic symptoms after Hurricane Katrina (Cohen et al., 2009).

The project used a three-tiered approach for children identified as having symptoms of a trauma-related disorder: (1) a universal intervention involving a 9-week classroom-based intervention that each week emphasized a specific theme in a group environment, permitting children to conceive of safe places to share their stories and develop coping strategies; (2) Cognitive-Behavioral Intervention for Trauma in Schools (CBITS) as a selected intervention for children with lingering symptoms; and (3) trauma-focused cognitive-behavioral therapy (TF-CBT), consisting of 12-16 individual sessions, for children with PTSD who did not respond to other school-based interventions (Cohen et al., 2009).

In the course of Project Fleur-de-lis™, a randomized trial of two of the interventions was undertaken (Jaycox et al., 2010). Participating children were randomized to receive either CBITS or TF-CBT. Unlike CBITS, the TF-CBT intervention was delivered outside the school (at Mercy Family Center). Even though taxi cab fare and free babysitting for siblings were provided, only 37 percent of the TF-CBT group attended the initial assessment (versus 98 percent for the CBITS group), and only 15 percent of the TF-CBT group had completed treatment by the time of follow-up (versus 91 percent for the CBITS group) (Jaycox et al., 2010). Although statistically and clinically significant improvements in PTSD symptoms were observed for students in both treatment groups, CBITS clearly was far more accessible to families who were unable or unwilling to participate in individual, clinic-based treatment that required parents to attend and bring children to appointments. The implication of these findings is that providing behavioral health treatment services for children in or near their schools may be one way to significantly increase uptake of those services after a disaster.

Other key lessons were learned from Project Fleur-de-lis™. First, obtaining funding for behavioral health screening and treatment programs in schools is difficult, which is troubling considering that children's behavioral health needs are complex and potentially life-altering and require substantial investment. Second, the trauma associated with Hurricane Katrina was only part of the problem (Cohen et al., 2009). The hurricane tended to exacerbate existing mental health issues in children exposed to previous traumas, such as community violence, domestic abuse, and child sexual abuse, indicating a need to be prepared to deal with trauma not related to the disaster when planning disaster behavioral health interventions.

In summary, these studies showed that school-based programs provide an important opportunity for identifying and addressing both disaster-related and longer-standing behavioral health problems in children exposed to trauma. However, if schools participate in such programs, they must be prepared to address a wide array of identified problems, including educational delay, severe mental illness, and comorbidities.

Treatment Programs (SAMHSA, 2013a) provides guidance for behavioral health treatment programs.[21] However, greater awareness of these important issues is needed within broader disaster response and recovery planning efforts through the education and involvement of emergency managers, social services organizations, and other key state and local stakeholders.

---

[21] *Disaster Planning Handbook for Behavioral Health Treatment Programs* is available at http://store.samhsa.gov/shin/content// SMA13-4779/SMA13-4779.pdf (accessed October 22, 2014).

Responders, Care Providers, and Recovery Workers

The mental health of responders (particularly in disasters that result in fatalities among these groups) and health care workers (Harvard School of Public Health, 2013), including behavioral health care providers, warrants special consideration. Organizations employing responders, health care workers, and recovery workers need to create behavioral health plans for offering support to workers during the course of trauma work. Responders and recovery workers should have pre- and post-deployment training on behavioral health risks and symptoms (offered through their employer or other community-based organization), and they should be monitored for symptoms both during and after their disaster deployment so that early intervention can be provided. Ensuring that workers' schedules provide adequate time to rest and unwind is crucial in preventing both burnout and compassion fatigue (Mendenhall, 2006). Training responders in psychological first aid prior to a disaster and then providing this supportive intervention to individuals or teams following their work in the field allows responders and rescue workers to both offer and accept support.

Behavioral health disaster plans should include the provision of a range of social and emotional supports, including individual, family, and group support, as well as educational presentations and literature. Employee assistance programs can be engaged in the provision of these supports. Support should continue to be offered to help workers recover from an event in the long term, keeping in mind that the signs of psychological trauma during and after a disaster may be delayed. These provisions might include working to connect individuals, families, and communities with resources needed to restore social and psychological functioning. SAMHSA and the National Institute of Environmental Health Sciences have collaborated on worker resiliency training that can be provided before and after disasters (NIEHS, 2015).[22]

BUILDING A MORE RESILIENT AND SUSTAINABLE BEHAVIORAL HEALTH SECTOR

Disasters offer an opportunity to strengthen the behavioral health sector (WHO, 2013), which too often exists in a fragile state even during normal times (Herrmann, 2014). The sector can be strengthened, for example, by enhancing both physical infrastructure and systems for delivering care. In the aftermath of a disaster, increased attention to mental health issues and the emergence of creative approaches to meeting disaster-related needs can be leveraged to transform long-term behavioral health care and reduce barriers to care (WHO, 2013). It is critical that this opportunity not be missed given the significant public health burden associated with mental illness and the essential role of behavioral health in the realization of a healthy, resilient community. Success will depend on an early commitment to building on the momentum of the acute post-disaster phase and planning for long-term sustainability.

Disasters often, of necessity, result in an expansion of community-based services and cross-sector collaboration (see Box 7-5). Leveraging relationships forged during a disaster can lead to better long-term integration of behavioral health services with other community services (medical care, education, and social services). Newly trained community members able to offer psychological first aid and other forms of psychosocial support also represent a valuable resource that can be maintained through ongoing training to increase system capacity and ensure resilience against future incidents. Community health workers, in particular, can play critical roles in addressing health disparities by helping to overcome barriers to access to care for underserved populations (see the discussion of community health workers in Box 6-13 in Chapter 6) (Springgate et al., 2011). Although short-term programs (e.g., crisis counseling programs) offered with outside assistance may help in meeting critical behavioral health capacity needs, programs that build long-term capacity need to be better supported. Philanthropic organizations often provide initial support to meet community behavioral health needs, but sustainability will require longer-term investments from local, state, and federal governments. Demonstration of the potential value of such investments, particularly

---

[22] For more information on worker resiliency training, see http://tools.niehs.nih.gov/wetp/index.cfm?id=2528 (accessed April 3, 2015).

BOX 7-5
Lasting Investments: Sustaining Mental Health Capacity After a Disaster

The destruction of health infrastructure in New Orleans by Hurricane Katrina and resultant gaps in capacity to meet health needs spurred the development of a novel partnership, REACH NOLA, that included community-based organizations (social service agencies, health clinics, and faith-communities) and academic institutions. Supported by funding from the Robert Wood Johnson Foundation and the American Red Cross, REACH NOLA developed a Mental Health Infrastructure and Training Project, aimed at promoting community recovery by increasing capacity for mental health service delivery (Meyers et al., 2011). Through the project, local health service providers were able to receive training and follow-up support on implementing evidence-based and novel approaches to mental health service delivery. Five years after Katrina, community health workers trained under the Mental Health Infrastructure and Training Project were still engaged in efforts to meet mental health and psychosocial needs in New Orleans (Springgate et al., 2011).

---

cost–benefit analysis, can be a powerful motivator for decision makers; consequently, greater attention needs to be paid to measurement of impact in terms of both individual well-being and fiscal efficiency.

Some disasters will necessitate the rebuilding of centers used for the delivery of health care services, including behavioral health services. If a presidential declaration of disaster is made, federal funds become available that can support the rebuilding of physical infrastructure (see Chapter 4). FEMA Public Assistance funds and, under some circumstances, block grant funds (Community Development Block Grant and Social Services Block Grant) can support the rebuilding of mental health facilities.[23] During significant rebuilding or new construction of physical infrastructure, opportunities to collocate services (e.g., psychiatric and primary care) should be examined by public and private partners to facilitate better access to care. Team-based approaches to care facilitated by collocation of services have been shown to be effective in meeting post-disaster mental health needs (see Box 7-6).

Finally, a community that has weathered a disaster should engage in post-disaster analysis of lessons learned and identification of opportunities for improvement. These lessons should be shared with other communities through state, regional, and national conferences, workshops, and discipline-specific professional meetings. Through cooperative and continuous assessment of the successes and challenges for behavioral health in disaster recovery, the behavioral health sector will be improved both for steady-state times and for disasters.

RESEARCH NEEDS

The evidence base to support behavioral health interventions after a disaster is distressingly inadequate, relying heavily on consensus expert opinion. Significant investment in research is critical to

- establish a more rigorous evidence base on the effectiveness of interventions that are currently used commonly for psychosocial support, including psychological first aid, crisis counseling, and psychoeducation (North and Pfefferbaum, 2013; Pfefferbaum et al., 2012);
- determine the effectiveness of current counselor training programs (i.e., the CCP);

---

[23] FEMA Public Assistance funds may only be used to support reconstruction of facilities for nonprofit organizations.

BOX 7-6
Increasing Resilience Through Integrated, Sustainable Mental Health Services

The Louisiana Mental and Behavioral Health Capacity Project was developed following the Deepwater Horizon oil spill to meet mental health needs in communities affected by the spill and earlier disasters. The project, funded by the Deepwater Horizon Medical Benefits Class Action Settlement, is a collaborative effort that includes the support and involvement of community stakeholders, providers, and five primary care clinics closest to affected communities. Prior to this project, the majority of affected communities had little access to behavioral health services, in part as a result of the exodus of medical professionals from Louisiana after Hurricane Katrina.

Under the Mental and Behavioral Health Capacity Project, an "interprofessional stepped-care collaborative" model for care is established with teams comprising primary care providers, mental health professionals, social workers, and care managers. Psychiatrists and psychologists are collocated within clinics with primary care providers, enabling the latter to become more familiar with mental health disorders and more confident about treating them. For more severe and complex cases, onsite mental health providers are available for assessment and treatment, or alternatively, treatment is managed by offsite providers through telemedicine. This model builds trust and allows patients to be treated in an effective and efficient manner. A recent study (Osofsky et al., 2014) showed that this continuity and collaboration between primary care providers and mental health clinicians reduces barriers to accessing care and decreases numbers of hospitalizations—benefits that may be related to earlier detection and intervention for mental health disorders. Reported results indicate broad community acceptance of these services, and clinical staff involved in the project report increased confidence in their ability to evaluate and treat mental health symptoms and face future disasters. This program could serve as a model for other communities at risk of disasters or those with little access to mental health clinicians.

SOURCE: Osofsky et al., 2014.

- better match interventions to specific target groups, including vulnerable populations such as children; and
- rigorously evaluate the effect of strengthening social networks on the incidence of post-disaster behavioral health disorders.

SUMMARY OF FINDINGS AND RECOMMENDATION

Through testimony and a review of the literature, the committee identified the following key behavioral health challenges related to disaster recovery:

- Even during steady-state times, behavioral health services may not meet a community's behavioral health needs, especially for underserved populations. These capacity issues are likely to be exacerbated by disaster.
- Current disaster behavioral health programs and funding focus primarily on the immediate response and early (months) recovery phases and not on addressing the long-term (years) behavioral health and emotional well-being of disaster survivors and responders.
- There is little financial support to help communities diagnose and treat new behavioral health disorders or preexisting ones that have been exacerbated after a disaster.

- The process for accessing current funding for psychosocial support (i.e., CCP and SERG funds) is overly burdensome.
- Little guidance exists on how to meet increased behavioral health needs that arise during the recovery period (after the immediate response phase) as a result of the disaster experience.
- Little training in trauma-informed behavioral health care exists for health care providers.
- First responders, as well as recovery workers, are vulnerable to PTSD and other psychiatric and substance use disorders, and few programs exist to provide mental health education and treatment for them.
- Behavioral health is not adequately integrated into the recovery efforts of other sectors (e.g., social services and housing).
- Attention to destigmatizing normal emotional reactions after disaster is inadequate.
- The effectiveness (and potential harm) of most current disaster behavioral health interventions is inadequately understood.
- Little is known about mechanisms for and benefits of integrating behavioral health interventions with existing (pre-disaster) assets and resources that are foundational to community resilience.

These ongoing challenges demonstrate that, despite increasing understanding of its importance to recovery and resilience, behavioral health has not been addressed systematically or consistently in disaster preparedness or post-disaster response and recovery efforts (Pfefferbaum et al., 2012). The committee concludes that behavioral health should be a higher priority for healthy community planning and integrated throughout the continuum of disaster preparedness, response, and recovery and across all sectors. Although behavioral health has been promoted as a critical concept in HHS reference materials and operational plans, the committee found no evidence of its widespread uptake outside of the health sector or of efforts to facilitate a coordinated, cross-sector approach to the delivery of adequate behavioral health services. The HHS Disaster Behavioral Health CONOPS, discussed previously in this chapter, represents a critical step forward, but the committee agrees with the findings of the Disaster Mental Health Subcommittee of the National Biodefense Science Board that a national policy is needed to overcome the fragmentation that currently impedes the horizontal and vertical coordination of behavioral health services and their integration into disaster preparedness, response, and recovery and with the disaster-related efforts of other sectors. Such a policy is also needed to establish roles and responsibilities and a clear incident command structure for all disasters irrespective of whether there is a presidential major disaster declaration.

Recommendation 8: *Develop a National Disaster Behavioral Health Policy.*

The U.S. Department of Health and Human Services and the Federal Emergency Management Agency should engage state and local governments, as well as private- and nonprofit-sector stakeholders, in the development of a national disaster behavioral health policy. This policy should delineate the roles, responsibilities, and authorities of the federal government for optimal integration of behavioral health services across the continuum of health care, public health, social services, and all other sectors (e.g., housing, public safety, education) before, during, and after a disaster or other emergency.

To support the implementation of this recommendation, the following steps should be taken at the federal level:

- Federal agencies responsible for funding and developing behavioral health policy should support and collaborate with behavioral and other health professional societies to enhance national understanding of the importance of behavioral health to the realization of healthy communities so that this agenda will be included more effectively in general community health planning.

- HHS should use its preparedness funding requirements and currently existing collaborative bodies (e.g., Disaster Behavioral Health Preparedness Forum, Federal Community Health Resilience Coalition), as well as other mechanisms, to overcome the fragmentation of disaster behavioral health services and stimulate their coordination and integration with health care, social support, emergency management, and information technology services.
- HHS should commission a study to analyze current federal behavioral health programs and generate recommendations for efforts at the federal level to address the long-term behavioral health needs of individuals and communities after a disaster or other emergency.

At the state and local levels, the following steps should be taken:

- State and local government disaster preparedness, response, and recovery officials should make the necessary efforts to ensure that behavioral health professionals at all levels are included in disaster preparedness planning and in emergency operations centers after a disaster.
- State and local government public health and mental health officials, supported by federal preparedness funding from the Hospital Preparedness Program (HPP) and Public Health Emergency Preparedness (PHEP) cooperative agreements, should work together and with other key community stakeholders, including state and local emergency managers, to integrate behavioral health into efforts to build community resilience and enhance planning for long-term behavioral health recovery. Opportunities to leverage other funding sources, such as the Substance Abuse Prevention and Treatment Block Grant, Community Mental Health Services Block Grant, and Social Services Block Grant, should be evaluated.
- Given the scale and range of mental health consequences associated with disasters and the need for local capacity to support long-term behavioral health recovery, the adequacy of the behavioral health workforce to meet disaster-related needs should be enhanced. Efforts to this end should include pre-disaster identification of trained professionals; training and exercising of support personnel; attention to licensure and credentialing requirements; and coordination of government mental health care systems, community- and faith-based organizations, and for-profit provider companies.

BEHAVIORAL HEALTH SECTOR RECOVERY CHECKLIST

The committee has identified two pre-event and seven post-disaster critical recovery priorities for the behavioral health sector that are inextricably linked to strengthening the health, resilience, and sustainability of a community. Action steps for each of these priorities are provided in the following checklist. Although behavioral health sector leaders will need to adapt these actions to the local context, this guidance provides an indicative set of concerns to be considered during recovery. The checklist illustrates how the following four key recovery strategies, identified as recurring themes at the beginning of this chapter, apply to individual priority areas:

- Integrate behavioral health activities and programming into other sectors (e.g., education, health care, social services) to reduce stand-alone services, reach more people, foster resilience and sustainability, and reduce stigma.
- Provide a spectrum of behavioral health services and use an approach based on stepped care (from supportive intervention to long-term treatment).
- Maximize the participation of the local affected population in recovery planning with respect to behavioral health, and identify and build on available resources and local capacities and networks (community, families, schools, and friends) in developing recovery strategies.
- Promote a sense of safety, connectedness, calming, hope, and efficacy at the individual, family, and community levels.

Pre-Event

Priority: Strengthen the Existing System with Day-to-Day Responsibility for Promoting Behavioral Health and Delivering Behavioral Health Services

Primary Actors[1]: Behavioral Health Authorities
Key Partners: Federal Agencies (including Substance Abuse and Mental Health Services Administration [SAMHSA] and Centers for Medicare & Medicaid Services [CMS]), State/Local Health Departments,[2] Social Services Agencies, Community- and Faith-Based Organizations; Education System, Judicial System

Key Recovery Strategies:

- Integrate behavioral health activities and programming into other sectors (e.g., education, health care, social services) to reduce stand-alone services, reach more people, foster resilience and sustainability, and reduce stigma.
- Maximize the participation of the local affected population in recovery planning with respect to behavioral health, and identify and build on available resources and local capacities and networks (community, families, schools, and friends) in developing recovery strategies.

Activities include but are not limited to:
- ☐ Integrate behavioral health into other community services, such as education and social services.
- ☐ Promote an increased understanding of the importance of behavioral health to individual health and a healthy community.
- ☐ Focus on building traits known to impart resilience to individuals (e.g., coping skills, social connectedness).

- -

Priority: Engage in Disaster Preparedness and Recovery Planning Activities

Primary Actors: Emergency Management Agencies, Behavioral Health Authorities, Disaster Relief Organizations (including the American Red Cross), Elected Officials and Community Leaders
Key Partners: State/Local Health Departments, Health and Medical System Partners, Community- and Faith-Based Organizations

Key Recovery Strategy:

- Maximize the participation of the local affected population in recovery planning with respect to behavioral health, and identify and build on available resources and local capacities and networks (community, families, schools, and friends) in developing recovery strategies.

---

[1] See Appendix F for further description of terms used to describe Primary Actors and Key Partners in this checklist.
[2] Throughout this checklist, "State/Local" is used for the purposes of brevity but should be inferred to include tribal and territorial as well.

Pre-Event

Activities include but are not limited to:
- ☐ Use available state and local data to identify at-risk populations susceptible to post-disaster mental health sequelae.
- ☐ Identify public and private organizations that provide behavioral health services.
- ☐ Ensure the participation of behavioral health stakeholders in state, regional, or local health care coalitions, and consider creating a disaster mental health task force or advisory group from within coalition membership.
- ☐ Ensure adequate continuity of operations plans for behavioral health authorities, organizations, and facilities providing behavioral health services. Plans should consider surge in demand arising from individuals who were not utilizing services before the disaster.
- ☐ Develop a local disaster behavioral health response team.
- ☐ Train community members and responders in universal behavioral health interventions (e.g., psychological first aid, American Red Cross's Coping in Today's World).
- ☐ Encourage interested behavioral health professionals to affiliate with a local disaster mental health response team (e.g., American Red Cross, Medical Reserve Corps) and to register in the Emergency System for Advance Registration of Volunteer Health Professionals or similar state registries so their credentials can be verified in advance of a disaster.
- ☐ Establish memorandums of understanding with community partners that could be tapped to provide behavioral health services after a disaster.
- ☐ Participate in drills and exercises.

Short-Term Recovery

Priority: Deliver Early Behavioral Health Interventions

Primary Actors: Behavioral Health Authorities, First Responders, Disaster Relief Organizations, Education System, Child Care Organizations
Key Partners: Health and Medical System Partners, Social Services Agencies, Community- and Faith-Based Organizations

Key Recovery Strategies:
- Maximize the participation of the local affected population in recovery planning with respect to behavioral health, and identify and build on available resources and local capacities and networks (community, families, schools, and friends) in developing recovery strategies.
- Promote a sense of safety, connectedness, calming, hope, and efficacy at the individual, family, and community levels.
- Provide a spectrum of behavioral health services and use an approach based on stepped care (from supportive intervention to long-term treatment).

Activities include but are not limited to:
- ☐ Apply population-level tools for rapid mental health triage that use known risk factors to better match need with available resources and appropriate level of services.
- ☐ Assess the behavioral health needs of the affected community.
- ☐ Use an outreach process to identify at-risk individuals who may be in need of further intervention.
- ☐ Activate response protocols for disaster behavioral health response teams.
- ☐ Provide support to first responders and other disaster relief workers to mitigate traumatization.
- ☐ Deliver universal interventions through mental health teams, first responders, and other disaster relief workers to
  - attend to practical needs of survivors,
  - connect survivors to additional community resources, and
  - enhance the ability of survivors to cope.

- -

Priority: Expand the Provider Pool to Meet Increased Demand for Behavioral Health Services

Primary Actors: Behavioral Health Authorities, Community- and Faith-Based Organizations, First Responders, Disaster Relief Organizations, Corrections System, Education System, Private Sector, Child Care Organizations
Key Partners: State/Local Health Departments, Law Enforcement Agencies, Judicial System, Social Services Agencies

Key Recovery Strategy:
- Integrate behavioral health activities and programming into other sectors (e.g., education, health care, social services) to reduce stand-alone services, reach more people, foster resilience and sustainability, and reduce stigma.

Short-Term Recovery

Activities include but are not limited to:
- ☐ Train paraprofessionals and community members (e.g., teachers) in the delivery of psychosocial support interventions.
- ☐ Mobilize and coordinate volunteer behavioral health workers and ensure that those from outside the community are linked with community groups familiar with local organizations, processes, and culture.
- ☐ If not done in advance of the disaster, verify credentials and licenses of volunteers.
- ☐ Engage the faith-based community to help survivors with grief, bereavement, and other emotional responses to the disaster.

Priority: Reestablish Services for Community Members with Preexisting Behavioral Health Disorders

Primary Actors: Behavioral Health Authorities
Key Partners: Health and Medical System Partners, State/Local Health Departments, Social Services Agencies, Community- and Faith-Based Organizations

Key Recovery Strategy:
- Provide a spectrum of behavioral health services and use an approach based on stepped care (from supportive intervention to long-term treatment).

Activities include but are not limited to:
- ☐ Ensure continuity of access to treatment for survivors in substance abuse and psychiatric programs.
- ☐ Use mobile services to reach patients without transportation access.

Intermediate- to Long-Term Recovery

Priority: Provide Ongoing Psychosocial Support

Primary Actors: Behavioral Health Authorities, Health and Medical System Partners, State/Local Health Departments

Key Partners: Disaster Relief Organizations, Education System, Community- and Faith-Based Organizations, Social Services Agencies

Key Recovery Strategies:
- Integrate behavioral health activities and programming into other sectors (e.g., education, health care, social services) to reduce stand-alone services, reach more people, foster resilience and sustainability, and reduce stigma.
- Provide a spectrum of behavioral health services and use an approach based on stepped care (from supportive intervention to long-term treatment).
- Maximize the participation of the local affected population in recovery planning with respect to behavioral health, and identify and build on available resources and local capacities and networks (community, families, schools, and friends) in developing recovery strategies.
- Promote a sense of safety, connectedness, calming, hope, and efficacy at the individual, family, and community levels.

Activities include but are not limited to:
- ☐ Continuously assess intermediate- and long-term behavioral health needs of the affected community.
- ☐ Incorporate behavioral health into a larger social recovery strategy.
- ☐ Normalize emotional reactions to the disaster through a social marketing campaign that uses a variety of media sources and public messaging focused on fostering an environment that makes it easy and acceptable for citizens to access resources.
- ☐ Promote activities designed to increase social connectedness (e.g., community dinners, school functions).
- ☐ Ensure that behavioral health services are accessible through one-stop shops and other locations that disaster survivors frequent.
- ☐ Ensure that behavioral health intervention programs are culturally and regionally appropriate.
- ☐ Identify survivors who are predisposed to more severe and persistent mental health problems as a result of preexisting traits (e.g., past trauma) or disaster-related adversities, and link them with appropriate services.
- ☐ Train community partners/crisis counselors in the delivery of evidence-based and evidence-supported psychosocial support interventions.
- ☐ Implement school-based psychosocial support and screening programs for children.
- ☐ Engage early childhood education centers (preschools, child care facilities) to extend the reach of psychosocial support interventions to children under 5 years.
- ☐ Engage community- and faith-based organizations to better reach adult populations, including vulnerable populations, that may not seek out behavioral health services.

Intermediate- to Long-Term Recovery

Priority: Expand the Provider Pool to Meet Increased Demand for Behavioral Health Services

Primary Actors: Behavioral Health Authorities, Disaster Relief Organizations
Key Partners: Health and Medical System Partners, State/Local Health Departments, Corrections System, Education System, Community- and Faith-Based Organizations, Private Sector, Child Care Organizations, Social Services Agencies

Key Recovery Strategies:
- Provide a spectrum of behavioral health services and use an approach based on stepped care (from supportive intervention to long-term treatment).
- Integrate behavioral health activities and programming into other sectors (e.g., education, health care, social services) to reduce stand-alone services, reach more people, foster resilience and sustainability, and reduce stigma.

Activities include but are not limited to:
- ☐ Train behavioral health practitioners to provide intermediate- and long-term mental health and substance abuse interventions.
- ☐ Train paraprofessionals and volunteers to identify people who may need support for mental health or substance abuse issues.

- -

Priority: Take Steps to Ensure the Behavioral Health of Responders, Care Providers, and Recovery Workers

Primary Actors: Behavioral Health Authorities, State/Local Health Departments, Health and Medical System Partners
Key Partners: Employers of Responders and Recovery Workers

Key Recovery Strategies:
- Integrate behavioral health activities and programming into other sectors (e.g., education, health care, social services) to reduce stand-alone services, reach more people, foster resilience and sustainability, and reduce stigma.
- Provide a spectrum of behavioral health services and use an approach based on stepped care (from supportive intervention to long-term treatment).

Activities include but are not limited to:
- ☐ Provide pre- and post-deployment training on behavioral health risks and symptoms.
- ☐ Engage employee assistance programs to provide support for workers.
- ☐ Monitor responders and recovery workers for symptoms of behavioral health problems and provide early interventions.

Intermediate- to Long-Term Recovery

Priority: Increase Community Resilience and Progress Toward a Healthy Community by Building Long-Term Capacity and Increasing Access to Services

Primary Actors: Behavioral Health Authorities, Health and Medical System Partners, Social Services Agencies
Key Partners: Education System, Community- and Faith-Based Organizations

Key Recovery Strategy:
- Integrate behavioral health activities and programming into other sectors (e.g., education, health care, social services) to reduce stand-alone services, reach more people, foster resilience and sustainability, and reduce stigma.

Activities include but are not limited to:
- ☐ Invest in maintaining psychosocial support skills acquired during recovery, and develop/offer training programs for community partners (clinics, schools) during steady-state periods.
- ☐ Collocate behavioral health services with primary care and/or social services when feasible.
- ☐ Leverage relationships forged during a disaster to increase long-term system capacity and integration of behavioral health services with other community services.
- ☐ Participate in an after-action process that includes analysis of lessons learned and identification of opportunities for improvement.
- ☐ Share lessons learned and opportunities for improvement with other communities through state, regional, and national conferences, workshops, and discipline-specific professional meetings so that other jurisdictions can benefit from recovery experiences.

REFERENCES

Adams, R. E., J. A. Boscarino, and S. Galea. 2006. Alcohol use, mental health status and psychological well-being 2 years after the World Trade Center attacks in New York City. *American Journal of Drug and Alcohol Abuse* 32(2):203-224.

Adams, R. E., C. R. Figley, and J. A. Boscarino. 2008. The compassion fatigue scale: Its use with social workers following urban disaster. *Research on Social Work Practice* 18(3):238-250.

AHA (American Heart Association). 2012. *Bringing behavioral health into the care continuum: Opportunities to improve quality, costs and outcomes.* http://www.aha.org/research/reports/tw/12jan-tw-behavhealth.pdf (accessed November 3, 2014).

All Right?. 2013. *A summary of the research behind the wellbeing campaign for Canterbury.* http://healthychristchurch.org.nz/media/100697/allrightresearchsummary.pdf (accessed September 22, 2014).

All Right?. 2014a. *Frequently asked questions.* http://img.scoop.co.nz/media/pdfs/1406/AllRightFAQs.pdf (accessed September 22, 2014).

All Right?. 2014b. *Our projects.* http://allright.org.nz/our-projects (accessed September 22, 2014).

All Right?. 2014c. *Starting a community conversation about wellbeing in post-earthquake Christchurch.* http://www.healthychristchurch.org.nz/media/111388/allrightbristolposter.pdf (accessed September 22, 2014).

All Right?. 2014d. *A summary of the All Right? campaign research findings.* http://allright.org.nz/media/uploads/AllRightResearchSummary_2_2.pdf (accessed September 22, 2014).

ARC (American Red Cross). 2010. *Coping in today's world. Psychological first aid and resilience for families, friends, and neighbors.* Washington, DC: ARC.

ARC. 2014. *Emergency service courses.* http://www.redcross.org/ma/boston/take-a-class/emergency-service-courses (accessed October 22, 2014).

ASPR (Office of the Assistant Secretary for Preparedness and Response). 2012. *Healthcare preparedness capabilities: National guidance for healthcare system preparedness.* Washington, DC: HHS.

ASPR. 2013. *Hospital Preparedness Program (HPP) measure manual: Implementation guidance for the HPP Program measures.* Washington, DC: HHS.

ASPR. 2014. *Disaster behavioral health: Current assets and capabilities.* http://www.phe.gov/Preparedness/planning/abc/Pages/dbh-capabilities.aspx (accessed July 9, 2014).

ASPR and ABC (At-Risk Individuals, Behavioral Health and Community Resilience). 2012. *At-risk individuals fact sheet.* http://www.phe.gov/Preparedness/planning/abc/Pages/at-risk.aspx (accessed November 3, 2014).

Berkowitz, S. J., R. Bryant, M. Brymer, J. Hamblen, A. Jacobs, C. Layne, R. Macy, H. Osofsky, R. Pynoos, J. Ruzek, A. Steinberg, E. Vernberg, and P. Watson. (National Center for Posttraumatic Stress Disorder and National Child Traumatic Stress Network). 2010. *Skills for Psychological Recovery (SPR).* http://www.nctsn.org/content/skills-psychological-recovery-spr (accessed April 3, 2015).

Birmes, P., J. P. Raynaud, L. Daubisse, A. Brunet, C. Arbus, R. Klein, L. Cailhol, C. Allenou, F. Hazane, H. Grandjean, and L. Schmitt. 2009. Children's enduring PTSD symptoms are related to their family's adaptability and cohesion. *Community Mental Health Journal* 45(4):290-299.

Brannen, D. E., R. Barcus, M. A. McDonnell, A. Price, C. Alsept, and K. Caudill. 2013. Mental health triage tools for medically cleared disaster survivors: An evaluation by MRC volunteers and public health workers. *Disaster Medicine and Public Health Preparedness* 7(1):20-28.

Brymer, M. J., A. K. Jacobs, C. M. Layne, R. S. Pynoos, J. I. Ruzek, A. M. Steinberg, E. M. Vernberg, and P. J. Watson. 2006. *Psychological first aid: Field operations guide, 2nd edition.* Washington, DC: NCTSN and NCPTSD.

CDC (Centers for Disease Control and Prevention). 2014. *Understanding suicide: Fact sheet.* http://www.cdc.gov/violenceprevention/pdf/suicide_factsheet-a.pdf (accessed December 3, 2014).

CDC. 2015. *Suicide and self-inflicted injury.* http://www.cdc.gov/nchs/fastats/suicide.htm (accessed April 2, 2015).

CDMHC (California Disaster Mental Health Coalition). 2011. *Resources for psychological first aid (PFA) and resilience.* http://www.cdmhc.org/ResourcesPsychologicalFirstAid.pdf (accessed April 3, 2015).

Chandra, A., and J. D. Acosta. 2010. Disaster recovery also involves human recovery. *Journal of the American Medical Association* 304(14):1608-1609.

Clements, B. 2014. *Public health and community recovery: Texas' experience.* Paper presented at IOM Committee on Post-Disaster Recovery of a Community's Public Health, Medical, and Social Services: Meeting Two, February 3, Washington, DC.

Cohen, J. A., L. H. Jaycox, D. W. Walker, A. P. Mannarino, A. K. Langley, and J. L. DuClos. 2009. Treating traumatized children after Hurricane Katrina: Project Fleur-de lis™. *Clinical Child and Family Psychology Review* 12(1):55-64.

Cross, W., C. Cerulli, H. Richards, H. He, and J. Herrmann. 2010. Predicting dissemination of a disaster mental health "train-the-trainer" program. *Disaster Medicine and Public Health Preparedness* 4(4):339-343.

CSTE (Council of State and Territorial Epidemiologists). 2013. *Disaster mental health surveillance at state health agencies: Results from a 2013 CSTE assessment.* Atlanta, GA: CSTE.

De Silva, M. J., K. McKenzie, T. Harpham, and S. R. A. Huttly. 2005. Social capital and mental illness: A systematic review. *Journal of Epidemiology and Community Health* 59(8):619-627.

Dirkzwager, A. J., L. Grievink, P. G. van der Velden, and C. J. Yzermans. 2006. Risk factors for psychological and physical health problems after a man-made disaster. Prospective study. *British Journal of Psychiatry* 189:144-149.

Ehring, T., S. Razik, and P. M. Emmelkamp. 2011. Prevalence and predictors of posttraumatic stress disorder, anxiety, depression, and burnout in Pakistani earthquake recovery workers. *Psychiatry Research* 185(1):161-166.

EMAC (Emergency Management Assistance Compact). 2015. *What is EMAC?* http://www.emacweb.org/index.php/learnaboutemac/what-is-emac (accessed April 2, 2015).

Fairbrother, G., J. Stuber, S. Galea, A. R. Fleischman, and B. Pfefferbaum. 2003. Posttraumatic stress reactions in New York City children after the September 11, 2001, terrorist attacks. *Ambulatory Pediatrics* 3(6):304-311.

FEMA (Federal Emergency Management Agency) and ARC. 2004. *Helping children cope with disaster.* http://www.redcross.org/images/MEDIA_CustomProductCatalog/m14740413_Helping_children_cope_with_disaster_-_English.pdf (accessed December 3, 2014).

FEMA. 2013. *Federal Emergency Management Agency Crisis Counseling Assistance and Training Program guidance.* http://www.dhhr.wv.gov/healthprep/programs/behavioralhealth/Documents/FEMA%20CCP%20Toolkit.pdf (accessed April 2, 2015).

FEMA. 2015. *Crisis Counseling Assistance & Training Program.* https://www.fema.gov/recovery-directorate/crisis-counseling-assistance-training-program (accessed April 2, 2015).

Flannelly, K. J., S. Roberts, and A. J. Weaver. 2005. Correlates of compassion fatigue and burnout in chaplains and other clergy who responded to the September 11th attacks in New York City. *Journal of Pastoral Care and Counseling* 59(3):213.

Flynn, B. W., and A. H. Speier. 2014. Disaster behavioral health: Legal and ethical considerations in a rapidly changing field. *Current Psychiatry Reports* 16(8):457.

Freedy, J. J., and W. M. Simpson. 2007. Disaster-related physical and mental health: A role for the family physician. *American Family Physician* 75(6):841-846.

Freeman Health System. 2012. *Ozark Center awarded grant by Missouri Foundation for Health.* http://www.freemanhealth.com/news/?sid=1&nid=176 (accessed November 3, 2014).

GAO (U.S. Government Accountability Office). 2008. *Catastrophic disasters: Federal efforts help states prepare for and respond to psychological consequences, but FEMA's crisis counseling program needs improvements.* GAO-08-22. Washington, DC: GAO.

GAO. 2015. *Mental health: HHS leadership needed to coordinate federal efforts related to serious mental illness.* GAO-15-375T. Washington, DC: GAO.

Gluckman, P. 2011. The psychosocial consequences of the Canterbury earthquake: A briefing paper. *Office of the Prime Minister's Science Advisory Committee.* http://cera.govt.nz/sites/default/files/common/christchurch-earthquake-briefing-psychosocial-effects-2011-05-10.pdf (accessed April 3, 2015).

Goodell, S. 2014. Health policy brief: Mental health parity. *Health Affairs.* http://www.healthaffairs.org/healthpolicybriefs/brief.php?brief_id=112 (accessed November 3, 2014).

Harvard School of Public Health. 2013. *Essential functions and considerations for hospital recovery.* Boston, MA: Harvard.

Healthy Christchurch. 2014a. *All Right? campaign update for February 2014.* http://www.healthychristchurch.org.nz/news/healthy-christchurch-notices/2014/2/all-right-campaign-update-for-february-2014 (accessed September 22, 2014).

Healthy Christchurch. 2014b. *All right? wellbeing campaign.* http://healthychristchurch.org.nz/priority-areas/wellbeing-and-community-resilience/all-right-wellbeing-campaign (accessed September 22, 2014).

Herrmann, J. 2014. *Perspectives on behavioral health recovery challenges from the field.* Paper presented at IOM Committee on Post-Disaster Recovery of a Community's Public Health, Medical, and Social Services: Meeting Five, August 14, Washington, DC.

HHS (U.S. Department of Health and Human Services). 1999. *Mental health: A report of the Surgeon General.* Rockville, MD: HHS.

HHS. 2013. *At-risk individuals.* http://www.phe.gov/Preparedness/planning/abc/Documents/at-risk-individuals.pdf (accessed April 2, 2015).

HHS. 2014. *HHS disaster behavioral health concept of operations.* http://www.phe.gov/Preparedness/planning/abc/Documents/dbh-conops-2014.pdf (accessed October 21, 2014).

Hobfoll, S. E., P. Watson, C. C. Bell, R. A. Bryant, M. J. Brymer, M. J. Friedman, M. Friedman, B. P. R. Gersons, J. T. V. M. de Jong, C. M. Layne, S. Maguen, Y. Neria, A. E. Norwood, R. S. Pynoos, D. Reissman, J. I. Ruzek, A. Y. Shalev, Z. Solomon, A. M. Steinberg, and R. J. Ursano. 2007. Five essential elements of immediate and mid-term mass trauma intervention: Empirical evidence. *Psychiatry: Interpersonal and Biological Processes* 70(4):283-315.

Hyde, P. S. 2014. *SAMHSA perspectives on behavioral health recovery challenges.* Paper presented at IOM Committee on Post-Disaster Recovery of a Community's Public Health, Medical, and Social Services: Meeting Five, August 14, Washington, DC.

Jaycox, L. H., J. A. Cohen, A. P. Mannarino, D. W. Walker, A. K. Langley, K. L. Gegenheimer, M. Scott, and M. Schonlau. 2010. Children's mental health care following Hurricane Katrina: A field trial of trauma-focused psychotherapies. *Journal of Traumatic Stress* 23(2):223-231.

Jaycox, L. H., S. H. Kataoka, B. D. Stein, A. K. Langley, and M. Wong. 2012. Cognitive behavioral intervention for trauma in schools. *Journal of Applied School Psychology* 28(3):239-255.

Johns Hopkins Bloomberg School of Public Health. 2014. *Psychological first aid (PFA).* http://www.jhsph.edu/research/centers-and-institutes/johns-hopkins-center-for-public-health-preparedness/training/PFA.html (accessed October 22, 2014).

Kessler, R. C., S. Galea, M. J. Gruber, N. A. Sampson, R. J. Ursano, and S. Wessely. 2008. Trends in mental illness and suicidality after Hurricane Katrina. *Molecular Psychiatry* 13(4):374-384.

Kinzie, J. D., J. K. Boehnlein, C. Riley, and L. Sparr. 2002. The effects of September 11 on traumatized refugees: Reactivation of posttraumatic stress disorder. *Journal of Nervous and Mental Disease* 190(7):437-441.

Layard, R., and A. Hagell. 2014. *Healthy young minds: Transforming the mental health of children.* Doha, Qatar: WISH.

Madrid, P. A., H. Sinclair, A. Q. Bankston, S. Overholt, A. Brito, R. Domnitz, and R. Grant. 2008. Building integrated mental health and medical programs for vulnerable populations post-disaster: Connecting children and families to a medical home. *Prehospital and Disaster Medicine* 23(4):314-321.

Massey, K. 2006. *Light our way: A guide for spiritual care in times of disaster.* Alexandria, VA: National Voluntary Organizations Active in Disaster.

Mendenhall, T. J. 2006. Trauma-response teams: Inherent challenges and practical strategies in interdisciplinary fieldwork. *Families, Systems, & Health* 24(3):357.

Meyers, D., C. E. Allen, III, D. Dunn, A. Wennerstrom, and B. F. Springgate. 2011. Community perspectives on post-Katrina mental health recovery in New Orleans. *Ethnicity & Disease* 21:S1–52.

Mitani, S., M. Fujita, K. Nakata, and T. Shirakawa. 2006. Impact of post-traumatic stress disorder and job-related stress on burnout: A study of fire service workers. *Journal of Emergency Medicine* 31(1):7-11.

MRC (Medical Reserve Corps). 2015. *About the Medical Reserve Corps.* https://www.medicalreservecorps.gov/pageViewFldr/About (accessed April 2, 2015).

National VOAD (Voluntary Organizations Active in Disaster). 2014. *National VOAD disaster spiritual care guidelines.* Alexandria, VA: National VOAD.

NBSB (National Biodefense Science Board). 2010. *Integration of mental and behavioral health in federal disaster preparedness, response, and recovery: Assessment and recommendations.* A report of the Disaster Mental Health Subcommittee of the National Biodefense Science Board. http://www.phe.gov/Preparedness/legal/boards/nprsb/meetings/Documents/dmhreport1010.pdf (accessed April 2, 2015).

NBSB. 2014. *National Biodefense Science Board community health resilience report.* Washington, DC: NBSB.

NCQA (National Committee for Quality Assurance). 2014. *The future of Patient-Centered Medical Homes: Foundation for a better health care system.* http://www.ncqa.org/Portals/0/Public%20Policy/2014%20Comment%20Letters/The_Future_of_PCMH.pdf (accessed April 2, 2015).

NCTSN (National Child Traumatic Stress Network). 2014a. *After the hurricane: Helping young children heal.* http://nctsn.org/sites/all/modules/pubdlcnt/pubdlcnt.php?file=/sites/default/files/assets/pdfs/Helping_Young_Children_Heal.pdf&nid=245 (accessed October 22, 2014).

NCTSN. 2014b. *Parent guidelines for helping children after a hurricane*. http://nctsn.org/sites/default/files/assets/pdfs/parents_guidelines_talk_children_hurricanes.pdf (accessed October 22, 2014).

NIEHS (National Institute of Environmental Health Sciences). 2015. *Resiliency: Worker Training Program*. https://tools.niehs.nih.gov/wetp/index.cfm?id=2528 (accessed April 3, 2015).

NIH (National Institutes of Health). 2014. *Featured topics: Mental health*. http://recovery.nih.gov/Stories/Featured_Topics.aspx?strSection=Topic&strName=Mental%20Health (accessed October 21, 2014).

Norris, F. H., and N. D. Bellamy. 2009. Evaluation of a national effort to reach Hurricane Katrina survivors and evacuees: The crisis counseling assistance and training program. *Administration and Policy in Mental Health* 36(3):165-175.

Norris, F. H., M. J. Friedman, and P. J. Watson. 2002. 60,000 disaster victims speak: Part II. Summary and implications of the disaster mental health research. *Psychiatry* 65(3):240-260.

Norris, F. H., J. L. Hamblen, and C. S. Rosen. 2009. Service characteristics and counseling outcomes: Lessons from a cross-site evalution of crisis counseling after Hurricanes Katrina, Rita and Wilma. *Administration and Policy in Mental Health and Mental Health Services Research* 36(3):176-185.

Norris, F. H., S. P. Stevens, B. Pfefferbaum, K. F. Wyche, and R. L. Pfefferbaum. 2008. Community resilience as a metaphor, theory, set of capacities, and strategy for disaster readiness. *American Journal of Community Psychology* 41(1-2):127-150.

North, C. S. 2010. A tale of two studies of two disasters: Comparing psychosocial responses to disaster among Oklahoma City bombing survivors and Hurricane Katrina evacuees. *Rehabilitation Psychology* 55(3):241-246.

North, C. S., and B. Pfefferbaum. 2013. Mental health response to community disasters: A systematic review. *Journal of the American Medical Association* 310(5):507-518.

North, C. S., S. J. Nixon, S. Shariat, S. Mallonee, J. C. McMillen, E. L. Spitznagel, and E. M. Smith. 1999. Psychiatric disorders among survivors of the Oklahoma City bombing. *Journal of the American Medical Association* 282(8):755-762.

North, C. S., L. Tivis, J. C. McMillen, B. Pfefferbaum, E. L. Spitznagel, J. Cox, S. Nixon, K. P. Bunch, and E. M. Smith. 2002. Psychiatric disorders in rescue workers after the Oklahoma City bombing. *American Journal of Psychiatry* 159(5):857-859.

North, C. S., B. Pfefferbaum, P. Narayanan, S. Thielman, G. McCoy, C. Dumont, A. Kawasaki, N. Ryosho, Y. S. Kim, and E. L. Spitznagel. 2005. Comparison of post-disaster psychiatric disorders after terrorist bombings in Nairobi and Oklahoma City. *British Journal of Psychiatry* 186:487-493.

Nucifora, F., A. M. Langlieb, E. Siegal, G. S. Everly, Jr., and M. Kaminsky. 2007. Building resistance, resilience, and recovery in the wake of school and workplace violence. *Disaster Medicine and Public Health Preparedness* 1:S33-S37.

Osofsky, J. D. 2014. *Helping young children and families cope with trauma*. http://www.nctsnet.org/sites/default/files/assets/pdfs/helping_young_children_and_families_cope_with_trauma.pdf (accessed October 22, 2014).

Osofsky, H. J., J. D. Osofsky, J. H. Wells, and C. Weems. 2014. Integrated care: Meeting mental health needs after the Gulf oil spill. *Psychiatric Services* 65(3):280-283.

Paget, N. 2014. *Perspectives on behavioral health recovery challenges from the field*. Paper presented at IOM Committee on Post-Disaster Recovery of a Community's Public Health, Medical, and Social Services: Meeting Five, August 14, Washington, DC.

Pfefferbaum, B. 2014. *Child Disaster Mental Health Services and Interventions*. Paper presented at IOM Committee on Post-Disaster Recovery of a Community's Public Health, Medical, and Social Services: Meeting Two, February 3, Washington, DC.

Pfefferbaum, B., D. E. Doughty, C. Reddy, N. Patel, R. H. Gurwitch, S. J. Nixon, and R. D. Tivis. 2002. Exposure and peritraumatic response as predictors of posttraumatic stress in children following the 1995 Oklahoma City bombing. *Journal of Urban Health* 79(3):354-363.

Pfefferbaum, B., J. Stuber, S. Galea, and G. Fairbrother. 2006. Panic reactions to terrorist attacks and probable posttraumatic stress disorder in adolescents. *Journal of Traumatic Stress* 19(2):217-228.

Pfefferbaum, B., B. W. Flynn, D. Schonfeld, L. M. Brown, G. A. Jacobs, D. Dodgen, D. Donato, R. E. Kaul, B. Stone, A. E. Norwood, D. B. Reissman, J. Herrmann, S. E. Hobfoll, R. T. Jones, J. I. Ruzek, R. J. Ursano, R. J. Taylor, and D. Lindley. 2012. The integration of mental and behavioral health into disaster preparedness, response, and recovery. *Disaster Medicine and Public Health Preparedness* 6(1):60-66.

Pfefferbaum, B., M. A. Noffsinger, L. H. Wind, and J. R. Allen. 2014. Children's coping in the context of disasters and terrorism. *Journal of Loss and Trauma* 9(1):78-97.

Phua, K. L. 2008. Post-disaster victimization: How survivors of disasters can continue to suffer after the event is over. *New Solutions* 18(2):221-231.

Pines, A., and E. Aronson. 1988. *Career burnout: Causes and cures*. New York: Free Press.

Pynoos, R. S., A. K. Goenjian, and A. M. Steinberg. 1998. A public mental health approach to the postdisaster treatment of children and adolescents. *Child and Adolescent Psychiatric Clinics of North America* 7(1):195-210, x.

Pynoos, R. S., A. M. Steinberg, and M. J. Brymer. 2007. Children and disasters: Public mental health approaches. In *Textbook of disaster psychiatry*, edited by R. J. Ursano, C. S. Fullerton, L. Weisaeth, and B. Raphael. Cambridge, MA: Cambridge University Press. Pp. 48-68.

Red River Resilience. 2010. *Know the facts of resilience*. http://www.redriverresilience.com/index.html (accessed October 22, 2014).

Rinard Hinga, B. D. 2015. *Ring of fire: An encyclopedia of the Pacific Rim's earthquakes, tsunamis, and volcanoes*. Santa Barbara, CA: ABC-CLIO.

Rose, S., J. Bisson, R. Churchill, and S. Wessely. 2002. Psychological debriefing for preventing post traumatic stress disorder (PTSD). *Cochrane Database of Systematic Reviews* (2):Cd000560.

Rosser, B. R. S. 2008. Working as a psychologist in the Medical Reserve Corps: Providing emergency mental health relief services in Hurricanes Katrina and Rita. *Professional Psychology: Research and Practice* 39(1):37-44.

Ruzek, J. I., M. J. Brymer, A. K. Jacobs, C. M. Layne, E. M. Vernberg, and P. J. Watson. 2007. Psychological first aid. *Journal of Mental Health Counseling* 29(1):17-49.

SAMHSA (Substance Abuse and Mental Health Services Administration). 2003. *Mental health all-hazards disaster planning guidance*. Rockville, MD: SAMHSA.

SAMHSA. 2013a. *Disaster planning handbook for behavioral health treatment programs*. http://store.samhsa.gov/shin/content//SMA13-4779/SMA13-4779.pdf (accessed October 22, 2014).

SAMHSA. 2013b. *Results from the 2012 national survey on drug use and health: Mental health findings*. Vol. NSDUH Series H-47, HHS Publication No. (SMA) 13-4805. Rockville, MD: SAMHSA.

SAMHSA. 2014a. *Crisis Counseling Assistance and Training Program (CCP)*. http://www.samhsa.gov/dtac/ccp (accessed October 22, 2014).

SAMHSA. 2014b. *Disaster Technical Assistance Center (DTAC)*. http://www.samhsa.gov/dtac (accessed October 22, 2014).

SAMHSA. 2015. *Substance abuse and mental health block grants*. http://www.samhsa.gov/grants/block-grants (accessed April 3, 2015).

Schreiber, M. D., R. Yin, M. Omaish, and J. E. Broderick. 2014. Snapshot from Superstorm Sandy: American Red Cross mental health risk surveillance in lower New York State. *Annals of Emergency Medicine* 64(1):59-65.

Secretary's Advisory Committee on National Health Promotion and Disease Prevention Objectives for 2020. 2010. *Healthy people 2020: An opportunity to address societal determinants of health in the U.S.* Washington, DC: HHS.

Singleton, C. 2014. *PHEP grantees' use of funds to improve health in communities post-disaster*. Paper presented at IOM Post-Disaster Recovery of a Community's Public Health, Medical, and Social Services: Meeting Six, October 2, Washington, DC.

The Sphere Project. 2015. *The Sphere Project in brief*. http://www.sphereproject.org/about/ (accessed April 3, 2015).

Springgate, B. F., A. Wennerstrom, D. Meyers, C. E. Allen, III, S. D. Vannoy, W. Bentham, and K. B. Wells. 2011. Building community resilience through mental health infrastructure and training in post-Katrina New Orleans. *Ethnicity & Disease* 21(3, Suppl. 1):S1-20-29.

Thienkrua, W., B. L. Cardozo, M. L. Chakkraband, T. E. Guadamuz, W. Pengjuntr, P. Tantipiwatanaskul, S. Sakornsatian, S. Ekassawin, B. Panyayong, A. Varangrat, J. W. Tappero, M. Schreiber, and F. van Griensven. 2006. Symptoms of posttraumatic stress disorder and depression among children in tsunami-affected areas in Southern Thailand. *Journal of American Medical Association* 296(5):549-559.

University of Rochester, the New York State Office of Mental Health, and the New York State Department of Health. 2005. *New York State County Disaster Mental Health Planning and Response Guide*. New York State Office of Mental Health. Rochester, NY: University of Rochester.

Vasterman, P., C. J. Yzermans, and A. J. Dirkzwager. 2005. The role of the media and media hypes in the aftermath of disasters. *Epidemiologic Reviews* 27(1):107-114.

Vlahov, D., S. Galea, H. Resnick, J. Ahern, J. A. Boscarino, M. Bucuvalas, J. Gold, and D. Kilpatrick. 2002. Increased use of cigarettes, alcohol, and marijuana among Manhattan, New York, residents after the September 11th terrorist attacks. *American Journal of Epidemiology* 155(11):988-996.

Walker, D. 2014. *Immediate, intermediate and long-term mental health response interventions for communities impacted by disaster.* Paper presented at IOM Committee on Post-Disaster Recovery of a Community's Public Health, Medical, and Social Services: Meeting Two, February 3, Washington, DC.

Wang, P. S., M. J. Gruber, R. E. Powers, M. Schoenbaum, A. H. Speier, K. B. Wells, and R. C. Kessler. 2008. Disruption of existing mental health treatments and failure to initiate new treatments after Hurricane Katrina. *The American Journal of Psychiatry* 165(1):34-41.

Watson, P. J., M. J. Brymer, and G. A. Bonanno. 2011. Postdisaster psychological intervention since 9/11. *American Psychologist* 66(6):482-494.

Weisler, R. H., J. G. T. Barbee, and M. H. Townsend. 2006. Mental health and recovery in the Gulf Coast after Hurricanes Katrina and Rita. *Journal of the American Medical Association* 296(5):585-588.

White, J. 2014. *Post-disaster social services and health outcomes in recovery.* Paper presented at IOM Committee on Post-Disaster Recovery of a Community's Public Health, Medical, and Social Services: Meeting Two, February 3, Washington, DC.

WHO (World Health Organization). 2011. *Psychological first aid: Guide for field workers.* http://www.who.int/mental_health/publications/guide_field_workers/en/ (accessed April 3, 2015).

WHO. 2013. *Building back better: Sustainable mental health care after emergencies.* Geneva, Switzerland: WHO.

Wisnivesky, J. P., S. L. Teitelbaum, A. C. Todd, P. Boffetta, M. Crane, L. Crowley, R. E. de la Hoz, C Dellenbaugh, D. Harrison, R. Herbert, H. Kim, Y. Jeon, J. Kaplan, C. Katz, S. Levin, B. Luft, S. Markowitz, J. M. Moline, F. Ozbay, R. H. Pietrzak, M. Shapiro, V. Sharma, G. Skloot, S. Southwick, L. A. Stevenson, I. Udasin, S. Wallenstein, and P. J. Landrigan. 2011. Persistence of multiple illnesses in World Trade Center rescue and recovery workers: A cohort study. *Lancet* 378(9794):888-897.

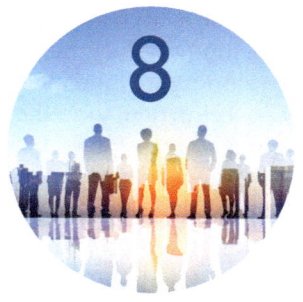

8

Social Services

Disasters are profoundly discriminatory.

—MacDonald, 2005

As a result of preexisting conditions in communities, disasters have disproportionate effects on certain subpopulations, particularly those of low socioeconomic status and other marginalized groups. Loss of meager resources, exacerbation of preexisting health conditions, and higher rates of prior trauma can lead to poor health outcomes in impoverished groups, including increased incidence of substance abuse (Cepeda et al., 2010a) and mental distress (Cepeda et al., 2010b). Social services[1] professionals act as advocates and service providers to underserved populations, enabling people to access critical goods and services and to become healthier and more self-sufficient. By ensuring access to needed resources, social services can help mitigate impacts of disasters on vulnerable populations.

Unfortunately, the social services sector has until only recently been largely excluded from preparedness and emergency management efforts (White, 2014). Events such as Hurricane Katrina that had devastating effects on vulnerable populations have demonstrated the importance of integrating social services into all other recovery activities, including but not limited to clinical care delivery, housing, economic and workforce development, and transportation. A RAND Corporation study on human services recovery 4 years after Hurricane Katrina found that nongovernmental organizations (NGOs) in Louisiana suffered from a lack of state and federal focus on human recovery and received little support for long-term case management. NGOs also reported that they were not integrated as partners in recovery planning and received little guidance on the implementation of human recovery plans (Chandra and Acosta, 2009). Yet successful human recovery depends on vertical integration and cross-sector coordination, collaboration, and communication—facilitated by technology and ongoing interagency relationships.

This chapter examines the impacts of disasters on the social services sector, the role the sector plays in advancing health in the community and reducing disparities, and the actions that various actors within the sector can take before and after disasters to ensure that the human needs of all community members,

---

[1] The terms "social services" and "human services" are used interchangeably in this chapter since both terms can be found throughout different reports, guidance materials, and other documents examined by the committee.

but especially the most vulnerable, are met. These activities, if undertaken, have the potential to yield significant positive impacts on recovery of community members and to make significant contributions to the creation of healthy communities. In developing its guidance, the committee identified the following key recovery strategies for the social services sector that should cut across all phases of the disaster cycle and that represent recurring themes throughout this chapter:

- Build on existing relationships and establish comprehensive plans for collaboration among social service funders and providers, community- and faith-based organizations, and advocates to ensure coordinated social service delivery through all phases of disaster planning and recovery.
- Integrate social services recovery plans into other disaster recovery services.
- Create compatible structures, policies, and procedures to promote the flow of funding and information across federal, state, and local systems.
- Provide support to reunite families and promote resilience through community programming designed to strengthen social support networks.
- Focus on restoring normalcy through key community services/activities, such as child care, elder care, foster care, mental health services, schools, housing, jobs, and transportation.
- Enhance efforts to increase accessibility and reach the most vulnerable populations to provide needed social services.
- Promote ongoing evaluation and continuous learning to advance social services efforts in achieving health community goals.

The chapter concludes with a checklist of key activities that the social services sector needs to perform during each of the phases of recovery.

SOCIAL SERVICES IN THE CONTEXT OF A HEALTHY COMMUNITY

As discussed in Chapter 2, social factors are an important determinant of health. The social services sector has close contact with members of the community who have been most disadvantaged by these factors; therefore, social services are one of the main tools for addressing the social determinants of health (e.g., access to healthy food, safe and supportive environments for children) and ensuring health equity (White, 2014). The social services system directly assists individuals and families that have insufficient resources to meet their needs—often as a result of systemic inequalities—and advocates for structural and policy changes aimed at alleviating the underlying causes of such inequalities. There is clear evidence of disproportionate health risks associated with low socioeconomic status. Lower income is associated with shorter life expectancy, worse self-reported health status, and greater occurrence of chronic diseases such as diabetes and heart disease (RWJF, 2008). Social service supports are vital in mitigating these effects, and higher rates of spending on social services are linked to better health outcomes (Bradley and Taylor, 2013). The portfolio of social services programs in the United States is diverse and covers the entire life course, from pregnancy to aging services. These services impact health outcomes through a number of mechanisms, such as nutrition, health care access, and injury prevention (see Table 8-1).

In a healthy community, the social services sector provides accessible, equitable, and high-quality services that support the social and economic well-being of all people, particularly the most vulnerable, enabling self-sufficiency and thereby preserving the dignity and respect of individuals and the community. Service delivery is not reactive and crisis-driven; rather, it mirrors the proactive and prevention-based approach now taking hold in the health care sector. Consumer-centric systems built on a "no wrong door" policy offer a full range of services and supports and an assessment process that evaluates client needs comprehensively. Thus, in a healthy community, social services are integrated—strategically and operationally—within the sector but also with public health, clinical care, behavioral health, housing, and community development services so that resources are used as efficiently as possible to address the social factors that drive health outcomes.

TABLE 8-1 Mechanisms by Which Social Services Programs Influence Health Outcomes

Social Services Program Type	Injury Risk	Health Services Access	Stress-Related	Economic Determinants	Behavioral Health	Environmental	Developmental
Economic Security (Cash Benefit)		X	◆	◆	X	◆	
Child Support		◆	X	◆	X		
Early Childhood	◆	X	◆		◆	◆	◆
Family Violence	◆	X	◆	X	◆	X	
Child Welfare	◆	◆	◆		◆	◆	◆
Nutrition			◆	◆			◆
Energy	X		◆	◆		◆	
Aging Services	◆	◆	◆	X	◆	◆	
Vulnerable Population Services	◆	◆	◆	◆	◆	◆	◆

NOTE: "X"s denote committee additions to the original figure.
SOURCE: Adapted from White, 2014.

Agenda setting for and implementation of social services are optimally effective if private, nonprofit, philanthropic, faith-based, and neighborhood stakeholders are integrated into the process. Unfortunately, few communities in the United States benefit from an integrated and sustainable social support system. In most communities, social services capacity is strained by a number of complex challenges, including fragmentation, which impedes access; lack of coordination of funding streams and service providers (Smith, 2008); fluctuating levels of funding; chronic workforce shortages; and, relatedly, overburdened case workers (AECF, 2003). In addition, silos have resulted from the proliferation of social service programs designed to meet the specialized needs of specific vulnerable populations and from multiple separate funding streams. Considerable inefficiency results as isolated programs end up servicing the same clients in the absence of systems for collaboration, information sharing, and coordination of funding (Smith, 2008).

In recent years, economic recession has resulted simultaneously in increased demand for services and major budget cuts, posing significant challenges to local government agencies that fund and provide community services, including social services. These and a number of other forces (aging populations and an increasing understanding of the link between economic vitality and social conditions such as poverty and homelessness) are driving interest in new approaches and models for social service delivery. Some social service agencies are following the lead of the business community and offering clients complete solutions rather than discrete services (Smith, 2008). Despite the improved efficiency of integrated systems, however, lack of political will and fiscal resources may impede a major overhaul. To restate a central theme of this report, although disasters pose significant challenges to communities by further straining already fragile systems, they also provide an opportunity to create healthy communities—in the present context, to achieve more integrated and sustainable models of social service delivery—by building on disaster-related collaborations and creative uses of relief and recovery funds.

DISASTER-RELATED SOCIAL SERVICES CHALLENGES

Disasters generate increased demands on all social services because of impacts on vulnerable populations, the creation of newly vulnerable populations, interrupted service delivery, and displacement of both providers and clients. Social service providers are called upon to mitigate the human impacts of disasters and fill the gaps in resources and capabilities. The same health determinants shown in Table 8-1 are relevant to the post-disaster context. For example, when schools and daycare centers are closed, children who have no safe place to play can be at increased risk of injury, and parents can experience added stress when there is no safe place to leave their child(ren) so they can return to work and begin restoring some normalcy to their lives (White, 2014). Post-disaster communities also experience increases in mental health and substance abuse issues (see Chapter 7), domestic violence, and child maltreatment (NJ DCF, 2013).

Disaster-related disruption of social services can impact health outcomes both directly and indirectly, and inadequate attention to the social service needs within a community will result in a greater post-disaster burden of poor health in the community. Depending on a disaster's nature and scope, it may both cause a surge in social service needs within the community (and perhaps in the surrounding areas), due to trauma and resource-related vulnerabilities, and diminish the sector's capacity to respond to those needs through loss of personnel and/or infrastructure. Service provision is further complicated in many disasters by damage to community infrastructure, including facilities of employers; schools; businesses essential to the fabric of the community, such as grocery stores and child care; and transit vehicles and routes. These losses have negative effects on food and job security for some disaster victims and tend to have disproportionate impacts on a community's already-vulnerable populations.

The roles of social service professionals immediately after a disaster are largely an extension of their pre-disaster functions (although case loads are significantly increased). After a disaster, two priorities emerge: ensuring continuity of services in the face of disaster-related disruptions and addressing disaster-related unmet needs (HHS, 2014a). Specific roles include but are not limited to

- reestablishing access to food, shelter, and clothing;
- facilitating access to needed medical providers, medications, equipment, and auxiliary services (in concert with clinical care organizations);
- reuniting displaced family members;
- facilitating access to federal disaster benefits (following presidentially declared disasters) by collecting and/or re-creating needed documentation;
- managing stress and behavioral health issues exacerbated by a disaster (in concert with NGOs and faith-based organizations); and
- coordinating with Social Security, Medicaid, and other entitlement programs regarding survivors' benefits.

It should be noted that many of these roles may begin during the response phase but continue into recovery, in some cases for years after the disaster. As the recovery progresses past the immediate crisis, opportunities exist for social services to evolve to incorporate holistic strategies targeted at achieving a healthy community.

Many barriers to access (e.g., physical impairment, location, hours of operation, language) need to be considered in planning for social services during the recovery period. For example, special attention is needed to ensure that messaging is culturally sensitive. Reaching the social service sector's diverse constituencies can be particularly difficult, and multiple avenues of communication are required. Low literacy, low English fluency, lack of computer access, and confusion related to stress must be taken into account. Existing pre-disaster communication mechanisms, such as those established by immigrant-serving organizations, are important tools for reaching non-English-speaking populations. Using respected spokespeople to target subpopulations can increase receptivity to important messages. As recovery progresses, the community needs easily accessible information regarding resources for rebuilding; a clearinghouse website such as the New Orleans area's GNOinfo.com provides a wide array of information in a centralized location to encourage self-help and resiliency.

Underpinning all of these considerations is the need to develop metrics for success and sustainable methods for measuring the effectiveness of chosen processes and interventions. Realistically, chronically limited resources and the difficulty of measuring outcomes make this task difficult. Recovery organizations focused on fundraising, volunteer management, and other aspects of recovery but with limited staff expertise for assessments may use other organizations to assist with this task. For example, Habitat for Humanity, among other housing organizations, may have the capacity to conduct a housing needs assessment. Such collaboration depends on the relationships among organizations and illustrates the importance of establishing such relationships prior to a disaster and sharing information.

Also important is for those involved in recovery processes to assist with identifying sources of capital and financing for rebuilding in ways that support a healthy community, incorporate lessons learned, and continuously measure progress toward healthy community goals. Whenever possible, communities that have faced disasters can disseminate information valuable in improving social services and share lessons learned so that other jurisdictions can benefit from their recovery experiences.

SOCIAL SERVICES SECTOR ORGANIZATION AND RESOURCES

Key stakeholders in the social services sector include agencies within the local, state, and federal levels of government, as well as nonprofit organizations, faith-based groups, and other private providers. A description of roles and responsibilities at each level and challenges related to integration of the social services provided follows in the sections below.

Federal Level[2]

Federal roles related to social services include funding, regulation, technical assistance, and coordination. Federal grant programs, primarily block grants, provide much of the day-to-day funding for state and local social service programs and can be leveraged after a disaster to support recovery efforts;[3] in the current fiscally constrained environment, however, this funding has been diminishing. Block grants often go to the states, and those funds are then allocated to support governmental and/or nongovernmental programs. Funding for Head Start programs is different in that it goes directly from the federal level to the service provider (ACF, 2015c). Although a number of federal agencies support community social services programs, the three major contributors are (1) the Administration for Children and Families (ACF) and (2) the Administration on Community Living[4] (both within the U.S. Department of Health and Human Services [HHS]), and (3) the Food and Nutrition Service within the U.S. Department of Agriculture, which funds the Special Supplemental Nutrition Program for Women, Infants, and Children (commonly known as WIC) and the Supplemental Nutrition Assistance Program (SNAP). One of the few federally funded

---

[2] A broader synopsis of legislation and federal policy related to disaster recovery and health security can be found in Appendix A.
[3] Federal block grants to support social services include the following:
- Community Development Block Grants (CDBGs), administered by the U.S. Department of Housing and Urban Development, are used to benefit low- or moderate-income people by ensuring affordable housing, providing services, and creating jobs (HUD, 2014).
- Social Services Block Grants (SSBGs), administered by the Administration for Children and Families, provide funds for services such as daycare, case management, and protective services for adults and children (ACF, 2015b).
- Community Services Block Grants (CSBGs), administered by the Administration for Children and Families, are intended to improve self-sufficiency and living conditions among low-income people by addressing such issues as employment, education, housing, nutrition, and health (ACF, 2015a).
- The Child Care and Development Fund (CCDF), administered by the Administration for Children and Families, provides working families with child care subsidies and improves the quality of child care (ACF, 2012).
- Community Mental Health Services Block Grants, administered by the Substance Abuse and Mental Health Services Administration, fund programs and centers that serve adults with serious mental illnesses and children with serious emotional disturbances (SAMHSA, 2015).
- The Family Violence Prevention and Services Act Program, administered by the Administration for Children and Families, provides funds for "emergency shelter and related assistance for victims of domestic violence and their children" (FYSB, 2015).
- Substance Abuse Prevention and Treatment Block Grants, administered by the Substance Abuse and Mental Health Services Administration, provide funds for substance abuse prevention and substance abuse disorder treatment and recovery for specific target populations (SAMHSA, 2015).
[4] The Administration for Community Living works to "maximize the independence, well-being, and health of older adults, people with disabilities, and their families and caregivers" (HHS, 2014a, p. 13).

disaster-specific human services programs is the Disaster Supplemental Nutrition Assistance Program, D-SNAP (White, 2014).

In the aftermath of a disaster, block grant funds can be made available for disaster recovery through either the congressional appropriation of additional disaster-specific funds or the reprogramming of current funds. Congress has appropriated billions of additional dollars for recovery through the Community Development Block Grant for Disaster Recovery (CDBG-DR) vehicle, which has broad latitude in terms of eligible expenses (HUD, 2014). Communities also have been permitted to reprogram their annual CDBG funds for disaster relief activities, and the U.S. Department of Housing and Urban Development (HUD) is statutorily authorized to suspend almost all program requirements in disaster areas (CRS, 2014). Congress has also appropriated supplemental funds to the Social Services Block Grant (SSBG) program three times in the past to help with recovery from natural disasters (CRS, 2012). SSBG funds appropriated specifically for disaster recovery (SSBG-DR) have fewer limitations than funds appropriated under the general SSBG program. Activities specifically permitted under SSBG-DR include food cards, child care vouchers, temporary housing, and repair or rebuilding of damaged facilities (including mental health facilities, child care centers, and other social service facilities) (ACF, 2013a). Following Hurricane Sandy, additional funding was provided for Head Start programs to cover costs of services (including behavioral health services for affected children) and renovation/repair of damaged facilities (ACF, 2013b).

In addition to funding, agencies provide technical assistance to help communities use their block grant funds for disaster recovery. For example, ACF released guidance on how funds from the Child Care Development Fund (CCDF) can be used flexibly after a disaster (e.g., paying for child care for displaced families or making minor repairs to child care facilities) (ACF, 2005).

Under the National Disaster Recovery Framework (NDRF, described in more detail in Chapter 3), social services fall under the Health and Social Services Recovery Support Function, which is coordinated by the Assistant Secretary for Preparedness and Response (ASPR) on behalf of the Secretary of HHS (FEMA, 2011). The Health and Social Services Recovery Support Function encompasses three key social services activities: (1) social services impacts, (2) disaster case management[5] and referral to social services, and (3) children's needs in disaster recovery. In 2014, ASPR released the *Disaster Human Services Concept of Operations (CONOPS)*, which provides the framework for coordination and guidance of HHS's federal-level social services activities before, during, and after a disaster (HHS, 2014a). It describes several coordinating structures for HHS operations related to social services during the preparedness, response, and recovery phases. The committee finds these efforts to create a "one HHS" enterprise with integration of social services into departmental responsibilities related to public health and medical care, behavioral health, environmental health, and responder health and safety to be commendable. However, the CONOPS does not address needs for interdepartmental coordination of federal social services support. Importantly, under the National Response Framework (NRF), human services,[6] temporary housing, and mass care fall under Emergency Support Function #6, which is led by the Federal Emergency Management Agency (FEMA) (FEMA, 2013). Thus, significant coordination between HHS and FEMA[7] is required to ensure a smooth transition in human services operations from response to recovery, and the development of a broader framework for coordination of social services activities is critical.

One additional gap the committee identified at the federal level is a lack of comprehensive federal

---

[5] Disaster case management is described in more detail later in this chapter.

[6] "Human services, for purposes of ESF #6, is defined as disaster assistance programs that help survivors address unmet disaster-caused needs and/or non-housing losses through loans and grants; also includes supplemental nutrition assistance, crisis counseling, disaster case management, disaster unemployment, disaster legal services, and other state and federal human services programs and benefits to survivors" (HHS, 2014a, p. 9).

[7] Disaster case management is another area requiring significant coordination between HHS and FEMA. Following a presidentially declared disaster with authorization for individual assistance under the Stafford Act, FEMA may also play a major role in directly supporting social services by funding disaster case management (DCM) services. One option for DCM, the Immediate Disaster Case Management program, is administered by the Administration for Children and Families in HHS. A Concept of Operations for the Federal Immediate Disaster Case Management program was released by HHS in 2012 and is available at https://www.acf.hhs.gov/sites/default/files/ohsepr/immediate_dcm_concept_of_operations_conops_october_2012_508_compliant.pdf (accessed April 3, 2015).

guidance for state and local social service organizations. Although there is some topic-specific guidance, such as ACF's guidance on developing task forces, general guidance (such as best practices) for these organizations is lacking.

State and Local Levels

All states have departments for social (or human) services, although multiple departments often share responsibility for these services. At the local level, many large cities, counties, and tribes have social service departments that cater to needs specific to their communities. Other communities have no social service department or are served by a higher level of government, and some social service departments offer only a limited range of services. Overall, these agencies provide regulation and enforcement, direct services, training, public awareness campaigns, and long-term planning for community social service needs.

State human service organizations provide oversight for local operations and are a prime funding source. Depending on the state, they impose various levels of regulation on local entities. Local operations depend highly on the state, but are nevertheless independent in developing creative solutions in times of disaster. In presidentially declared disasters, in which supplemental funding through Social Services Block Grants is available, those funds pass through the state to local operations (ACF, 2014).

Countless nonprofits and faith-based organizations operate around the country, focusing on separate areas of social services needs (GuideStar, 2014; Pipes and Ebaugh, 2002). These organizations often receive government funding to support their work, especially during and after disasters and other emergencies. Faith-based organizations and nonprofits play a critical role in social service delivery because they often fill gaps in government services. They also provide an outlet for the involvement of community volunteers and residents in social service delivery. Philanthropy plays a significant role in the social services sector as well. Donations to human services organizations made up 12 percent of all charitable giving in 2013, totaling more than $40 billion (National Philanthropic Trust, 2014).

Cross-Sector Collaboration

Leaders of all social service organizations can have positive impacts on the health of their community following a disaster through leadership, intraorganizational collaboration, and teamwork throughout the community. However, the fragmentation that exists during steady-state times poses significant challenges to coordination among social service providers after a disaster. And although many documents promoting improved disaster recovery stress the importance of cross-sector collaboration, such partnering often is difficult to achieve. Human services agencies and organizations are notoriously understaffed. As one human services provider in Pennsylvania stated, "Every day is an emergency for us" (Hipper et al., 2013, p. 14). In addition to limited staffing, most agencies are hampered by a general lack of sufficient resources, have differences in eligibility definitions, have different perspectives on strategies based on their focus, and receive no added funding for collaboration. They also may distrust other organizations and see the demands of collaboration as threatening to their organizational autonomy.

Communication among social service professionals (both intra- and interagency) during recovery planning and implementation needs to emphasize purposive, collaborative decision making and program implementation with the goal of building the community's short- and long-term health and well-being. Regularly scheduled meetings of social service and other providers was important to the sharing of information and coordination of service delivery in post-Katrina New Orleans.[8] Building a culture of teamwork and acceptance among collaborators is an ongoing process greatly aided by frequent multimodal communication.

Empowerment of vulnerable populations in recovery also is critical. Organizations should identify vulnerable populations and their potential needs before a disaster strikes and institutionalize meaningful

---

[8] Personal communication, J. Kelly, CEO Kingsley House, to L. Usdin, committee member, regarding post-Katrina recovery of social service, September 2013.

participation of these groups in planning efforts. Research investigating how early identification and support of vulnerable populations can reduce long-term needs and psychological consequences associated with disasters would be helpful in making the case for these identification and inclusion efforts. Social service professionals can act as advocates for vulnerable populations, working with key community partners to ensure that their needs are met both before and after disasters. Such community partners include but are not limited to planning, housing, community development, and public health departments; schools; employment agencies; health care organizations; and their respective partner organizations in the for-profit, nonprofit, and philanthropic sectors. Many of these organizations have goals in common (or at least compatible) with social service providers, as well as relevant experience and resources. Social service agencies seeking to form or enhance cross-sector partnerships are most effective when they understand and leverage preexisting administrative arrangements, processes, advisory bodies, and funding streams operating at the local level instead of attempting to create new structures that compete for scarce financial, time, and staff resources. One-off projects implemented outside of existing structures typically lack longevity as a result of insufficient buy-in.

Organizations need to determine the level and type of integration most appropriate to their local circumstances. A universal need, however, is for agencies—and professionals within them—to build an understanding of partnering organizations and professions, including the rules and constraints under which they operate. Cross-training is one way to accomplish this goal. Social service leaders also should be attuned to opportunities to share their expertise and their sensitivity to diverse needs to inform recovery efforts in other sectors. For highly vulnerable populations, a greater degree of integration is warranted, while for less vulnerable populations, looser linkages between organizations may be more appropriate (Leutz, 1999).

Planning Departments, Community Development Entities, and Housing

City planners (also often called community planners or urban and regional planners) develop comprehensive plans that guide long-term private- and public-sector land development. These plans affect residential and business growth patterns and the associated infrastructure, all of which in turn affect the neighborhoods and services available to residents. Planning processes employed during steady-state times and after disasters typically provide for community participation (see the discussion in Chapter 3 on public engagement), which can be leveraged by social service organizations to discuss the needs of their client populations (Enarson and Fordham, 2001). Planning departments and community development entities are logical partners with social services departments in pre-disaster planning.

The community development sector shares goals with social services—both aim to help low-income populations improve self-sufficiency and access to services and amenities. Although there are important exceptions, community development generally uses "place-based" strategies (e.g., affordable housing, public transit systems; see Chapter 9) as opposed to the "people-based" approaches of the social services sector. The community development sector does its work to alleviate poverty and revitalize neighborhoods through planning processes that would (and in some communities already do) benefit from collaboration and coordination with health and human services agencies (Erickson and Andrews, 2011).

Housing service organizations work on such issues as homelessness, access to affordable housing, and eviction prevention. These organizations are closely linked to social services, as both aim to help low-income populations meet basic needs and maintain self-sufficiency. Clients of housing service organizations may be particularly vulnerable during and after a disaster as a result of closure of public housing or shelters, as well as a lack of resources to secure alternative housing. (Disaster-related housing issues are discussed in Chapter 10.)

Public Health, Behavioral Health, and Clinical Care Delivery

The client populations served by social services every day are the same populations that are at risk for adverse health outcomes after a disaster (i.e., the socially vulnerable). Public health and social service organizations have an interest in working collaboratively to find mechanisms for mitigating these adverse outcomes. Likewise, the behavioral health and health care sectors need to work in tandem with social service organizations, as both mental and physical health issues can be exacerbated or caused by a disaster, and the populations served by social services are particularly at risk for these outcomes. Collaboration among social services, public health, behavioral health, and clinical care can markedly improve the health and well-being of individuals and communities affected by a disaster by coordinating care, improving the client experience, and reducing the burden on each individual organization. For example, The Jesse Tree, a social service organization in Galveston, Texas, partners with the public health department, clinical care providers, and mental health providers. Its clients can receive services as varied as classes in chronic disease management, referrals to federal assistance programs, glucose screening, and case management all under one roof. After Hurricane Ike, The Jesse Tree and its partners continued to work together to meet the emergent and ongoing needs of the community. Community health workers such as those at The Jesse Tree can provide "a community-based system of care and social support" that links social services with health care (CDC Division of Diabetes Translation, 2003) and promotes a healthy community approach to recovery. (The Jesse Tree is used as a case study later in this chapter.)

PRE-DISASTER SOCIAL SERVICES SECTOR PRIORITIES

In keeping with a key theme of this report, the committee emphasizes that the speed and success of social services recovery after a disaster depend heavily on pre-disaster planning both within the social services sector and collaboratively across sectors. The committee identified three key pre-disaster priorities in which the social services sector should be engaged to support pre-disaster recovery planning efforts:

- Establishing Forums for Coordination and Collaboration Before and After Disasters
- Establishing Mechanisms for Information Sharing After Disasters
- Planning for Fluctuations in Social Services Workforce Needs

Establishing Forums for Coordination and Collaboration Before and After Disasters

Social service providers have limited resources to fulfill their missions even in non-disaster times. Thus, it is important to integrate pre-disaster planning into existing planning processes instead of creating additional processes. Organizations aiming to improve planning for social services recovery can build on existing community leadership and coordinating entities. These entities take many different forms, such as advisory groups and collaboratives. Often there are multiple coordinating entities in a community that work on specialized issues (e.g., child welfare, homelessness, domestic violence). If a community-level forum does not already exist, leaders should consider forming one to foster cross-sector coordination for purposes of (1) defining resources, roles, and responsibilities in recovery; (2) appropriately sharing client information among service providers; and (3) maximizing access to recovery resources, information, and activities. In addition, these forums provide a central clearinghouse and communication base for updated information on each organization's key contacts and provide up-to-date information for all partners. Forums also are important arenas for the development of structures, policies, and procedures that facilitate a culture of collaboration and promote information sharing. Memorandums of understanding and mutual-aid agreements specifying disaster-related resources, roles, and responsibilities are useful mechanisms for formalizing these relationships. It is critical that all essential partners be identified and invited to participate in such forums.

Voluntary Organizations Active in Disaster (VOAD) and Community Organizations Active in Disaster (COAD) (described in Box 4-1 in Chapter 4) are common forums for collaborating on disaster issues related to human needs. Involvement of local health departments in COAD can help ensure that health considerations are better integrated into local planning efforts and that essential health and social services are prioritized in post disaster recovery. VOAD and COAD usually are involved in the formation of long-term recovery committees. These groups—which can go by a number of different names, including long-term recovery groups and unmet needs committees—link recovery resources to the unmet needs of

---

BOX 8-1
Considerations for Coordination of Long-Term Recovery Committee Activities

Coordination in the context of long-term recovery committees (LTRCs) is fundamentally different from the coordination that occurs among stakeholders involved in early recovery efforts (e.g., those conducting damage assessment, setting up response centers, and reestablishing vital services). First responder agencies are for the most part seasoned in disaster response, their roles are defined, and it is not unusual for many of these organizations to have previous experience working together. They also operate within the "honeymoon" phase of the recovery process, when optimism and good will prevail despite concerns over the magnitude of the task ahead. While conflicts are common among agencies, a process and institutional context for handling these matters are in place. LTRCs are being organized and/or activated during the initial recovery phase, but their work can extend to several years or more after the event, with a period of disillusionment arising from the inevitable delays associated with the recovery process.

The job of the LTRC entails a series of complex tasks such as recruiting and housing volunteer groups, assessing unmet needs, coordinating construction, establishing a case management strategy, and coordinating public and donated funds. The forum provided by the LTRC is a natural place for questions to be raised and concerns expressed by a cross section of stakeholders. In this context, and given the diversity of participants, spirited debate can be expected. It is often said that a disaster does not resolve underlying issues within a community, and such issues predictably emerge as the recovery process proceeds.

LTRC membership consists of funding agencies, faith-based groups, responder agencies, and many other interested organizations, including local community groups. Such diversity in membership and differing interests within the group pose unique challenges for LTRCs. Funding organizations frequently want assurances that the recovery is well organized and proceeding satisfactorily, while community groups are concerned with the changes in their community and the many unmet needs of residents. Additionally, constituencies have differing styles of debate, dialogue, and decision making, which adds to the challenges of long-term recovery efforts. When these issues are identified and handled, the long-term recovery process proceeds more smoothly in terms of both process and production. But when these issues go unresolved or are handled only partially, resulting problems with low trust levels and ongoing conflict can impede or even derail the recovery effort. Thus, special attention needs to be given to ensuring that a full voice and participation are afforded to a representative cross section of the community.

---

community members "in order to ensure that even the most vulnerable in the community recover from disaster" (National VOAD, 2012, p. 6). These important coordinating entities (discussed further in Box 8-1) are composed of members of nonprofits, governmental organizations, faith-based entities, and businesses, and they can be structured in many different ways depending on such factors as local needs, available resources, and community history.

Establishing Mechanisms to Facilitate Record and Information Sharing After Disasters

Development of an institutionalized cross-agency record-sharing arrangement before a disaster facilitates post-disaster social services recovery (see Box 8-2). Most social service clients are eligible for, and use, a wide variety of services; with proper attention to confidentiality and consent, information and documentation collected by one service provider can be shared with others.[9] This allows service providers

---

[9] The American Red Cross has an exemption from requirements of the Health Insurance Portability and Accountability Act (HIPAA) during certain emergencies. This legal caveat enables them to provide family members of disaster victims with some basic information that generally would not be allowable (HHS, 2014b).

to see the full picture of community services and resources used by clients, thereby helping to reduce over-lapping services and service gaps. It also frees up time that would otherwise be spent on intake interviews for other case management activities and reduces stress on disaster survivors associated with multiple intake processes. As noted earlier, moreover, disaster survivors often are mobile (i.e., they may relocate, temporarily or permanently, to other jurisdictions). Allowing documentation and case management notes collected by agencies in one jurisdiction to follow clients to sister agencies in different jurisdictions avoids the need for those agencies to start over with new intake and qualification processes, and it gives them a more comprehensive understanding of client needs and progress already made. Finally, because service providers typically change over time following a disaster—with national early responder organizations augmenting local organizations in early recovery, then transferring cases to local agencies for longer-term management—record sharing avoids the loss of data between organizations. Establishing such a system prior to a disaster is key in light of the chaos and emergent demands on time and resources following a disaster.

The first step in creating a shared system is to develop an understanding of existing social service data sources, reports, and relationships and to explore opportunities for access to electronic records. As mentioned above, strategies for dealing with challenges to the sharing of information/reports need to be explored and developed. During the pre-event stage, post-disaster data needs can be identified. Sharing an information plan with all partners makes it possible to develop a comprehensive system for meeting information demands after a disaster.

Planning for Fluctuations in Social Services Workforce Needs

One of the most difficult challenges prior to a disaster is anticipating social services resource needs after such an event. Disasters have differential impacts depending on the extent of infrastructure and housing damage, as well as the number of people impacted. Despite this uncertainty, communities need to consider before a disaster strikes the array of services that may be needed and how they can be provided. Pre-disaster planning requires clear articulation of who will recruit and train staff and volunteers so that public and private agencies and organizations will be familiar with their roles and responsibilities in advance of a crisis. The training needs to cover mental health needs, as well as special post-disaster issues, such as accessing benefits. Pre-disaster planning also should include memorandums of understanding among governmental and private agencies, local hospitals, NGOs, schools and child care centers, faith-based organizations, and other groups, specifying disaster-related roles, responsibilities, and duties. Continuity of operations plans can facilitate rapid recovery after a disaster, promote the concepts of a healthy communities approach, and provide guidance on social service impacts for medical service personnel and emergency management partners. More research is needed on how the social services sector can anticipate the impact of a disaster on the workforce, maintain a healthy workforce, and optimize functioning after a disaster.

When a disaster strikes, communities may need more intake workers, grief counselors, and other paraprofessionals. Not only must previously vulnerable populations be reached, but disasters create newly vulnerable populations that must be identified. Communities that have developed a rapid assessment capacity for identifying social service needs consistent with state and local emergency response and recovery plans are better situated to identify and serve the expanded pool of vulnerable populations.

The number of available providers fluctuates during different phases of disaster recovery. In the immediate post-disaster period, communities may experience a loss of providers because providers themselves are affected by the disaster and are either displaced or incapable of offering their usual services. The surge of untrained volunteers can further drain professional resources because providers must spend time supervising and training them. As the recovery progresses, providers may experience burnout and need breaks, and volunteer support will diminish. This oscillation in workforce capacity should be planned for in advance. Potential ways to preserve or expand the social service workforce capacity after a disaster include

BOX 8-2
Information Systems in Social Services Recovery

Coordinated Assistance Network

The Coordinated Assistance Network (CAN) is a multiorganizational partnership among many disaster relief organizations in the United States, including the Red Cross and United Way (CAN, 2014a). CAN was founded following the September 11, 2001, terror attacks to allow for information sharing across disaster relief organizations, thereby improving the quality, efficiency, and management of response to a disaster. The network was piloted during the 2004 Florida hurricanes and has played a role in the response to other major disasters, including Hurricane Sandy (2012), the Oklahoma City tornadoes (2013), and the Deepwater Horizon oil spill (2010) (CAN, 2014c). CAN's website (www.can.org) features an extensive cloud-based database system that is used to collect data on the experiences of clients in the wake of a disaster (CAN, 2014b). The database is open to any relief organization operating in the United States that chooses to use it, but CAN's client data must remain confidential within the user network. For more information about CAN, see http://www.can.org/images/CommunityIntro.pdf (accessed April 4, 2015).

Efforts to Outcomes™

Efforts to Outcomes™ is software designed to help nonprofits collaborate and share data across organizations. The software can track and analyze demographic data, manage referrals, assess needs and progress, identify and track trends, and monitor and assess program and staff effectiveness (Social Solutions, 2014). Boulder County, a user of Efforts to Outcomes, finds that it allows multiple divisions in the county government to share data and coordinate services. For example, when individuals seek service, their data need be entered into the system only once, and providers across the collaborative are informed (Microsoft Case Studies, 2010).

Parkland Center for Clinical Innovation (PCCI) Pieces™

There is increasing focus on incorporating sociodemographic information (e.g., education, employment, and financial resource strain) into electronic health records (IOM, 2014) to support both individual- and population-level health interventions. Such information also has value in the planning for and response to disasters, particularly with respect to identifying and serving at-risk populations. PCCI, a nonprofit organization in Dallas specializing in the development of real-time predictive and surveillance analytics for health care, has created Pieces™, software designed to identify patients at high risk for experiencing an adverse event by detecting clinical and social risk factors in the electronic health record system. PCCI also has developed an information exchange portal that captures social health components important to public health preparedness and response. The aim is to include more than 400 community organizations that provide a range of social services, including food and nutrition assistance, shelter, transportation assistance, housing assistance, and financial support. The information exchange portal uses technology to provide coordination of care for patients moving throughout the various health and social sectors. Connie Chan, project director at PCCI, reports that many of the benefits of health information technology, including information exchange portals, not only are useful during daily operations but also can provide extra benefit during disasters or emergencies (Chan, 2013).

- preventing burnout by rotating workers through difficult assignments, assisting caseworkers with child care or other services that may have been disrupted, or offering peer support;
- recruiting professionals from other communities and states, which may require emergency licensure of professionals[10];
- integrating providers from relief groups such as the American Red Cross, the Salvation Army, Church of the Brethren, and other National Voluntary Organizations Active in Disaster (National VOAD) members;
- integrating staff and volunteers from existing community groups, including clergy/faith leaders and other community leaders;
- exploiting cross-cutting opportunities for accreditation;
- developing systems for including spontaneous volunteers;
- maintaining up-to-date lists of translators and bilingual providers to help reach non-English-speaking vulnerable populations; and
- engaging providers from retired professional groups.

As noted above, organizations may be inundated with volunteers who need to be trained to support the provision of social services; the use of untrained spontaneous volunteers is not a viable option since it raises liability issues (Sauer et al., 2014). Pre-disaster training programs can reduce the burden associated with post-disaster "just-in-time" training needs. More research is needed, however, to elucidate the training needed to support the social services system in a disaster and to clarify which tasks are appropriate for volunteers and how NGOs and faith-based organizations can be mobilized in planning efforts. Some communities have found it helpful for a single local organization to register and coordinate volunteer workers. A clearinghouse for volunteers also can help during the chaos following a disaster. Hands On, for example, is a national group that establishes procedures and systems for coordinating untrained volunteer efforts. Such clearinghouses require clear standards covering issues that include

- the need for volunteers to have a basic background check;
- how volunteer hours can be tracked for possible credit against FEMA's local match requirement for public assistance funds;
- issues of training and liability for spontaneous untrained volunteers to minimize safety risks; and
- the need for regular, coordinated communication with volunteers (e.g., training opportunities, updates, news).

Several resources can help in addressing the need for increased social services workforce capacity after a disaster. These resources include but are not limited to

- FEMA Crisis Counseling Assistance and Training Program funding for counselor training (for psychosocial support services),
- SSBG-DR-funded education and training programs,
- hotlines such as the Substance Abuse and Mental Health Services Administration's (SAMHSA's) Disaster Distress Helpline and the National Domestic Violence Hotline that provide around-the-clock access to skilled counselors,
- local and national philanthropic foundations committed to employment initiatives, and
- businesses seeking to invest in community workforce development.

---

[10] For more information on state licensure requirements for disaster volunteer social workers, see http://www.socialworkers.org/ldf/legal_issue/200509.asp?back=yes (accessed April 2, 2015).

THE CONTINUUM OF POST-DISASTER SOCIAL SERVICES INTERVENTIONS

Social service organizations have key roles to play throughout the post-disaster recovery process. Immediately after a disaster, these organizations, particularly if they are already embedded in the community, can meet individuals' basic needs, provide psychosocial support, and initiate case management to connect people with resources available to meet their myriad recovery needs. As recovery efforts continue into the intermediate and long terms, social service organizations can continue case management, offer ongoing psychosocial support, and help people manage their chronic conditions.

As discussed previously, ensuring access to services is a critical part of meeting the post-disaster needs of low-income and other vulnerable populations. Access has many dimensions, including physical location and accessibility to those with handicaps, hours of operation, and availability of materials and services in needed languages (SAMHSA, 2012). Since disaster victims often have multiple needs following a disaster—including food, housing, medical care, medical prescriptions and equipment, behavioral health support, cash assistance, transportation, and child care—efficiency in providing those services is paramount in enabling communities to begin recovery quickly. Early coordination through a joint recovery information system staffed by representatives of all engaged sectors can facilitate access to needed services. In particular, people are more likely to access food and auxiliary services before seeking behavioral health care because of the stigma associated with the latter and the perceived urgency of other matters. Providing disaster victims with a "one-stop shop" for social service, behavioral health, and other needs decreases the time required to travel between offices; eases the difficulty of transport and the stress of visiting multiple sites; and minimizes stigma related to seeking services, particularly for behavioral health.

FEMA and the Red Cross often establish multipurpose centers after disasters to help survivors access disaster benefits and a range of services (see Box 8-3). Another approach is to bring the services to survivors. Residents of temporary housing, for example, may require several kinds of assistance. The Human Services Campus developed in Joplin, Missouri, after the 2011 tornado illustrates the benefits of collocating these services and reaching people where they are. This community center, located at a FEMA temporary housing site, housed 40 local agencies, including legal aid and crisis counseling. It helped survivors access services, especially those who had lost vehicles in the storm and would have had difficulty traveling to multiple sites for services (Missouri Department of Mental Health, 2013; Rodriguez, 2013).

The committee identified three early critical services that represent priorities for the social services sector in the early recovery period, including

- meeting basic human needs (e.g., food shelter);
- initiating disaster case management; and
- providing psychosocial/behavioral health support for survivors.

In the intermediate- and long-term recovery periods, social services efforts should focus on providing ongoing social support and building client self-sufficiency. Each of these priority areas are discussed in the following sections.

EARLY POST-DISASTER SOCIAL SERVICES RECOVERY PRIORITIES

Meeting Basic Human Needs

An early priority for social service organizations is to coordinate with mass recovery sites to provide victims with basic needs: food, shelter, clothing, and medical prescriptions and supplies, as well as social services. To the extent possible in the context of a crisis, it is important to attend to special needs, such as meals with appropriate nutritional content for individuals with medical conditions (e.g., diabetes).

Although mass care is considered a response phase function, needs for assistance in obtaining basic resources can extend well into the recovery phase, depending on survivors' personal assets and the scope

---

BOX 8-3
Example of Collocation: Multi-Agency Resource/Relief Center

On May 29, 2011—just seven days after the tornado in Joplin, Missouri—the American Red Cross opened the doors to a Multi-Agency Resource/Relief Center where more than 30 partner agencies joined to provide services. Together, these local, state, and federal agencies partnered with the Red Cross to listen to survivor stories, verify each family's damage and needs, and record the documentation necessary to open more than 1,500 recovery cases.

Over the course of 15 days, the Multi-Agency Resource/Relief Center became the one-stop shop for survivor assistance: agencies coming to the survivor rather than the survivor needing to navigate to the varied locations of multiple agencies. Working together, these agencies helped more than 5,000 people, not only by offering financial assistance, legal services, and replacement driver's licenses and social security cards, but also by providing hot meals and moments of comfort. For those families that lost loved ones, the center facilitated access to an integrated care team made up of a caseworker, nurse, behavioral health professional, and chaplain, who met separately with each family to offer condolence, guide them compassionately through the assistance process, and ensure that they obtained additional assistance for funeral related expenses. There were specific services for veterans, children, seniors and those with disabilities. The Department of Family Services replaced food stamps and provided Disaster-Supplemental Nutrition Assistance Program (D-SNAP) assistance. Faith-based organizations provided shuttle services using church vans. Medical and mental health personnel listened, assisted, and counseled. Federal Emergency Management Agency (FEMA) specialists helped families submit applications for federal assistance and explained the opportunity to receive benefits and the necessary application processes.

Beyond the provision of these critical services, the Multi-Agency Resource/Relief Center became a gathering place for survivors. It was where neighbors reconnected with neighbors, and where families could get respite from the tragedy.

SOURCE: Meeds, 2013.

---

of the disaster. Experience with past disasters has shown that survivors' families, neighbors, and other members of personal support networks play critical roles in helping to meet basic human needs (Aldrich, 2012). It is when these capabilities and resources are overwhelmed (e.g., when members of personal support networks themselves require assistance) that auxiliary assistance is especially needed. The first and most critical step in supporting social networks is to reunite families, neighbors, and those with social ties who have been separated. At the community level, this work typically occurs in congregate settings, and it is important for a wide range of social service and other providers to develop a basic knowledge of mass care services. State emergency management agencies offer Community Mass Care/Emergency Assistance G108 courses periodically to build this knowledge base (National Mass Care Strategy, 2014).

Responsibilities of the social services sector in helping to meet basic human needs immediately following a disaster include an effective communication system that provides accurate mapping of available resources; multimodal, multi-language communications for both those in need of and those who wish to provide services and supplies; and a tracking system that monitors increases in mental health disorders, domestic violence, and other disaster-impacted issues. Messages about available resources and services can be integrated into general emergency management messages. It is also during this early phase that social service providers can begin to help individuals and families access disaster benefits by helping them compile needed portfolios of information.

Initiating Disaster Case Management

Although providing for short-term survival needs such as food, shelter, and clothing is often accomplished in congregate settings, concurrent with and after this process, one-on-one case management is the primary strategy for determining and addressing the myriad recovery needs of individuals and families. Disaster case managers provide clients with access to the resources and programs of multiple relief agencies, as well as financial assistance depending on the resources available to the individual, including existing savings, level of family income, and homeowner's and other insurance. The disaster case management process entails:

- identifying disaster survivors' needs using metrics developed in the pre-disaster phase;
- developing viable individual or family recovery plans that allow for long-term recovery even after the disaster case management program expires in the disaster area (FEMA, 2014);
- reconnecting survivors to essential services (including legal assistance, if needed);
- identifying new services needed and newly vulnerable populations resulting from the disaster; and
- helping survivors move toward a healthier lifestyle.

Individuals and families with minimal financial resources and insurance require more assistance and support. The elderly (particularly the frail elderly); people with disabilities; those who are underinsured, uninsured, and financially fragile; children in foster care or under the care of protective services; those who are medically vulnerable, such as those with acute or chronic illnesses; homeless families; and the mentally ill all have special needs that require additional casework coordination and attention. Case management for vulnerable populations frequently involves additional efforts at outreach; coordination with a wide range of agencies and organizations so these individuals can achieve stable living arrangements; and restoration and improvement of services tailored to ensuring that they can live as independently as possible. Many socially vulnerable people are enrolled in government assistance programs prior to a disaster; as a result of this ready access to their information, social service providers can more easily furnish them with information on special disaster benefits. On the other hand, many clients may require special assistance to re-create documentation lost as a result of the disaster.

In the event of a presidential disaster declaration, the Stafford Act authorizes FEMA to fund the Disaster Case Management Program. This program provides assistance in accessing disaster-specific federal benefits and works with the local long-term recovery committee to address needs not met by other programs. In the absence of this federally funded program, a similar disaster case management program can be run by a local entity, such as a VOAD, and can help identify sources of additional funding for social services. Additional resources with further information on disaster case management can be found in Appendix C.

Case managers often work for an organization that is contracted by the state to provide case management services and may not be linked to the community or work in concert with local social services agencies. Further, case managers change over time, which complicates recovery and adds to frustrations for many disaster survivors, who must relate the facts of their case repeatedly and produce documentation for different service providers. Therefore, as discussed earlier, strategies for facilitating the collection and sharing of case information are essential, as is working closely with strong community supports, such as schools, neighborhood associations, community centers, civic groups, and faith-based organizations.

Providing Psychosocial/Behavioral Health Support for Survivors

Early psychosocial support interventions, such as psychological first aid (discussed in more detail in Chapter 7), can be provided by a number of professional and trained individuals, including mental health and social service professionals, volunteers (retired professionals and trained volunteers), representatives of faith-based groups, and community members (e.g., teachers). Social service organizations can play a key role in several ways: providing psychosocial support directly; making referrals; or reaching out to individuals in community settings, such as schools and community centers. As discussed above, after a disaster, people are likely to visit a social service organization to meet basic needs such as food or shelter. When these organizations take that opportunity to offer psychosocial support, they can mitigate the behavioral health effects of disasters and facilitate individual and community recovery. Faith-based organizations also can play a role in providing early support, particularly when they are already integrated into the community. (See Chapter 7 for more discussion of psychosocial support, including emotional and spiritual care.)

INTERMEDIATE- TO LONG-TERM RECOVERY PRIORITIES

As community-level early needs are addressed—which may take months depending on the scope of loss—the social service sector begins working toward reestablishing normalcy, although often with sorely depleted resources and increased needs among clients. The majority of national disaster relief funds are focused on meeting short-term needs, with few notable exceptions following extreme disasters.[11] Long-term recovery needs must be met primarily through local resources or reprogramming of existing federal funds (e.g., SSBG funds), although supplemental appropriations through the SSBG-DR program have been used to support mental health and social services.[12] Social service departments can help communities identify how needs will be met once external resources have diminished. This includes efforts to move the social service delivery model to one that embraces a healthy community approach.

Although most individuals require social service supports for only a short time following a disaster, many unmet needs remain; in some cases, survivors may be subject to long-term displacement, job loss, and loss of family or other social supports. These needs are the focus of longer-term case management, which continues from the early recovery period and aims to assist individuals and families in achieving the fullest possible recovery. The emphasis during the long-term recovery phase is on helping to replace losses; adjust to changes in life circumstances; restore suitable permanent housing that is safe, sanitary, and secure; and support self-sufficiency and a healthy lifestyle. When gaps exist between an individual's resources and recovery needs, work is directed toward documenting those needs, assessing costs, and applying for assistance. Issues that can arise during the long-term recovery period that require a case manager's attention include financial problems, health issues, job loss, stress-related domestic issues, and emotional problems. For individuals and families that continue to need support after exhausting funds from FEMA's individual assistance grants[13] (when authorized) and other federal and state disaster resources, their cases are referred to the local long-term recovery committee, which reviews cases and distributes funds according to need and availability. However, these committees are often not permanent and may dissolve when donated funds are exhausted.

Providing Ongoing Psychosocial Support

Management of chronic post-disaster stress is of central concern in the months—and often years—following a disaster. The stress caused by evacuation, relocation, and disruption of routines continues to affect people even if their homes and the community's physical infrastructure are restored to normal quickly. This post-disaster stress, along with the grief associated with catastrophic loss, is a normal response that

---

[11] Following the September 11, 2001, terrorist attacks and Hurricane Sandy, the American Red Cross allocated a portion of the donations it received for a recovery grant program (ARC, 2014; The Urban Institute, 2006).

[12] After Hurricane Sandy, Congress enacted a nearly $475 million supplemental appropriation for the Social Services Block Grant to be devoted to social, health, and mental health services for individuals and to repair, renovate, and rebuild health care facilities, mental hygiene facilities, and child care and other types of social service facilities. Additional post-Sandy supplemental funds were made available through the Family Violence Prevention and Services program and Head Start, as well as a SAMHSA Emergency Response Grant (ACF, 2013b; HHS, 2012).

[13] Individual assistance funds from FEMA may be made available after a presidential disaster declaration and have a broad range of eligible uses, including but not limited to housing repair, temporary housing costs, medical and dental costs not covered by insurance, and child care costs. These grants are capped at approximately $30,000 per individual or household and generally are limited to a period of 18 months (CRS, 2012) (see also Chapter 4).

requires psychosocial support. As mentioned earlier, an early warning tracking system can aid in monitoring increases in behavioral health problems. Chapter 7 addresses in detail behavioral health issues that may be exacerbated by post-disaster stress, as well as clinical and nonclinical interventions for dealing with these issues.

The community may benefit from a public messaging campaign that normalizes the stress of a disaster and helps overcome fears of stigma associated with help-seeking behavior. The "All Right?" campaign in New Zealand (see Box 7-3 in Chapter 7) is an example of success with this type of messaging. Psychosocial support also can be provided by family, neighbors, faith communities, and other nonprofessional volunteers. Use of these sources of support strengthens social networks and community cohesion and alleviates the burden on a behavioral health system that may be sorely taxed following a disaster.

Building Client Self-Sufficiency and Managing Chronic Medical Conditions

Long-term goals for recovery should include interventions to build clients' capacity for resilience and self-care (and thus reduce future strain on resources). Through partnerships between community or neighborhood groups and social service providers, communities can develop plans for self-help support groups facilitated by professionals or appropriately trained lay volunteers. These groups can assist in the exchange of information about recovery resources and encourage individual recovery and resilience.

Job loss resulting from closure or relocation of businesses is a major barrier to individual and community recovery following a disaster. However, the recovery process itself may require a large number of workers, which presents an opportunity to address unemployment and assist low-income populations in the community. Partnerships between workforce development and social services agencies can promote both training that includes recognition of the social determinants of health and local hiring to fill recovery-related positions and help support client self-sufficiency. Academic institutions may also be key partners. After Hurricane Katrina, for example, Dillard University's Minority Worker Training Program[14] worked with United Steelworkers to launch the initiative "A Safe Way Back Home," which was designed to train local low-income and minority neighborhood residents to dispose of waste and replace soil on properties in New Orleans (NIEHS, 2014). Similar training was provided through the Minority Worker Training Program after the Deepwater Horizon oil spill and Hurricane Sandy. Providing valuable environmental cleanup skills represents a sustainable approach to helping those in underserved and disadvantaged communities.

As discussed in Chapter 1, chronic conditions such as diabetes, hypertension, asthma, and many others are increasingly common in U.S. communities. Disaster-related disruption of care routines can lead to health crises, even among people whose chronic conditions were previously well controlled (Kessler, 2007). Thus, another important area for capacity building interventions is chronic disease self-management. The committee heard testimony that, both in non-disaster times and following a disaster, many social service clients experience repeated flare-ups of chronic conditions. Complicating this pattern is a behavioral health component: people with other chronic diseases are more likely to suffer from depression (Chapman et al., 2005), and depression is closely linked with substance abuse (Regier et al., 1990). These health issues complicate many aspects of employment and family life, so building clients' capacity to manage their chronic conditions—while traditionally understood as a health care responsibility—is a function that social service organizations can undertake in partnership with health care professionals and organizations to help reduce reliance on the social safety net in the long term. Outside of the disaster context, chronic disease self-management classes have shown great promise for improving patient outcomes, although only anecdotal evidence is available regarding these interventions during disaster recovery (see Box 8-4).

Community health workers (CHWs) can play a critical role in helping to manage chronic disease after a disaster (see the discussion of CHWs in Box 6-3 in Chapter 6). CHWs are laypersons—not trained

---

[14] The Minority Worker Training Program is a program funded by the National Institute of Environmental Health Sciences at the National Institutes of Health. The program is designed to recruit and train young minority individuals who live in communities with contaminated properties to work in construction and environmental remediation.

BOX 8-4
Chronic Disease Management Assistance from The Jesse Tree, Galveston, Texas

The Jesse Tree is a faith-based organization that connects Galveston, Texas, residents with basic necessities (food, medications) and essential services (medical and social services). One way in which The Jesse Tree serves the community is by offering chronic disease self-management classes. These classes use a Chronic Disease Self-Management Program developed by the Patient Education Research Center at Stanford University School of Medicine, which is designed to help patients manage their chronic health problems and control their symptoms (Stanford School of Medicine, 2014). The classes cover conditions including diabetes, hypertension, and chronic diseases generally, as well as stress management and relaxation training. In addition to these classes, The Jesse Tree offers such services as blood pressure screenings and glucose checks, and helps people apply for food stamps, Medicare, and the Children's Health Insurance Program.

The Chronic Disease Self-Management Program designed by Stanford and offered by The Jesse Tree has been found to result in better self-management skills, improved health outcomes, more appropriate health care utilization, and reduced costs and hospitalizations (CDC and National Council on Aging, 2008). For example, a review of studies on the program found that it results in

- better quality of life,
- better psychological well-being,
- less fatigue,
- more exercise and healthier eating,
- better communication with physicians,
- improved self-reported health, and
- slightly fewer visits to hospitals and physicians (CDC and National Council on Aging, 2008).

When Hurricane Ike struck Galveston, The Jesse Tree lost $2.5 million in facilities and supplies. With the help of donors, it reopened and responded to the needs of the Galveston residents, providing food, medical supplies, and help with applications for disaster assistance benefits (The Jesse Tree, 2015). Chronic disease management classes were offered to help those whose medical conditions had been exacerbated by the disaster get them under control.

---

medical professionals—who are members of the community and usually share ethnicity, language, culture, and socioeconomic status with those they serve (HRSA, 2011). They can help manage chronic disease in many ways: educating patients on self-management; administering health screenings, such as blood pressure tests; facilitating and coordinating care by primary care providers; providing social support to patients and caregivers; and helping patients follow a self-management plan (CDC, 2011). After a disaster, CHWs are especially vital because they are present and integrated into the community, and they can help support chronic disease management while primary care providers are occupied with treating more acute medical needs. Their use to manage chronic disease has been shown to increase patients' knowledge of their disease and ability to self-manage, improve individual health outcomes, decrease mortality, and reduce visits to emergency departments and hospitalizations (CDC, 2011).

SPECIAL CONSIDERATIONS FOR CHILDREN AND THE ELDERLY

Although the social services sector routinely addresses the needs of vulnerable populations, children and the elderly are especially vulnerable groups that require special consideration during pre-disaster planning and after an event.

Children and Youth

Part of the challenge of addressing the needs of children and youth relates to the diffuse nature of the systems that service this population—comprising a number of sectors, including education/child care, pediatrics, child welfare authorities, social services, family violence prevention and services, and community- and faith-based groups (ACF, 2013a). After a disaster, it is critical for community leaders to focus on children's needs, working with school districts, Head Start, and other child-focused organizations to help them return to normal routines as soon as possible (DHS, 2012). A children and youth task force can be used to bring together all relevant agencies, organizations, and professionals to pool resources and jointly develop a strategic approach to meeting the needs of this vulnerable population. Such a task force can develop strategies for identifying children most likely to be vulnerable following a disaster by working with existing public assistance programs, and it can serve as a source of information about child-related services after a disaster. If a children and youth task force is in place, it can be used to coordinate efforts to meet the needs of these groups. Where such a task force is not already in place, leaders should consider forming one, as it has been shown to be a successful model for meeting children's post-disaster needs[15] (White, 2014).

In addition to the recovery needs of children themselves, quick return of school programs and child care is vital to community recovery overall (see Box 8-5). The committee heard from speakers at the federal and community levels that the lack of child care following a disaster poses significant challenges to individual and community recovery; as noted earlier, parents who are unable to find child care cannot return to work or meet other daily needs, and children may be exposed to unsafe environments (Nolen, 2014; White, 2014). As discussed in Chapter 7, schools also are important in enabling children to have access to behavioral health interventions after a disaster. Yet while significant progress has been made in integrating behavioral health services into schools, this is not the case for early childhood programs such as Head Start (White, 2014), although supplemental funding for Head Start programs made available after Hurricane Sandy was used to fund behavioral health services for affected children (ACF, 2013b). Better integration of behavioral health and social services is needed to ensure that interventions reach the youngest and most vulnerable children. Mitigation measures (e.g., structural hardening) that minimize the duration of school closures are critical to ensuring that children have safe places to be and access to needed services after a disaster. Although such measures are best carried out in advance, post-disaster reconstruction may be an important opportunity to build safer and stronger schools.

Despite the availability of small business loan programs at the federal and state levels, child care businesses often struggle to recover because of high start-up costs and a lack of licensed providers. Long-term lack of affordable child care was noted more than a decade following the Grand Forks flood (Gerber, 2006). Moreover, child care providers often have low incomes and may be in need of assistance themselves after a disaster. Further, licensing requirements for child care facilities are complex, and compliance requires time and resources, both of which are in short supply following a disaster. Thus, disaster pre-planning might include the development of mechanisms for post-disaster rapid assessment of the status of child care centers; temporary waivers of requirements, such as those for vaccination; processes for assisting centers in attracting resources and rebuilding; and strategies for recruiting and training new staff. A child care recovery group can be formed under a children and youth task force to address this critical need. This group can work with child care advocates to set priorities for ensuring the most inclusive response to a disaster and for making infrastructure investments that strengthen safety and resilience at schools and child care sites.

---

[15] Guidelines on developing children and youth task forces are available at www.acf.hhs.gov/sites/default/files/ohsepr/childrens_task_force_development_web.pdf (accessed July 2, 2014).

BOX 8-5
The Role of School Systems in Recovery: Case Study of Joplin, Missouri

In the event of a disaster, schools play a vital role in contributing to the overall recovery of a community. The quick return of school programs, as well as schools' role in promoting the mental and behavioral health of children following disasters, facilitates a community's resilience and efforts to rebuild.

The tornado that struck Joplin, Missouri, a rural community with a population of approximately 50,000, in May 2011 occurred at the close of the school year. The tornado directly affected 18,000 residents and severely damaged nine of the city's 18 schools. Less than 48 hours after the disaster, however, city officials publicly declared a commitment to starting the 2011-2012 school year on time. The city made a concerted effort to locate and contact all children associated with the school system, both to offer assistance and to coordinate future school activities. Summer school enrollment was expanded, and for the first time, transportation to summer school was provided, allowing parents to address post-disaster concerns with their children safely under the protection of schools. Joplin's post-disaster interventions, as part of this effort to restore school services as soon as possible, spurred on the overall recovery of the community. The early decision to reopen on time may have encouraged families to stay in the community; despite the displacement of 30 percent of Joplin residents, few ultimately left the community. The city achieved a 95 percent retention rate in student re-enrollment for the 2011-2012 academic year, only slightly below average.

Beyond encouraging families to remain in the community, schools played a vital role in promoting children's behavioral health. Joplin's summer school program emphasized both children's safety and emotional well-being. Following the disaster, school staff were trained on behavioral health issues. Counseling sessions took place at schools in the following year, with as many as 25 percent of students at some schools participating, an intervention that also facilitated the referral of children to community providers if needed. Further discussion of school-based behavioral health programs can be found in Chapter 7.

Joplin's post-disaster school-based interventions demonstrate the extent to which schools can promote the recovery and resilience of their community. Furthermore, school-based programs encourage a community to engage in its own recovery, and schools themselves can offer visible recovery milestones, reopening on schedule, for example. Consequently, incorporating school systems into preparedness, response, and recovery planning and activities is critically important.

SOURCE: Kanter and Abramson, 2014; NCDP, 2013.

The Elderly

Many challenges are unique to the elderly during disaster recovery. First, they encompass a diverse range of circumstances—from those living in nursing homes needing comprehensive supportive services to active, able older adults who live independently but in some cases are isolated from their communities. The impacts of disasters on different subpopulations of the elderly are varied and require different strategies. A comprehensive plan of support for the elderly does not exist in part because of a lack of supportive networks. The geriatric education centers that once existed lost their funding and have disappeared (Brown, 2014), so there are no logical hubs for the provision of information and services for the elderly that are especially needed during disaster recovery.

In addition to the lack of infrastructure support, it is rare for relief workers or crisis counselors to receive specialized training for working with the elderly after a disaster (Brown, 2014). This gap is exacerbated by special issues that arise from the unique vulnerabilities of older adults (e.g., being prey to unscrupulous contractors and scammers, limited mobility leading to service access issues).

To better meet the disaster-related needs of older adults, social service departments can develop specialized materials and training for emergency and other disaster recovery workers. The previously mentioned strategy of collocation or centralized disaster recovery services will be especially effective for the elderly, as will all strategies designed to promote stronger social networking within communities. As communities change over the years, many elderly who have aged in place no longer know their neighbors, so strategies that strengthen neighbor-to-neighbor communications and social bonds not only diminish this isolation in normal times but also can provide lifelines to help the elderly prepare for and deal with disasters. Further, if communities develop disaster recovery forums/coordinating bodies, these entities can promote pre-disaster programming that identifies opportunities for elderly people to provide their varied expertise as volunteers during recovery.

BUILDING A MORE RESILIENT AND SUSTAINABLE SOCIAL SERVICES SECTOR

The recovery process itself can provide a foundation for building a stronger social services system by leveraging new resources, lessons learned, and partnerships developed in the aftermath of a disaster to achieve greater capacity and interoperability. The recovery period may present opportunities to restructure service provision within the community, particularly in the case of major disasters that have destroyed significant portions of local infrastructure. If infrastructure must be rebuilt, collocation of agency offices can be used to facilitate client access and cross-agency collaboration. Regardless of infrastructure conditions, however, social service providers should use all available opportunities to advocate for decisions that facilitate integration of services and a healthy community approach to recovery. Integration of social services with other community services is a powerful tool for building local partnerships aimed at improving the community's health.

Long-term recovery committees, although traditionally focused on case management, are diverse in makeup and focus, and they may serve as a natural platform for integration at the local level. Communities may identify other, more viable structures for their context. As discussed earlier in this chapter, integration can take many forms; local social service agencies are in the best position to determine what level and type of integration is both helpful for the clients they serve and attainable within the community's existing administrative arrangements.

Consistent with the traditional view of social services, this chapter has focused heavily on people-oriented strategies for improving social well-being. However, the committee recognizes that long-term strategies for achieving lasting transformation must also target the physical, social, and economic environments associated with defined geographic areas that contribute to social vulnerability. These "place-based strategies," which often fall in the realm of community development, are discussed in Chapter 9.

RESEARCH NEEDS

In the process of developing its guidance and recommendation specific to social services, the committee noted that further research is needed to address the following questions:

- How does early identification of and support for vulnerable populations reduce long-term psychological consequences or long-term recovery needs?
- How can the social services system maintain a healthy workforce and optimize its utilization after disaster? What percentage of workers can an agency expect to lose as a result of trauma, loss, burnout, or family needs?
- What training do event-based volunteers need to be able to support the social services system? What types of tasks are appropriate for volunteers? How can faith-based and other NGOs be mobilized in pre-disaster recovery planning?
- What strategies can be promoted to facilitate information sharing during and after disasters?
- What are the long-term impacts to beneficiaries of government assistance and their families when a disaster causes disruptions in benefits?

SUMMARY OF FINDINGS AND RECOMMENDATION

The current provision of post-disaster social services is fragmented and episodic and lacks flexibility, with components of the system too often working in isolation. Further, social services are not adequately integrated with other sectors, such as emergency management and public health, at the state and local levels. This fragmented structure creates a lack of continuity of care and reduces the ability of governmental and nongovernmental organizations at all levels to provide effective services, resulting in inefficiency and suboptimal health outcomes. Although HHS's Human Services CONOPS is a commendable step forward in terms of coordination at the federal level, the lack of federal guidance for coordination of activities and resources at the state and local levels remains a critical gap. The committee concludes that an integrated social services recovery framework is needed to enable intra- and intersector coordination that can meet post-disaster human recovery needs and link effective practices to funding sources.

Recommendation 9: *Develop an Integrated Social Services Recovery Framework.*

The U.S. Department of Health and Human Services should lead the development of an integrated post-disaster social services framework that more effectively meets human services needs during recovery.

The following steps should be taken to enable the development of the framework:

- ASPR should commission a study to analyze federal programs related to disaster recovery social services and to generate recommendations for decreasing duplication and fragmentation, streamlining processes, and optimally meeting the needs of the affected populations.
- Based on the results of this study, ASPR should work with federal and nonfederal partners—including but not limited to FEMA, HHS (including ACF, SAMHSA, and the Health Resources and Services Administration), HUD, the U.S. Department of Agriculture, the U.S. Department of Education, the U.S. Department of Veterans Affairs, the American Red Cross, and other appropriate nongovernmental organizations—to create a framework linking current and future funding sources, policies, and regulations to the recommended strategies for optimizing social services after disasters.
- The multiple federal agencies and nongovernmental organizations that provide day-to-day funding for human services and funding to support social services during recovery (including those agencies cited above) should condition funding on the creation by each state or municipality (in cases where large municipalities receive funding directly) of an integrated strategy for social service delivery. This strategy should be designed to facilitate the accessibility of these services through such means as collocation of services and data portability for disaster survivors.
- Departments responsible for human/social services within states and municipalities should serve as the coordinators for operationalizing the above strategy and coordinating faith-based and other nongovernmental organizations, and related state agencies implementing the post-disaster social services framework.

SOCIAL SERVICES SECTOR RECOVERY CHECKLIST

The committee has identified three pre-event and five post-disaster critical recovery priorities for the social services sector that are inextricably linked to strengthening the health, resilience, and sustainability, of a community. Action steps for each of these priorities are provided in the following checklist. Although social services leaders will need to adapt these actions to the local context, this guidance provides an indicative set of concerns to be considered during recovery. Although the committee has suggested a primary actor for each priority area, it is recognized that individual circumstances in each community will influence the actual choice of a lead entity. The checklist illustrates how the following seven key recovery strategies, identified as recurring themes at the beginning of this chapter, apply to individual priority areas:

- Build on existing relationships and establish comprehensive plans for collaboration among social service funders and providers, community- and faith-based organizations, and advocates to ensure coordinated social service delivery through all phases of disaster planning and recovery.
- Integrate social services recovery plans into other disaster recovery services.
- Create compatible structures, policies, and procedures to promote the flow of funding and information across federal, state, and local systems.
- Provide support to reunite families and promote resilience through community programming designed to strengthen social support networks.
- Focus on restoring normalcy through key community services/activities, such as child care, elder care, foster care, mental health services, schools, housing, jobs, and transportation.
- Enhance efforts to increase accessibility and reach the most vulnerable populations to provide needed social services.
- Promote ongoing evaluation and continuous learning to advance social services efforts in achieving health community goals.

Pre-Event

Priority: Establish Forums for Coordination and Collaboration for Disaster Planning and Recovery

Primary Actors[1]: Social Services Agencies
Key Partners: Disaster Relief Organizations, Education System, State/Local Health Departments,[2] Community Development Organizations, Housing Agencies, Transportation Agencies, Health and Medical System Partners, Emergency Management Agencies, Community- and Faith-Based Organizations, Private Sector

Key Recovery Strategies:
- Build on existing relationships and establish comprehensive plans for collaboration among social service funders and providers, community- and faith-based organizations, and advocates to ensure coordinated social service delivery through all phases of disaster planning and recovery.
- Integrate social services recovery plans into other disaster recovery services.
- Create compatible structures, policies, and procedures to promote the flow of funding and information across federal, state, and local systems.

Activities include but are not limited to:
- ☐ Identify program areas within social services where alignments and relationships exist.
- ☐ Identify existing cross-sector, cross-agency collaborations that can be leveraged for recovery planning.
- ☐ Identify essential partners that are not yet but need to be collaborating and work to engage them.
- ☐ Establish relationship with urban and regional planning and community development organizations to integrate disaster recovery planning into ongoing planning efforts.
- ☐ Identify/update key contacts within each partner organization and develop a communication system (based on the above four activities).
- ☐ Integrate representatives of vulnerable populations and elected officials and community leaders in collaborative efforts.
- ☐ Educate elected officials and community leaders, in conjunction with urban and regional planners, on the elements of a healthy and resilient community and the important opportunity to use recovery efforts to achieve healthy community goals.
- ☐ Integrate forums into the National Disaster Recovery Framework to leverage activities/resources/contacts.
- ☐ Develop structures, policies, and procedures to facilitate collaborative efforts, promote information sharing, and foster compatible cultures within partner organizations (including the development of memorandums of understanding [MOUs] and mutual-aid agreements, where appropriate).
- ☐ Enhance regulatory and accreditation requirements for more intensive pre-event recovery planning by local and state social services agencies, health and medical system partners, behavioral health authorities, public health agencies, and local and state emergency management agencies using standard criteria.

---

[1] See Appendix F for further description of terms used to describe Primary Actors and Key Partners in this checklist.
[2] Throughout this checklist, "State/Local" is used for the purposes of brevity but should be inferred to include tribal and territorial as well.

Pre-Event

☐ Pre-identify priority essential services to be provided during recovery and areas in which recovery resources can be used to develop new programs for improving social services.

- -

Priority: Establish Mechanisms to Facilitate Record and Information Sharing After Disasters

Primary Actors: Social Services Agencies
Key Partners: Health and Medical System Partners, Behavioral Health Authorities, Community Development Organizations, Housing Agencies, Community- and Faith-Based Organizations, Community Data Centers

Key Recovery Strategies:
- Build on existing relationships and establish comprehensive plans for collaboration among social service funders and providers, community- and faith-based organizations, and advocates to ensure coordinated social service delivery through all phases of disaster planning and recovery.
- Integrate social services recovery plans into other disaster recovery services.
- Create compatible structures, policies, and procedures to promote the flow of funding and information across federal, state, and local systems.

Activities include but are not limited to:
☐ Review all existing social services data sources and relationships.
☐ Examine opportunities for access by social services agencies to electronic records from clinical and other relevant service agencies and organizations, community- and faith-based organizations, and providers.
☐ Develop strategies for addressing current challenges to sharing information in post-disaster scenarios.
☐ Determine key metrics to be used after a disaster to measure social services needs and resources required to move toward a healthy community model.
☐ Develop disaster social services data needs related to metrics in the pre-disaster environment.
☐ Proactively engage in planning for information technology infrastructure to connect data sets relevant to social services, and develop data-sharing policies across agencies and organizations.
☐ Define how current analyses and reports can support recovery planning, and develop new reports to inform recovery planning if needed.
☐ Share data with disaster recovery planners, elected officials and community leaders, governmental agencies, community- and faith-based organizations, and the community.

- -

Priority: Plan for Fluctuations in Social Services Workforce Needs

Primary Actors: Social Services Agencies

Pre-Event

Key Partners: Disaster Relief Organizations (including American Red Cross), Community- and Faith-Based Organizations, Community Development Organizations, Behavioral Health Authorities, Education System

Key Recovery Strategies:
- Build on existing relationships and establish comprehensive plans for collaboration among social service funders and providers, community- and faith-based organizations, and advocates to ensure coordinated social service delivery through all phases of disaster planning and recovery.
- Enhance efforts to increase accessibility and reach the most vulnerable populations to provide needed social services.
- Integrate social services recovery plans into other disaster recovery services.
- Promote ongoing evaluation and continuous learning to advance social services efforts in achieving health community goals.

Activities include but are not limited to:
- ☐ Provide caseworker training on special post-disaster issues (e.g., insurance and mortgage issues, loss of documentation), as well as typical social services needs (which will be amplified after a disaster).
- ☐ Provide cross-training for multiorganizational staff, volunteers, and partners.
- ☐ Create policies and systems to support the social services workforce during/after disasters to mitigate strain on these workers.
- ☐ Promote disaster mental health training and psychological first aid to help staff identify stressors in themselves and coworkers.
- ☐ Create guidance and training materials addressing disaster impacts on social services, as well as the value of a healthy community approach.
- ☐ Exercise and train for recovery activities.
- ☐ Exploit cross-cutting activities for accreditation and social services emergency planning.
- ☐ Develop social services department continuity of operations plans that enable impacted jurisdictions to rapidly overcome damage and engage in recovery efforts by using social services department staff or social services staff from other jurisdictions and volunteers.
- ☐ Identify sources that can supplement the social services workforce, and develop MOUs with community- and faith-based organizations with relevant social services skills.
- ☐ Identify sources for post-disaster financial support for social services, including businesses seeking to invest in community workforce development.
- ☐ Identify potential new vulnerable populations based on experience with past disasters.
- ☐ Promote and develop capacity for rapid assessment of social services consistent with local and state emergency response and recovery plans, and provide training on post-disaster community assessments.
- ☐ Train health and medical system partners and emergency management agencies regarding social services assessments during recovery efforts, with special consideration for vulnerable and difficult-to-reach populations, such as the elderly and immigrants.
- ☐ Routinely include social services personnel in local, regional, state, and national disaster exercises.
- ☐ Develop standards for communication with and vetting, coordination, and tracking of volunteers, and develop plans for preventing post-disaster burnout.

Short-Term Recovery

Priority: Conduct Impact Assessments and Establish Critical Social Services to Meet Basic Human Needs

Primary Actors: Social Services Agencies
Key Partners: State/Local Health Departments, Housing Agencies, Private Sector, Community- and Faith-Based Organizations

Key Recovery Strategies:
- Build on existing relationships and establish comprehensive plans for collaboration among social services funders and providers, community- and faith-based organizations, and advocates to ensure coordinated social service delivery through all phases of disaster planning and recovery.
- Integrate social services recovery plans into other disaster recovery services.
- Provide support to reunite families and promote resilience through community programming designed to strengthen social support networks.
- Focus on restoring normalcy through key community services/activities, such as child care, elder care, foster care, mental health services, schools, housing, jobs, and transportation.
- Enhance efforts to increase accessibility and reach the most vulnerable populations to provide needed social services.
- Promote ongoing evaluation and continuous learning to advance social services efforts in achieving health community goals.

Activities include but are not limited to:
- ☐ Participate in a recovery joint information system staffed by representatives from all engaged sectors.
- ☐ Assess the impact of the disaster on social services and resources needed using metrics developed in the planning phase.
- ☐ Coordinate with mass recovery sites to provide social services that meet survivors' basic needs (food, shelter, clothing, and medical prescriptions and supplies).
- ☐ Maintain early warning tracking systems to monitor increases in mental health, domestic violence, and other disaster-impacted issues.
- ☐ Establish guidelines for promoting accessibility of social services for all residents.
- ☐ Develop multimodal communication strategies for people in need of services and people who want to donate or volunteer (in multiple languages).
- ☐ Map available resources for:
  - shelter and housing,
  - food and water distribution,
  - medical care,
  - medical supplies and medications,
  - basic living supplies, and
  - behavioral health support.
- ☐ Develop a communication system to provide information on these resources.
- ☐ Identify opportunities for generating additional resources.
- ☐ Coordinate with other disaster-related activities and resources (e.g., housing coalition, medical providers/advocates, schools, transportation).
- ☐ Focus on reuniting families, neighbors, and those with social ties who have been separated.
- ☐ Provide ongoing training for social services providers on post-disaster mass care services.

Short-Term Recovery

☐ Integrate social services messages with general emergency management messages related to ongoing recovery efforts, focusing on accessibility for items/services that meet basic human needs.

- -

Priority: Facilitate Access to Disaster Assistance Resources and Provide Disaster Case Management

Primary Actors: Social Services Agencies
Key Partners: State/Local Health Departments, Health and Medical System Partners, Emergency Management Agencies, Community- and Faith-Based Organizations

Key Recovery Strategies:
- Build on existing relationships and establish comprehensive plans for collaboration among social service funders and providers, community- and faith-based organizations, and advocates to ensure coordinated social service delivery through all phases of disaster planning and recovery.
- Integrate social services recovery plans into other disaster recovery services.
- Create compatible structures, policies, and procedures to promote the flow of funding and information across federal, state, and local systems.
- Provide support to reunite families and promote resilience through community programming designed to strengthen social support networks.
- Focus on restoring normalcy through key community services/activities, such as child care, elder care, foster care, mental health services, schools, housing, jobs, and transportation.
- Enhance efforts to increase accessibility and reach the most vulnerable populations to provide needed social services.
- Promote ongoing evaluation and continuous learning to advance social services efforts in achieving health community goals.

Activities include but are not limited to:
☐ Activate or consider forming a long-term recovery committee to assist in decision making on the allocation of funding for meeting the unmet needs of individuals and families.
☐ Reach out to vulnerable and low-income families with information on disaster benefits and services using client contact information from governmental assistance programs such as Temporary Assistance for Needy Families, Head Start, and the local housing authority.
☐ Develop strategies for reaching the expanded population of vulnerable people created by the disaster.
☐ Work closely with community supports such as schools, neighborhood associations, community centers, civic groups, and faith-based organizations, all of which play a major role in creating an environment in which problems are readily identified and access to services is facilitated.
☐ Contact legal services organizations and private legal practitioners with appropriate expertise to assist with benefit eligibility issues.
☐ Identify and provide local resources to assist people with difficulty in producing the documents required to qualify for governmental and nongovernmental relief programs.

Short-Term Recovery

(Documentation often is destroyed or unavailable because of such issues as relocation, and federal disaster relief programs do not allow funds to be used for obtaining new copies of documents.)

☐ Work with immigrant support groups to assist immigrant populations that may not seek assistance because of fear of deportation. Undocumented families are ineligible for Federal Emergency Management Agency (FEMA) Individual Assistance, so they are susceptible to especially difficult recovery.

☐ Recruit bilingual volunteers, have signage in all languages represented in the community, and provide telephone translation/interpreter services.

☐ As the recovery process continues, intake workers and disaster case managers identify those households with unmet needs to be referred to the long-term recovery committee.

☐ Implement special measures to help clients overcome barriers to access to disaster assistance resources.

☐ Tap community- and faith-based organizations to disseminate information about available resources.

☐ Create a website to serve as a clearinghouse for community resources, information, and key contacts for assistance.

☐ Collocate service providers in the same facility, if possible.

☐ Collect and compile service restoration timelines from key social services and health and medical system partners.

Intermediate- to Long-Term Recovery

Priority: Promote Social Services Strategies That Can Help Clients Manage Chronic Health Conditions and Build Self-Sufficiency

Primary Actors: Social Services Agencies
Key Partners: State/Local Health Departments, Housing Agencies, Behavioral Health Authorities, Health and Medical System Partners, Federal Agencies (including SAMHSA and ACF), Community- and Faith-Based Organizations

Key Recovery Strategies:
- Build on existing relationships and establish comprehensive plans for collaboration among social service funders and providers, community- and faith-based organizations, and advocates to ensure coordinated social service delivery through all phases of disaster planning and recovery.
- Create compatible structures, policies, and procedures to promote the flow of funding and information across federal, state, and local systems.
- Provide support to reunite families and promote resilience through community programming designed to strengthen social support networks.
- Focus on restoring normalcy through key community services/activities, such as child care, elder care, foster care, mental health services, schools, housing, jobs, and transportation.
- Enhance efforts to increase accessibility and reach the most vulnerable populations to provide needed social services.
- Promote ongoing evaluation and continuous learning to advance social services efforts in achieving health community goals.

Activities include but are not limited to:
- ☐ As external resources leave the community, identify how the community will meet needs internally, including building secondary surge capacity.
- ☐ Identify sustainable strategies for moving people toward independence.
- ☐ Maintain early warning and tracking systems to monitor increases in mental health disorders, domestic violence, and other disaster-impacted issues.
- ☐ Provide psychosocial and behavioral screening and support through community institutions such as schools, child care centers, elder day care, and health centers.
- ☐ Identify new funding sources—either those that are recovery related or those that are general and can be used to meet recovery goals.
- ☐ Institute strategies designed to strengthen social networks in the community.
- ☐ Develop a community messaging campaign that helps people identify early warning signs of psychosocial/mental health problems and overcome stigma associated with help-seeking behaviors.
- ☐ Build, strengthen, and seek funding for community health worker training programs.
- ☐ Provide support for initiating and sustaining self-help support groups through partnerships between community groups and social services agencies.
- ☐ Develop partnerships among workforce development programs, community colleges, universities, and social services to train and promote hiring of local people to fill recovery-related positions, including community health workers who can assist in chronic disease self-management.
- ☐ Coordinate with health care programs to help reduce reliance on safety-net programs through chronic disease self-management.

Intermediate- to Long-Term Recovery

☐ Develop greater social services workforce capacity in the community to address the social determinants of health and move toward a healthy community model.
☐ Build resiliency by regularly updating organizational and community plans.

- -

Priority: Address the Unique Needs of Children and the Elderly

Primary Actors: Social Services Agencies
Key Partners: State/Local Health Departments, Child Care Organizations, Foster Care and Elder Care Organizations, Urban and Regional Planning Agencies, Education System, Transportation Agencies, Housing Agencies, Community- and Faith-Based Organizations, Health and Medical System Partners (including Nursing Homes)

Key Recovery Strategies:
- Create compatible structures, policies, and procedures to promote the flow of funding and information across federal, state, and local systems.
- Provide support to reunite families and promote resilience through community programming designed to strengthen social support networks.
- Focus on restoring normalcy through key community services/activities, such as child care, elder care, foster care, mental health services, schools, housing, jobs, and transportation.
- Enhance efforts to increase accessibility and reach the most vulnerable populations to provide needed social services.
- Promote ongoing evaluation and continuous learning to advance social services efforts in achieving health community goals.

Activities include but are not limited to (for each care system [child care, foster care, elder care]):
☐ Bring together partner organizations for needs assessment, planning, and implementation, including
  – social services agencies that ensure the availability of resources;
  – state agencies responsible for licensing and administration of subsidy programs for low-income families;
  – local providers of care, including faith-based institutions;
  – local and national funders (e.g., United Way, private foundations, community foundations);
  – local resource and referral agencies;
  – behavioral health professionals to work with sites to deal with disaster-related trauma in staff and clients;
  – community volunteers; and
  – private-sector organizations that need child care services to get the workforce back.

In conjunction with other post-disaster planning efforts and partner organizations:
☐ Determine the status of existing centers and service sites; needs based on the post-disaster environment; and community assets that can be used to support sites in the short term.

Intermediate- to Long-Term Recovery

☐ Consider temporarily waiving some requirements for facilities to enable their reopening.

☐ Identify a process for seeking and applying public and private funding to restore damaged sites or build new ones.

☐ Establish a process for selecting sites that need to be rebuilt.

☐ Use existing information from government assistance programs to follow up with displaced residents and notify them about services.

☐ Work with disaster recovery communication networks to disseminate information about services, job opportunities, and training.

☐ Design/provide training to facilitate the recruitment of new staff and volunteers for sites (based on post-disaster criteria established by state agencies).

☐ Identify priorities needing immediate advocacy to ensure the most inclusive response to the disaster, and identify advocacy allies.

☐ Inform about and advocate for infrastructure investments that will strengthen safety and resilience, such as improved construction standards and energy-efficient standards/ construction.

- -

Priority: Reorganize the Social Services System Toward a Healthy Community Model by Integrating New Strategies and Lessons Learned

Primary Actors: Social Services Agencies

Key Partners: State/Local Health Departments, Housing Agencies, Behavioral Health Authorities, Health and Medical System Partners, Federal Agencies (including SAMHSA and ACF), Community- and Faith-Based Organizations

Key Recovery Strategies:

- Integrate social services recovery plans into other disaster recovery services.
- Enhance efforts to increase accessibility and reach the most vulnerable populations to provide needed social services.
- Promote ongoing evaluation and continuous learning to advance social services efforts in achieving health community goals.

Activities include but are not limited to:

☐ Assist with identifying sources of capital and financing for rebuilding in ways that promote meeting the social service needs of a healthy community.

☐ Participate in an after-action process, including analysis of lessons learned and identification of opportunities for improvement.

☐ Continuously measure progress toward healthy community goals and adapt recovery plans accordingly.

☐ Use state, regional, and national conferences, workshops, and discipline-specific professional meetings to share lessons learned and opportunities for improvement so that other jurisdictions can benefit from recovery experiences.

☐ Disseminate information regarding opportunities for improved social services to the social services sector and other groups, such as the council of mayors, city managers, city councilors, emergency management agencies, and urban and regional planning agencies.

REFERENCES

ACF (Administration for Children and Families). 2005. *Flexibility in spending CCDF funds in response to federal or state declared emergency situations.* http://www.acf.hhs.gov/sites/default/files/occ/im0503_0.pdf (accessed August 8, 2014).

ACF. 2012. *Child Care and Development Fund.* http://www.acf.hhs.gov/programs/occ/resource/child-care-and-development-fund (accessed April 3, 2015).

ACF. 2013a. *SSBG Q&As Hurricane Sandy supplemental FY 2013.* http://www.acf.hhs.gov/programs/ocs/resource/ssbg-qas-2013-sandy-supplemental (accessed August 5, 2014).

ACF. 2013b. *Superstorm Sandy.* http://www.acf.hhs.gov/superstorm-sandy (accessed March 3, 2015).

ACF. 2014. *Social Services Block Grant program (SSBG).* http://www.acf.hhs.gov/programs/ocs/programs/ssbg (accessed August 5, 2014).

ACF. 2015a. *About Community Services Block Grants.* http://www.acf.hhs.gov/programs/ocs/programs/csbg/about (accessed April 3, 2015).

ACF. 2015b. *About SSBG.* http://www.acf.hhs.gov/programs/ocs/programs/ssbg/about (accessed April 3, 2015).

ACF. 2015c. *What we do.* http://www.acf.hhs.gov/programs/ohs/about/what-we-do (accessed April 3, 2015).

AECF (Annie E. Casey Foundation). 2003. *The health of the human services workforce.* http://www.aecf.org/m/resourcedoc/aecf-HealthHumanServicesWorkforce-2003.pdf (accessed November 5, 2014).

Aldrich, D. P. 2012. *Building resilience: Social capital in post-disaster recovery.* Chicago, IL: University of Chicago Press.

ARC (American Red Cross). 2014. *Long-term recovery grants for Superstorm Sandy.* http://www.redcross.org/images/MEDIA_CustomProductCatalog/m39840088_NNJ-sandy-recovery-grants-sheet-sep2014.pdf (accessed November 6, 2014).

Bradley, E. H., and L. A. Taylor. 2013. *The American health care paradox: Why spending more is getting us less.* New York: Public Affairs.

Brown, L. 2014. *Older adults and post-disaster recovery.* Paper presented at IOM Committee on Post-Disaster Recovery of a Community's Public Health, Medical and Social Services: Meeting Two, February 3, Washington, DC.

CAN (Coordinated Assistance Network). 2014a. *Our partners.* http://www.can.org/our-partners (accessed November 5, 2014).

CAN. 2014b. *Our tools.* http://www.can.org/our-tools (accessed November 5, 2014).

CAN. 2014c. *Supported disasters.* https://can.communityos.org/cms/disasters (accessed November 5, 2014).

CDC (Centers for Disease Control and Prevention). 2011. *Addressing chronic disease through community health workers: A policy and systems-level approach.* http://www.cdc.gov/dhdsp/docs/CHW_brief.pdf (accessed August 11, 2014).

CDC and National Council on Aging. 2008. *Review of findings on Chronic Disease Self-Management Program (CDSMP) outcomes: Physical, emotional & health-related quality of life, healthcare utilization and costs.* http://patienteducation.stanford.edu/research/Review_Findings_CDSMP_Outcomes1%208%2008.pdf (accessed August 15, 2014).

CDC Division of Diabetes Translation. 2003. *Community health workers/promotores de salud: Critical connections in communities.* http://www.cdc.gov/diabetes/projects/pdfs/comm.pdf (accessed November 5, 2014).

Cepeda, A., A. Valdez, C. Kaplan, and L. E. Hill. 2010a. Patterns of substance use among Hurricane Katrina evacuees in Houston, Texas. *Disasters* 34(2):426-446.

Cepeda, A., J. M. Saint Onge, C. Kaplan, and A. Valdez. 2010b. The association between disaster-related experiences and mental health outcomes among drug using African American Hurricane Katrina evacuees. *Community Mental Health Journal* 46(6):612-620.

Chan, C. 2013. *The Dallas Information Exchange Portal: New technologies for public health preparedness.* Paper presented at IOM Forum on Medical and Public Preparedness for Catastrophic Events: The Impact of the Affordable Care Act on U.S. Preparedness Resources and Programs: An IOM Workshop, November 18-19, Washington, DC.

Chandra, A., and J. D. Acosta. 2009. *The role of nongovernmental organizations in long-term human recovery after disaster: Reflections from Louisiana four years after Hurricane Katrina.* Santa Monica, CA: RAND Corporation.

Chapman, D. P., G. S. Perry, and T. W. String. 2005. The vital link between chronic disease and depressive disorders. *Preventing Chronic Disease.* http://origin.glb.cdc.gov/pcd/issues/2005/jan/04_0066.htm (accessed November 6, 2014).

CRS (Congressional Research Service). 2012. *Social Services Block Grant: Background and funding.* Washington, DC: CRS, Library of Congress.

CRS. 2014. *Community Development Block Grants and related programs: A primer.* Washington, DC: CRS, Library of Congress.

DHS (U.S. Department of Homeland Security). 2012. *Supplemental resource: Children in disasters guidance.* Washington, DC: DHS.

Enarson, E., and M. Fordham. 2001. Lines that divide, ties that bind: Race, class, and gender in women's flood recovery in the US and UK. *Australian Journal of Emergency Management* 15(4):43-53.

Erickson, D., and N. Andrews. 2011. Partnerships among community development, public health, and health care could improve the well-being of low-income people. *Health Affairs (Millwood)* 30(11):2056-2063.

FEMA (Federal Emergency Management Agency). 2011. *National disaster recovery framework.* Washington, DC: FEMA.

FEMA. 2013. *National response framework.* Washington, DC: U.S. Department of Homeland Security.

FEMA. 2014. *Fact sheet: Disaster case management.* https://s3-us-gov-west-1.amazonaws.com/dam-production/uploads/1400186513405-1e9c8c2fb88eb30d399d0e1345c56885/FactSheet%20DCM%20-%20April%202014.pdf (accessed November 5, 2014).

FYSB (Family and Youth Services Bureau). 2015. *Family Violence Prevention and Services Program.* http://www.acf.hhs.gov/programs/fysb/programs/family-violence-prevention-services (accessed March 25, 2015).

Gerber, S. 2006. Disaster recovery for low-income people: Lessons from the Grand Forks flood. *Community Dividend* (September). http://www.minneapolisfed.org/publications_papers/pub_display.cfm?id=2198 (accessed November 6, 2014).

GuideStar. 2014. *Directory of charities and nonprofit organizations.* http://www.guidestar.org/nonprofit-directory/human-services.aspx (accessed November 5, 2014).

HHS (U.S. Department of Health and Human Services). 2012. *Hurricane Sandy—public health situation updates.* http://www.phe.gov/newsroom/Pages/situpdates.aspx (accessed March 3, 2015).

HHS. 2014a. *Disaster Human Services Concept of Operations (CONOPS).* Washington, DC: HHS.

HHS. 2014b. *HIPAA privacy in emergency situations.* Washington, DC: HHS.

Hipper, T., A. Orr, and E. Chernak. 2013. *Ensuring the delivery of human services in disasters: A white paper for Southeastern Pennsylvania.* http://unitedforimpact.org/uploads/about/publications-and-reports/HSA-White-Paper.pdf (accessed November 5, 2014).

HRSA (Health Resources and Services Administration). 2011. *Community health workers evidence-based models toolbox.* http://www.hrsa.gov/ruralhealth/pdf/CHWtoolkit.pdf (accessed August 11, 2014).

HUD (U.S. Department of Housing and Urban Development). 2014. *Community Development Block Grant Disaster Recovery program.* https://www.hudexchange.info/cdbg-dr (accessed March 23, 2015).

IOM (Institute of Medicine). 2014. *Capturing social and behavioral domains in electronic health records: Phase 1.* Washington, DC: The National Academies Press.

The Jesse Tree. 2015. *About us.* http://www.jessetree.net/about-us.asp (accessed February 26, 2015).

Kanter, R. K., and D. Abramson. 2014. School interventions after the Joplin tornado. *Prehospital and Disaster Medicine* 29(2):214-217.

Kessler, R. C. 2007. Hurricane Katrina's impact on the care of survivors with chronic medical conditions. *Journal of General Internal Medicine* 22(9):1225-1230.

Leutz, W. N. 1999. Five laws for integrating medical and social services. *Milbank Quarterly* 77(1):77-110.

MacDonald, R. 2005. How women were affected by the tsunami: A perspective from Oxfam. *PLoS Medicine* 2(6):e178.

Meeds, D. 2013. *Joplin pays it forward.* http://joplincc.com/Joplin%20Pays%20It%20Forward%20-%20Community%20Leaders%20Share%20Our%20Recovery%20Lessons.pdf (accessed February 26, 2015).

Microsoft Case Studies. 2010. *Boulder County: County deploys collaborative social services tool, wait times drop from weeks to hours.* http://www.microsoft.com/casestudies/Case_Study_Detail.aspx?CaseStudyID=4000008098 (accessed November 5, 2014).

Missouri Department of Mental Health. 2013. *Stories from healing Joplin.* http://dmh.mo.gov/docs/opla/storiesfromhealingjoplin.pdf (accessed November 5, 2014).

National Mass Care Strategy. 2014. *Training and exercises.* http://nationalmasscarestrategy.org/resource-center/training-and-exercises (accessed November 6, 2014).

National Philanthropic Trust. 2014. *Charitable giving statistics.* http://www.nptrust.org/philanthropic-resources/charitable-giving-statistics (accessed November 5, 2014).

National VOAD (Voluntary Organizations Active in Disaster). 2012. *Long term recovery guide.* Alexandria, VA: National VOAD.

NCDP (National Center for Disaster Preparedness). 2013. *At the crossroads of long-term recovery: Joplin, Missouri six months after the May 22, 2011.* New York: Earth Institute, Columbia University.

NIEHS (National Institute of Environmental Health Sciences). 2014. *Minority Worker Training Program: Guidance on how to achieve successes and best practices.* http://www.niehs.nih.gov/research/supported/dert/programs/peph/materials/assets/docs/minority_worker_training_program_guidance_on_how_to_achieve_successes_and_best_practices.pdf (accessed November 6, 2014).

NJ DCF (State of New Jersey Department of Children and Families). 2013. Domestic violence and disasters. http://nj.gov/dcf/home/Domestic%20Violence%20and%20Disasters%20with%20Sources.pdf (accessed April 3, 2015).

Nolen, A. 2014. *A Health in All Policies approach to disaster recovery: Lessons from Galveston.* Paper presented at IOM Committee on Post-Disaster Recovery of a Community's Public Health, Medical, and Social Services: Meeting Four, June 13, Washington, DC.

Pipes, P. F., and H. R. Ebaugh. 2002. Faith-based coalitions, social services, and government funding. *Sociology of Religion* 63(1):49-68.

Regier, D. A., M. E. Farmer, D. S. Rae, B. Z. Locke, S. J. Keith, L. L. Judd, and F. K. Goodwin. 1990. Comorbidity of mental disorders with alcohol and other drug abuse. Results from the Epidemiologic Catchment Area (ECA) Study. *Journal of the American Medical Association* 264(19):2511-2518.

Rodriguez, J. 2013. *How legal aid of Western Missouri is helping the community recover from the Joplin tornado.* http://povertylaw.org/communication/advocacy-stories/rodriguez (accessed November 5, 2014).

RWJF (Robert Wood Johnson Foundation). 2008. *Overcoming obstacles to health.* Princeton, NJ: RWJF. http://www.rwjf.org/content/dam/farm/reports/reports/2008/rwjf22441 (accessed October 12, 2014).

SAMHSA (Substance Abuse and Mental Health Services Administration). 2012. *Cultural awareness: Children and disasters.* http://www.samhsa.gov/sites/default/files/podcasts-cultural-awareness-presentation.pdf (accessed November 5, 2014).

SAMHSA. 2015. *Substance abuse and mental health block grants.* http://www.samhsa.gov/grants/block-grants (accessed April 3, 2015).

Sauer, L. M., C. Catlett, R. Tosatto, and T. D. Kirsch. 2014. The utility of and risks associated with the use of spontaneous volunteers in disaster response: A survey. *Disaster Medicine and Public Health Preparedness* 8(1):65-69.

Smith, M. 2008. *Building an interoperable human services system: How Allegheny County transformed systems, services and outcomes for vulnerable children and families.* http://www.alleghenycounty.us/uploadedFiles/DHS/SOC_Building_Interoperable_Human_Services_System-10-30-08.pdf (accessed November 5, 2014).

Social Solutions. 2014. *ETO collaborate.* http://www.socialsolutions.com/case-management-software-products/human-services-database-software (accessed November 5, 2014).

Stanford School of Medicine. 2014. *Stanford Patient Education Research Center.* http://patienteducation.stanford.edu (accessed August 14, 2014).

The Urban Institute. 2006. *Findings from a survey of 9/11-affected clients served by the American Red Cross September 11 Recovery Program.* http://www.urban.org/UploadedPDF/411335_redcross_survey.pdf (accessed November 6, 2014).

White, J. 2014. *Post-disaster social services and health outcomes in recovery.* Paper presented at IOM Committee on Post-Disaster Recovery of a Community's Public Health, Medical, and Social Services: Meeting Two, February 3, Washington, DC.

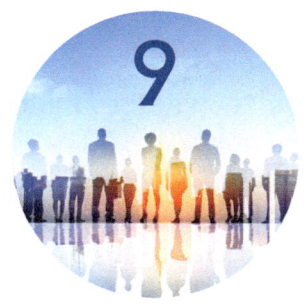

Place-Based Recovery Strategies
for Healthy Communities

Consider that Detroit, an area of 139 square miles and over 900,000 citizens, has just five grocery stores. An apple a day may help keep the doctor away but that assumes you can find an apple in your neighborhood.

—James Marks, Robert Wood Johnson Foundation (Marks, 2009)

As discussed in Chapter 2, the concept of "place matters" has grown in recent years, with many health departments and community groups around the country realizing the connection between health status and social determinants such as transportation, housing, and education. As noted by the Robert Wood Johnson Foundation in *Time to Act*, "place-based differences in health are strongly linked with differences in people's incomes, educational attainment, and racial or ethnic group" (RWJF, 2014, p. 32). The World Health Organization defines social determinants of health more broadly as "the conditions in which people are born, grow, live, work and age, including the health system. These circumstances are shaped by the distribution of money, power and resources at global, national and local levels, which are themselves influenced by policy choices. Social determinants of health are mostly responsible for health inequities—the unfair and avoidable differences in health status seen within and between countries" (WHO, 2014).

As an example of action to combat some of these place-based health inequities, the Boston Public Health Commission operationalized the concept in 2010 when it launched an interactive "What's Your Health Code" website to show the variations in health throughout the city depending on the neighborhood and to bring awareness to health equity needs (Boston Public Health Commission, 2010). Other cities have employed various place-based strategies,[1] some of which are discussed throughout this chapter, to improve the physical and social environments in communities in hopes of improving the health status of their residents (see Box 9-1 for differences between place-based and people-based interventions). "Place-based policies leverage investments by focusing resources in targeted places and drawing on the compounding effect of well-coordinated action. Effective place-based policies can influence how rural and metropolitan

---

[1] It is important to note that although place-based strategies are geographically targeted, they are not limited to alterations of the physical environment. Place-based strategies often also address the social and economic environments of a community.

BOX 9-1
Place- Versus People-Based Interventions

Although there are a number of ways to define place- versus people-based interventions, the terms are used here as follows:

Place-based—encompasses "real estate- and infrastructure-based activities, including affordable housing preservation and development, commercial development, green space set-asides and improvements, and community facilities including charter schools, health centers, day and elder care centers, and community centers devoted to other community activities and gatherings; transit, communications, and energy improvements."

People-based—encompasses "child care and job training and placement to enable adults to work and improve their incomes, savings and homeownership programs to help people build assets (but not tied to housing development or rehabilitation), early childhood interventions and charter school services intended to narrow educational achievement gaps, small business development and lending for economic development, community policing and safety, community organizing, and social case work to address special needs like addiction or disabilities or reentry after incarceration."

People-based interventions are discussed in more detail in Chapter 8.

SOURCE: Belsky and Fauth, 2012, p. 76.

areas develop, and how well they function as places to live, work, operate a business, preserve heritage, and more. Such policies can also streamline otherwise redundant and disconnected programs" (The White House, 2009).

While coordinated, place-based initiatives are strong in theory and academic support, they can be difficult to achieve in practice because of the need for robust collaboration across community agencies, as well as sometimes-significant reallocation of funding. Disaster recovery also requires multi-agency coordination and long-term planning, but it can sometimes be accompanied by more funding and fewer restrictions. Combining these areas of practice and intertwining their goals and policies can have an increased collective impact on a community's progress toward becoming healthy, resilient, and sustainable. This chapter outlines the evidence behind these theories while highlighting real-life examples that illustrate the effect these types of initiatives can have in practice—both in normal times and during recovery from a disaster.

During this study and throughout its deliberations, the committee identified key place-based recovery strategies that appear as recurring themes throughout this chapter and cut across multiple sectors involved in planning, transportation, sustainability, health, and community development. Application of these strategies, which apply to multiple pre- and post-disaster activities, will facilitate the protection and promotion of health as a community works to meet physical, social, and infrastructure needs after a disaster:

- Reduce health disparities and improve access to essential goods, services, and opportunities.
- Preserve and promote social connectedness.
- Use a systems approach to community redevelopment that acknowledges the connection among social, cultural, economic, and physical environments.
- Seek holistic solutions to socioeconomic disparities and their perverse effects on population health through place-based interventions.
- Rebuild for resilience and sustainability.

- Capitalize on existing planning networks to strengthen recovery planning, including attention to public health, medical, and social services, especially for vulnerable populations.

The chapter concludes with a checklist of key activities that need to be performed during each of the phases of recovery.

A SYSTEMS VIEW OF A HEALTHY COMMUNITY

As discussed in Chapter 2, viewing a community from a systems perspective can help in considering options for rebuilding and holistic recovery. Healthy behaviors do not occur in isolation within a community, so it is important to consider connections among a society's social, cultural, economic, and physical elements. Simply building a park and a walking trail for residents may not be successful if the trail is not well lit or the park is in an area plagued by crime. In addition to examining how these different systems intersect, it is important to consider how residents in a community are able to access those systems. Rebuilding after a disaster is an opportunity to give these elements a fresh look.

There is growing consensus on the elements that help build a healthy and sustainable community (see Box 2-2 in Chapter 2). This chapter examines some of those elements in the context of the physical and social environments of a community. Specifically, these elements can include clean air, parks and green spaces, a sustainable transportation grid promoting active living, access to nutritious food and clean water, safe communities free of violence, and accessible and integrated community services that can contribute to increased social cohesion. How communities are structured and how public transportation, health care, and social services are built within a city often can dictate the level of access residents have to these and other community services and features. When these elements are not present in a community or their integration is not well designed, making access strained or difficult, adverse health effects can result. The following section expands on this evidence.

The Impact of Place on Health

The environment in which a person lives influences health in countless ways. The natural and built environments of a community can promote the health of its residents by providing opportunities for physical activity, clean air and water, safe roadways, and access to healthy food and essential services; as noted above, the absence of these elements can hinder health. The physical environment is heavily influenced by a community's social environment. Neighborhoods with high concentrations of racial minorities or low-income families tend to lack elements that promote health, such as opportunities for activity, and contain elements that hinder health, such as pollution from highways or factories.

Physical Activity and the Environment

Regular physical activity can help reduce or maintain body weight; reduce the risk of cardiovascular disease, diabetes, and some cancers; improve mental health; and increase life expectancy (CDC, 2011). Unfortunately, fewer than half of U.S. adults meet the recommended guideline of 150 minutes of moderate activity per week (CDC, 2014a). Chronic diseases associated with a lack of physical activity plague millions of Americans: more than one-third of adults and 17 percent of children are obese (Ogden et al., 2014), 29.1 million have diabetes (CDC, 2014c), and one in four deaths each year are due to heart disease (Murphy et al., 2013). Inactivity's burden on the health care system is sizable, with one study estimating the aggregate national cost of overweight and obesity at $113.9 billion (Tsai et al., 2011).

Communities that include parks, sidewalks, and public transit give residents opportunities to be active and can make activity safer and more appealing (Williams, 2007). For example, physical activity levels are higher for people who live near recreational facilities—parks, playgrounds, sports facilities (Sallis et al., 2012)—or whose neighborhood sidewalks are well maintained (Kwarteng et al., 2013). Walking and biking for transportation are increased when neighborhoods are more densely populated, use a grid pattern, and have commercial areas within walking distance (Transportation Research Board, 2005). People who use public transportation are more active than those who do not, and 29 percent of those who use transit meet the recommended activity level of 150 minutes per week by simply walking to and from transit (Sallis et al., 2012).

When the Austin, Texas, airport was relocated in 1999, the community of Mueller, Texas, was left with 700 acres of what could have been unused space (Mueller, 2014). Instead, Mueller is being redeveloped as a mixed-use urban village as a joint project with the city of Austin. Following a Texas A&M study sponsored by the American Institute of Architects, researchers found that nearly three of four residents reported more physical activity after joining the new community. They found that such elements as sidewalks, parks, open space, and bike routes, along with diverse uses and destinations, supported more physical and social activity (ULI, 2013).

Air and Water Pollution

John Snow famously demonstrated the link between environment and health when he mapped the public wells in his London neighborhood along with the location of cholera deaths. Noticing a cluster around one particular well, he lobbied local authorities to remove the handle from the pump, and the outbreak subsided. Today, environmental threats to communities include particulate air pollution associated with motor vehicle traffic and industrial facilities, and poor water quality related to stormwater management.

Air becomes polluted with particles when mechanical or chemical processes—such as construction, agriculture, or burning of fossil fuels in cars or factories—create tiny particles of chemicals, metals, and other pollutants that are inhaled. This pollution is linked to short- and long-term health issues including respiratory and cardiovascular diseases, cancer, inflammation of lung tissue, exacerbation of asthma, infant mortality, and decreased life expectancy (State of the Air, 2013). The air quality of a community is influenced by its characteristics; for example, industrial plants or large agriculture operations in a community will produce particulate pollutants, while motor vehicles contribute to more than 50 percent of the air pollution in urban areas (CDC, 2009). Altering the built environment of a community to eliminate or diminish these elements may reduce pollution. For example, to accommodate the visitors to the 1996 Olympic Games, Atlanta developed an extensive public transportation system, encouraged telecommuting, and closed the downtown to private automobiles. As a result, peak weekday morning traffic was reduced by 22.5 percent, and there were measurable decreases in air levels of ozone, carbon monoxide, and nitrogen dioxide. During this time period, the number of children seeking acute care or hospitalization for asthma events was significantly reduced (Friedman et al., 2001). This example starkly demonstrates the close relationship among environment, pollution, and health and suggests that changes in the community environment can have an immediate impact on residents' health. Using "green," or environmentally friendly, infrastructure also can lower air temperatures, which is valuable in tightly packed urban areas that suffer from the "urban heat island" effect (ASLA, 2010). Another study found that large numbers of trees and green spaces throughout a city can reduce the local air temperature by 1-5 degrees Celsius (McPherson, 1994).

The water quality in a community is affected in part by stormwater management. Stormwater runoff can pollute drinking and recreational water with harmful pathogens such as *Cryptosporidium*, *Giardia*, and *E. coli*, as well as pollutants such as heavy metals, insecticides, and excess nitrogen. While community drinking water is usually treated, several common microorganisms are resistant to treatment and remain in the water (Gaffield et al., 2003). These waterborne pathogens can cause illness and death. In Milwaukee, for example, an outbreak of *Cryptosporidium* spread via the public water supply and sickened 403,000 people (Mac Kenzie et al., 1994) and contributed to the deaths of 54 people (Hoxie et al., 1997). Contamination by stormwater runoff is more likely when a community has large impervious surface areas, such as roads and parking lots (Gaffield et al., 2003). Runoff can be controlled, and water contamination reduced, by adding such features as green parking lots, grassed swales, permeable pavement, and vegetation. These types of "green infrastructure" allow stormwater to be absorbed by the ground rather than into the city water system or a nearby waterway. A program in Michigan, for example, diverted roof downspouts into yards rather than into the sewer system. This simple change reduced the flow of stormwater into sewers by up to 62 percent, thus reducing both the cost of water treatment and potential contamination (Kaufman and Wurtz, 1997). Green absorbent infrastructure, while aesthetically pleasing, also can be the most cost-effective way to manage stormwater, in addition to appreciating in value over time and providing multiple uses (Francis, 2010). Elements such as rain gardens or green roofs can mitigate flooding and pollution of the aquifer. One inch of rainwater hitting 1 acre of asphalt produces 27,000 gallons of stormwater over the course of 1 hour (Elmendorf, 2008).

Injuries Associated with Unsafe Streets

Millions of people are injured or killed each year on the nation's roads. In 2013, 26,491 drivers or passengers and 5,552 pedestrians or cyclists died in traffic crashes (NHTSA, 2014). While many of these injuries and deaths are attributable to individual error, some are due to unsafe road conditions, including roadway design, maintenance, and such features as lighting and crosswalks. A study by the National Highway Traffic Safety Administration (NHTSA) found that 16.3 percent of motor vehicle crashes involved at least one roadway-related factor—roadway condition, view obstruction, geometry of the road, narrow shoulder or road, or missing traffic signs (NHTSA, 2008). Another NHTSA study found that 24 percent of nonfatal pedestrian injuries were due to tripping on cracked or uneven sidewalks, and 13 percent of nonfatal cyclist injuries occurred because the roadway was not in good repair (NHTSA, 2012). Pedestrian safety can be improved not only by maintaining sidewalks but also by using crosswalks with traffic signals, raised medians, and traffic-calming measures such as curb extensions and lane reductions (FHWA, 2005). In short, the condition and design of a community's roads can contribute greatly to the safety and well-being of its residents.

Hazard Risk

The natural and built features of a community can dramatically affect its ability to withstand and recover from disasters. Natural protective land features such as sand dunes, wetlands, and barrier islands can blunt the impact of a storm or hurricane and protect inland areas from flooding and damage. The design of the built environment—including homes, buildings, and infrastructure—is a critical factor in the health and safety of residents during and after a disaster. It has been said that "earthquakes don't kill people—buildings do" (FEMA, 2014a). Residences and buildings that are well built and well maintained can help keep residents safe from seismic activity, fire, flooding, and strong winds. In addition, if facilities such as water treatment and power plants are not sufficiently disaster-resilient, the loss of these critical services can make disaster response and recovery even more difficult. For example, millions of residents in New York City lost power during Hurricane Sandy as a result of storm-related damage and flooding. Many residents—including those in the city's public housing—were without power for more than 2 weeks, during which time they lacked electricity for such essentials as heat and medical devices (Rexrode and Dobnik, 2012).

Health Disparities

Health disparities are "preventable differences in the burden of disease, injury, violence, or opportunities to achieve optimal health that are experienced by socially disadvantaged populations" (CDC, 2013a). Socially disadvantaged populations—such as those of lower socioeconomic status or racial minorities—bear a disproportionate burden of disease and death. African Americans, for example, have higher rates of premature death, infant mortality, obesity, and homicide than their white counterparts, and poor people are more likely to suffer from asthma, diabetes, and poor self-rated health (CDC, 2013c). These disparities are due in part to differences in the communities in which people live (LaVeist et al., 2011). Neighborhoods populated primarily by racial minorities and/or low-income families are less likely to have a retail outlet offering healthy food (Grimm et al., 2013), more likely to be in close proximity to a highway (and thus pollution) (Boehmer et al., 2013), less likely to have access to recreational facilities (Gordon-Larsen et al., 2006), and more likely to have high rates of street violence (Prevention Institute, 2011). These neighborhoods also have less access to health and other essential services, and their housing, infrastructure, and roads may be poorly built or maintained.

By almost every measure, neighborhoods with concentrations of low-income people and racial minorities tend to be less conducive to health than other neighborhoods, and this difference is exhibited in the disparities in their health outcomes. Babies born in the suburbs of Maryland and Virginia have a life expectancy 6 to 7 years longer than those born a few miles away in Washington, DC (RWJF, 2014). Children who live in low-income urban neighborhoods are more likely to suffer from asthma than their counterparts in bordering neighborhoods (Olmedo et al., 2011). These health disparities might be diminished by efforts to change the environment of the neighborhood through policies designed to improve housing, transit, infrastructure, sources of pollution, and access to healthy food and health care (Lee and Rubin, 2007).

A Systems Approach for Health Improvement

While the natural and built environments have direct effects on population health and the social determinants of health, it is important to consider the socioeconomic systems that operate within those environments. There are obvious relationships between the shape, pattern, and composition of physical environmental features and socioeconomic systems. When it is necessary to rebuild or repair a community's physical infrastructure, including residences and businesses, it makes sense to do so in concert with strategies addressing the services and systems that operate there. In New Orleans after Hurricane Katrina, for example, major repairs were needed for many features of the health care infrastructure. In light of more serious underlying problems represented by low metrics of population health, however, the community and its health care leadership fashioned a whole new approach, a reconfiguration of the entire system, instead of simply rebuilding those buildings that had been damaged by the storm and subsequent flooding. Thus, physical environments and human systems within those environments determine success in striving for a healthy community.

Well-being is a general metric of how well the community functions, how smoothly its systems perform. Social and health disparities typically arise when system performance wanes or, rarely, in the event of a disaster. Significantly, many federal and other government programs address issues of socioeconomic system failure. Those same programs, to varying degrees, are forced into "overdrive" when a disaster strikes—old problems are exacerbated and new problems arise. One example concerns crime, especially violent crime that has a severe negative effect on health. A contributor to crime is poor community design. A partial remedy for crime is to design streets, sidewalks, businesses, and housing to incorporate impediments to criminal behavior and to increase social observance of public places through increased social activity and stronger social capital. Also needed, however, is attention to crime prevention systems such as crime analysis, effective policing, and new inducements for those who may be inclined to pursue crime. Obvious linkages are education, employment, poverty, behavioral health, and a variety of social service initiatives pertaining to substance abuse, teen pregnancy, gambling addiction, and early childhood development. In this context, it is not sufficient simply to restore the community to its prior state after a disaster. Achieving a safe environment promises major co-benefits for health, especially for vulnerable populations.

These relationships are crucially important after a disaster, and they affect the pace of recovery because these fundamental risks in society's systems are ever present, but they are stressed and exacerbated by a disaster. The committee heard testimony, for example, on the toxic effect of temporary housing on children as a result of relocation, change of schools, and other disruptions (Redlener, 2014). Restoring the natural and built environments after a disaster is an important step, but attention must also be paid to system weaknesses. Importantly, this is a challenge already well recognized because communities of all sizes must wrestle with the high cost of servicing neighborhoods dominated by disparities in the socioeconomic system. Addressing blight, poverty, low educational attainment, commercial decline, joblessness, and the full range of negative influences from deteriorated housing is the mission of community development (supported in part by the U.S. Department of Housing and Urban Development's [HUD's] Community Development Block Grant). Communities with experience in system remedies are well suited to bridging the gap between concerns for the natural and the built environment and the social and economic functions within those environments.

Box 9-2 highlights a real-world example of a community using this type of systems planning in its disaster recovery. Springfield, Massachusetts, came together as a community following a tornado in 2011 that destroyed areas of the city and used a "nexus" framework for an integrated approach to recovery project planning. Since creating the plan and executing the plan are fundamentally different and also can be separated by a period of months or even years, it will be important to monitor how Springfield's plan becomes operational to see whether the community's needs are truly met when competing financial priorities arise. Coordinated implementation of the plan elements is necessary so that each element is not implemented as an individual project, which could lead to inefficiencies and gaps in execution.

Contemporary Approaches to Healthier and More Resilient and Sustainable Communities

Revisiting the "duality of use" concept, many agencies and organizations outside the health sector also are thinking about sustainable, long-term planning for communities. As it happens, many of the smart growth strategies recommended by the U.S. Environmental Protection Agency (EPA) for achieving sustainability also can have positive impacts on community health as well as mitigate the impacts of a disaster.

As discussed earlier, environmental quality has both direct and indirect effects on population health. Major improvements in water quality in the nation's streams and lakes have been made since the 1970s. Planning for better infrastructure for wastewater treatment has lowered concentrations of toxic material. In some extreme cases—such as Love Canal in New York and Times Beach in Missouri—homes have been relocated away from hazards because of explicit health risks. Community plans also have become more health conscious. Transportation planning has integrated measures of environmental effects on the population, including emissions, noise, safety, and elements that facilitate pedestrian and bicycle travel for both recreational and commuting trips. Themes such as smart growth represent an attempt to balance social and economic objectives. EPA's report on creating equitable, healthy, and sustainable communities describes smart growth as "a range of strategies for planning and building cities, suburbs, and small towns in ways that protect the environment and public health, support economic development, and strengthen communities" (EPA, 2013, p. 4). The Partnership for Sustainable Communities, an initiative of the U.S. Department of Transportation (DOT), HUD, and EPA, is the centerpiece of the nation's new approach (DOT et al., 2014), empowered by three factors: (1) coordinated financing, (2) planning mandates, and (3) technical assistance. While this notion of development and interaction with the environment goes back decades, new ways of incorporating sustainable strategies and elements into homes, public centers, parks, and other sections of a community have increased in recent years.

Accompanying this shift is guidance and renewed energy from EPA and such groups as the Partnership for Sustainable Communities and the American Society of Landscape Architects. In 2009, through a partnership with local government councils, EPA developed smart growth guidelines for sustainable design and development for communities striving to achieve future growth that results in stronger neighborhoods, protected open space and watersheds, and healthier and more affordable homes (EPA, 2009). These strategies, coupled with "green" initiatives—environmentally friendly approaches that can range from building practices to product labeling to chemical engineering—can lead to a more resilient, sustainable community. These practices, although created with sustainability in mind, can have an impact on the health of a population. For example, people in communities with abundant green space tend to be healthier (Maas et al., 2006). Cities incorporating green infrastructure into their planning often find

---

BOX 9-2
Building the Community Nexus

Significant social and financial costs are associated with siloed approaches to community planning and the resultant inefficiency. For communities looking to design a more collaborative and systematic approach, particularly in the process of rebuilding following a disaster, the "nexus" concept may serve as a guideline for meeting the comprehensive needs of community members. These needs, which include a community's most crucial quality-of-life resources, fall into six domains:

- **the physical domain**, which includes a community's built and natural resources;
- **the cultural domain**, which includes those aspects of a community related to individual and collective values;
- **the social domain**, which governs well-being and includes a community's health and human services;
- **the economic domain**, which works to maintain a healthy balance among a community's financial, human, and environmental capital;
- **the organizational domain**, which encompasses programs and services such as community clubs, civic societies, and city and county school boards and councils; and
- **the educational domain**, which covers the span from early childhood education to college, as well as workforce training programs.

It is the nexus of interactions among these domains that will best serve to promote a community's overall well-being and health.

The nexus planning framework is a highly integrated model in which a nexus of planning exists for the people, programs, and places involved in the provision of public services and programs. A fully developed nexus site will serve as the place where a variety of community services and amenities—such as grocery stores, farmer's markets, parks, libraries, child care centers, and schools—are situated, coordinated, and administered to best address and serve the needs of the community. Importantly, the approach transcends physical design,

---

that the environmental benefits justify the up-front costs and are worthwhile for day-to-day needs, such as by reducing energy use, filtering air and water pollutants, and preserving wildlife habitats. Preserving habitats to ensure healthy ecosystem functioning can have a positive impact on the dense urban and suburban environments in which more than 80 percent of the U.S. population lives (USDA, 2014). For those concerned about hazard mitigation and resiliency, such strategies as green roofs, rain gardens, and porous concrete can help manage stormwater runoff, alleviate flooding, and prevent aquifer pollution after a hurricane or other disaster.

Again, however, many of these ideas are attractive in theory and in the planning stages, but they are sometimes challenging to execute. To overcome such barriers, federal agencies are using programmatic incentives to drive sustainable change in communities that aligns with national strategic priorities. Leadership in Energy & Environmental Design (LEED) for Neighborhood Development (LEED-ND), for example, is "a rating system that incorporates principles of smart growth, New Urbanism, and green building into a voluntary framework for sustainable neighborhood planning and design" (HUD, 2012). To incentivize the use of this framework, "HUD recently incorporated LEED-ND into all of its grant funding through the General Section and required LEED-ND certification for Choice Neighborhoods Planning Grant recipients" (HUD, 2012). Other federal support and community grants with this type of focus on green development and smart growth strategies can help communities manage hazards in a cost-effective way while realizing other benefits for social and physical well-being.

and also integrates program design and policy tools. For example, joint use agreements can expand access to amenities by enabling the community to use school facilities such as gyms, auditoriums, and libraries during evenings and weekends. The result is not only a more sustainable community but also a more equitable one— vehicle ownership is no longer a prerequisite for accessing community amenities and services. The opportunity for increased physical activity benefits all community members.

In Springfield, Massachusetts, redevelopment under a nexus framework is under way in response to a devastating tornado that tore through the city on June 1, 2011. In the aftermath of this disaster, citizens came together to develop a community-driven plan called Rebuild Springfield, with both residents and stakeholders working collaboratively inside the nexus framework. Among the recommendations prioritized as part of this plan is putting schools and libraries at the center of a nexus approach to provide a wide range of community services and programs. One proposed approach for catalyzing this process is the development of partnerships between public library branches and educational institutions.

Springfield has been designated as a "Gateway City," a title given to formerly thriving industrial cities now showing promise as regional economic and cultural centers. Many recommendations of the Rebuild Springfield plan take into account and celebrate Springfield's cultural diversity. The redevelopment proposal emphasizes the need to better connect the community, both physically and culturally. This will be accomplished with improved transportation systems, as well as efforts to increase access to cultural amenities through coordinated outreach.

Rebuild Springfield represents a unique example of a planning project developed entirely around the nexus framework and domains. While implementation of Springfield's plan is still in progress, there are numerous examples of completed nexus sites whose positive impact on their communities can already be observed. In Houston, Texas, the Baker-Ripley Neighborhood Center was completed in 2010 and serves as a true neighborhood nexus site. The center includes an elementary school, a public library, a farmer's market, parks, business facilities, and a community health center. Since its completion, the center has become a vibrant community hub, providing a vast number of services for a previously underserved community.

SOURCES: Bingler, 2011, 2014; Springfield Redevelopment Authority, 2012.

DISASTER IMPACTS ON COMMUNITY SYSTEMS: IMPLICATIONS FOR HEALTH AND RECOVERY

Following a disaster, the short-term impacts on community systems and overall health generally are well known, often receiving significant media coverage. Initial concerns include impeded access to goods and services—including food and supplies and ambulance services—because of impassable roads or nonfunctioning transit. Another concern is impaired functioning of critical infrastructure that provides clean water to the community and power to important buildings such as hospitals. Environmental degradation that can exacerbate existing conditions (e.g., asthma) or cause new ones may be less apparent in the immediate aftermath of a disaster. After Hurricane Sandy, for example, "Floodwaters, massive storm runoff, wind damage, and loss of electricity combined to cause wastewater treatment plants up and down the mid-Atlantic coast to fail. These failures sent billions of gallons of raw and partially treated sewage into the region's waterways, impacting public health, aquatic habitats, and resources" (Hurricane Sandy Rebuilding Task Force, 2013, p. 27).

By the time long-term disaster impacts start to manifest in a community, the media cameras usually are long gone, and many downstream consequences go unnoticed until the situation reaches a threshold. Occasionally, commercial buildings or housing projects are too damaged to be repaired easily, so they are abandoned or shifted further down the priority list. The result can be an increase in blight and associated crime, causing the community to break up and individuals to scatter across a state or region. Positive health effects of the social capital that existed in the neighborhood may be at risk. Because disasters often cause disproportionate hardship for vulnerable populations and low-income neighborhoods, recovery planning requires careful demographic analysis. Post-disaster reconstruction and relocations are steep hurdles for individuals and families. Upgraded construction codes, mitigation requirements, and changes in actuarial insurance rates are major challenges for elderly and fixed-income individuals, for example. Neighborhood changes and the loss of hospitals, physicians, grocery stores, and pharmacies can exacerbate the hardships faced by residents even if temporary housing is provided. Rarely do recovery plans address all of these needs, nor can restoration of full community services be accomplished immediately, leaving the population in dire straits at a time when all forms of stress and uncertainty are at their highest levels. This is an important unmet need. If a family is displaced from its affordable housing but wants to stay in the community, there may be limited options for doing so. All of these scenarios lead to further deterioration of the social determinants of health.

It is possible to overcome these challenges, although as Robert Olshansky from the University of Illinois testified to the committee, intensive planning is required to rebuild a city successfully after a disaster (Olshansky, 2014). Building a city under normal circumstances is highly complex, with many different actors involved. Added complexity arises during disaster recovery as a result of the compression of time in which the same set of tasks must be accomplished. Despite the added challenges, this planning process should be guided by a shared goal of helping people create settlements that are healthy and safe places to live that provide viable livelihoods, and that enable convenient access to all of the things they need. Sudden loss creates opportunities for reorganizing the elements of a community—not just facilities, but also services. As discussed earlier, disaster-related challenges provide an opportunity to approach community redevelopment in ways that improve health and social well-being. It is important to note, however, that the extent of need and opportunities for community redevelopment will depend on the pattern and extent of the damage caused by a disaster. Every disaster may not present the opportunity to revamp the community or undertake long-term planning. For example, tornados usually leave the foundations or basements of buildings intact, so the most economical solution often is to build on the preexisting base, keeping the same footprint.

ORGANIZATIONAL STRUCTURES AND RESOURCES FOR HEALTHY COMMUNITY PLANNING AND REDEVELOPMENT

Federal Level[2]

In steady-state times, a number of federal agencies provide funding and technical assistance to support the development of the built and natural environments. A comprehensive review of these resources is beyond the scope of this report, but the relevant agencies and funding sources related to community development and rebuilding are briefly reviewed here. As mentioned earlier, the major federal agencies whose policies and funding shape the built and natural environments in the United States came together in 2009 to form the Partnership for Sustainable Communities. Through the efforts of DOT, HUD, and the EPA, "more than 1,000 communities in all 50 states, Washington, D.C., and Puerto Rico have received more than $4 billion in grants and technical assistance to help them grow and improve their quality of life" (DOT et al., 2014, p. 2).

Individually, the agencies within the partnership also are major funding sources for sustainable community building. DOT offers the Transportation Investment Generating Economic Recovery (TIGER) Discretionary Grant program that enables applicants to invest in road, rail, transit, or port projects. Applicants must describe the benefits of their proposed project for "five long-term outcomes: safety, economic competitiveness, state of good repair, livability and environmental sustainability" (DOT, 2015).

In response to community demands from around the country, EPA's Office of Sustainable Communities launched the Building Blocks for Sustainable Communities Program. This program offers targeted technical assistance to selected communities using tools that already have demonstrated widespread results.

---

[2] A broader synopsis of legislation and federal policy related to disaster recovery and health security can be found in Appendix A.

To illustrate some of the topic areas within the program, the topics highlighted for the 2015 program are listed below, showing overlap among sustainable objectives for cities, hazard mitigation needs, and healthy community elements:

- bikeshare planning,
- supporting equitable development,
- infill development for distressed cities,
- sustainable strategies for small cities and rural areas, and
- flood resilience for riverine and coastal communities (EPA, 2014).

HUD offers the Community Development Block Grant (CDBG) program, alluded to earlier, which provides funds for addressing a wide range of community needs. Specifically, grantees must use at least 70 percent of the funding for projects directed at low- or moderate-income populations and encourage citizen participation (HUD, 2015). The program provides annual funding to state and local entities, but it also is flexible enough to provide assistance following a presidentially declared disaster, subject to the availability of a congressional supplemental appropriation.

HHS also has a role in healthy community development. The Centers for Disease Control and Prevention's (CDC's) Built Environment and Health Initiative (also known as the Healthy Community Design Initiative) works to improve community design decisions by linking them with public health surveillance, utilizing such tools as the health impact assessment (HIA), building partnerships with key decision makers in the community, and conducting research and translating its results into best practices. The initiative funded and supported 34 HIAs in 2011 and continued to fund 6 local, county, and state entities' HIAs from 2011 to 2014. Data from the HIAs have been used to develop health-focused frameworks in communities in Nebraska, North Carolina, and Oregon (CDC, 2013b). Additionally, the Patient Protection and Affordable Care Act (ACA) authorized the Community Transformation Grant Program through the CDC, aimed at helping communities design changes to their built and social environments to address chronic diseases[3] (CDC, 2014b).

After a disaster, a number of different federal funding mechanisms come into play. When a disaster exceeds the capacity of the state or locality to respond, a presidential disaster declaration can bring in federal aid under the Robert T. Stafford Disaster Relief and Emergency Assistance Act[4] (CRS, 2014; see also Chapter 4). The National Disaster Recovery Framework (NDRF, described in detail in Chapter 3), serves as a conceptual guide for recovery planning at all levels of government and is intended to improve coordination of federal recovery resources (FEMA, 2014b). Similar to the Emergency Support Functions (ESFs) of the National Response Framework (NRF), the NDRF introduces six Recovery Support Functions (RSFs), each designated to a different lead federal agency:

- **Community Planning and Capacity Building**—Federal Emergency Management Agency,
- **Economic**—U.S. Department of Commerce,
- **Health and Social Services**—U.S. Department of Health and Human Services,
- **Housing**—U.S. Department of Housing and Urban Development,
- **Infrastructure Systems (including transportation)** —U.S. Army Corps of Engineers, and
- **Natural and Cultural Resources**—U.S. Department of the Interior (FEMA, 2014b).

Under the NDRF, a FEMA official functions as the federal disaster recovery coordinator and for presidentially declared disasters, FEMA also provides public assistance and hazard mitigation funding for repair and restoration of public (and some nonprofit) infrastructure where needed. Although HUD leads

---

[3] Funding for the Community Transformation Grant Program was eliminated by Congress in the Fiscal Year 2014 Omnibus package.
[4] 42 U.S.C. § 5121 et seq.

the Housing RSF, it is also an important funder for major disasters if Congress makes a supplemental appropriation through HUD's CDBG program for Disaster Recovery (CDBG-DR) as a vehicle to aid rebuilding efforts and to provide the start-up funds necessary to initiate the recovery process. Since such funding may support a wide range of recovery activities, it enables HUD to better assist communities that otherwise might not recover because of limited resources and to prevent them from experiencing the long-term health impacts discussed previously (HUD, 2014). However, as discussed in Chapter 3, HUD's community development function has not adequately been integrated into the NDRF.

The framework aspires to better utilization of existing resources; however, it does not yet clearly capture the contemporary healthy community and sustainable development practices that are being led by CDC and the Partnership for Sustainable Communities. As discussed in Chapter 3, the NDRF needs to be upgraded to reflect these prior achievements and their relevance to disaster circumstances. Combined, these additional themes of integration and transformation could foster a major advance in the nation's capacity for disaster recovery.

State and Regional Levels

As discussed in Chapter 3, states and regional entities have key roles in recovery, and in many cases, they are the grantees for federal grant programs in the case of a presidentially declared disaster. State emergency management agencies, for example, are the grantees for FEMA Public Assistance and Hazard Mitigation Grant Programs, and they must work closely with community planning entities to manage mitigation activities. For optimal vertical integration, state agencies need to align with the NDRF structure and, in doing so, should ensure that their state-level entities with everyday responsibilities for urban or regional planning and development are incorporated into the RSF structure and understand their roles. For long-range transportation planning, for example, there are transportation planning and policy assets and personnel at both state and regional levels that need to be incorporated into long-term recovery planning following a disaster to see projects through to fruition. The state should not rely on the emergency operations personnel that may have represented that sector during the immediate response to fulfill an ESF.

In contrast to the strong state-local relationships designed into financial, technical, and operational systems funded by DOT, HUD, and EPA for steady-state community planning, disaster recovery is a process that often reveals a mismatch between state and municipal governments. Because of the infrequency of disaster occurrences and the absence of strong policy foundations, states, cities, and counties do not have regular opportunities to share information or practice how to address recovery issues that arise during disasters. Strategies of redevelopment, economic incentives, and neighborhood revitalization are inherently in the municipal domain and may not be well understood by state agency personnel. After Hurricanes Katrina, Rita and Ike, both Louisiana and Texas experienced tumultuous reorganizations of their disaster recovery programs midstream, with legislative and media investigations of disharmony (Kirkland, 2012). States need to organize and align their RSF structure with both the national and the local level to ensure that events from past disasters are not repeated.

Since some planning—particularly for transportation and economic development—takes place primarily at the regional (substate) level, it is important for those organizations to be included in the development of recovery plans, especially as their functions may align with the NDRF structure. Metropolitan planning organizations (MPOs) play a large role in organizing and executing transportation planning throughout a defined urban area of one or more counties and sometimes a multistate region. Since they already exist, with defined leadership, processes, and networks, they often can play an important role in making recovery decisions for transportation- and development-related issues. In Washington's Puget Sound region, for example, the 2014 Transportation Recovery Annex recommends including MPOs in a transportation stakeholder forum for the development of regional transportation recovery policies (Washington Emergency Management Division, 2014). Because the Economic Development Administration serves as the coordinating agency for the Economic RSF (EDA, 2015), organizing the regional economic development districts to align with the NDRF structure also can facilitate the recovery process for a community. By becoming involved in recovery at the regional level, the economic development districts can provide important on-the-ground knowledge and awareness to the federal RSF lead and ensure that national recovery decisions are being made with the most accurate economic information available.

Local Level

Comprehensive plans created at the local level drive land use policy and community investments in infrastructure, but different locally derived structures for developing and implementing policies for health exist across the country. In Pinellas County, Florida, for example, the health department is actively engaged with other departments in addressing the needs of blighted and deteriorated neighborhoods, followed by redevelopment with new, safe construction enabled by HUD grants and interagency collaboration. King County in Washington is taking a similar approach through its Communities of Opportunity program (see Box 2-8 in Chapter 2). Yet there are virtually no known research cases that address how this kind of demonstrated capacity of health and social service agencies at the local level to achieve high levels of collaboration around development policies translates to better post-disaster recovery. It is reasonable to assume that this approach can offer distinct advantages and that better plans will result when health, medical, and social services are viewed holistically among themselves and with other community policies of a recovery plan.

Like state and regional entities, local government agencies need to align with the NDRF structure and appoint or identify representatives to coordinate with their state, regional, and federal counterparts. Such arrangements should be put in place before a disaster. While recommendations and guidelines may come from the state or national level, ultimately it is often up to the local government to decide how to reinvest in its community. As discussed throughout this chapter, there are many ways to leverage strategies and the energy and interest of community leaders to bring about positive change at the local level.

Nonprofits, Philanthropies, and the Private Sector

Nonprofit organizations and businesses have a vested interest in rebuilding in the communities in which they work and with which they feel a connection, and therefore, they also should be included in discussions at the local government level to facilitate and execute recovery planning. Philanthropies can be important funders for redevelopment to address the needs of underserved populations, especially those groups, such as the Rockefeller Foundation and the Robert Wood Johnson Foundation, that support resilience building and improvement of the social determinants of health in their day-to-day work. Following a disaster, having their added funding along with expertise in focusing health interventions on vulnerable populations also can aid in long-term recovery. After a disaster, nonprofit organizations such as Architecture for Humanity provide pro bono design services through their membership. These groups need to be engaged proactively in recovery planning to ensure that recovery activities are seamless across the spectrum of a community.

Nonprofit institutions and the private sector also can play a role in financing recovery and supporting public health outcomes. The Reinvestment Fund is a Community Development Financial Institution (CDFI) that serves people who might otherwise be disconnected from the credit system (TRF, 2015). CDFIs use federal resources, such as incentives, tax credits, and bond guarantees, to serve low-income people and communities that lack access to affordable financial services and products (U.S. Department of the Treasury, 2014). This sector also is experiencing a change in focus, with increased awareness of the nexus between healthy and productive communities. In recognition of this nexus, one nonprofit CDFI, the Low Income Investment Fund, has been taking a more holistic approach that involves not only building affordable housing in a neighborhood but also building and supporting high-performing schools, health clinics, and recreational facilities with access to public transit (IOM, 2014b). While some might be skeptical that larger banking institutions would invest in these kinds of community development projects, the Community Reinvestment Act,[5] passed in 1977, mandates that banks reinvest in low-income communities from which they take deposits. They are graded on their performance in this regard and so are incentivized to strive for higher rankings. Tax credit incentives through the New Markets Tax Credit also are spurring investors to revitalize impoverished areas. Established as part of the Community Renewal Tax Relief Act of 2000,[6] it has helped jump-start community development and is used to capitalize lending institutions that finance small businesses and help address the social determinants of health in low-income neighborhoods (Erickson and Andrews, 2011).

Collaboration and Coordination

During steady-state periods, mechanisms for collaboration and coordination are necessary because of the interconnected nature of the various facets of community planning (e.g., land use and transportation). These mechanisms are essentially systematic arrangements for professional teams and advisory groups to carry out analysis and program development that includes plans, projects, and budgets. Some groups, such as MPOs, are more familiar and comfortable with working together than others because they operate together routinely. For others, it is important to assess the ability to work together on short notice in the event of a disaster demanding multisector recovery planning. Such an assessment needs to consider the ability to collaborate across sectors and whether the partners are familiar with each other's language and terminology. With the emergence of many new opportunities for partnerships with the health sector, the question arises of what collaboration among various sectors would look like. In a 2013 study conducted for the Robert Wood Johnson Foundation's Commission to Build a Healthier America, the researchers wanted to measure the degree to which cross-sector collaboration occurs between health and other sectors, whether such collaborations have positive effects, and what the indicators of positive collaboration are (Mattessich and Rausch, 2013). They report that respondents frequently cited major benefits of collaboration such as pooling resources and dividing risk. They also note that skilled leadership was identified as one of the top three factors for a successful collaboration, yet at the national level, no single formal network exists to unify this newly emerging field of cross-sector collaboration aimed at improving health (Mattessich and Rausch, 2013). Finally, they emphasize the importance of "building the evidence base for cross-sector initiatives that effectively improve health by creating environments that protect and actively promote health" (Mattessich and Rausch, 2013, p. 10). Determining how to acquire and share the evidence needed to make the case for joint investments can make partnerships between the health sector and entities involved in the design of the physical environment even more attractive and widespread. If such integrated initiatives can be shown to save medical costs downstream, health management and affordable care organizations may have an even greater incentive to collaborate (Erickson and Andrews, 2011). New networks can create an opportunity for breaking down silos to achieve shared goals across sectors. Opportunities for such collaborations are discussed in the sections below.

Planning and Design

Although community planning as a field was created in large part in response to public health needs (e.g., addressing sanitation issues), the fields of public health and planning have since diverged. There is growing recognition, however, that these two sectors cannot continue to operate in isolation (Ricklin et al., 2012). Health concerns increasingly are falling within the scope of planning departments, and the public health field has discovered the power of comprehensive plans, social capital and cohesion, and other planning tools for altering the physical and social environments that impact health. As discussed earlier in this chapter, decisions being made about community design, land use, and transportation are

---

[5] Community Reinvestment Act of 1977, Public Law 95-128, 91 Stat. 1147, Title VIII of the Housing and Community Development Act of 1977, 12 U.S.C. § 2901 et seq.

[6] Community Renewal Tax Relief Act of 2000, incorporated into Public Law 106-554.

having effects on air and water quality, physical activity, exposure to contaminated industrial sites, and other important determinants of health.

Recognizing this linkage, New York City established a working group in 2010 comprising design organizations; academics; and city agencies involved in health, city planning, transportation, and construction. The group was tasked with developing Active Design Guidelines—"evidence-based and best-practice strategies for increasing physical activity in the design and construction of neighborhoods, streets, and buildings" (Lee, 2012, p. 5). Likewise, the American Institute of Architects has established a New Design and Health Agenda, and in 2014 it held a summit focusing on how public health officials and designers can intersect (AIA, 2014). Planners are beginning to understand the impact they can have on public health, and some public health departments are even hiring planning professionals to advise communities on healthy designs. Likewise, planners would benefit from data and metrics that are available to public health departments to understand where interventions would best be implemented. A recent example of such partnerships is King County Board of Health's adoption of "Planning for Healthy Communities" guidelines in 2011. These guidelines are intended to inform land use and transportation planners about strategies that could have an effect on all residents of King County, Washington, based on actual causes of death and illness (King County, 2011).

Community Development Entities

Recent years also have seen increased collaboration between the community development sector and the public health sector as greater understanding of their shared goals reveals opportunities to coordinate or combine their individual funding streams. As with the planning and green infrastructure sector, community development entities are realizing that the benefits of their efforts extend to health. At an Institute of Medicine (IOM) workshop on financing population health, Raphael Bostic, the Judith and John Bedrosian Chair in Governance and the Public Enterprise at the Sol Price School of Public Policy, University of Southern California, said he believes a reset is occurring in the way people think about community development and population health (IOM, 2014b). He attributed this reset in part to demonstration projects in the housing and urban development sectors revealing the largest effect on health benefits:

> For example, the Moving to Opportunity program, in which low-income families were given vouchers that enabled them to move out of areas with concentrated poverty, produced marked improvements in stress-related outcomes, depression, obesity, and diabetes. "That was a wake-up call," Bostic said. "When the demonstration started, health was not even on the radar screen." (IOM, 2014b, p. 27)

Erickson and Andrews (2011) also argue that through the ACA, federally qualified health centers should coordinate more closely with community development entities. If medical clinics were able to connect more easily and seamlessly with a network with existing links to funders, social services, and other community organizations, divisions between sectors could be further broken down.

The increased awareness of shared goals between the community development and health sectors is encouraging but represents only a first step. The Robert Wood Johnson Foundation's Commission to Build a Healthier America recommends that the United States fundamentally change its approach to revitalizing neighborhoods by fully integrating health into community development (RWJF, 2014). By extending the concept of "health" into the neighborhoods where people live, play, and work, both sectors can think more broadly about potential interventions and desired outcomes to build healthier communities.

Transportation

Transportation has long been associated with public health with respect to prevention of injuries related to vehicle crashes and safety laws such as those mandating the use of seatbelts. However, DOT and the Federal Highway Administration (FHWA) also have been involved in policies related to health, and increasingly are regarding healthy outcomes as an important part of their objective in creating livable, sustainable communities. In 2012, they created a Health in Transportation Working Group to examine their policies and regulations on health issues, as well as ways to incorporate health into transportation planning and educate both internal and external stakeholders (FHWA, 2015).

Awareness of this connection occurred at the state level in Massachusetts. In 2009, a strong transportation reform law designed to consolidate disparate services in the state led to the development of the Healthy Transportation Compact, an interagency group chaired by the secretary of transportation and secretary of health and human services at the state level. Its goal is to collaborate on the potential health effects of transportation decisions. Examples of the group's initiatives include:

- Mass in Motion Program (a statewide program that promotes opportunities for active living);
- Municipal Wellness Grants (distributed at the local level so communities can increase opportunities and customize initiatives to their needs); and
- Safe Routes to School (which promotes healthy alternatives for children to travel to school) (IOM, 2014a).

PRE-DISASTER PRIORITIES

Creating a Healthy Community Vision for Recovery

Prior to a disaster, when there is time to think through priorities, leaders can take various actions to create and promote a healthy vision for recovery should a disaster strike. Holding community planning and visioning workshops—also called charrettes—is a good way to obtain input from residents with which to prioritize needed actions, and it also can secure buy-in for projects or developments. Such visioning exercises may have been conducted in the past, either as a coordinated effort or by separate groups. As discussed in Chapter 3, building on these efforts and being as inclusive as possible can ensure less pushback by those who contributed previously and may shorten the timeline for action if work has already been done or processes designed.

In these efforts, it is important to engage the health sector. The health sector is a source of data and information that may be difficult to find elsewhere (e.g., from community health assessments); it has connections with various community networks; and it brings a different perspective on strategies for building stronger communities. The vision and goals created from these workshops should be incorporated into the overall comprehensive plan for a town or city, as discussed in Chapter 3.

Organizing for Disaster Recovery Planning

Each sector has its own roles and responsibilities in recovery planning that need to be laid out, but a forum also is needed to identify and create synergy among the various projects and programs being planned. There may often be overlap or shared goals across projects within a community, and being aware of those projects and their goals before a disaster will facilitate streamlining recovery in a coordinated manner should such an event occur. It is difficult to plan what every sector's actions will be during pre-event recovery planning, since most communities are at risk of several different types of disasters with varying impacts. Nonetheless, it is important to plan the operations and identify roles and contingencies. As part of its project to update its 1998 report, *Planning for Post-Disaster Recovery*, the American Planning Association created an annotated Model Pre-event Recovery Ordinance designed to guide communities in preparing prior to a disaster so they can better manage the recovery process. This guidance includes advising communities to create a recovery management organization prior to a disaster (APA, 2014a).

As discussed earlier, the representatives for the RSFs in community recovery will need to be different from those leading the ESFs. In some cases there may be some overlap but, generally, different expertise is needed to address long-term needs versus those associated with the emergency response. As discussed in Chapter 3, jurisdictions need to leverage existing community structures that promote an integrated approach. There is no value to building a new network of people and processes that will be used only in the aftermath of a disaster. Structures and networks already in place are familiar with their target audiences, stakeholders, and potential vendors and partners for rebuilding. After a tornado demolished much of Joplin, Missouri, in 2011, City Manager Mark Rohr attributed some of the success of the town's recovery, including the development of the Citizens Advisory Recovery Team (CART), to activities initiated in 2001 to revitalize the downtown area. Rohr suggested that the community's history of engagement in downtown revitalization served as a precursor to the CART's mission to consider and outline a long-term disaster recovery strategy (Abramson and Culp, 2013). By building on a holistic vision, especially one already known and shared among stakeholders, sectors in a community can determine how they can best work together to realize that vision for their neighborhood, town, or city during recovery.

Conducting Vulnerability and Capacity Assessments

In addition to creating a vision for recovery and organizing sectors and stakeholders for recovery management, it is important for communities to conduct assessments of their vulnerable infrastructure, populations, and locations; take inventory of their assets; and understand their capacity limitations that would be stressed during the recovery process. For example, rebuilding and redevelopment will likely necessitate a massive amount of permitting so communities should assess in advance their capacity to meet this surge in need rapidly and smoothly. Capacity assessments of physical assets alone will be insufficient; the workforce needed to provide the increased services required after a disaster must also be assessed, and alternatives explored if it is inadequate. Having memorandums of understanding in place and processes for waiving regulations and collaborating across sectors prior to an event can facilitate recovery. Pinellas County, Florida, in its recent post-disaster redevelopment plan (PDRP), described its capacity assessment as follows:

> The purpose of the Pinellas County Institutional Capacity Analysis is to examine the capacity of the county to facilitate redevelopment in the context of the goals and objectives of this plan. "Capacity" in the context of this plan is not focused on physical assets (i.e., number of fire trucks, ambulances, etc.). Instead, capacity is assessed to determine if the framework exists to implement the goals and actions in the PDRP, such as programs, agencies, organizations (and their associated staffs) and other tools. The assessment is intended to determine the robust programs and resources that strongly support post-disaster redevelopment, programs that exist but could be improved to better support post-disaster redevelopment goals, and the weakness or gaps where programs or plans could be implemented to improve the County's capacity to recover in the long term. (Pinellas County, 2012, p. 4-55)

In addition to capacity, a strong understanding of a community's vulnerabilities is needed to inform recovery planning. Although these kinds of analysis often focus on critical infrastructure, social vulnerability is increasingly being evaluated in the risk management process (see Chapter 2 for discussion on social vulnerability). The Pinellas County PDRP, for example, includes a socioeconomic profile (Pinellas County, 2012) as a component of its vulnerability assessment. Digital technologies are enabling emergency managers and health officials alike to identify areas with high social vulnerability. While geographic information systems (GIS) often are used in emergencies to map flood plains or key assets that can be deployed, they also can be used to map public health and social services data to show community and government officials where vulnerable neighborhoods may be following a disaster. In New Orleans, the health department, using data from the Centers for Medicare & Medicaid Services (CMS), created a map of residents who were oxygen dependent and would need immediate assistance in the case of lost power. The CMS data were found to be 93 percent accurate, giving the health department a clear picture to start with in the event of an emergency (DeSalvo et al., 2014). Similarly, King County, Washington, used GIS software to map socioeconomic factors in the county that are associated with health risks (see Figure 9-1). Such data are invaluable to the effective targeting of resources to areas of need after a disaster.

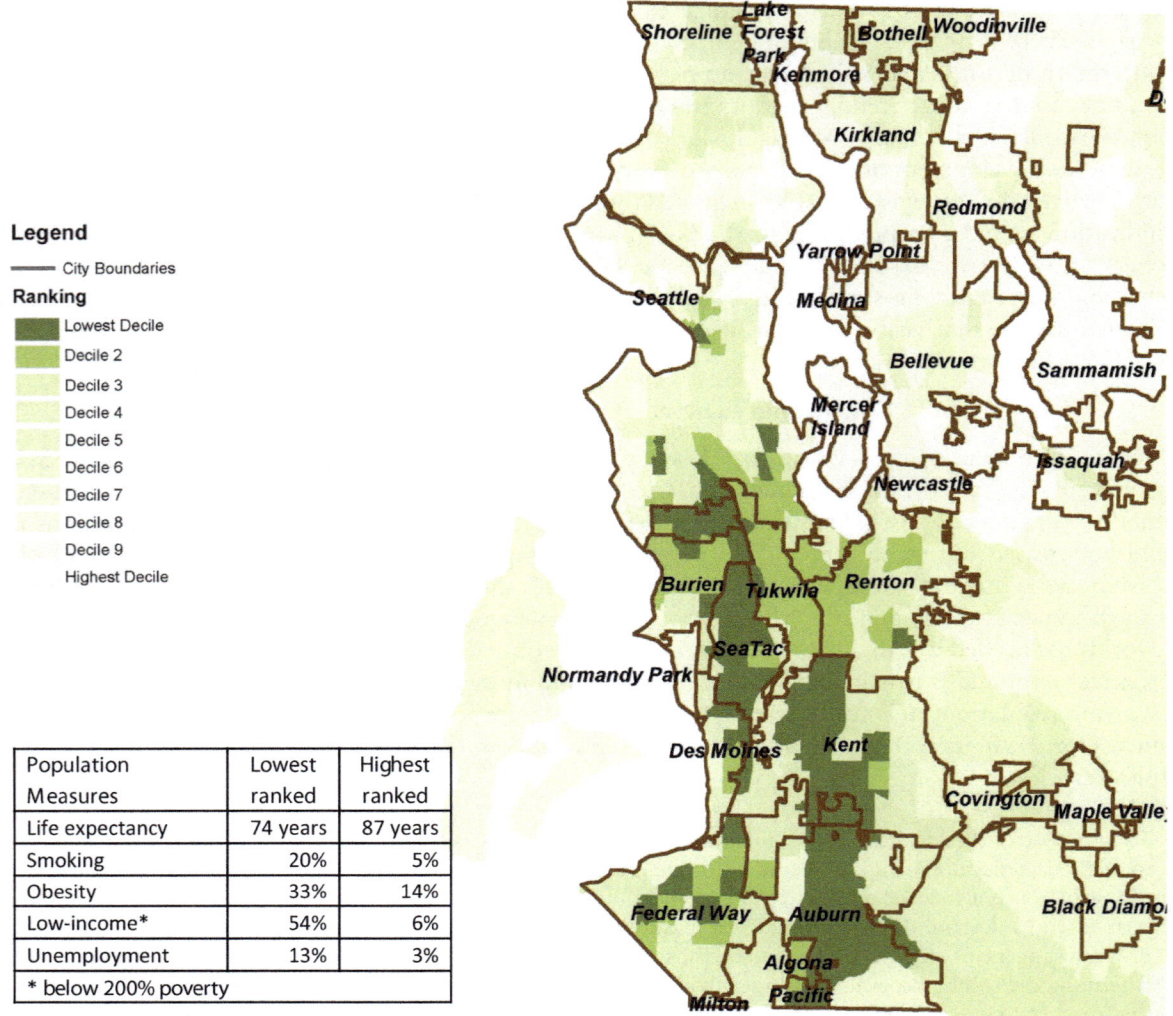

Population Measures	Lowest ranked	Highest ranked
Life expectancy	74 years	87 years
Smoking	20%	5%
Obesity	33%	14%
Low-income*	54%	6%
Unemployment	13%	3%
* below 200% poverty		

FIGURE 9-1 Geographic information systems data from King County, Washington, show clustering of vulnerabilities from the convergence of health risk factors (dark green).
SOURCE: King County. 2014. *Health and Human Services transformation plan and communities of opportunity.* King County, Washington. Available at http://www.kingcounty.gov/exec/HHStransformation/coo.aspx.

EARLY POST-DISASTER RECOVERY PRIORITIES

The early recovery period often overlaps with and runs parallel to the disaster response phase. During this time, communities assess the extent of the disaster-related damage and begin restoration efforts. Although it is tempting to postpone considerations related to rebuilding in ways that support health, resilience, and sustainability, without these goals in mind, early restoration efforts may be undertaken in a manner that impedes future betterment opportunities.

Assessing Disaster Impacts on Community Systems

In the early stages of disaster recovery, it is important to conduct an impact assessment. This assessment will dictate what resources are needed, how the available funding will best be allocated, as well as what players and stakeholders need to be engaged quickly. As mentioned previously, if a tornado destroys a neighborhood or private businesses, much of the recovery can be funded by private insurance, and a robust effort to overhaul the social fabric of a community will not be warranted. However, if public facilities are affected, infrastructure is destroyed past the point of repair, or an already declining area is heavily impacted, it will be necessary to assess the impacts quickly and facilitate the community's transition from disaster response to disaster recovery planning—not waiting until the response ends to plan the recovery needs.

Restoring Critical Infrastructure and Remediating Immediate Health Threats

Following an impact assessment, early restoration operations needed for the short term, including those addressing infrastructure, land use, and environmental management, should be conducted. A comprehensive examination of the restoration phase of recovery is beyond the scope of this report, but the sections below highlight restoration needs related to protecting health.

Infrastructure and Transportation

In the initial phases of recovery, communities should address post-disaster challenges of transportation access in a prioritized manner. FEMA Public Assistance funds often cover emergency repair of public infrastructure and debris removal. However, debris removal can be a rate-limiting step for recovery activities and is critical to restoring access to goods and services that are essential to health. With the passage of the Sandy Recovery Improvement Act of 2013,[7] FEMA developed a pilot program to incentivize rapid debris removal. Upon receiving a debris management plan prior to a declared disaster, FEMA will provide a one-time incentive of a 2 percent cost share adjustment for the first 90 days of debris removal activities, beginning the first day of the declared incident period, provided the plan is implemented for that disaster (FEMA, 2014c).

Selection of an appropriate site for dumping of debris is important to prevent potential health risks to nearby or future populations. Historically, careful site selection has not occurred, leading to issues of environmental justice (Allen, 2007). In light of the increased emphasis on green infrastructure and design discussed earlier in this chapter, a community also may want to consider a recycling program for debris, which could lessen the workload of disposal as well as contain costs. Through the FEMA pilot program, costs of sorting debris for a recycling program are eligible for reimbursement.

Reopening roads is another key recovery priority and can impact health. In setting criteria for reopening roads and restoring power, access roads to hospitals and other medical and ancillary facilities (e.g., pharmacies) should have priority. The need for alternative transit routes should be evaluated as well. If large temporary housing sites are set up in an area outside typical access routes, for example, community leaders may need to ensure that they are serviced by public transit so those temporarily displaced residents without access to personal vehicles can access essential goods and services as well as employment.

Another critical early priority is the restoration of utilities and communications systems. For example, water treatment facilities need to be up and running to prevent illness from contaminated water supplies and power is essential to health facilities and individuals requiring electricity-dependent medical equipment. Reestablishment of communication infrastructure is important for continued use of health information systems after a disaster, particularly for providers using cloud-based record storage. For those organizations that established backup measures in advance of the disaster (e.g., power generators, physical servers at nearby sites) as part of resilience-building efforts, such systems can be used until critical infrastructure is restored, thereby protecting against adverse health outcomes.

---

[7] Sandy Recovery Improvement Act of 2013, 113th Congress, H.R. 219 (January 29, 2013).

Land Use

Although there is often pressure to get a community "back to normal" after a disaster, it is important to discourage immediate rebuilding in potentially hazardous areas. A moratorium on immediate rebuilding may be the best option when there has been a great deal of destruction so that authorities and building owners can explore the advantages and disadvantages of rebuilding in the same location. Instituting a building moratorium also can prevent unscrupulous contractors who come into the affected community from taking advantage of people who have been traumatized and are willing to pay the first person who offers to help them get their home and life back. Following the Cedar Rapids, Iowa, floods in 2008, the city developed a model that required anyone doing repair or reconstruction in the city to first visit city hall and become certified as qualified and trustworthy (Schwab, 2014).

On the other hand, it is also important to examine options holistically and to consider the downstream effects a moratorium could have. Low-income housing often tends to be in vulnerable (e.g., low-lying) areas of a community. Delays in rebuilding public housing could add even more strain to parts of a community that are in great need (APA, 2014b). An extreme consequence could be increasing homelessness for residents and families who are unable to find affordable housing options. With this in mind, if a moratorium is deemed necessary while authorities examine mitigation strategies, particular attention should be given to temporary housing needs to ensure that vulnerable populations are provided for. (Temporary housing needs are explored in further detail in Chapter 10.) Many actions that should be taken at the local level are described in the American Planning Association's model recovery ordinance described earlier in this chapter.

Environmental Management

Another early recovery priority is securing public sites contaminated with hazardous materials. It is important for municipal leadership to understand that this is a priority even if no immediate health effects are noticed. Following removal of hazardous materials, immediate environmental remediation should be executed to ensure that these materials do not pose a risk to the community in the months or years to follow.

INTERMEDIATE- TO LONG-TERM RECOVERY: OPPORTUNITIES TO ADVANCE HEALTHIER AND MORE RESILIENT AND SUSTAINABLE COMMUNITIES

The health promotion strategies discussed in this section are evidence-based but communities will need to determine what is appropriate to their local conditions and community vision. Communities should inventory their prior plans to identify opportunities to apply disaster-related resources to meet previously agreed-upon objectives. If those plans focus on safe access to healthy foods, for example, the recovery plan might include locating new or rebuilding retail grocery businesses or farmer's markets in areas with demonstrated need. However, it is important to remember that the severity of the disaster may dictate what is possible with respect to strategies and desired outcomes of recovery. In cases of widespread damage, comprehensive initiatives such as mixed-use and transit-oriented development are possible, but if the impact is not as widespread and the corresponding recovery funding is more limited, smaller-scale initiatives, such as creating buffer areas around rivers, may be more practical.

In many cases, farsighted approaches focusing on long-term health, resilience, and sustainability will require an upfront investment. Incentives may be necessary to overcome aversion to added costs and complexity. In Hillsborough County, Florida, for example, the post-disaster redevelopment plan recommends the use of financial incentives for preestablished healthy community priorities such as giving permitting preference to redevelopment plans that incorporate walkable streets or green infrastructure (Hillsborough County Government, 2010).

Developing Transportation and Land Use Strategies

As discussed earlier, transportation and land use strategies can impact health status in a variety of ways, including promotion of active lifestyles; injury reduction; improved access to essential goods, services, and employment; promotion of social cohesion; and improved environmental sustainability (e.g., reduced vehicle emissions). A well-thought-out, transit-oriented design can achieve multiple health benefits for the residents of a neighborhood or town. Developing such a design prior to a disaster can create an opportunity for a community to allocate recovery funds in a balanced and comprehensive manner when rebuilding. As an example, Atlanta, Georgia—typically regarded as a commuter city with urban sprawl—is currently engaged in a project to revitalize its "Beltline" and decrease dependence on vehicles. Once completed, the Atlanta project will have developed 33 miles of multiuse trails, 1,300 acres of parks, and 5,600 units of affordable housing, linking 45 neighborhoods through enhanced transit (ULI, 2013). Even if the funds needed to execute the entire plan are not available prior to a disaster, envisioning such a plan, identifying vendors, and determining implementation methods during steady-state times can allow for quick action toward becoming more sustainable and creating healthy, livable environments following a disaster. To implement such improvements after a disaster, the cross-sector collaboration discussed throughout this report is essential.

A number of strategies can be employed to build more livable and active communities after a disaster. Historically, many cities and towns have been zoned to keep residential and commercial areas separate, but there is now increased awareness that zoning for mixed-use development creates more walkable and bikeable communities, which have been increasing in demand in recent years. Traffic-calming measures, such as speed bumps or pedestrian islands, also have been shown both to increase pedestrian and bicycle safety and to increase active travel (Winters et al., 2010). The introduction or expansion of public transportation systems has a positive effect on active travel as well (What Works for Health, 2010). More accessible transit options in a community also support the "aging in place" concept—enabling seniors to stay at home and provide for themselves.[8]

While improved streetscape design, zoning regulations, and mixed-use development can contribute to a much more active population, also key to success is combining physical infrastructure improvements with social programs. Walking school buses and Safe Routes to School programs, for example, are designed to give children better active options for getting to school. California's Safe Routes to School program helped communities build and improve sidewalks, street crossings, and traffic controls, and an evaluation of the program found that as a result, more children were walking and cycling to school (Transportation Research Board, 2005). Such programs are important because simply improving infrastructure and widening sidewalks will not result in more children being active. If streets are still unsafe, or there is no chaperone to ensure a timely arrival, many parents may still choose the school bus as a better option.

Developing Community Development Strategies

Post-disaster neighborhood revitalization represents one of the largest opportunities to improve long-term health outcomes and community resilience. As discussed in Chapter 2, the social determinants of health (e.g., housing, education, poverty) are in most cases also the determinants of social vulnerability to disasters. During post-disaster redevelopment, one of the greatest opportunities to improve both community health status and social vulnerability is to leverage the recovery funds that often become available to address the needs of low-income individuals and families—most notably CDBG-DR funding, but possibly also economic development and rural development funds. A number of place-based strategies can address blight and reduce socioeconomic and health disparities through interventions that provide access

---

[8] AARP recently developed a disaster recovery toolkit that provides policy information, tools, and resources for building more livable communities after disasters, available at http://www.aarp.org/livable-communities/tool-kits-resources/info-2015/disaster-recovery-tool-kit.html (accessed April 9, 2015).

BOX 9-3
Transit-Oriented Development and Zoning and
Planning in Mission Bay, San Francisco

The Mission Bay development in San Francisco is a good example of how a station area plan was combined with tax increment financing (TIF) and a novel inclusionary housing strategy to create value for both the master developer and the broader community. In this case, the station area plan is, in fact, a redevelopment plan for an area with multiple transit providers, including CalTrain commuter rail service, electric buses, and MUNI METRO light rail, all of which co-terminate and share a common intermodal facility.

Mission Bay is a 303-acre redevelopment project along San Francisco's waterfront, adjacent to both that transit facility and to SBC Park, which is the San Francisco Giants baseball stadium. At the start of the planning process, the area was owned almost entirely by Catellus, a real estate company spun off to shareholders in 1990 to develop property owned by Santa Fe Pacific Corporation. The project area will eventually include over 6,000 residential units, 5 million square feet of corporate offices and biotech space, a new campus for the University of California, San Francisco, a hotel and conference center, 750,000 square feet of retail, and 49 acres of parks and open space. So far, nearly 40 percent of the housing is complete or under construction, along with much of the new University of California, San Francisco, campus.

As part of the development agreement with the San Francisco Redevelopment Agency (SFRA), Catellus agreed to dedicate 14 parcels to the SFRA for the purpose of developing affordable housing. The SFRA then competitively selected developers and provided both land and TIF funds to build mixed-use affordable housing complexes throughout the development. Catellus and the SFRA created a unique land dedication and funding strategy that enabled 28 percent of the housing—which will be created in both standalone affordable housing developments and as part of larger market-rate condominium developments—to be affordable to very low-, low-, and moderate-income households. For example, Rich Sorro Commons is a 100-unit rental apartment development with a 40-child Head Start program and 10,000 square feet of ground floor retail. Around the corner, the SFRA provided land and TIF funds to Mercy Housing California to develop a 100-unit senior care community with a local library on the ground floor. These two developments are sandwiched among a half-dozen market-rate condominium developments that include a grocery store and thousands of square feet of local retail.

SOURCE: Excerpted from Shoemaker, 2006, p. 17.

---

to such resources as affordable housing, employment, nutritious food, and health services. Some of these strategies are discussed below.

Housing, discussed in more detail in Chapter 10, is one of the greatest and most immediate needs after a disaster and can be particularly challenging for already vulnerable populations. Communities need to take steps to prevent former low-income residents from being forced out of their neighborhoods (sometimes called disaster gentrification) and ensure that they have access to essential services, community amenities (e.g., libraries), and centers of employment. Initiatives ensuring that a certain percentage of newly constructed housing is affordable and near transit centers can prevent some of the health inequities described earlier. Low-income populations are often most in need of public transportation, but market prices may exclude these vulnerable populations, necessitating creative market interventions. Mission Bay in San Francisco, California (see Box 9-3), for example, created affordable housing and community elements such as a Head Start program and a senior care community, accessible via multiple transit routes, reducing the parking burden in the area and allowing people of all income levels to obtain goods and services safely and easily.

Although evidence on the health benefits of mixed-income housing is inconclusive (as discussed further in Chapter 10), reducing dense clusters of vulnerable populations in segregated areas of a city may have other benefits in terms of reduced social vulnerability. Where mixed-income housing is incorporated into mixed-use developments, there may be added benefits. A report by the Urban Land Institute, *Housing in America*, highlights an example of an unexpected consequence of mixed-use development:

> A study of the 1995 heat wave in Chicago found that residents—particularly vulnerable populations, including low-income individuals and the elderly—were at lower mortality risk during the heat wave if they lived in neighborhoods with "dense commercial activity" and "streets with more vibrant social ecologies." This reduced risk was attributed to the fact that residents without air conditioning were more readily able to seek relief from high temperatures in local stores. A dense mix of uses and pedestrian-friendly environments enabled the neighborhood's most vulnerable residents to seek shelter from the extreme heat. (ULI, 2014, p. 8)

Education campaigns regarding these benefits can help stem concerns among some buyers and residents about rent control and tax breaks for certain income levels when mixed-income developments are being planned.

Another disaster-related challenge associated with housing is the problem of blighted, abandoned buildings—which, according to Pat Morrissy, executive director of Housing and Neighborhood Development Services, Inc., often can be one of the most significant contributors to a neighborhood's demise, affecting health, crime rates, fire potential, and market values (Mallach, 2006). Two years after Hurricane Katrina, the New Orleans Redevelopment Authority developed the Lot Next Door Program. This program gives the neighboring businesses or owners the opportunity to buy the "lot next door" property for fair market value (New Orleans Redevelopment Authority, 2014). Vacant lots also can be transformed into community gardens that not only reduce blight but also provide access to fresh produce. A community development council in Philadelphia, for example, realized the effect abandoned buildings and lots were having and partnered with the Pennsylvania Horticultural Society to start a vacant land management program in the late 1990s. By 2004 they had reclaimed more than 600 of the vacant lots, planting trees and reselling many of the lots to homeowners for gardens and side yards. They also developed a community garden center and worked to create .75-acre urban farm on another abandoned site, which now sells produce to top area restaurants (Mallach, 2006). Within 10 years, the program had tremendous impact, again showing the multitude of benefits thoughtful redevelopment and environmental management can have in addressing issues of the social determinants of health.

Many vulnerable neighborhoods lack access to nutritious food even before a disaster. Taking the opportunity to address this gap in a long-term recovery process can improve health, resilience, and sustainability. A global program called Urban Farming, for example, began working in Detroit, Michigan, to encourage people to start gardens, grow their own food, and incorporate healthy eating into their lifestyle. In addition to improving nutritional status and reducing reliance on unsustainable food systems, such measures also serve as a disaster risk reduction strategy by improving food security (ULI, 2013). Another example of access to healthy food is the Fresh Food Retailer Initiative in New Orleans, started in 2011 to increase the number of fresh food markets in low-income neighborhoods and communities. While the problem of inadequate access to healthy food existed prior to Hurricane Katrina, it was exacerbated by that event, and the program provided welcome assistance to the neighborhood (ULI, 2013).

The community development sector employs a variety of complementary approaches to improve access of low-income populations to community services and amenities. After a disaster, this could entail strategic placement of new schools and community health clinics near public and affordable housing developments. Changes to land use policies can be complementary to reconstruction of physical infrastructure. Joint-use agreements that enable community members to use school facilities (libraries, pools, athletic fields) during non-school hours, for example, can provide opportunities for recreation in a safe environment and reduce disparities associated with unequal access to community amenities. In addition to the physical health benefits, creating a school-centered community site that supports different kinds of extracurricular activity may also enhance social cohesion in a community, contributing to closer social connections among neighbors and greater awareness of and engagement in community issues. As discussed throughout this report, social cohesion can have positive effects on people's stress levels and mental health.

Redevelopment designs that address community needs holistically are difficult to fashion and complicated to implement. The obvious goal of such designs would be to reconfigure land uses such that residential developments such as assisted living facilities, independent living facilities, senior housing, and affordable housing are situated in a pattern that aligns with business services and employment centers. Most communities lack administrative and management capacity to plan and carry out such ambitious initiatives in a short time, however, and special surge resources are needed to carry them out in a compressed timeframe after a disaster. Disasters that result in widespread devastation, such as the Joplin, Missouri, tornado, may offer special opportunities to replace outmoded pre-disaster land use patterns in creative ways. The case of the C.J. Peete housing redevelopment following Hurricane Katrina exemplifies many of the concepts of approaching the recovery of a community holistically to promote a healthy and sustainable future (see Box 9-4). Coming together after a disaster with multiple parties to consider the implications of the damage and the options available for addressing it is an important part of successful recovery planning.

Developing Environmental Management Strategies

Green, or environmentally responsible, strategies generally focus on environmental sustainability and associated benefits, such as reduced energy consumption and cost, but they also have demonstrated parallel health benefits. When air quality is better, for example, asthma attacks are reduced, which leads in turn to reductions in health care costs and absenteeism from school (Kats, 2006). Typically, green infrastructure is understood as entailing such elements as rain gardens, green roofs, wetlands, and walking trails. However, the design of physical structures also can play a role in encouraging healthy behaviors and promoting healthy environments.

Indoor Environments

A study conducted by McGraw Hill Construction, commissioned by the American Institute of Architects, found that decisions about building design, construction, and operations are critical to the well-being of building occupants and demonstrated the strong role buildings can play within the surrounding communities (McGraw Hill Construction, 2014). Indoor environments with poor air quality can contribute to adverse health effects and, in turn, to more doctor visits, higher medical bills, and even cost to employers (Loftness et al., 2007). Sustainable building design depends on material selection, which can impact not just air quality but also health issues related to whether the materials selected promote mold, toxicity in fires, or cancer-causing fibers (Dainoff, 1990). Examples discussed below illustrate health impacts in schools and economic impacts in neighborhoods, but this topic is explored further with regard to housing in Chapter 10.

Outdoor Environment

The American Society of Landscape Architects (ASLA) offers examples of and strategies for green infrastructure and design that not only can mitigate future hazards in a community but also have positive economic benefits. "In the typical market, an additional 1 point increase in [a community's] walk score was associated with between a $700 and $3,000 increase in home values" (Cortright, 2009, p. 2). The use of less impervious surfaces such as rain gardens, porous concrete, or green roofs can be more sustainable, prevent stormwater runoff and water pooling, and make a community more resilient to storms or floods.

The High Line Park in New York City is an example of the combined use of green infrastructure and community development, focused on revitalizing an abandoned railroad track running through Manhattan. A neighborhood group advocated for its preservation and reuse as public open space. Through zoning amendments and competitive green design, the park now spans over 20 blocks, with more phases to follow (ASLA, 2013). There are many layers within the "living roof" on the elevated rail line, which will help

---

BOX 9-4
New Orleans' C.J. Peete Public Housing Redevelopment

Even before Hurricane Katrina flooded New Orleans, the neighborhood of Central City was suffering—the neighborhood was racially segregated and poor, and lacked the services and opportunities that might help residents escape poverty. The large public housing development, C.J. Peete, was in the process of being demolished, with only half of the original 1,403 units remaining and the previous residents having been displaced. After the storm, C.J. Peete was largely undamaged, but the city's housing authority chose to take the storm as an opportunity to demolish it and redevelop the housing facilities.

The Annie E. Casey Foundation joined with other philanthropic and community organizations to support the redevelopment of C.J. Peete and the revitalization of the Central City neighborhood. Along with a for-profit developer and its nonprofit community development subsidiary, the foundation and its partners followed a guiding framework of "holistic community redevelopment and transformation." This framework, rather than focusing solely on rebuilding the physical structures of the neighborhood, gave equal priority to all elements of a healthy community, including: affordable mixed-income housing, authentic resident engagement, good schools, jobs and job training, integrated services, access to transportation, and building the capacity of residents and community organizations. Flexible funding from a variety of sources allowed the project to fund some of these unconventional objectives.

Many residents had lived in C.J. Peete for generations and were deeply rooted in the community, and some opposed the plan to demolish and rebuild. The developer took the time to get residents on board and to engage them meaningfully in the process. First, the developer's nonprofit subsidiary spent substantial time reaching out to displaced residents, stabilizing families, and providing case management and referrals to services. Residents were offered training in leadership skills, job training, and literacy and financial management classes. Second, the developer involved the residents in the planning of the new community, holding conversations about residents' priorities, hopes, and needs, and residents weighed in on decisions that affected them. The developer and the residents signed memorandums of understanding, and when tensions arose, the developer addressed residents' concerns. Some residents even helped build the new development—after a 13-week construction training program, 29 new jobs were filled by low-income neighborhood residents.

Six years after the hurricane, the end result of this process was Harmony Oaks, a mixed-income housing development that, along with the surrounding Central City neighborhood, includes a new elementary school; a park; a business incubator; and a community center with Head Start, a health clinic, a playground, and offices for state services. Almost 400 Harmony Oaks residents have received employment training and assistance, and the employment rate has risen 42 percent since the project began. One success story encapsulates the unique impact of Harmony Oaks: the building's first resident, who had lived in C.J. Peete, received case management for 3 years, became certified as a nurse, found a steady job, and moved into Harmony Oaks as a market-rate renter.

SOURCE: AECF, 2013.

---

filter stormwater runoff and prevent pooling of water and flooding. Considerable planning for long-term sustainability was conducted as well, resulting in the use of special long-lasting concrete to reduce waste caused by later replacements and the selection of native, drought-resistant plant species capable of withstanding the specific microclimate. Additionally, plans are being made to harvest rainwater from nearby buildings to reduce environmental impact (ASLA, 2013). In addition to its function as green infrastructure, the placement and design of High Line Park also encourage elements of a healthy community described throughout this report, such as active lifestyles and positive community interaction, which can contribute to increased social cohesion. The park also has been incorporated into the local school curriculum, and a "youth corps" program was created to employ teenagers in tending the park landscape and facilitating park-related educational and community engagement efforts (ASLA, 2014).

In September 1999, flooding caused by Hurricanes Dennis and Floyd devastated the town of Kinston, North Carolina. More than three-quarters of homes in the flood plain and many businesses were damaged or completely destroyed. In its recovery strategy, the town decided to take a two-pronged approach encompassing community redevelopment and hazard mitigation strategies discussed throughout this chapter. The objectives were to reduce the impacts of future floods while revitalizing existing neighborhoods and businesses to increase self-sufficiency and promote long-term sustainability. To accomplish the first objective, they used GIS mapping to identify flood-prone areas and determine which areas were suitable for development and which should remain as buffers and open space. To protect social networks, residents from the same neighborhoods were relocated together. In addition, they developed a cooperative green infrastructure plan with the nearby University of North Carolina at Chapel Hill and a conservation non-profit to create different types of green space, allowing for all types of recreation as well as promotion of heritage tourism (Natural Hazards Center, 2006).

Incorporating Hazard Mitigation, Resilience, and Sustainability Planning

Disaster risk reduction or hazard mitigation can increase resilience in a community and decrease the impact of future events (NRC, 2012). As climate change brings increasing numbers of disasters of increased severity, as well as sea-level rise and coastal erosion, many communities across the nation, and indeed worldwide, have been taking a closer look at their needs and vulnerabilities (NRC, 2014). Hazard mitigation is particularly critical for facilities and other infrastructure that need to remain functional after a disaster, including hospitals (see Chapter 6), emergency operations centers, public safety facilities, and utilities. Both structural and nonstructural mitigation strategies are available, each with their advantages and disadvantages (NRC, 2012). Structural options include levees; floodwalls; dams; floodways; impact-resistant construction materials; and elevation of critical elements such as rails, highways, and homes. Nonstructural options include buyouts or natural defenses such as coastal sand dunes or wetlands, similar to some of the green design elements described previously. When feasible, communities should select redevelopment areas outside of known hazards areas (e.g., flood zones[9] and man-made pollution such as busy highways), and they may consider discouraging rebuilding in hazard zones by withholding public funds for reconstruction. However, telling a community it needs to move is much easier in policy than in practice, and these kinds of discussions can be highly political and contentious (benefits and challenges related to buyouts are discussed in Box 9-5). Even if moving a community appears necessary because of concerns about coastal resilience, simply relocating infrastructure may not result in successful transplantation. In many cases, communities will lean toward employing structural and nonstructural mitigation measures to build resilience before attempting to move. In the event of a presidentially declared disaster, funding for mitigation measures is available from FEMA (Hazard Mitigation Grant Program and Section 406 Stafford Act mitigation funds) and, following a supplemental appropriation, HUD's CDBG-DR.

While there are many strategies for hazard mitigation, the national or even regional vision to undertake these important efforts often is lacking. According to a recent report of the National Research Council (2014, p. 6), "Studies have reported benefit-cost ratios between 5:1 and 8:1 for nonstructural and design strategies that reduce the consequences of flooding, but between 2004 and 2012, federal funds for such strategies were only about 5 percent of disaster relief funds." That report notes further that "the vast majority of funding for coastal risk-related issues is provided only after a disaster occurs, through emergency supplemental appropriations" (NRC, 2014, p. 4). Thus, as with many other sources of disaster funding, these issues receive little attention and funding prior to a disaster. Even once funding is available, often only a very small percentage is allocated for mitigation and risk reduction efforts.[10] However,

---

[9] FEMA has been modifying flood plain maps and 100-year flood projections and evacuation zones, which may help direct funding for mitigation strategies to certain areas and may alter eligibility for participation in the National Flood Insurance Program (FEMA, 2015a).

[10] As discussed in Chapter 4, Section 406 of the Stafford Act authorizes funding to be used for mitigation measures during rebuilding as long as it will contribute to protection from subsequent events.

BOX 9-5
Managed Retreat: Benefits and Challenges Related to Buyouts

Difficult choices are ahead in the years to come as climate change threatens to result in sea-level rise, coastal erosion, and more severe storms. Although communities have started implementing a variety of structural and nonstructural adaptive strategies to harden infrastructure and increase resilience in waterside communities, it will not be possible or financially feasible for some to adequately protect public safety and property using these measures.

Hazardous events such as Hurricane Sandy have spurred greater interest in the use of buyout programs to facilitate a managed retreat from flood-prone areas. The Federal Emergency Management Agency's (FEMA's) Hazard Mitigation Grant Program and the Department of Housing and Urban Development's (HUD's) Community Development Block Grant for Disaster Recovery are two funding sources commonly used to finance buyouts, and homeowners generally are offered prestorm market value for their homes. Both programs require that the acquired properties not be redeveloped but remain as open space with such functions as recreation and/or environmental management (e.g., wetlands).

Because of the contentiousness surrounding government acquisition of private property, such buyout programs often are voluntary. For targeted areas with high risk, incentives can be used to encourage homeowners to relocate. In New York, for example, 10 percent of fair market house value was offered as an incentive for residents in targeted areas, who received an additional 5 percent if they relocated within the same county. While these kinds of incentives are valuable motivators, homeowners in some cases will resist or be unable to accept a buyout (if, for example, they owe far more on their mortgage than the prestorm market value). In such cases, governments may consider exercising eminent domain to ensure that all or most properties in a high-risk area are relocated. Despite the distinct possibility of public outcry, this may be necessary to protect the lives of residents and the responders responsible for rescue operations, to reduce expenditures of public funds associated with recovery needs, and to create more effective environmental conservation areas.

SOURCE: Bova-Hiatt et al., 2014.

FEMA's National Mitigation Framework, created in 2013, represents a major step forward for mitigation and disaster risk reduction at the national level, and states and regions need to follow suit. The FEMA framework describes mitigation roles within a community to embed risk management within community priorities and plans (e.g., critical infrastructure, land use, capital improvement, sustainability, recovery, health improvement) (FEMA, 2015b). Seven core capabilities in the framework and an example of a critical task for each are listed below:

- **"Threats and Hazard Identification.** Build cooperation between private and public sectors by protecting internal interests but sharing threats and hazard identification resources and benefits.
- **Risk and Disaster Resilience Assessment.** Perform credible risk assessments using scientifically valid and widely used risk assessment techniques.
- **Planning.** Incorporate the findings from assessment of risk and disaster resilience into the planning process.
- **Community Resilience.** Recognize the interdependent nature of the economy, health and social services, housing infrastructure, and natural and cultural resources within a community.
- **Public Information and Warning.** Target messages to reach organizations representing children, individuals with disabilities or access and functional needs, diverse communities and people with limited English proficiency.

- **Long-Term Vulnerability Reduction.** Adopt and enforce a suitable building code to ensure resilient construction.
- **Operational Coordination.** Capitalize on opportunities for mitigation actions following disasters and incidents" (FEMA, 2015b).

Unfortunately, disasters themselves are one of the most powerful motivators for instituting hazard mitigation strategies. Once municipalities and states have been exposed to the debilitating effects and costs of disasters, leaders often are more likely to focus on reducing exposures for future incidents. After Hurricane Sandy in 2012, for example, Governor Cuomo convened a NYS2100 Commission to review the vulnerabilities of the state's infrastructure systems and make recommendations for increasing the state's resilience in five different areas: transportation, energy, land use, insurance, and infrastructure finance (NYS 2100 Commission, 2013). The commission developed several cross-cutting recommendations, as well as recommendations specific to each of the sectors, focused both on the recovery process and on mitigation of future hazards and decreased vulnerability. The nine cross-cutting recommendations, listed below, highlight the integration needed across systems:

- Protect, upgrade, and strengthen existing systems.
- Rebuild smarter: ensure replacement with better options and alternatives.
- Encourage the use of green and natural infrastructure.
- Create shared equipment and resource reserves.
- Promote integrated planning and develop criteria for integrated decision making for capital investments.
- Enhance institutional coordination.
- Improve data, mapping, visualization, and communication systems.
- Create new incentive programs to encourage resilient behaviors and reduce vulnerabilities.
- Expand education, job training, and workforce development opportunities. (NYS 2100 Commission, 2013, p. 12-13)

Hurricane Sandy also spurred the launch of Rebuild by Design, a competition funded by HUD through a supplemental congressional appropriation to challenge local and global designers to develop innovative large-scale infrastructure solutions to build resiliency in the impacted region. The case study in Box 9-6 is an example of natural hazard mitigation efforts developed in the context of this competition.

Given the physical, psychological, economic, and social consequences of disasters, recommendations for leveraging long-term recovery planning to build healthier communities need to encompass hazard mitigation and risk reduction to protect against the effects of future disasters. Hazard mitigation plans (like health improvement plans) need to be incorporated into a community's comprehensive plan, not created in isolation. Hazard mitigation plans most commonly are developed by the emergency management sector, but those efforts should be supplemented by the multiple sectors and stakeholders mentioned throughout this chapter to ensure cross-sector involvement and streamlined goal setting. Health sector (public health, behavioral health, health care) stakeholders have a clear role in advocating for mitigation actions that will protect against future disaster-related physical and psychological trauma and can help inform mitigation decisions through health impact assessments (see Box 3-6 in Chapter 3). Further, the health sector can work with the emergency management sector to educate the broader community about the importance of reducing social vulnerability as part of a larger disaster risk reduction strategy.

Complementary Approaches

Problems faced by a community often are multifaceted. As a result, complementary investments are needed to address complex challenges and achieve synergies. For example, preserving undeveloped buffer zones around rivers that present a flood hazard can mitigate future disasters but also can provide rec-

BOX 9-6
Rebuild by Design Case Study: Living with the Bay, Nassau County, New York

The damage from Hurricane Sandy was caused primarily by storm surge. Unfortunately, however, storm surge is not Long Island's only water-related threat. Because groundwater is insufficiently recharged, for example, saltwater intrusion is contaminating the aquifer. And Long Island faces serious threats from sea-level rise, stormwater, and wastewater. The latter two threats are a major source of pollution: unfiltered stormwater runoff entering the bay by way of the region's rivers and creeks threatens the bay's ecology. Effluent from the Bay Park Sewage Treatment Plant—which is currently released in the bay—exacerbates nitrogen levels that cause harmful algae blooms, hypoxia, and excessive seaweed growth, and that also deteriorate salt marshes that could otherwise help protect Long Islanders from storm surge. To address these challenges, Nassau County, New York, formulated a plan for making the South Shore more resilient.

Strategies for the Ocean Shore: Sediment Flow

The drowning of the marshland will be stopped only when plates grow along with sea-level rise, and for this purpose, the plan includes a multifaceted approach to recovering the region's sediment system. Overall, this strategy is focused on using the available amount of sediment within the active system in a smart way so that it can move around the system and strengthen it, with sediment from outside the active system being added to allow the area to grow along with the rising sea level.

Strategies for the Barrier Island: The Smart Barrier

As a result of their location and topography, Long Island's barrier islands are vulnerable to sea-level rise and storm surge. The plan includes the addition of protective infrastructure that would also serve as a landscape amenity, ensuring access to the bay shore and providing a place where stormwater can be stored, cleaned, and replenished.

Strategies for the Marsh: The Eco-Edge

Urban development has negatively affected Nassau County's wetlands, which play a critical role in buffering coastal communities. The plan includes the development of new marsh islands that would reduce wave action, improve the bay ecology, and provide new recreational opportunities.

Strategies for the Lowlands: Slow Streams

Flooding from coastal surges and stormwater inundation threatens the areas around southern Nassau's north-south tributaries. The plan addresses these threats—along with other problems such as water quality and ecological recovery—through a series of interconnected interventions designed to transform rivers into green-blue corridors that would simultaneously store and filter water and provide public space and space for new urban development.

SOURCE: Rebuild by Design, 2014.

reation areas if used for trails. This is often the case with environmental management efforts and green designs. The ecology created can mitigate many hazards, improve air quality, and moderate temperature while also contributing to healthy communities by promoting active lifestyles and vibrant community centers and activities. At the same time, it is important to remember that addressing just the physical infrastructure of a community cannot bring about healthy, resilient, and sustainable communities; reducing social vulnerabilities is critical as well for both health improvement and disaster risk reduction. This essential synergy reinforces the emphasis throughout this report on collaboration across sectors and with multiple stakeholders. Table 9-1 provides a summary of strategies that can be employed in this kind of complementary approach.

TABLE 9-1 Summary of Strategies for Healthy Community Planning

Guidance Area	Rationale	Healthy Community Planning Strategies
Transportation and Land Use	Community design that promotes active lifestyles, injury reduction, and social cohesion while improving access to goods and services and encouraging environmental sustainability can enhance the community's overall health.	• Provide safe routes for schoolchildren to walk or bike to school through sidewalk improvements, street crossings, and traffic-calming controls. • Improve streetscape designs and zoning regulations to increase a community's activity levels in a safe and an inviting environment. • Focus on mixed-use development incorporating transit-oriented designs that are safely accessible by pedestrians and cyclists to reduce public dependence on cars. • Organize multiuse centers, such as schools and athletic facilities, to be used as community resources after school hours.
Community Development	Developing placed-based strategies targeting community redevelopment can provide access to such resources as affordable housing, employment, nutritious food, and health services that can reduce socioeconomic and health disparities.	• Ensure that a percentage of redeveloped housing is kept affordable and near transit centers. • Provide education on the benefits of mixed-income housing for the community as a whole. • Address abandoned buildings and vacant lots in neighborhoods to create a safe and welcoming environment. • Make nutritious food readily available and easily accessible by locating grocery stores closer to communities and encouraging partnerships with local farms to bring produce to corner stores. • Provide easier access to health services and community centers by locating them near transit stops and places where residents regularly visit, such as schools, senior centers, and public housing.
Environmental Management	Community design that focuses on environmental sustainability can have a lasting impact on air, water, food, and soil quality, contributing to a healthier environment as well as making a community more resilient to disasters.	• Incorporate designs that focus on environmental sustainability and are beneficial to community health, such as relocating highways away from residential areas to reduce air and noise pollution. • Encourage innovative planning and development of open public space and impervious surfaces through green infrastructures such as rain gardens and "living roofs" that help prevent flooding and pooling of water. • Reduce energy consumption and cost by planting more trees and developing more green spaces, which can decrease air temperatures and reduce the use of air conditioners in urban areas.

TABLE 9-1 Continued

Guidance Area	Rationale	Healthy Community Planning Strategies
Hazard Mitigation	Disaster risk reduction or hazard mitigation can increase resilience in a community and reduce the health, social, and economic impacts of future emergencies.	• Incorporate risk-based strategies. • Identify threats and hazards with both the private and the public sector. • Understand who and where vulnerable populations are and their specific needs. • Incorporate both structural and nonstructural hazard mitigation practices in planning (e.g., natural buffer zones, sand dunes, levees, floodwalls, dams). • Select redevelopment areas outside of known hazard (e.g., flood-prone) areas when feasible.

The committee found both domestic and international examples of communities taking advantage of the synergies of complementary approaches. Following the floods in Iowa in 2008, for example, the city of Cedar Rapids developed a recovery plan that addressed hazard mitigation, active lifestyles, and the need to reduce social vulnerability through affordable housing (see Box 9-7). And in Sendai City, Japan, measures taken to create energy self-sufficient neighborhoods contributed to both sustainability and disaster risk reduction (see Box 9-8).

BOX 9-7
Cedar Rapids: Complementary Post-Disaster Investments
for Improved Health, Resilience, and Sustainability

In June 2008, Cedar Rapids, Iowa, experienced a record-setting flood causing an estimated $6 billion in damages that affected more than 5,000 residential properties and 20,000 residents. The flood damaged not only residential properties but also many of the city's main public service buildings. Just months before the flood occurred, however, the city council and manager had engaged the community in an inclusive process of developing a shared vision for the city's future. This existing engagement process, the resultant community vision, and a related effort to adopt a systems approach to government operations all enabled the community to come together quickly after the flood around a plan for what their new community would look like. The plan included such goals as encouraging active, healthy lifestyles; ensuring equitable redevelopment; building resource-efficient and resilient buildings; and protecting the city against future floods by rebuilding outside of flood-prone areas.

An immediate need for the city after the flood was to find housing for the 20,000 displaced residents. Temporary housing was offered through the help of the Federal Emergency Management Agency (FEMA), rental communities, and property managers. The city's long-term plan was to build affordable housing for residents of all income levels. Consistent with pre-disaster plans, redevelopment was focused on making the community more compact and urban by offering an array of options, including multifamily housing rebuilt in denser neighborhoods closer to downtown. By educating the community on the benefits of higher-density neighborhoods, Cedar Rapids was able to avoid much of the "not in my backyard" attitude that can often impede equitable development initiatives. Developers received tax incentives, both state and local, for plans with a focus on mixed-use development. A request for proposals was submitted for city-owned parcels located outside the 100-year flood plain; this competitive process ensured that the city received high-quality proposals from local developers. These projects were joint ventures between the city and the developers. Development companies were encouraged to use resilient designs (e.g., raising buildings off the ground and having parking spaces on the first floor) to increase sustainability and flood resistance.

continued

BOX 9-7 Continued

The city was able to move residents through voluntary property acquisitions—the city purchased about 1,400 properties, helping homeowners move on from the disaster, both physically and financially. Public resources for rebuilding were not given for parcels located within the 100-year flood plain to discourage redevelopment in areas at higher risk of future damage. Community development funds were awarded from the U.S. Department of Housing and Urban Development's Community Development Block Grant program, which granted $300 million for recovery and rebuilding, with a focus on low- and middle-income households and the Home Investment Partnership fund. Low-income housing tax credits also were used to rebuild affordable multifamily units. City staff met regularly with local housing groups to determine which neighborhoods needed improvement to be considered high-functioning and equitable.

To encourage the community members to live healthy, active lifestyles, part of the recovery plan focused on providing connectivity and walkability from the planned housing developments to make the downtown core more accessible. Included in steps toward attaining this goal was the addition of a large green space area that was acquired through the city-purchased voluntary property acquisitions program. In a good example of an approach yielding multiple simultaneous benefits, a flood protection strategy created by city staff, stakeholders, and residents included a levy and floodwall system with some floodable greenway, which allowed the community to keep enjoying the accessible downtown area as well as the Cedar River.

Key to the success of Cedar Rapids' recovery was the fact that the community already had in place initiatives aimed at increasing density in the downtown area and building housing near municipal services and employment centers. After the flood, these initiatives were accelerated and integrated into the community's comprehensive plan, Envision CR, helping the community focus not on just the immediate disaster response but also on investing in the city's recovery and future goals 15 to 20 years down the line.

As a result of its efforts to use the disaster recovery process to build back healthier by increasing physical activity, social connectedness, and a sense of belonging as a community, Cedar Rapids is now a Blue Zones Community and was awarded the 2014 National Civic League's All-American City Award.

SOURCE: ULI, 2014.

BOX 9-8
Complementary Approaches to Achieving Resilience and Sustainability in Sendai City, Japan

After the Great East Japan Earthquake and subsequent typhoon devastated a coastal area of Sendai City in Japan, Kokusai Kogyo Co., Ltd., a private civil engineering consulting firm, led an environmentally friendly property development project that also incorporated disaster risk reduction strategies (UNISDR, 2013). The firm was responsible for developing one of the city's mass relocation areas and, conscious of the hardships the survivors (particularly those dependent on electricity for medical equipment) had experienced as a result of power loss after the disaster, included in its plan for the development a goal of energy self-sufficiency. Kokusai Kogyo was able to achieve this goal by obtaining government subsidies to offset the added costs of implementing these innovative disaster risk reduction measures; thus, public–private partnerships were essential to the success of the initiative. "The disaster resilient, low-carbon-footprint, nature-embracing Green Community Tagonishi, designed with the comfort of its residents in mind, has garnered attention as the embodiment of a new and positive direction in the reconstruction of disaster-affected areas and urban renewal" (UNISDR, 2013, p. 7).

RESEARCH NEEDS

In the process of developing its guidance and recommendations specific to place-based recovery strategies, the committee noted the need for research to address the following questions:

- How do high levels of collaboration at the local level among the community development and health and social services sectors to examine problems holistically translate to better post-disaster recovery?
- How does the built environment impact social cohesion, behavioral health, and well-being, and how can this knowledge be transformed into resilience-building strategies?
- What are the best ways to incorporate healthy community outcomes into transportation planning? Are there best practices for educating both internal and external stakeholders in this area?
- What risk-based strategies can be employed during recovery planning to reduce the physical, psychological, economic, and social consequences of future disasters?

SUMMARY OF FINDINGS AND RECOMMENDATIONS

This chapter has presented a number of strategies that integrate public health and social services goals with other community systems involved in place-based redevelopment. Each of these strategies builds on a prior investment in planning. For decades, metropolitan and rural areas—supported by the programs of the agencies now comprising the Partnership for Sustainable Communities—have been implementing community redevelopment plans of all kinds, many of them comprehensive in nature, which can serve as the foundation for an integrated approach to disaster planning and recovery. While major disasters can facilitate widespread redevelopment and improvements, even more isolated instances of flooding or storm surge, for example, can present opportunities to formulate and execute a vision of recovery, particularly one focused on reducing concentrations of poverty and improving other social determinants of health.

In most cases, communities dealing with disaster recovery fail to recognize the opportunities for advancing such a vision. Two federal departments, HUD and HHS, place great emphasis on this transformative aspect of community investments, and their respective socioeconomic programs have broad untapped potential to bolster disaster recovery in most communities. Proportionately, only a small fraction of the nation's local governments are affected by disasters, but nearly all of them are and indeed have for decades engaged in HUD- and HHS-funded programs that target similar objectives. Unfortunately, those initiatives (at federal, state and local levels) have not been adequately integrated into the disaster recovery planning process.

Disasters often necessitate significant efforts to restore the physical infrastructure of a community, including repair of roads and bridges, reconstruction of housing and other buildings, repair of public works, and restoration of natural resources. Rather than rebuilding to a prior state, the recovery process offers a unique opportunity to mitigate against future hazards and create environments intentionally designed to support health. Such strategies focus on healthier housing and community features that enhance active lifestyles and improve equitable access to critical goods (e.g., healthy food), community services (e.g., medical care), and amenities (e.g., libraries, schools). A well-planned recovery also attends to the economic vitality of the affected area, fostering commercial revitalization, industrial and business development, and greater employment opportunities, thereby improving financial prospects for both residents and businesses. To ensure that these opportunities are not missed, planning and design, housing, community development, and environmental and public health professionals should be engaged in the development of pre- and post-disaster recovery strategies, which should be linked to community plans for improving health and social well-being developed in advance of a disaster. Communities that have such plans in hand when a disaster strikes are better equipped to undertake recovery more quickly with the long-term objectives of health, resilience, and sustainability. Given that the pool of resources for recovery is limited, creative uses of funds that simultaneously meet multiple objectives can improve the efficiency of recovery and leverage opportunities to integrate health considerations. Such opportunities deserve special attention in disaster recovery plans.

Recommendation 10: *Design for Healthy Post-Disaster Communities.*

State and federal agencies (the Federal Emergency Management Agency, the U.S. Department of Transportation, the U.S. Department of Housing and Urban Development, the U.S. Environmental Protection Agency, the U.S. Department of Health and Human Services, and others), acting alone or as components of the federal Partnership for Sustainable Communities, should ensure through funding requirements that the use of federal community development and disaster recovery and preparedness funds optimizes the built environment in support of healthy communities by creating places that protect against health threats, promote good health, and address unmet social needs.

Local and state planning entities should develop a team-based approach to integrated recovery planning aligned with the policies and processes of the Partnership for Sustainable Communities so as to maximize efficiency in the use of federal resources to enhance smart growth, equity, hazard mitigation, resilience, sustainability, and other elements necessary to the creation of healthy communities. Priority areas for funding should specifically address the following essential health-enhancing requirements that are pertinent to the community's needs as laid out in pre- and post-disaster health improvement and comprehensive plans:

- physical activity-enhancing infrastructure that includes trails, bike paths, sidewalks, and parks and recreational spaces, as well as walkable, mixed-use neighborhood designs; and
- comprehensive transportation infrastructure and land use policies that ensure the accessibility of healthy food retail outlets, employment, health and social services, schools, and community amenities such as libraries and community centers for all residents.

Optimal health, social well-being, and safety are dependent on avoiding or reducing the impacts of disasters by using best practices of hazard mitigation, including both structural and nonstructural (e.g., zoning and land use) standards and strategies. Forward-looking strategic plans, improved infrastructure, and stronger construction codes need to be used in combination to address identified community vulnerabilities, thereby reversing the nation's trend toward higher disaster losses and the attendant human misery and social and economic costs, as well as preparing the nation for the potential effects of climate change.

Recommendation 11: *Mitigate Against Future Health Hazards.*

Building on the National Mitigation Framework, federal agencies, led by the Federal Emergency Management Agency, should immediately intensify their efforts, undertaken collectively and supported by aligned funding eligibility requirements, to ensure that all critical infrastructure and facilities—such as hospitals (public and private), nursing homes, fire stations, and public utilities—constructed after a disaster are designed and built with a level of protection that better ensures post-disaster safety and functionality essential to protecting health and recovering more quickly. When feasible, they should be located outside of known hazard zones. Additionally, requirements should ensure that existing critical infrastructure and facilities restored with federal recovery funds are upgraded to the new standards.

PLACE-BASED RECOVERY STRATEGIES CHECKLIST

The committee has identified two pre-event and six post-disaster critical recovery priorities for the planning, community development, environmental management, and transportation sectors that are inextricably linked to strengthening the health, resilience, and sustainability of a community. Action steps for each of these priorities are provided in the following checklist. Although leaders of these sectors will need to adapt these actions to the local context, this guidance provides an indicative set of concerns to be considered during recovery, and also identifies potentially new and different stakeholders that should be included as partners. The checklist illustrates how the following five key recovery strategies, identified as recurring themes at the beginning of this chapter, apply to individual priority areas:

- Reduce health disparities and improve access to essential goods, services, and opportunities.
- Preserve and promote social connectedness.
- Use a systems approach to community redevelopment that acknowledges the connection among social, cultural, economic, and physical environments.
- Seek holistic solutions to socioeconomic disparities and their perverse effects on population health through place-based interventions.
- Rebuild for resilience and sustainability.
- Capitalize on existing planning networks to strengthen recovery planning, including attention to public health, medical, and social services, especially for vulnerable populations.

Pre-Event

Priority: Organize for Future Disaster Recovery Planning

Primary Actors[1]: Elected Officials and Community Leaders, Emergency Management Agencies
Key Partners: Urban and Regional Planning Agencies, State/Local Health Departments,[2] Community Development Organizations, Social Services Agencies, Housing Agencies, Community- and Faith-Based Organizations

Key Recovery Strategy:
- Capitalize on existing planning networks to strengthen recovery planning, including attention to public health, medical, and social services, especially for vulnerable populations.

Activities include but are not limited to:
- ☐ Hold community planning and visioning workshops (charrettes).
- ☐ Consider adopting a model recovery ordinance to help organize for short- and long-term recovery.
- ☐ Identify agencies and/or individuals as designated leads for Recovery Support Functions (RSFs) following a disaster.
  - – Consider contingencies for when specific groups should or should not be included based on the type and severity of a disaster and recovery needs.
- ☐ Create a plan for debris management for Federal Emergency Management Agency (FEMA) incentive eligibility.
  - – Identify vendors for selection when needed following a disaster.

- -

Priority: Conduct Vulnerability and Capacity Assessments

Primary Actors: Elected Officials and Community Leaders, Emergency Management Agencies, Urban and Regional Planning Agencies
Key Partners: State/Local Health Departments, Chamber of Commerce, Private Sector, Community- and Faith-Based Organizations

Key Recovery Strategies:
- Capitalize on existing planning networks to strengthen recovery planning, including attention to public health, medical, and social services, especially for vulnerable populations.
- Rebuild for resilience and sustainability.

Activities include but are not limited to:
- ☐ Review comprehensive emergency management plans, community health assessments, and other information sources on community vulnerability and risk.

---

[1] See Appendix F for further description of terms used to describe Primary Actors and Key Partners in this checklist.
[2] Throughout this checklist, "State/Local" is used for the purposes of brevity but should be inferred to include tribal and territorial as well.

Pre-Event

☐ Use risk assessment tools to simulate damage and measure the effects of different disaster events.
☐ If available, use geographic information systems (GIS) to map the socioeconomic profile of communities.
  – Analyze results and prioritize specific needs of different locations during the recovery phase.
☐ Assess planning and regulatory capacity, the status of programs, and potential impacts on post-disaster redevelopment.
  – Examine for gaps or weaknesses.
☐ Assess political will for long-term recovery and redevelopment.
☐ Assess fiscal capacity for projects.
  – Determine which redevelopment projects already have seed funding and which require new money for completion.

Short-Term Recovery

Priority: Assess Disaster Impacts on Community Systems

Primary Actor: Emergency Management Agencies
Key Partners: Environmental Health Agencies, Community Development Organizations, Public Works and Utilities, Housing Agencies, Social Services Agencies

Key Recovery Strategy:
- Use a systems approach to community redevelopment that acknowledges the connection among social, cultural, economic, and physical environments.

Activities include but are not limited to:
- ☐ Assess the extent of damage to public facilities, roads, and hospitals.
- ☐ Project the types of expanded capacity needed to facilitate rapid recovery.
  - – Determine needs for previously arranged memorandums of understanding.
  - – Determine needs for waiving regulations to speed recovery.
- ☐ Consider the need for a moratorium on immediate rebuilding.

- -

Priority: Restore Critical Infrastructure and Remediate Immediate Health Threats

Primary Actors: Emergency Management Agencies, Urban and Regional Planning Agencies, Public Works and Utilities
Key Partners: Environmental Health Agencies, Federal Agencies (including the Environmental Protection Agency and the U.S. Army Corps of Engineers), Private Sector (including Environmental Remediation and Debris Removal Vendors)

Key Recovery Strategy:
- Rebuild for resilience and sustainability.

Activities include but are not limited to:
- ☐ Implement the debris management plan (if created prior to the event).
  - – Perform site selection to ensure environmental justice when dumping.
- ☐ Examine changes to FEMA 100-year flood maps to confirm that rebuilding locations are appropriate.
- ☐ Prioritize reopening of roads required for access to medical facilities.
- ☐ Ensure that public transportation is available to residents of temporary mass relocations sites.
- ☐ Restore critical infrastructure including water treatment facilities, power, and communication infrastructure.
- ☐ Remediate indoor and outdoor environments contaminated with toxic pollutants.

Intermediate- to Long-Term Recovery

Priority: Develop Transportation and Land Use Strategies to Improve Health

Primary Actors: Urban and Regional Planning Agencies, Transportation Agencies
Key Partners: State/Local Health Departments, Education System

Key Recovery Strategies:
- Reduce health disparities and improve access to essential goods, services, and opportunities.
- Preserve and promote social connectedness.
- Use a systems approach to community redevelopment that acknowledges the connection among social, cultural, economic, and physical environments.
- Seek holistic solutions to socioeconomic disparities and their perverse effects on population health through place-based interventions.
- Rebuild for resilience and sustainability.
- Capitalize on existing planning networks to strengthen recovery planning, including attention to public health, medical, and social services, especially for vulnerable populations.

Activities include but are not limited to:
- ☐ Inventory prior plans for transit-oriented development to promote active living.
- ☐ Review 1-year, 5-year, and long-term transportation and land use plans in the disaster context.
- ☐ Develop schedules for the implementation of transportation recovery actions that align with all other recovery plan elements.
- ☐ Identify opportunities to stimulate recovery and overcome access disparities.
- ☐ Review existing bus and rail lines between vulnerable neighborhoods and common commercial and retail centers.
- ☐ Target disadvantaged neighborhoods where access upgrades will stimulate investments.
- ☐ Explore alternative pedestrian and cycling strategies for both recreation and commuting purposes.
- ☐ Promote trail investments through discretionary programs such as the U.S. Department of Transportation's (DOT) Transportation Investment Generating Economic Recovery (TIGER) program.
- ☐ Review and upgrade development standards and zoning and subdivision regulations for resiliency.

- -

Priority: Develop Community Development Strategies to Reduce Health and Socioeconomic Disparities

Primary Actors: Community Development Organizations, Housing Agencies, Social Services Agencies
Key Partners: Urban and Regional Planning Agencies, State/Local Health Departments, Federal Agencies (including HUD), Private Sector (including Architects, Designers, and Developers), Community- and Faith-Based Organizations

Intermediate- to Long-Term Recovery

Key Recovery Strategies:
- Reduce health disparities and improve access to essential goods, services, and opportunities.
- Preserve and promote social connectedness.
- Use a systems approach to community redevelopment that acknowledges the connection among social, cultural, economic, and physical environments.
- Seek holistic solutions to socioeconomic disparities and their perverse effects on population health through place-based interventions.
- Rebuild for resilience and sustainability.
- Capitalize on existing planning networks to strengthen recovery planning, including attention to public health, medical, and social services, especially for vulnerable populations.

Activities include but are not limited to:
- ☐ Assess and categorize existing and proposed revitalization programs for commercial areas.
- ☐ Review priorities for vulnerable neighborhoods, blight, social indicators, and unmet needs.
- ☐ Promote community use of schools and facilities after school hours.
- ☐ Ensure that affordable housing is maintained in areas where established communities exist and social networks are preserved.
- ☐ Consider pilot projects or partnerships to provide better access to nutritious food for underserved areas.
- ☐ Examine the potential for integrating health care providers into community areas to provide better access.
- ☐ Evaluate potential partnerships between federally qualified health centers and community development organizations.
- ☐ Evaluate and build upon collaborations with community- and faith-based organizations.
- ☐ Explore partnerships to encourage community gardens, educational opportunities, and employment.
- ☐ Encourage the creative use of architecture, engineering, and landscape architecture in recovery plans to serve multiple purposes.
- ☐ Educate the community on the benefits of mixed-income housing, and explore options and incentives for affordable housing in new residential buildings.
- ☐ Explore opportunities for open green space and trees.

- -

Priority: Develop Environmental Management Strategies to Improve Environmental Quality and Sustainability

Primary Actors: Urban and Regional Planning Agencies, Public Works and Utilities, Environmental Health Agencies

Key Partners: Private Sector (including Landscape Architects), Community- and Faith-Based Organizations, Community Development Organizations

Intermediate- to Long-Term Recovery

Key Recovery Strategies:
- Rebuild for resilience and sustainability.
- Use a systems approach to community redevelopment that acknowledges the connection among social, cultural, economic, and physical environments.

Activities include but are not limited to:
- ☐ Consider using green infrastructure to improve sustainability and health.
- ☐ Determine plant species and supplies that can be sourced locally and are suitable for the climate.
- ☐ Integrate stormwater management planning into the recovery plan.
- ☐ Incorporate flood plain studies, mitigation plans, and buyout opportunities.
- ☐ Evaluate watershed area planning.
- ☐ Review and incorporate regulatory standards, ordinances, and subdivision designs.

- -

Priority: Incorporate Hazard Mitigation, Resilience, and Sustainability Planning into a Recovery Strategy

Primary Actors: Urban and Regional Planning Agencies, Emergency Management Agencies, Environmental Health Agencies, Coastal and Hazard Agencies
Key Partners: Conservation Groups and Agencies, Water Resource Agencies, Federal Agencies (including FEMA and the U.S. Department of Agriculture), Education System

Key Recovery Strategy:
- Rebuild for resilience and sustainability.

Activities include but are not limited to:
- ☐ Assess long-term damage and areas of future vulnerability.
- ☐ Merge hazard mitigation into comprehensive planning, together with strategies for resilience and sustainability.
- ☐ Consider such options as stormwater utility fees to augment funding for recovery efforts and future mitigation practices.
- ☐ Review and upgrade development standards, zoning, and subdivision regulations to support innovative site designs and resilient infrastructure.
- ☐ Consider structural and nonstructural options for hazard mitigation and the cost-benefit ratio of potential efforts, including
  - – brownfield redevelopment;
  - – riparian buffers, retention basins; and
  - – green infrastructure.
- ☐ Ensure compliance with Planning Advisory Service 560 recommendations on integration with the comprehensive plan.
- ☐ Set priorities for reducing risk, reducing damages, and planning for recovery.
- ☐ Maximize use of the Hazard Mitigation Grant Program (HMGP) to fund crucial investments/buyouts.
- ☐ Maximize use of Stafford Act Section 406 Mitigation during recovery and redevelopment.

REFERENCES

Abramson, D. M., and D. Culp. 2013. *At the crossroads of long-term recovery: Joplin, Missouri six months after the May 22, 2011 tornado.* http://academiccommons.columbia.edu/catalog/ac%3A166312 (accessed December 3, 2014).

AECF (Annie E. Casey Foundation). 2013. *Investing in New Orleans: Lessons for philanthropy in public housing redevelopment.* Baltimore, MD: AECF.

AIA (American Institute of Architects). 2014. *AIA establishes new design and health agenda.* http://www.aia.org/practicing/AIAB103676 (accessed December 3, 2014).

Allen, B. L. 2007. Environmental justice and expert knowledge in the wake of a disaster. *Social Studies of Science* 37(1):103-110.

APA (American Planning Association). 2014a. *Model pre-event recovery ordinance.* https://www.planning.org/research/postdisaster/pdf/modelrecoveryordinance.pdf (accessed December 3, 2014).

APA. 2014b. *Post-disaster recovery briefing papers.* https://www.planning.org/research/postdisaster/briefingpapers (accessed February 22, 2014).

ASLA (American Society of Landscape Architects). 2010. *Leveraging the landscape to manage water.* http://www.asla.org/sustainablelandscapes/Vid_Watermanagement.html (accessed December 3, 2014).

ASLA. 2013. *High Line Park.* http://www.asla.org/sustainablelandscapes/highline.html (accessed March 25, 2015).

ASLA. 2014. *High Line Park: New York City, New York, U.S.A.* http://www.asla.org/sustainablelandscapes/pdfs/High_Line_Fact_Sheet.pdf (accessed December 3, 2014).

Belsky, E. S., and J. Fauth. 2012. Crossing over to an improved era of community development. In *Investing in what works for America's communities: Essays on people, place and purpose*, edited by N. O. Andrews and D. J. Erickson. San Francisco, CA: Federal Reserve Bank of San Francisco and Low Income Investment Fund. Pp. 72-103.

Bingler, S. 2011. Building the community nexus: A community centered approach to planning and design. *Educational Facility Planner* 45(3):35-37.

Bingler. 2014. *Nexus case studies: Design, engagement and planning.* Portland, OR: Concordia.

Boehmer, T. K., S. L. Foster, J. R. Henry, E. L. Woghiren-Akinnifesi, and F. Y. Yip. 2013. Residential proximity to major highways—United States, 2010. *Morbidity and Mortality Weekly Report Supplements* 62(03):46-50.

Boston Public Health Commission. 2010. *Take Action.* http://www.bphc.org/wyhc/Pages/TakeAction.aspx (accessed December 3, 2014).

Bova-Hiatt, L., M. Millea, and J. Redente. 2014. *Rising waters and storm resiliency.* Paper presented at The Land Use Law Center's 13th Annual Land Use and Sustainable Development Conference: Transitioning Communities, New York.

CDC (Centers for Disease Control and Prevention). 2009. *Respiratory health & air pollution.* http://www.cdc.gov/healthyplaces/healthtopics/airpollution.htm (accessed December 3, 2014).

CDC. 2011. *Physical activity and health.* http://www.cdc.gov/physicalactivity/everyone/health/index.html#LiveLonger (accessed December 3, 2014).

CDC. 2013a. *Adolescents and school health: Health disparities.* http://www.cdc.gov/healthyyouth/disparities (accessed December 3, 2014).

CDC. 2013b. *CDC's built environment and health initiative.* http://www.cdc.gov/nceh/information/built_environment.htm (accessed March 30, 2015).

CDC. 2013c. CDC health disparities and inequalities report—United States, 2013. *Morbidity and Mortality Weekly Report Supplements* 62(3):1-187.

CDC. 2014a. *Facts about physical activity.* http://www.cdc.gov/physicalactivity/data/facts.html (accessed December 3, 2014).

CDC. 2014b. *Investing in healthier communities.* http://www.cdc.gov/nccdphp/dch/programs/communitytransformation (accessed December 3, 2014).

CDC. 2014c. *National diabetes statistics report, 2014.* http://www.cdc.gov/diabetes/pubs/statsreport14/national-diabetes-report-web.pdf (accessed December 3, 2014).

Cortright, J. 2009. *Walking the walk: How walkability raises home values in U.S. cities.* Cleveland, OH: CEOs for Cities.

CRS. 2014. *Congressional primer on responding to major disasters and emergencies.* Washington, DC: CRS, Library of Congress.

Dainoff, M. J. 1990. Ergonomic improvements in VDT workstations: Health and performance effects. In *Promoting health and productivity in the computerized office: Models of successful ergonomic interventions*, edited by S. L. Sauter, M. J. Dainoff, and M. J. Smith. London: Taylor & Francis. Pp. 49-67.

DeSalvo, K., N. Lurie, K. Finne, C. Worrall, A. Bogdanov, A. Dinkler, S. Babcock, and J. Kelman. 2014. Using Medicare data to identify individuals who are electricity dependent to improve disaster preparedness and response. *American Journal of Public Health* 104(7):1160-1164.

DOT (U.S. Department of Transportation), EPA (U.S. Environmental Protection Agency), and HUD (U.S. Department of Housing and Urban Development). 2014. *Partnership for sustainable communities: Five years of learning from communities and coordinating federal investments.* Washington, DC: DOT, EPA, and HUD.

DOT. 2015. *About TIGER grants.* http://www.dot.gov/tiger/about (accessed March 25, 2015).

EDA (U.S. Economic Development Administration). 2015. *Disaster Recovery.* http://www.eda.gov/about/disaster-recovery.htm (accessed April 9, 2015).

Elmendorf, B. 2008. *Managing natural resources: A guide for municipal commissions.* State College: Pennsylvania State University.

EPA. 2009. *Smart growth guidelines for sustainable design and development.* http://www.epa.gov/smartgrowth/sg_guidelines.htm (accessed December 3, 2014).

EPA. 2013. *Creating equitable, healthy, and sustainable communities: Strategies for advancing smart growth, environmental justice, and equitable development.* Washington, DC: EPA.

EPA. 2014. *Building blocks for sustainable communities.* http://www.epa.gov/smartgrowth/buildingblocks.htm (accessed December 3, 2014).

Erickson, D., and N. Andrews. 2011. Partnerships among community development, public health, and health care could improve the well-being of low-income people. *Health Affairs (Millwood)* 30(11):2056-2063.

FEMA (Federal Emergency Management Agency). 2014a. *The importance of building codes in earthquake-prone communities fact sheet.* http://www.fema.gov/media-library-data/1410554614185-e0da148255b25cd17a5510a80b0d9f48/Building%20Code%20Fact%20Sheet%20Revised%20August%202014.pdf (accessed December 3, 2014).

FEMA. 2014b. *National disaster recovery framework: Overview.* https://www.fema.gov/national-disaster-recovery-framework-overview (accessed December 3, 2014).

FEMA. 2014c. *Public assistance alternative procedures pilot program guide for debris removal (Version 2).* Washington, DC: FEMA.

FEMA. 2015a. *Coastal frequently asked questions.* https://www.fema.gov/coastal-frequently-asked-questions (accessed April 9, 2015).

FEMA. 2015b. *National mitigation framework.* https://www.fema.gov/national-mitigation-framework (accessed April 9, 2015).

FHWA (Federal Highway Administration). 2005. *Safety effects of marked versus unmarked crosswalks at uncontrolled locations: Final report and recommended guidelines.* McLean, VA: DOT.

FHWA. 2015. *Health in Transportation Working Group.* http://www.fhwa.dot.gov/planning/health_in_transportation/workgroup/ (accessed April 9, 2015).

Francis, S. E. 2010. *Gray to green: Jumpstarting private investment in green stormwater infrastructure.* http://www.sbnphiladelphia.org/images/uploads/EIP_GrayToGreen_final_lowres.pdf (accessed December 3, 2014).

Friedman, M. S., K. E. Powell, L. Hutwagner, L. M. Graham, and W. G. Teague. 2001. Impact of changes in transportation and commuting behaviors during the 1996 summer olympic games in Atlanta on air quality and childhood asthma. *Journal of the American Medical Association* 285(7):897-905.

Gaffield, S. J., R. L. Goo, L. A. Richards, and R. J. Jackson. 2003. Public health effects of inadequately managed stormwater runoff. *American Journal of Public Health* 93(9):1527-1533.

Gordon-Larsen, P., M. C. Nelson, P. Page, and B. M. Popkin. 2006. Inequality in the built environment underlies key health disparities in physical activity and obesity. *Pediatrics* 117(2):417-424.

Grimm, K. A., L. V. Moore, and K. S. Scanlon. 2013. Access to healthier food retailers—United States, 2011. *Morbidity and Mortality Weekly Report Supplements* 62(03):20-26.

Hillsborough County Government. 2010. *Post-disaster redevelopment plan.* http://www.hillsboroughcounty.org/index.aspx?nid=1795 (accessed November 3, 2014).

Hoxie, N. J., J. P. Davis, J. M. Vergeront, R. D. Nashold, and K. A. Blair. 1997. Cryptosporidiosis-associated mortality following a massive waterborne outbreak in Milwaukee, Wisconsin. *American Journal of Public Health* 87(12):2032-2035.

HUD. 2012. *U.S. Department of Housing and Urban Development: Leveraging LEED-ND as a sustainability tool.* http://www.usgbc.org/Docs/Archive/General/Docs10503.pdf (accessed December 3, 2014).

HUD. 2014. *Community Development Block Grant Disaster Recovery program.* https://www.hudexchange.info/cdbg-dr (accessed December 3, 2014).

HUD. 2015. *Questions and answers about HUD.* http://portal.hud.gov/hudportal/HUD?src=/about/qaintro (accessed April 9, 2015).

Hurricane Sandy Rebuilding Task Force. 2013. *Hurricane strategy rebuilding strategy: Stronger communities, a resilient region.* Washington, DC: HUD.

IOM (Institute of Medicine). 2014a. *Applying a health lens to decision making in non-health sectors: Workshop summary.* Washington, DC: The National Academies Press.

IOM. 2014b. *Financing population health improvement: Workshop summary.* Washington, DC: The National Academies Press.

Kats, G. 2006. *Greening America's schools: Costs and benefits.* http://www.usgbc.org/Docs/Archive/General/Docs2908.pdf (accessed March 30, 2015).

Kaufman, M. M., and M. Wurtz. 1997. Hydraulic and economic benefits of downspout diversion. *JAWRA Journal of the American Water Resources Association* 33(2):491-497.

King County. 2011. *Planning for healthy communities.* King County, WA: King County Board of Health.

Kirkland, G. 2012. *U.S. Department of Housing and Urban Development Office of Inspector General Audit Report: The State of Texas did not follow requirements for its infrastructure and revitalization contracts funded with CDBG disaster recovery program funds.* https://www.hudoig.gov/sites/default/files/documents/audit-reports//2012-fw-1005.pdf (accessed April 12, 2015).

Kwarteng, J. L., A. J. Schulz, G. B. Mentz, S. N. Zenk, and A. A. Opperman. 2013. Associations between observed neighborhood characteristics and physical activity: Findings from a multiethnic urban community. *Journal of Public Health* 36(3):358-367.

LaVeist, T., K. Pollack, R. Thorpe, R. Fesahazion, and D. Gaskin. 2011. Place, not race: Disparities dissipate in Southwest Baltimore when blacks and whites live under similar conditions. *Health Affairs* 30(10):1880-1887.

Lee, K. K. 2012. Developing and implementing the active design guidelines in New York City. *Health Place* 18(1):5-7.

Lee, M., and V. Rubin. 2007. *The impact of the built environment on community health: The state of current practice and next steps for a growing movement.* Los Angeles, CA: The California Endowment.

Loftness, V., B. Hakkinen, O. Adan, and A. Nevalainen. 2007. Elements that contribute to healthy building design. *Environmental Health Perspectives* 115(6):965-970.

Maas, J., R. A. Verheij, P. P. Groenewegen, S. de Vries, and P. Spreeuwenberg. 2006. Green space, urbanity, and health: How strong is the relation? *Journal of Epidemiology and Community Health* 60(7):587-592.

Mac Kenzie, W. R., N. J. Hoxie, M. E. Proctor, M. S. Gradus, K. A. Blair, D. E. Peterson, J. J. Kazmierczak, D. G. Addiss, K. R. Fox, J. B. Rose, and J. P. Davis. 1994. A massive outbreak in Milwaukee of cryptosporidium infection transmitted through the public water supply. *New England Journal of Medicine* 331(3):161-167.

Mallach, A. 2006. From eyesores to assets: CDC abandoned property strategies. *Shelterforce Online* (146). http://www.nhi.org/online/issues/146/researchupdate.html (accessed December 3, 2014).

Marks, J. S. 2009. Why your zip code may be more important to your health than your genetic code. *The Huffington Post.* http://www.huffingtonpost.com/james-s-marks/why-your-zip-code-may-be_b_190650.html? (accessed April 8, 2015).

Mattessich, P. W., and E. J. Rausch. 2013. *Collaboration to build healthier communities: A report for the Robert Wood Johnson Foundation Commission to Build a Healthier America.* http://www.rwjf.org/content/dam/farm/reports/surveys_and_polls/2013/rwjf406479 (accessed November 18, 2014).

McGraw Hill Construction. 2014. *The drive toward healthier buildings: The market drivers and impact of building design on occupant health, well-being and productivity.* Washington, DC: Dodge Data & Analytics.

McPherson, E. G. 1994. Cooling urban heat islands with sustainable landscapes. In *The ecological city: Preserving and restoring urban biodiversity*, edited by R. H. Platt, R. A. Rowntree, and P. C. Muick. Boston, MA: University of Massachusetts Press. Pp. 161-171.

Mueller. 2014. *About us.* http://www.muelleraustinonline.com/about.php (accessed December 3, 2014).

Murphy, S. L., J. Xu, and K. D. Kochanek. 2013. Deaths: Final data for 2010. *National Vital Statistics Reports* 61(4):1-118.

Natural Hazards Center. 2006. *Holistic disaster recovery: Ideas for building local sustainability after a natural disaster.* Fairfax, VA: Public Entity Risk Institute.

New Orleans Redevelopment Authority. 2014. *Lot next door 3.0.* http://www.noraworks.org/lnd3 (accessed December 3, 2014).

NHTSA (National Highway Traffic Safety Administration). 2008. *National motor vehicle crash causation survey: Report to Congress.* Washington, DC: DOT.

NHTSA. 2012. *National survey of bicyclist and pedestrian attitudes and behavior.* Washington, DC: DOT.

NHTSA. 2014. *2013 motor vehicle crashes: Overview.* Washington, DC: DOT.

NRC (National Research Council). 2012. *Disaster resilience: A national imperative.* Washington, DC: The National Academies Press.

NRC. 2014. *Reducing coastal risk on the east and gulf coasts.* Washington, DC: The National Academies Press.

NYS 2100 Commission. 2013. *Recommendations to improve the strength and resilience of the empire state's infrastructure.* New York: The Rockefeller Foundation.

Ogden, C. L., M. D. Carroll, B. K. Kit, and K. M. Flegal. 2014. Prevalence of childhood and adult obesity in the United States, 2011-2012. *Journal of the American Medical Association* 311(8):806-814.

Olmedo, O., I. F. Goldstein, L. Acosta, A. Divjan, A. G. Rundle, G. L. Chew, R. B. Mellins, L. Hoepner, H. Andrews, S. Lopez-Pintado, J. W. Quinn, F. P. Perera, R. L. Miller, J. S. Jacobson, and M. S. Perzanowski. 2011. Neighborhood differences in exposure and sensitization to cockroach, mouse, dust mite, cat, and dog allergens in New York City. *Journal of Allergy and Clinical Immunology* 128(2):284-292.

Olshansky, R. 2014. *Post-disaster recovery: How to rebuild cities in compressed time.* Paper presented at IOM Committee on Post-Disaster Recovery of a Community's Public Health, Medical, and Social Services: Meeting Two, February 3, Washington, DC.

Pinellas County. 2012. *Pinellas County post-disaster redevelopment plan.* Pinellas County, FL: Pinellas County.

Prevention Institute. 2011. *Fact sheet: Links between violence and health equity.* http://www.preventioninstitute.org/component/jlibrary/article/id-311/127.html (accessed December 3, 2014).

Rebuild by Design. 2014. *Living with the bay: A comprehensive regional resiliency plan for Nassau County's South Shore.* http://www.rebuildbydesign.org/project/interboro-team-final-proposal (accessed December 3, 2014).

Redlener, I. 2014. *Post-disaster recovery: Restoring lives, fast.* Paper presented at IOM Committee on Post-disaster Recovery of a Community's Public Health, Medical, and Social Services: Meeting Two, February 3, Washington, DC.

Rexrode, C., and V. Dobnik. 2012. Hurricane Sandy: New Jersey, New York still struggle with power outages. *The Huffington Post.* http://www.huffingtonpost.com/2012/11/11/hurricane-sandy-new-jersey-york-power-outage_n_2113856.html (accessed April 8, 2015).

Ricklin, A., A. Klein, and E. Musiol. 2012. *Healthy planning: An evaluation of comprehensive and sustainability plans addressing public health.* Chicago, IL: APA.

RWJF (Robert Wood Johnson Foundation). 2014. *Time to act: Investing in the health of our children and communities.* Princeton, NJ: RWJF.

Sallis, J. F., M. F. Floyd, D. A. Rodríguez, and B. E. Saelens. 2012. Role of built environments in physical activity, obesity, and cardiovascular disease. *Circulation* 125(5):729-737.

Schwab, J. 2014. *Post-disaster recovery plans: Types and purposes.* Paper presented at IOM Committee on Post-Disaster Recovery of a Community's Public Health, Medical, and Social Services: Meeting Two, February 3, Washington, DC.

Shoemaker, D. 2006. *Tools for mixed-income TOD.* http://community-wealth.org/sites/clone.community-wealth.org/files/downloads/tool-CTOD-mixed-income_0.pdf (accessed November 30, 2014).

Springfield Redevelopment Authority. 2012. *Rebuild Springfield.* Springfield, MA: Springfield Redevelopment Authority.

State of the Air. 2013. *Particle pollution.* http://www.stateoftheair.org/2013/health-risks/health-risks-particle.html (accessed December 3, 2014).

Transportation Research Board. 2005. *Does the built environment influence physical activity?: Examining the evidence.* Washington, DC: National Academy of Sciences.

TRF (The Reinvestment Fund). 2015. *About.* http://www.trfund.com/about/ (accessed April 9, 2015).

Tsai, A. G., D. F. Williamson, and H. A. Glick. 2011. Direct medical cost of overweight and obesity in the USA: A quantitative systematic review. *Obesity Reviews* 12(1):50-61.

ULI (Urban Land Institute). 2013. *Intersections: Health and the built environment.* Washington, DC: ULI.

ULI. 2014. *Housing in America: Integrating housing, health, and resilience in a changing environment.* Washington, DC: ULI.

UNISDR (United Nations International Strategy for Disaster Reduction). 2013. *Private sector strengths applied: Good practices in disaster risk reduction from Japan.* http://www.unisdr.org/files/33594_privatesectorstrengths applied2013di.pdf (accessed March 15, 2015).

U.S. Department of the Treasury. 2014. *About the CDFI Fund.* http://www.cdfifund.gov/who_we_are/about_us.asp (accessed December 3, 2014).

USDA (U.S. Department of Agriculture). 2014. *Urban wildlife.* http://www.fs.fed.us/research/wildlife-fish/themes/ urban-wildlife.php (accessed December 3, 2014).

Washington Emergency Management Division. 2014. *Puget Sound transportation recovery annex.* http://mil.wa.gov/ uploads/pdf/PLANS/transportationrecoveryannexnew.pdf (accessed December 3, 2014).

What Works for Health. 2010. *Physical environment—housing & transit.* http://whatworksforhealth.wisc.edu/factor. php?id=126 (accessed December 3, 2014).

The White House. 2009. *Developing effective place-based policies for the FY 2011 budget.* http://www.whitehouse. gov/sites/default/files/omb/assets/memoranda_fy2009/m09-28.pdf (accessed March 4, 2015).

WHO (World Health Organization). 2014. *Social determinants of health.* http://www.wpro.who.int/topics/social_ determinants_health/en (accessed December 1, 2014).

Williams, C. 2007. *The built environment and physical activity: What is the relationship?* Princeton, NJ: RWJF.

Winters, M., M. Brauer, E. M. Setton, and K. Teschke. 2010. Built environment influences on healthy transportation choices: Bicycling versus driving. *Journal of Urban Health* 87(6):969-993.

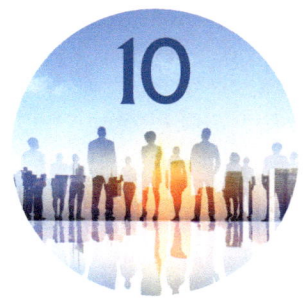

Healthy Housing

*The connection between health and the dwelling of the population
is one of the most important that exists.*

—Florence Nightingale (Lowry, 1991)

As discussed in Chapter 2, housing is a fundamental element of a healthy community. A healthy community ensures the availability of safe, decent, and affordable housing that supports the health of its occupants. Homes are intended to provide shelter from the elements, especially during and after disasters; to provide privacy; and to ensure safety from the outside world (APHA and NCHH, 2014). In many communities, however, housing guidelines and codes have failed to advance and to reflect the way individuals interact with their homes (Krieger and Higgins, 2002). Furthermore, housing regulations often do not adequately take into account modern health issues, including chronic diseases such as asthma, depression, and injuries. Retrofitting housing to meet healthy housing standards can be expensive; however, costs are significantly decreased if these elements can be incorporated during the building of new residences or during substantial rehabilitation of damaged homes and apartment buildings. Therefore, the rebuilding effort that follows a disaster offers an important opportunity to improve community health by providing access to and creating healthy housing.

The U.S. Department of Housing and Urban Development (HUD) recognized this opportunity after Hurricane Sandy by requiring that federally funded rebuilding comply with green healthy housing standards (discussed in further detail below). However, the housing sector also must overcome a number of disaster-related challenges. Following a disaster, health hazards within homes must be mitigated, and those displaced or made homeless require immediate access to temporary housing that provides safe shelter and a place of belonging while homes are being rebuilt. As community recovery proceeds, individuals need permanent, affordable replacement housing. Both the temporary and the permanent housing stock needs to be built with health in mind: "A healthy home is sited, designed, built, renovated, and maintained in ways that support the health of residents" (HHS, 2009).

This chapter addresses the role of housing in advancing health; the impacts of disasters on the housing sector; and actions that housing sector leaders at the federal, state, and local levels can undertake across

369

the disaster continuum to strengthen communities by providing access to healthy housing. In developing its guidance on healthy housing, the committee identified key recovery strategies that appear as cross-cutting themes throughout this chapter and apply to multiple pre- and post-disaster activities. Application of these strategies will facilitate the protection and promotion of health as a community works to meet housing needs after a disaster:

- Protect survivors and recovery workers from health hazards associated with unhealthy or unsafe housing.
- Preserve and promote social connectedness in plans for immediate response, short-term housing, and long-term rebuilding.
- Consider needs for access to health and social services during all phases of housing recovery.
- Incentivize the use of healthy and/or green criteria for the rebuilding of homes, buildings, and neighborhoods.
- Engage community members, including representatives of and advocates for vulnerable populations, in the development of post-disaster housing plans to ensure that the needs of all community members are met.

The chapter concludes with a checklist of key activities that the housing sector needs to perform during each of the phases of recovery.

HOUSING IN THE CONTEXT OF A HEALTHY COMMUNITY

Housing is a well-documented determinant of health, and the burden of disease associated with inadequate housing is large (WHO, 2011). Substandard housing impacts multiple dimensions of health, including chronic disease and mental health. For example, asthma is associated with improper mold abatement (Zock et al., 2002), pest infestations, and dampness (Krieger and Higgins, 2002), while exposure to toxins such as asbestos (Landrigan, 1998) and radon (Lubin and Boice, 1997) can cause cancer. Exposure to lead in older housing continues to be a major concern, particularly with regard to the health of children (Jacobs, 1995), because of its known effects on brain development (NTP, 2012; Rodier, 1995). Mental health also is affected by housing. Housing of better structural quality has been shown to increase self-efficacy, optimism, and life satisfaction and to decrease anxiety and depression (WHO, 2011), while housing issues such as pest infestation, dampness, and cold have been correlated with poorer mental health (Duvall and Booth, 1978; Elton and Packer, 1986; Evans et al., 2000, 2003; Gifford and Lacombe, 2006; Halpern, 1995; Weich and Lewis, 1998; Wilner et al., 1962).

In addition to direct impacts of poor housing conditions on health, deterioration of individual, family, and community well-being results from secondary impacts such as the burden of medical expenses associated with resultant health conditions. The magnitude of the impacts of housing conditions on health is illustrated by the following examples:

- Radon in homes causes 21,000 lung cancer deaths per year (EPA, 2012).
- More than 24 million homes have significant lead-based paint hazards that put children at risk of the irreversible effects of lead poisoning, including brain damage, seizures, and death (Jacobs et al., 2002).
- Home injuries are the leading cause of death for young children (Nagaraja et al., 2005).
- In 2013, nonfatal falls sent 2.5 million adults over age 65 to the emergency room (CDC, 2014).

Unfortunately, most communities in the United States face challenges in their housing sector that result in some individuals and families living in housing environments that are not optimally supportive of health. For example, many residences fail to meet key principles of healthy housing, including proper ventilation (both adequate fresh air and its distribution), moisture and mold control, proper maintenance, integrated pest management, avoidance of toxic chemicals and agents, safety (free of injury hazards), accessibility, cleanliness, and adequate lighting (HHS and HUD, 2006). These challenges are especially common among the poor and other vulnerable populations, but they may impact anyone in a community. Many residences have more than one health hazard, and some risk factors are directly linked (Jacobs, 2011). For example, energy-inefficient housing is more prone to dampness and thus mold. As a result, multiple risk factors may have additive effects on health (WHO, 2011).

Remediation of health hazards in homes can have substantial impacts on health and quality of life. The Centers for Disease Control and Prevention (CDC) and the National Center for Healthy Housing recently reported evidence that certain housing interventions improve health based on clinical, self-report, and/or environmental data (DiGuiseppi et al., 2010; Jacobs et al., 2010; Krieger et al., 2010; Sandel et al., 2010). For example, the National Inner City Asthma study showed through a randomized controlled trial that children in an intervention group that received remediation of exposure to dust mites, cockroaches, pets, rodents, and mold suffered from asthma symptoms fewer days compared with children in the control group. This result was observed during the intervention year and throughout the year afterward. In addition, the intervention group had reduced levels of allergens in the residential environment (Morgan et al., 2004). Other benefits observed in the intervention group included significant reductions in the disruption of caretakers' plans and quality of life, caretakers' and children's loss of sleep, and missed school days, as well as significantly fewer unplanned trips to the emergency department or clinic due to asthma. For every 2.85 children treated, there was one less unscheduled visit at the 1-year follow-up (Morgan et al., 2004). The evidence that housing interventions improve asthma also has been systematically reviewed by the CDC (Crocker et al., 2011). This systematic review, which included 20 studies targeting children and adolescents, found that the time with symptoms was reduced by 0.8 days per 2 weeks (equivalent to 21.0 symptom-days per year); missed school days were reduced by 12.3 per year; and the number of asthma acute care visits was reduced by 0.57 per year (Crocker et al., 2011). Another review yielded similar findings (Krieger et al., 2010).

Housing Standards That Promote Health

Physical changes to the nation's housing supply are an ongoing process. Two important recent developments are relevant to disaster-related housing recovery operations: (1) the issuance in 2014 of the National Healthy Housing Standard (APHA and NCHH, 2014), which is an update of the 1986 *Housing and Health: Recommended Minimum Housing Standards from the American Public Health Association*; and (2) the issuance of "green" housing standards. The National Healthy Housing Standard covers duties of owners and occupants, structural concerns, noise, crowding, injury prevention, chemical safety, smoke and carbon monoxide alarms, lighting and electrical issues, safety, ventilation and moisture, and contaminants. "The Standard constitutes minimum performance standards for a safe and healthy home" (APHA and NCHH, 2014).

Green building is "the practice of creating structures and using processes that are environmentally responsible and resource-efficient throughout a building's life-cycle from siting to design, construction, operation, maintenance, renovation and deconstruction. . . . Green buildings are designed to reduce the overall impact of the built environment on human health and the natural environment" (EPA, 2014). In recent years, a plethora of green standards for construction practices have appeared. These include Enterprise Green Communities, the ICC-700 National Green Building Standard, the U.S. Environmental Protection Agency's (EPA's) Indoor AirPlus, and Leadership for Energy & Environmental Design (LEED). Each program has different criteria, a different method for calculating whether a project meets the criteria, and different criteria for different types of housing project (e.g., multifamily or single-family). For example, LEED has four levels of certification: Certified, Silver, Gold, or Platinum, and certification can be for family homes, neighborhoods, existing building operations, interior design, or new building construction (USGBC, 2009). The Enterprise Green Communities standard has mandatory health requirements. Table 10-1 shows some examples of criteria used by Enterprise Green Community and LEED.

TABLE 10-1 Examples of Green Building Criteria

	Enterprise Green Communities[a]	Leadership for Energy & Environmental Design (LEED)[b] (new construction and major renovations)
Location	Open spaces Access to fresh food Walkability Public transportation access Environmental remediation	Bicycle storage Protection or restoration of habitat Brownfield redevelopment Fuel-efficient vehicles Reduction of light pollution
Materials	Construction waste management Low/no volatile organic compounds (VOCs)/formaldehyde Local or salvaged materials	Recycling for residents Percentage of existing structures maintained Reused or recycled materials
Interior environment	Mold prevention Radon mitigation Integrated pest management Smoke-free building	Minimizing or eliminating tobacco smoke Controllability of thermal system
Water	Water-conserving fixtures Reuse of rain- or greywater Stormwater management	Water-efficient landscape Innovative wastewater technologies
Energy and Ventilation	ENERGY STAR certification or American Society of Heating, Refrigerating, and Air-Conditioning Engineers (ASHRAE) standards Efficient lighting	ASHRAE standards Renewable energy Refrigerant management
Other	Fully accessible units	Views of outdoors and daylight

[a] The criteria listed are a representative sample of technical requirements included in the Enterprise Green Communities criteria. To achieve Enterprise Green Communities certification, projects must implement certain mandatory measures, as well as achieve a set number of optional points. New construction projects must achieve 35 optional points, substantial rehab projects 30 optional points, and moderate rehab projects 30 optional points (Enterprise, 2011).

[b] The LEED Green Building Rating System for New Construction helps professionals improve building quality and reduce impact on the environment. The criteria listed are a representative sample of prerequisites and additional green standards that project teams can implement to gain points toward obtaining LEED certification. There are 69 possible points, with a range of certification levels (Certified: 40-49 points, Silver: 50-59 points, Gold: 60-79 points, and Platinum: 80 points and above) (USGBC, 2009).
SOURCE: Enterprise, 2011; USGBC, 2009.

Another housing program employing standards relevant to post-disaster reconstruction is the Resilience STAR™ program. This pilot project by the U.S. Department of Homeland Security is modeled after the EPA's ENERGY STAR certification program. The designation will be given to structures that are built to withstand damage from disasters, using criteria from the Insurance Institute for Business & Home Safety's FORTIFIED program. The FORTIFIED criteria cover building or retrofitting roofs, soffit vents, entry and garage doors, chimneys, and foundations (Insurance Institute for Business & Home Safety, 2012). The committee found no studies showing improved health outcomes associated with the FORTIFIED criteria, indicating a need for further evaluation.

Green Housing Standards and Health

Energy conservation often is the driving force behind the adoption of "green" building standards in residential structures, but it also has been bolstered by the promise of ancillary environmental health benefits for the building occupants. According to the World Health Organization (WHO), for example, the annual burden of mortality due to cold homes can be estimated conservatively at 30 percent of excess winter deaths in Europe (Rudge, 2011). Beyond the straightforward impact of thermal improvements, energy conservation can plausibly be related to health because it often includes the following: repair or replacement of heating and cooling equipment to increase efficiency and reduce the generation of pollutants such as carbon monoxide; improvement of ventilation to remove contaminants; air sealing and improvement of building envelopes, which often can reduce moisture leaks from the exterior; and reduced moisture incursion (WHO, 2011). Further, increased energy efficiency and resultant reductions in household energy costs leave individuals with more income to spend on other essentials, such as food and medicine. The "Heat or Eat" study found that families whose energy costs were lowered as a result of receiving fuel assistance had a reduced odds ratio both of being at aggregate nutritional risk for growth problems and of hospitalization (Frank et al., 2006). Results of one recent study suggest that more than 30 housing elements typically included in green standards could plausibly be associated with health outcomes (Jacobs et al., 2014a). These elements include high-efficiency furnaces, programmable thermostats, absence of carpeting in kitchens and bathrooms, foundation waterproofing, radon and lead testing and mitigation, and doors and windows that reduce air infiltration and water penetration.

Evidence of positive health outcomes associated with rebuilding housing in compliance with green standards is robust. Improvements in general self-reported health, respiratory health (notably asthma), mental health, and other health outcomes following both new construction and housing rehabilitation that comply with green building standards have been found in numerous studies (see Table 10-2). Most of these studies relied primarily on self-reported health, using structured interview data collection instruments. Substantial evidence, however, indicates that self-reported health is correlated with other, more objective measures, such as clinical outcomes (Burstrom and Fredlund, 2001; Halford et al., 2012; Idler et al., 2000; Krokstad et al., 2002; Li et al., 2011; Mansson and Rastam, 2001; Marmot et al., 1995; Miilunpalo et al., 1997; Pietilainen et al., 2011; Singh-Manoux et al., 2007).

There appear to be no studies to date showing that use of green building standards in the context of post-disaster rebuilding also promotes better health, but there is little reason to expect different results. Further research is needed to assess the link between health outcomes and housing reconstruction that complies with green building standards in the post-disaster context.

DISASTER-RELATED HOUSING CHALLENGES

Depending on their nature and the pattern of damage, disasters can create significant challenges for the housing sector, including residential health hazards that need to be mitigated, strain on capacity, and displacement. A significant long-term issue that can impact both individual and community recovery and well-being is the loss of affordable housing (sometimes referred to as disaster gentrification).

Disaster-Related Health Hazards

Disasters can cause significant damage to homes, resulting in increased exposure to new threats and exacerbation of existing threats. Common examples include safety hazards from debris and health hazards such as high levels of mold and microbial products associated with allergies, asthma, and other respiratory conditions (IOM, 2004; Krieger, 2010; Wilson et al., 2010). High concentrations of microbial toxins and allergens result from microbial growth under conditions of dampness and inadequate ventilation, both of which can be prevalent in the indoor environment after a disaster. There have been reports of very high levels of exposure to mold and bacterial toxins among both occupants and recovery workers who repair moisture and mold problems in housing (Chew et al., 2006). Additionally, post-disaster use of temporary housing that has chemical contaminants such as high levels of formaldehyde has been associated with respiratory problems, sensitization, and other adverse health outcomes (Murphy et al., 2013). Moisture control, ventilation, and chemical source control are therefore essential elements for healthy housing in the context of disaster recovery (HHS, 2009).

TABLE 10-2 Summary of Literature Showing Improvements in Health Due to Green Housing Interventions

Intervention	Results	Source
Special ventilation systems in new homes	Significant improvements in throat irritation, cough, fatigue, and irritation	Leech et al., 2004
Insulation of existing homes	Significant improvements in self-rated health and self-reported wheezing; fewer sick days from school and work; fewer visits to doctors and fewer hospital admissions for respiratory conditions	Howden-Chapman et al., 2007
Weatherization	Improvement of adult general health score and self-reported sinusitis, hypertension, use of asthma rescue medication, and overweight	Wilson et al., 2014
Green public housing	Adults: Lower prevalence of angina, hay fever, sinusitis; significantly better mental health measures for sadness, nervousness, restlessness, hopelessness, and "everything being an effort"	Jacobs et al., 2014a
	Children: Lower prevalence of hayfever, headaches, and respiratory allergies; more reporting excellent, very good, or good health	
	Asthmatic children: Lower frequency of symptoms, less difficulty staying asleep, less use of prescription inhaler	
Green housing rehabilitation	Reduced cockroach, mouse, and dust mite allergens; more adults reporting excellent, very good, or good health	Jacobs et al., 2014b
"Breathe easy home" (BEH)	More asthma-symptom-free days after 1 year in a BEH; decrease in proportion of residents with urgent asthma-related clinical visits in a 3-month period; significant improvements in (FEV1) and percent with well-controlled asthma, rescue medication use, days with limited physical activity due to asthma, nights with asthma symptoms, and number of asthma attacks	Takaro et al., 2011

Strain on Capacity

The sudden destruction of large proportions of a community's housing stock as the result of a disaster places a considerable burden on the housing sector during recovery. Repair, rehabilitation, and new construction of housing stock that would otherwise take years must be accomplished at a greatly accelerated pace to meet needs for both human and economic recovery. Governmental housing agencies can be overwhelmed by such tasks as inspection, permitting, and oversight; there may also be insufficient labor and materials within a community to meet reconstruction needs. Construction contractors and subcontractors from outside the community may come in to assist, but this creates an additional need to check that they hold the proper licenses and certifications to ensure that they can perform the work properly and safely, as well as to help prevent fraudulent, incorrect, and unhealthy building practices and noncompliance with codes.

Displacement and the Need for Healthy Temporary Housing

After a disaster, individuals frequently require short- and sometimes long-term temporary housing. Following Hurricane Katrina, for example, more than 400,000 individuals were displaced from their homes (Geaghan, 2011), while more than 12,000 were displaced following the Loma Prieta earthquake in 1989 (CA Department of Conservation, 2013; Lew, 1990). Although many displaced survivors seek short-term shelter with relatives and friends, others may go to emergency congregate shelters established in the immediate aftermath of an event by local governments, the American Red Cross, or others. Such emergency shelters often close within a few weeks following a disaster, but repair and replacement of lost housing stock can take several years (Marin County Sheriff, 2003). Evidence shows that longer-term temporary housing needs to be established as soon as possible to enable rapid community recovery, mitigate the potential spread of disease, prevent avoidable injuries, and avoid potential adverse behavioral health outcomes that occur when large numbers of individuals are housed in shelters for extended periods of time. Displaced children who lived in a shelter after Hurricane Katrina, for example, experienced increased trauma symptoms and were more likely to be referred for mental health services as compared with displaced children who lived elsewhere (Osofsky et al., 2009). These findings are consistent with previous research on the mental health effects of living in shelters after Hurricane Andrew (Sattler et al., 1995).

Following a disaster, survivors in most cases prefer to stay in their original communities—next to their schools, jobs, and neighbors. If adequate housing is not made available, however, residents will leave the community, temporarily or permanently, further disrupting social networks and degrading the community and its economy. Communities with limited housing stock are at particular risk (Association of Bay Area Governments, 2014). Moreover, secondary impacts of long-term displacement include increases in psychological distress (Freedy and Simpson, 2007), posttraumatic stress symptoms in children (Lonigan et al., 1994), and violence (Marin County Sheriff, 2003; Rezaeian, 2013). Therefore, communities need to establish plans ahead of disasters to guide how temporary housing will be provided for survivors for the months to years following a disaster and how needs for permanent housing will be met. Even if temporary housing is provided for a timely manner, it is important to recognize that (1) displacement disrupts people's social networks, (2) survivors are likely to be more vulnerable than they were prior to the disaster, and (3) the availability of community resources will be limited.

Loss of Affordable Housing

Low-cost housing, including rental properties, tends to be concentrated in older buildings and more vulnerable locations. For these reasons, it is often affected disproportionately by disasters (Florida Department of Community Affairs, 2010). Not only are these homes more likely to be destroyed, they are also less likely to be rebuilt. After Hurricane Katrina, housing recovery varied significantly by housing type—single-family dwellings were rebuilt or repaired more quickly than multifamily units, and many rental housing investors chose simply not to rebuild and to "take their investment money elsewhere" (McIntosh, 2013). This loss of affordable housing—coupled with an increase in demand for such housing—created a dearth of housing options for lower-income residents, and many simply did not return to New Orleans (AlJazeera America, 2013). Consequently, failure to plan adequately for replacement of low-income housing will further widen the affordability gap and may result in the permanent loss of residents, with attendant workforce and tax base losses.

HOUSING SECTOR ORGANIZATION AND RESOURCES

Government agencies, nongovernmental organizations, and private businesses all play key roles in ensuring that safe and affordable housing is available to support the health of all members of a community. Through their specific responsibilities, each has a function that may be utilized to ensure the availability of resilient healthy housing after a disaster. However, given the myriad functions of each of these components in the housing sector, strong pre- and post-disaster coordination is required to ensure that housing is rebuilt in a healthy, resilient, and sustainable manner.

Federal Level[1]

At the federal level, multiple agencies—including HUD, the U.S. Department of the Treasury, and the U.S. Department of Agriculture (Rural Housing Service)—provide funding for housing (primarily for low-income housing) and perform oversight functions. Many of the federal programs may, with the infusion of additional resources, help meet post-disaster housing needs. For example, the U.S. Department of the Treasury administers low-income housing tax credit programs and related mortgage bond programs with the states. These funds are important sources of capital for reconstructing low-income housing after a disaster, and they also often specify housing standards and codes that must be complied with, including fair housing regulations. HUD's HOME Investment Partnerships Program (HOME) also is designed to create affordable housing for low-income people. HOME offers grants to states and localities with which to construct, buy, or rebuild affordable housing or to provide direct rental assistance. In the event of a disaster, a grantee may request that HOME funds be expedited or that program requirements be modified to facilitate recovery (HUD, 2014e). HUD's Office of Public and Indian Housing provides financial assistance for low-income housing across the country, which encompasses both conventional public housing and vouchers for privately owned low-income housing, and these programs can sometimes be used to provide temporary housing assistance in the disaster recovery context.

The Federal Emergency Management Agency (FEMA) and HUD are the primary players in disaster-specific preparedness and recovery, as relates to shelters and housing. Immediately after a disaster, FEMA and its partners (including the American Red Cross) coordinate sheltering assistance through Emergency Support Function (ESF) #6—Mass Care, Emergency Assistance, Housing, and Human Services—under the National Response Framework. FEMA and HUD partner to provide interim housing assistance, which generally falls in the period of transition from ESF #6 to the Housing Recovery Support Function (RSF) under the National Disaster Recovery Framework (NDRF, described in more detail in Chapter 3). For issues related to permanent housing, HUD has lead responsibility as the coordinating agency for the Housing RSF.

Disaster-specific funding provided by FEMA and HUD is an important resource for post-disaster recovery. FEMA's Hazard Mitigation Grant Program provides funding to state governments for the implementation of long-term hazard mitigation measures, including property acquisition, structure elevation, floodproofing, and retrofitting of existing structures (FEMA, 2013a). FEMA's Individual Assistance program provides financial assistance for temporary housing, as well as for repairs or replacements not covered by insurance (FEMA, 2015). FEMA's Public Assistance program provides money to states and communities for rebuilding infrastructure, such as roads, utilities, and public transportation facilities. Although the Public Assistance funds cannot be used specifically for housing, the repair and reconstruction of infrastructure are vital to the success of housing efforts. In the event of a supplemental congressional appropriation, HUD's Community Development Block Grant for Disaster Recovery (CDBG-DR) (discussed in more detail in Chapter 4) is a significant source of funds for assisting homeowners with repairs and new construction after a disaster. At least half of CDBG-DR funds, which are distributed through the state or local government, must be used to benefit low- or moderate-income people (unless a waiver is granted), and may be used for a range of efforts, including

- purchasing damaged properties within a flood plain and relocating those residents;
- rehabilitating homes and buildings damaged by a disaster; and
- assisting homeowners with down payments, interest rate subsidies, and loan guarantees (FEMA, 2013a).

In past disasters such as Hurricane Sandy, FEMA and HUD have jointly implemented the Disaster Housing Assistance Program (DHAP). This program provides such assistance as rent subsidies, security deposit assistance, and utility deposit assistance for displaced residents (HUD, 2014c).

---

[1] A broader synopsis of legislation and federal policy related to disaster recovery and health security can be found in Appendix A.

In 2009, FEMA released the *National Disaster Housing Strategy*, which outlines the nation's current approach to post-disaster housing and describes a new direction for meeting disaster housing needs (FEMA, 2009a). It lays out roles and responsibilities at all levels and includes a detailed description of disaster housing programs. The strategy emphasizes the importance of collaboration among government, nongovernmental organizations, and the private sector. At the federal level, interagency collaboration on the strategy's implementation is facilitated by the FEMA-led National Disaster Housing Task Force, and an implementation plan for the strategy was released in 2010. The strategy identifies the challenges to the current system and establishes six goals for a new framework for disaster housing:

1. Help affected residents and communities meet their own housing needs and return to self-sufficiency as quickly as possible.
2. Organizations must understand and fulfill their fundamental responsibilities and roles, and coordinate their efforts across sectors.
3. Housing assistance must be responsive to the complex needs of disaster victims, including those with special needs (e.g., those with disabilities, children, pets), and be culturally and linguistically appropriate and accessible.
4. Organizations must build their own capabilities, and know how to request assistance if it is needed, in order to provide a broad range of housing options.
5. Disaster housing assistance must be integrated with related community support services (e.g., case management or support for the elderly) and long-term recovery efforts.
6. Organizations must jointly plan for housing needs following the full range of potential disasters that may occur, from small-scale to catastrophic events (FEMA, 2009a).

One of the areas for improvement addressed by the National Disaster Housing Strategy is interim disaster housing. The strategy notes the importance of identifying alternatives to traditional interim housing, such as travel trailers, manufactured homes, or existing vacant units. FEMA launched the Joint Housing Solutions Group in 2006 to research, evaluate, and identify these potential alternatives. The Joint Housing Solutions Group developed a Housing Assessment Tool that analyzes alternative housing according to four criteria: range of use, livability, timeliness, and cost. The Joint Housing Solutions Group, which includes experts from HUD, the National Institute of Building Sciences, and multiple FEMA divisions, provides expertise and ground support to FEMA's disaster housing operations (FEMA, 2009a).

State and Local Levels

Several types of state and local housing agencies are involved in providing housing services and regulating housing construction. They include the following:

- Housing authority—The local housing authority typically is an independent local organization, with commissioners appointed by the local elected public official or tribal leader. The housing authority often owns housing, such as public housing, and also provides vouchers and other subsidies to low-income tenants and homeowners and low-income housing providers. There are wide differences in how housing authorities are organized across the country, but all receive funding through HUD's Public and Indian Housing program.
- Homeless services—These are local housing agencies that provide services for those who are unable to acquire housing, with support from HUD's Emergency Solutions Grant program and others.
- Zoning/permitting—These local departments regulate the types and locations of housing, as well as how modifications to that housing are made, through permitting, inspections, codes, and other means.
- State housing department and state housing finance agencies—Most housing is regulated by local jurisdictions, not at the state level, with important exceptions, such as the provision of low-income

housing tax credits. The state housing department typically is the entity that oversees housing in rural areas, while city housing agencies oversee housing in urban and suburban areas, although there are exceptions.

Nongovernmental and Philanthropic Organizations

Nongovernmental and philanthropic organizations have a critical role to play by representing community voices, particularly those of vulnerable residents, and by filling gaps not addressed by government programs or private investments. National-level philanthropies such as the Annie E. Casey Foundation have been important funders of post-disaster revitalization efforts, particularly for underserved areas. Further, community-based organizations such as tenants' associations and tenants' unions ensure that community members have a voice in how housing is rehabilitated and built, and they can help facilitate interactions with private and public housing providers. The multifamily building community has many organizations that advocate on behalf of its members and can be a powerful force throughout the recovery process. Examples of such organizations include the National Multifamily Housing Council, National Leased Housing Association, Council of Large Public Housing Authorities, National Association of Housing and Redevelopment Officials, and National Apartment Association, all of which could play a significant role in rebuilding and promoting successful recovery. Community development corporations are local nonprofit organizations or quasi-governmental entities that provide and develop low-income housing, often with the support of subsidies such as low-income housing tax credits. Organizations such as Habitat for Humanity and Rebuilding Together use volunteers to build or rehabilitate low-income housing, while Architecture for Humanity provides pro bono design services after disasters. These nongovernmental organizations need to be actively engaged in post-disaster recovery efforts to ensure optimal functioning as part of a coordinated effort instead of a series of disconnected projects.

Private Businesses

Private businesses play a key role in recovery and can sometimes be more nimble than government agencies, but, as described below, neighborhood redevelopment will require close coordination between private and public sector stakeholders. Insurance companies have a large role in providing financing for recovery when homes have been damaged or destroyed by a disaster. However, certain kinds of damage (e.g., damage due to flooding) may not be covered, leaving homeowners to fend for themselves. Coordination between insurance companies and local and state government insurance commissions is essential because insurance companies may provide settlements or funds for reconstruction of housing before determinations have been made about whether (and where) rebuilding should occur and which standards and codes should apply. Once these determinations have been made, replacement costs may be impacted, and insurance settlements may no longer be adequate. Likewise, private developers may undertake acquisition and other preconstruction activities before the parameters of reconstruction have been set, making early coordination with local government essential. Builders and contractors bring essential skills to the rebuilding context, and special efforts may be needed to ensure that a reliable, trained workforce is available to carry out rebuilding efforts. Finally, lending and finance organizations, such as banks, mortgage institutions, underwriters, and others, play an essential role in providing needed capital as well as in specifying how private funds can be used for which activities. Public–private partnerships ensure that key decisions in the recovery process are made out by all responsible parties in a coordinated manner.

Partnering Organizations and Cross-Sector Collaboration

As stated in the National Disaster Housing Strategy, success in disaster housing requires "genuine collaboration and cooperation among the various local, State, tribal, and Federal partners, nongovernmental organizations, and the private sector to meet the needs of all disaster victims" (FEMA, 2009a). One potential mechanism for this type of collaboration between housing and non-housing sectors is a disaster housing task force (discussed in more detail below) that brings together the various players with key roles in disaster housing response and recovery.

Emergency Management

Non-housing organizations can provide important support and advice on housing provision and reconstruction. Emergency management personnel typically are involved in determining which housing solution for a given disaster is most appropriate, such as sheltering in place or evacuation, and providing security for temporary and short-term shelters. They also need to be involved in efforts to transition displaced individuals from shelters to alternative housing options.

Health and Social Services Sectors

The involvement of state or local public health and environmental health professionals is critical to meeting the housing-related needs of disaster victims. First, health and environmental health departments can provide surveillance to identify potential health issues related to housing, such as mold, carbon monoxide poisoning, or disaster-related health hazards (e.g., toxic chemicals). Second, public health can provide or coordinate health care in interim housing, such as medical need shelters. Finally, representatives of public health must be at the table to assess the health risks and benefits of various housing recovery strategies. For example, they may suggest healthy housing criteria for rebuilding, or propose innovative ways of incorporating health into community rebuilding, such as including bike paths or recreational facilities. The social services sector also is a key partner in housing recovery because displaced people need essential services, and social services professionals can help integrate service provision with interim housing.

Planning and Community Development

Urban and regional planning agencies are involved in determining the advisability of rebuilding (or not rebuilding) in certain areas affected by a disaster, as well as adapting housing and building codes to promote resilient and sustainable housing. Community development organizations can help create a long-term vision for a community that encompasses the voices and perspectives of all community residents, including low-income and vulnerable populations, and can help ensure that the building of affordable housing has priority in recovery efforts. Plans and relationships necessary to engage these sectors in housing recovery should be developed in advance of a disaster.

Engaging the Community in Housing Recovery

The community is an integral partner in housing recovery. In addition to housing agencies and housing providers, community-based organizations need to be involved in housing decisions. This can be achieved by involving such organizations as tenant unions, building associations, neighborhood associations, and advocates for low-income housing in the recovery planning process. Working through these community-based groups can help reach vulnerable populations by leveraging the existing connections between community groups and these populations. Low-income populations in particular are at risk of exclusion from decisions that impact them. In Galvestson, Texas, for example, residents who were displaced by Hurricane Ike's destruction of the community's public housing units were excluded from the recovery process because input was sought only from those still living in Galveston (Nolen, 2014). As a result, the public housing on the island was very nearly not rebuilt. Involving community-based organizations and seeking input from all sectors of the population can make housing recovery plans more fair, equitable, and sustainable.

PRE-DISASTER HOUSING SECTOR PRIORITIES

The ability of a community to recover quickly from a disaster depends in part on pre-disaster preparation. Before a disaster strikes, a community can work to identify how a disaster might affect its housing needs and what resources and policies will be needed for recovery. Having a post-disaster recovery plan in place enables a community to respond more quickly and to leverage the resources it already has more efficiently.

Establishing a Disaster Housing Task Force

Because timelines are compressed and resources are often scarce following a disaster, a community needs to establish a disaster housing task force[2] before a disaster strikes to begin establishing plans and identifying potential resources to guide recovery. Prior to a disaster, this task force is responsible for

- performing vulnerability assessments;
- developing an understanding of existing resources of the salient organizations; and
- developing plans, programs, and procedures to enable rapid rebuilding of healthy housing.

Representation on this task force should include a broad range of agencies and community organizations. In Marin County, California, for example, the task force included representatives from 16 different local government agencies, each with a specific set of responsibilities (see Box 10-1). However, the committee believes that the local health department should not only serve on the task force and assist in the delivery of medical and behavioral health care but also should ensure that all actions taken by the task force are based on information about what will best serve the community's immediate- and long-term health needs. Further, displaced individuals often require an array of human services with which health department personnel may not be familiar, so it is important that both health and human services expertise be represented on the task force. In addition to local government agencies, the task force should coordinate with relevant federal agencies, such as HUD, FEMA, and the U.S. Department of Health and Human Services (HHS) to ensure optimal vertical integration.

Conducting Vulnerability and Capacity Assessments

A primary pre-disaster function of a disaster housing task force is to acquire knowledge about the community's current housing stock. This knowledge greatly improves the ability of a community to plan for and recover from a disaster (HUD, 2007). Knowing current housing conditions enables a community to plan for temporary housing needs, prepare to assist residents with post-disaster repairs and rebuilding, and make policy decisions that will result in the redevelopment of a more resilient and sustainable community. Before a disaster, data should be gathered on the housing stock in the community, the vulnerabilities of the housing, vacancy rates, the proportions of rental and owner-occupied residences, and the suitability of various properties for temporary or long-term housing after a disaster. Many different strategies can be used to perform housing vulnerability assessments, depending on the risks the community faces. Hillsborough County, Florida, for example, which is most likely to experience hurricanes, uses a methodology that categorizes residential parcels by wind and flood vulnerability (Hillsborough County Government, 2010). This analysis provided Hillsborough County planners with data showing that about 22 percent of the county's housing stock was located in the 100-year flood plain. Knowing where clusters of vulnerable houses are located helps county planners determine where temporary shelters are more likely to be required, for example. This information also may assist a community in identifying priority redevel-

---

[2] This task force can go by many names, including housing recovery technical advisory committee and housing solutions task force.

BOX 10-1
Example of Agency-Specific Responsibilities in a Post-Disaster Housing Task Force: Marin County, California

- *Marin County Community Development Agency:* Lead the Post-Disaster Housing Task Force (Task Force). Coordinate local, state, and federal disaster housing programs including the Federal Emergency Management Agency's (FEMA's) Individuals and Households Program and those managed by the Small Business Administration (SBA) and the U.S. Department of Housing and Urban Development (HUD). Estimate the need for temporary housing. Develop and recommend temporary housing sites to governing boards.
- *Building and Safety Division of the Community Development Agency:* Serve on the Task Force. Coordinate the inspection of damaged buildings—develop detailed reports. Establish criteria for reoccupying damaged buildings. Provide technical support to building owners; coordinate access to licensed contractors; review and permit permanent repairs. Establish criteria for plan checks and permitting of temporary structures. Advise on temporary housing site selection. Review the need for temporary exemptions from building codes.
- *Marin Housing Authority:* Serve on the Task Force. Coordinate local, state, and federal individual and public assistance disaster housing programs. Establish criteria for determining eligibility for post-disaster housing. Develop resources to assist victims in relocating from emergency shelters to temporary housing. Coordinate for the appointment of caseworkers as necessary.
- *Marin County Health and Human Services:* Serve on the Task Force. Coordinate the delivery of social, mental health, public health services and emergency medical services to interim and temporary housing tenants.
- *Marin County Public Works:* Serve on the Task Force. Advise on temporary housing site selection. Coordinate the development and delivery of services to temporary housing sites.
- *Marin County Sheriff, Office of Emergency Services:* Serve on the Task Force as available. Facilitate coordination with state and federal disaster relief agencies and community-based organizations. Coordinate the development and adoption of emergency proclamations and ordinances as necessary.
- *Marin County Sheriff:* Serve on the Task Force. Advise on site selection and law enforcement/crime prevention issues. Coordinate the delivery of law enforcement and crime prevention services.
- *Marin County Fire:* Serve on the Task Force. Advise on site selection and fire suppression/safety issues. Coordinate the delivery of fire suppression and emergency medical services.
- *Marin County Counsel:* Advise on site selection and legal issues including eminent domain and the State Redevelopment Law. Expedite review of loans and contracts.
- *Marin County Parks:* Advise on site selection.
- *Marin County Office of Education:* Advise on site selection.
- *Marin County Economic Commission:* Advise on site selection involving property of private companies and represent the needs of employers.
- *Marin County Auditor:* Serve on Task Force. Review financial budget and track expenditures. Coordinate with state and federal disaster relief programs.
- *Marin County Community Relations Manager:* Serve on Task Force. Conduct outreach to media, victims, and general public.
- *Incorporated Cities and Towns:* Serve on the Task Force as necessary. Internal departments have the same responsibilities as the corresponding County departments listed above.
- *American Red Cross (ARC):* Serve on the Task Force. Assist in the transition from emergency shelters to interim and temporary housing. Assist in coordinating the establishment and use of a Rental Housing Replacement Revolving Fund.
- *Marin Operational Area Recovery Committee:* Develop and coordinate overall recovery effort. Define the mission and direct the efforts of the Task Force as necessary.

SOURCE: Excerpted from Marin County Sheriff, 2003, pp. 4-5.

opment areas. For example, areas with houses that have lead-based paint or asbestos might be slated for major renovation after a disaster to mitigate those hazards.

Not only is it important to conduct an assessment of housing vulnerabilities; communities such as Hillsborough County also perform institutional capacity assessments to determine what capabilities exist within the community to promote rebuilding and guide the development of policies that may promote the effectiveness of these capabilities during recovery (Hillsborough County Government, 2010). This assessment includes an inventory of different organizations and the roles and expertise of each. This assessment needs to include a determination of which manufactured housing vendors would be capable of providing the type of temporary units that would be needed for on-site and group temporary housing sites in the event of a disaster. Based on this determination, formal relationships may be established with different vendors, but as highlighted by the case of Hillsborough County, these relationships should be flexible so that if a particular vendor does not have the necessary stock in a timely manner, the community can move on to another vendor.

Identifying Pre-Disaster Plans, Programs, and Procedures

Prior to a disaster, the disaster housing task force should establish an inventory of existing local plans, ordinances, programs, and procedures relevant to housing during long-term recovery (Hillsborough County Government, 2010). After a disaster, the task force will be able to use this inventory to locate resources and identify opportunities for rebuilding. An example of an inventory, developed by Hillsborough County, is shown in Table 10-3. Opportunities to leverage existing programs to rebuild housing should be examined.

Planning for Siting of Temporary Housing

Emigration of residents from communities that have been struck by a disaster (and have experienced the resultant social and economic impacts, such as revenue loss, blight, and disruption of social networks) may be reduced by facilitating the timely and efficient transition of displaced individuals from shelters to temporary housing. Communities vulnerable to disasters should work with state and federal partners and use existing guidance (APA, 1998; ARC, 1998) in developing plans to guide where and how temporary housing is to be established. Potential sites can be designated in advance, or communities can develop criteria for temporary housing sites and apply those criteria to the post-disaster selection of sites after considering the extent and location of damage. To protect health and promote well-being, sites should

- be free of health hazards (e.g., contamination) and not subject to further safety and health risks (e.g., flooding); and
- adequately support those without access to private vehicles (near public transportation and/or in walkable distance from essential community amenities and employment centers).

In selecting group sites for long-term temporary housing, possibilities for conversion to permanent affordable housing units should be considered. Long-term temporary housing requires a significant investment in infrastructure (e.g., roads, utilities) that can be capitalized on during the construction of permanent housing (Florida Department of Community Affairs, 2010). Collaboration with urban and regional planning agencies and the community is essential to identifying appropriate locations for siting of temporary housing.

EARLY POST-DISASTER HOUSING RECOVERY PRIORITIES

When a disaster has resulted in damage to the physical infrastructure of a community, meeting survivors' short- and long-term housing needs is one of the most fundamental aspects of recovery. Immediately following a disaster, the impacted community should convene its disaster housing task force. The task force

TABLE 10-3 Hillsborough County, Florida, Pre-Disaster Housing Recovery: Primary Plans, Programs, and Procedures

Plan/Program/Procedure	Purpose	Lead Entity
Affordable Housing Density Bonuses	Encourages developers to build at higher density, promoting efficient use of land and preservation of open space	Hillsborough County Planning and Growth Management; Hillsborough County Affordable Housing Department
Community Development Block Grant	Provides communities with resources to address a wide range of unique community development needs	Hillsborough County Affordable Housing Department; City of Tampa Growth Management and Development Department
Density Bonuses/Transfer of Development Rights Program	Promote development in specific areas	Hillsborough County Planning and Growth Management; Hillsborough County City-County Planning Commission
Disaster Temporary Housing Plan	Formation, membership, and tasks of the Disaster Temporary Housing Committee; temporary housing criteria, and siting criteria	Disaster Temporary Housing Committee
Hillsborough County Land Development Code, Section 6	Temporary housing regulations	Hillsborough County Planning and Growth Management
HOME Investment Partnership Program	Develops affordable housing for low- and moderate-income citizens	Hillsborough County Affordable Housing Department
Homeowner Rehabilitation Program	Provides assistance to homeowners to meet minimum housing standards	Hillsborough County Affordable Housing Department; City of Tampa Growth Management and Development Department
Neighborhood Stabilization Program	Stabilizes communities that have suffered from foreclosures and abandonment through the purchase and redevelopment of foreclosed and abandoned homes and residential properties	Hillsborough County Affordable Housing Department
Post-Disaster Redevelopment Ordinance 93-20 Section 5 Procedures	Determination of damage, build-back policy, moratoria, and emergency repairs	Hillsborough County Redevelopment Task Force
Community Land Trust	Provides access to affordable housing in high cost, service-industry dependent areas while keeping housing affordable for future residents	Florida Community Land Trust Institute
Homelessness Prevention and Rapid Re-Housing Program	Provides financial assistance and services to prevent individuals and families from becoming homeless	Homeless Coalition of Hillsborough County; City of Tampa Growth Management and Development Department
State Housing Initiatives Partnership	Incentive to produce and preserve affordable housing for low- and moderate-income families	Hillsborough County Affordable Housing Department; City of Tampa Growth Management and Development Department

SOURCE: Hillsborough County Government, 2010.

will be responsible, in part, for determining the need for interim and long-term housing and identifying the necessary resources. As the response phase abates, the early recovery priorities are

- assessing housing needs;
- preventing unnecessary displacement;
- protecting homeowners and recovery workers against health risks; and
- providing short- and long-term temporary housing that meets health and human service needs.

The sections below review the health considerations that should be incorporated into decision making during recovery to prevent unintended negative health consequences and to promote health and well-being as communities work to meet post-disaster housing needs for survivors.

Assessing Housing Needs

Assessment (including quantification) of housing needs is an important first step in promoting housing recovery after a disaster. It includes data collection and analysis from sources that include the Census Bureau, preliminary damage assessments, shelters, and the community directly (e.g., evaluation of the extent of damage to housing stock) (FEMA, 2009b). Online databases, such as the National Shelter System (NSS) and FEMA's Housing Portal, can be used to help identify available housing.

An early decision that must be made in the immediate aftermath of a disaster is whether the existing housing or building stock will be adequate to house the displaced, new temporary units will be needed, or displaced populations should be transferred to nearby cities with adequate housing. This determination depends in part on pre-disaster vacancy rates and the suitability of vacant properties. To increase efficiency, these data should be gathered during pre-disaster assessments. Immediately after a disaster, HUD or a local entity should survey the entire HUD-assisted and HUD-owned housing inventory in and near the jurisdiction to determine the vacant units and vouchers available for providing temporary housing for displaced families (FEMA, 2009b).

If housing resources within an affected region cannot meet all of the community's housing needs, alternatives may include relocation outside of the community, although this solution may impede the community's recovery since it will further disrupt social support systems and may have long-term consequences for the community's viability. Furthermore, tensions can arise in host communities where large numbers of survivors relocate. Other solutions include the use of rental housing beyond the affected area, which can be facilitated through HUD's Housing Choice Voucher program (Section 8); immediate repair assistance so that damaged homes and rental housing can be made habitable; and the use of transitional shelters and temporary housing units (FEMA, 2009b).

Preventing Unnecessary Displacement

Displacement of people from their homes after a disaster—whether they go to a shelter, a relative's house, or temporary housing—has effects on health, and it also disrupts social connections that are integral to community functioning (Spokane et al., 2012). Evidence on the health effects of displacement is scarce because of a lack of pre-disaster data, an emphasis on short-term recovery, and the ambiguity of an appropriate follow-up period (Uscher-Pines, 2009). It is clear, however, that displacement is associated with psychological morbidity (including anxiety and depression), and there are indications that displaced individuals may experience a decrease in general health status and an increase in health care utilization (Uscher-Pines, 2009). Therefore, preventing unnecessary displacement after a disaster may prevent some negative health outcomes.

Rapid Repairs Programs

The need for temporary housing may decrease greatly if communities quickly assess and properly repair moderately damaged buildings to avoid unnecessary displacement of people from their homes (Marin County Sheriff, 2003). The community itself often is in the best position to make quick repairs. After Hurricane Sandy, for example, New York City implemented a program that provided free repairs so that residents could remain in or quickly return to their homes. The Rapid Repairs Program deployed thousands of contractors, electricians, plumbers, and construction workers around the city to restore heat, power, and water to more than 20,000 residences (NYC, 2013). This first-of-its kind program helped New Yorkers return quickly to a sense of normalcy while reducing the demand for large-scale temporary sheltering. New York State and FEMA built on the success of Rapid Repairs by developing the Sheltering and Temporary Essential Power (STEP) pilot program, which provided similar services for areas outside of New York City. Once Rapid Repairs had wound down, the state released federal funds to reimburse the city for the costs incurred by the program (New York State Governor, 2013).

The role of the government in facilitating repairs to housing will depend on the nature of the disaster and the demographics of the impacted area. As noted earlier, for example, damage from a tornado that strikes a residential neighborhood may be covered largely by private insurance, whereas floods and earthquakes often are not covered unless a separate policy (e.g., a National Flood Insurance Program policy) was purchased. Experience from past disasters has shown that many homeowners (and often the most vulnerable, such as the elderly and low-income individuals) do not have adequate housing insurance, limiting rapid rebuilding capacity.

Foreclosure Relief

Another approach to preventing unnecessary displacement is to provide foreclosure relief to homeowners suffering short-term financial difficulties as a result of the disaster (Hurricane Sandy Rebuilding Task Force, 2013). The Hurricane Sandy Rebuilding Strategy recognizes the need to prevent responsible homeowners from being displaced and experiencing foreclosure while recovering from a disaster. Upon instruction from HUD or other regulatory bodies, mortgage servicers can temporarily halt foreclosure on homes with Federal Housing Administration (FHA) and other government-insured mortgages (HUD, 1994, 2000, 2002, 2009b, 2014a).[3] Similarly, mortgage service providers can provide relief to those without government-insured mortgages. Foreclosure relief gives servicers extra time to confirm the intent and ability of the mortgagee to repair the home, resume regular mortgage payments, and retain ownership (FEMA, 2009b). However, different mortgage companies have differing policies and guidelines, sometimes causing confusion within impacted communities. Therefore, pre-disaster coordination between the financial and housing sectors and the government can enable more consistent application of waivers. Further, mortgage relief is a key mechanism for providing incentives to rebuild in a way that enhances housing resiliency and compliance with healthy housing standards. Financial institutions, developers, and contractors also have key roles to play in enforcing decisions on which areas should not contain rebuilt housing, as well as on the quality of rebuilt housing and its compliance with green and healthy housing standards.

Protecting Homeowners and Recovery Workers Against Health Risks

In any effort to conduct repairs, the health and safety of recovery workers must be protected. A training system will be needed to ensure that workers, including volunteers wishing to aid in recovery operations, have the knowledge, skills, and equipment to do their work safely. All workers involved in housing and other building recovery and immediate repair/stabilization should be trained in how to identify potential mold, asbestos, lead-based paint, and injury hazards in homes they are seeking to repair and in how to

---

[3] 61 F.R. 35020 § 203.614 Special forbearance. Vol. 61, No. 120, Jul. 3, 1996.

control those hazards for both themselves and future occupants (e.g., mitigation practices). Measures to protect recovery workers also include provision of personal protective equipment, such as protective clothing, goggles, and fit-tested respirators, as well as plans for handling any work-related injuries expeditiously, including on-site first aid capacity. A wealth of information resources on worker protection during disasters is available through the National Clearinghouse for Worker Safety and Health Training, which is maintained by the National Institute of Environmental Health Sciences (NIEHS).[4] NIEHS also offers training for response and recovery workers through its worker education and training program. After Hurricane Sandy, for example, NIEHS mobilized its worker education and training resources to support cleanup efforts (NIEHS, 2013). Guidance on mold mitigation in the context of disasters is available from many sources, including the National Center for Healthy Housing (2008) and the EPA (2010).

While multifamily housing often has property management personnel responsible for repairs and maintenance, owners of single-family housing are more likely to adopt a "do it yourself" attitude. Such homeowners, especially those whose houses have sustained minimal damage, may attempt to repair and remediate damages themselves. Therefore, homeowners need ready access to information on how to protect themselves from injury or illness as they repair their homes. For example, homeowners need information about identifying and mitigating lead-based paint, mold, and asbestos hazards, as well as injury prevention practices such as turning off the electricity when there is standing water or avoiding carbon monoxide poisoning from the indoor use of gas-powered tools or generators. This type of information can be provided to homeowners in pamphlets available at disaster recovery centers, home repair stores, and other places where homeowners may seek information. Homeowners also can utilize the resources of HUD's Office of Healthy Homes and Lead Hazard Control, which has developed a disaster recovery portal providing information about how housing-related hazards can be exacerbated by a disaster and how to identify and address them[5] (HUD, 2014d).

Providing Short- and Long-Term Temporary Housing That Meets Health and Human Service Needs

When displacement cannot be avoided, temporary housing must be found for residents affected by a disaster. This short- and long-term temporary housing must be adequate to support the health of its occupants. Tent cities, vacation trailers, special event and conference centers, hotels and motels, railroad cars, shipping containers, covered stadiums, and cruise ships are all examples of temporary short-term solutions that should not be used to meet intermediate- and long-term housing needs during recovery because of potential health impacts associated with both physical and social environments (FEMA, 2009b).

Following the sheltering operations of the initial response phase, decisions must be made about options for interim housing for displaced individuals. Generally, there are three options:

- leveraging the appropriate existing buildings in either impacted or host communities;
- setting up temporary housing units (not vacation trailers) that FEMA may purchase and deploy (these may be placed on a homeowner's property if feasible); and
- using community sites to provide temporary housing—usually a last resort because it is dependent on the location, design, and infrastructure of the site selected and on whether the community finds it acceptable to use the site for more permanent housing (FEMA, 2009b).

The first option can involve FEMA's Multi-Family Lease and Repair Program (MLRP), which works to make better use of existing vacant multifamily property units in impacted or host communities. The MLRP

---

[4] The National Clearinghouse for Worker Safety and Health Training is available online at http://tools.niehs.nih.gov/wetp/index.cfm (accessed June 15, 2015).

[5] HUD's disaster recovery portal can be found at http://portal.hud.gov/hudportal/HUD?src=/program_offices/healthy_homes/disasterrecovery (accessed June 15, 2015).

provides funding to property owners for repairs to existing properties in exchange for the owners' making units available to individuals and households eligible for FEMA assistance (FEMA, 2013b). This program provides an "opportunity to minimize cost and reduce recovery time when the temporary housing needs are expected to be extensive and where local, affordable and accessible rental resources are insufficient to meet the permanent housing need" (FEMA, 2009b, p. 68). Many jurisdictions already have inadequate affordable healthy housing options, and repairing existing residential or commercial buildings can increase housing availability and affordability in many urban areas. The repairs should ensure that the units comply with the National Healthy Housing Standard developed by the American Public Health Association and the National Center for Healthy Housing. Applicable housing and energy codes also should be observed.

The second option entails the use of housing units that can lend themselves to becoming permanent residences, either in whole or in part. This option can involve the use of private sites where nearby housing will be restored.

The third option involves the use of community sites for temporary housing. As noted, this is usually a last resort because it is dependent on the location, design, and infrastructure of the site selected.

The degree to which any of these three options proves feasible will depend largely on the extent to which the affected or host communities are willing to allow "temporary housing" to become "permanent housing" (FEMA, 2009b). If commercial and private facilities fail to meet the community's housing needs, factory-built housing may be an alternative. Such housing should be placed in community site configurations, and the layout should include communal common areas to promote social interaction and to provide play areas for children. Factory-built housing typically is used to meet temporary housing needs. These manufactured homes, therefore, generally are located on commercial pads or sites developed specifically for such a purpose, although they also can be placed in existing commercial temporary sites. Alternatively, factory-built units may be placed on private sites so that homeowners can remain on their personal property as they repair or rebuild their permanent home (FEMA, 2009b).

HUD (through local housing authorities and others) can sell or lease housing it owns to displaced individuals at a discounted price. To minimize rebuilding time and reduce costs, federal-, state-, and local government-owned housing should be considered a primary option following a disaster. Additionally, the U.S. General Services Administration (GSA) can be used to acquire leases from private landowners. At the state and local levels, governments are responsible for identifying vacant land they own (FEMA, 2009b). These strategies help ensure that the short- and long-term housing needs of affected communities can be met adequately and quickly following a disaster.

Ensuring Safety and Health in Temporary Housing

Although emergency situations in which large numbers of individuals and families are displaced may require creative solutions to ensure that basic sheltering needs are met in the immediate aftermath, requirements for temporary housing that will be used to meet longer-term needs (months to years) should be significantly more stringent. If mobile vacation trailers are used for temporary housing (although this is not recommended), residents should be transferred from them as quickly as possible because they are not manufactured for long-term occupancy, and there is evidence that their use compromises occupants' health as a result of inadequate indoor air quality (e.g., formaldehyde) and inadequate space (CDC, 2010). Manufactured housing should comply with the National Healthy Housing Standard and should not include components that off-gas hazardous substances. Such housing also may require special siting and construction considerations, such as tie-downs in tornado areas and seismic designs in earthquake zones. The adequacy of housing with regard to health can be assessed using various tools, including the Housing Habitability checklist in Box 10-2 and the CDC/HUD Healthy Housing Inspection Manual, which also is available in a computerized ACCESS database suitable for laptops and tablets.

Key principles of healthy housing that should be applied to temporary post-disaster housing include proper ventilation (both adequate fresh air and its distribution), moisture and mold control, maintenance,

BOX 10-2
Health and Safety Checklist for Temporary Housing

All short- and long-term temporary housing should comply with the following checklist:

1. *Structure and materials*: The structures must be structurally sound so as to pose no threat to the health and safety of the occupants and to protect the residents from hazards.
2. *Access*: Structures must provide alternative means of egress in case of fire or other emergency.
3. *Space and security*: All residents must be afforded adequate space and security for themselves and their belongings. All residents must be provided with an acceptable place to sleep.
4. *Interior air and environmental quality*: Every room or space must be provided with natural or mechanical ventilation. Structures must be free of pollutants in the air and on surfaces at levels that threaten the health of residents. Particular attention should be paid to the location of generators to ensure that combustion products, such as carbon monoxide, do not enter the air in the living area.
5. *Water supply*: The water supply must be free from contamination.
6. *Sanitary facilities*: Residents must have access to sufficient sanitary facilities that are in proper operating condition, can be used in privacy, and are adequate for personal cleanliness and the disposal of human waste.
7. *Thermal environment*: The housing must have adequate heating and/or cooling facilities in proper operating condition.
8. *Illumination and electricity*: The housing must have adequate natural or artificial illumination to permit normal indoor activities and to support the health and safety of residents. Sufficient electrical sources must be provided to permit the use of essential electrical appliances while ensuring safety from fire.
9. *Food preparation and refuse disposal*: All food preparation areas must contain suitable space and equipment to store, prepare, and serve food in a sanitary manner.
10. *Sanitary condition*: The housing and any equipment must be maintained in a sanitary condition.
11. *Fire/carbon monoxide safety*: Both conditions below must be met to meet this standard.
    a. Each unit must include at least one battery-operated or hard-wired smoke detector/alarm and carbon monoxide detector/alarm, in proper working condition, on each occupied level of the unit. Smoke detectors must be located, to the extent practicable, in a hallway adjacent to a bedroom. If the unit is occupied by hearing-impaired persons, each bedroom occupied by such a person must have a detector with an alarm system designed for the hearing-impaired.
    b. The public areas of all housing must be equipped with a sufficient number of detectors, but at least one for each area. Public areas include, but are not limited to, laundry rooms, day care centers, hallways, stairwells, and other common areas.
12. *Lead exposure*: In units built before 1978, when lead-based paint was banned, and in which a household with a child or pregnant woman intends to reside, a visual assessment and/or lead-based paint risk assessment/inspection should be conducted. Visual assessment means looking for, as applicable (1) deteriorated paint (chipping, loose, crumbling); (2) visible surface paint dust, debris, and residue; and (3) the completion or failure of a hazard reduction measure as part of a risk assessment or clearance examination.
13. New or temporary housing should not be located on newly or previously contaminated sites, such as brownfield or Superfund sites, unless those sites have been remediated.

SOURCE: Adapted from HUD, 2009a.

integrated pest management, avoidance of toxic chemicals and agents, safety (free of injury hazards), accessibility, cleanliness, and adequate lighting (HHS and HUD, 2006).

Supporting Social Connectedness

As discussed earlier in this chapter, the selection of sites for long-term temporary housing will have a significant impact on the experiences of those who are living there, and thus on its success. For example, temporary housing should be located near places of employment or transportation routes that can provide access to places of employment. Location, access, and mitigation of vulnerabilities are critical, but communities also need to consider other variables that can improve health outcomes, including how best to maintain social networks and ensure access to health care and social services.

One option for minimizing the negative impacts of relocation is to locate temporary housing on a person's original property—for example, to place a trailer next to a house that is being repaired. If residents remain on their own property, their lives are minimally disrupted, and existing social networks and neighborhood cohesiveness are maintained. When it is necessary to establish temporary housing such as a trailer park, a common choice for transitional housing, the park can be designed in a way that supports social connectedness. In Figure 10-1, for example, the park on the left shows a typical arrangement: trailers are aligned in rows, with the door of one facing the side of another, and there are no communal spaces or walking paths. The park on the right shows an alternative design: trailers are arranged in groups of four around common courtyards, and paths are placed around the park to encourage social interaction and casual contact (Spokane et al., 2012).

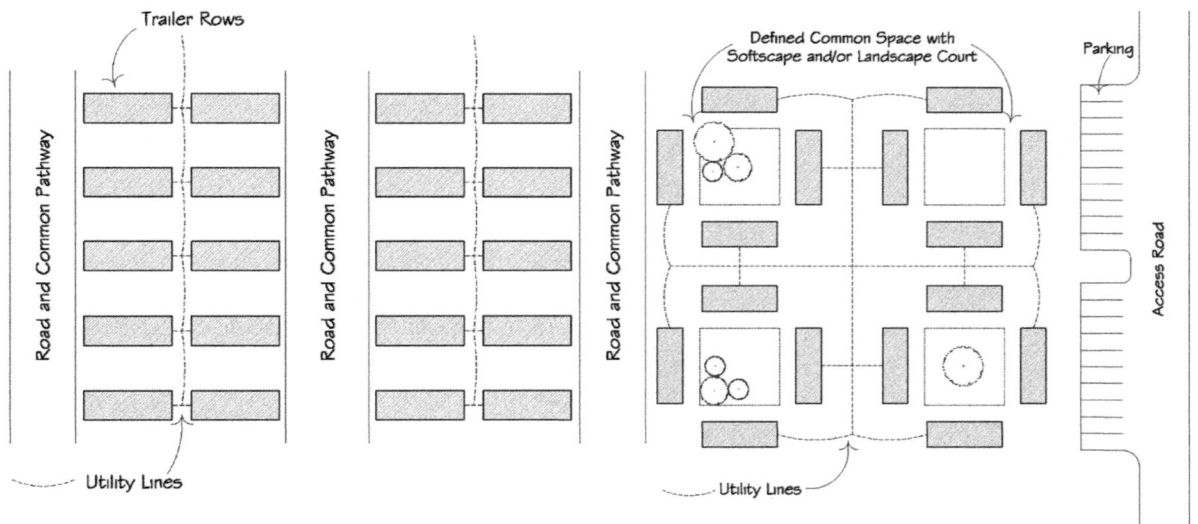

FIGURE 10-1 Alternative arrangements of post-disaster temporary housing.
NOTE: The figure on the left shows the typical arrangement of Federal Emergency Management Agency (FEMA) trailers after Hurricane Katrina, which provided little space and opportunity for social interaction among residents, in contrast to the proposed arrangement on the right, where a quad-style layout is designed to promote social connectedness.
SOURCE: Spokane et al., 2012. Reprinted with permission from SAGE Publications.

Ensuring Access to Needed Health and Human Services

As individuals are displaced from their homes for increasing periods of time, the need for community and social services tends to rise (FEMA, 2009a). Consequently, human services need to be integrated into disaster housing recovery efforts, and they may need to be offered on-site or nearby. These services—sometimes called "wraparound services"—include health care, schools, daycare, social services, public transportation, and employment counseling. The provision of these services can help expedite recovery and speed the transition to a permanent housing solution. After the tornado in Joplin, Missouri, for example, the Red Cross opened a multi-agency resource center that served as a one-stop shop for survivor assistance, offering myriad resources under one roof: financial assistance, legal services, hot meals, health care, counseling, and help with government assistance programs (Meeds, 2013). When wraparound services are offered within or near temporary housing sites, displaced individuals and families can better access the resources they need to recover, and community recovery is expedited.

SPECIAL CONSIDERATIONS FOR VULNERABLE POPULATIONS

When transitioning disaster survivors from emergency shelters to short- and long-term temporary housing, special care must be taken for vulnerable populations. As emphasized throughout this report, disasters affect vulnerable populations disproportionately—damages rarely are evenly distributed, and the families that are hardest hit are often socially, culturally, or economically vulnerable before the disaster (Spokane et al., 2012). Furthermore, vulnerable populations without resources such as insurance or assistance are less able than others with these resources to repair or rebuild properly, and they are more likely to be placed in long-term group trailer housing. After Hurricane Katrina, for example, 80 percent of owners had a trailer placed on their own home site, whereas around 80 percent of renters were moved to group sites (Spokane et al., 2012). The renters who were low-income, unemployed, elderly, or disabled were more likely to stay in the group sites longer. As stated in Chapter 3, a recovery plan that addresses the special needs of vulnerable populations—and preferably includes these residents in the planning process—is critical to the recovery of the entire community. Meeting the needs of vulnerable populations may require pre- and post-disaster coordination among emergency management, social services, health care, the housing sector, and others.

Survivors with Disabilities and Special Medical Needs

People with disabilities and medical issues have unique needs in sheltering operations. Special-needs and medical shelters may be established to provide care that is normally provided in nursing homes or hospitals, but advance planning is essential to ensure that medical personnel and volunteers can adequately meet the medical needs of the shelter residents (ADA, 2007). Medicare- and Medicaid-certified nursing homes are required to have emergency plans and to train staff in providing emergency services; however, a recent study found that these plans have major gaps, and nursing home administrators (more than 70 percent of those surveyed) report significant challenges in preparing for a disaster (HHS, 2012). Under the Americans with Disabilities Act, emergency shelter programs must not exclude or deny benefits to those with disabilities—shelter must be available that is physically accessible to people with disabilities, including those in wheelchairs (ADA, 2007). Such needs will also need to be accommodated in temporary housing arrangements.

The Homeless

The homeless are especially vulnerable to the impacts of disasters. They are among the most difficult to reach with any pre-disaster information-gathering systems, and the lack of baseline information is cited as one of the primary problems encountered in disasters (Runkle et al., 2012). In addition, homeless persons are four times more likely than the general population to suffer from severe mental illness—20-25 percent of the U.S. homeless population suffers from severe mental illness, whereas only 6 percent of Americans are severely mentally ill (National Coalition for the Homeless, 2009). Compounding these problems are higher addiction rates, social isolation, lack of income, lack of transportation, and limited means of communication for people who lack a permanent residence.

The same issues that create difficulties in helping the homeless prepare for disasters persist during recovery. Without addresses, homeless people cannot be contacted by relief organizations or file for benefits. If homeless populations are disconnected before disasters, the impact of the disaster often puts them farther out of reach of disaster recovery safety nets. Disasters also create newly homeless populations as a result of a multitude of factors, including lost employment, destruction of affordable housing, and associated rent increases. The city of New Orleans serves as an example of such issues and the challenges they pose to successful disaster recovery. According to a 2010 report on homelessness in New Orleans after Hurricane Katrina, the rate of homelessness in the city had nearly doubled 5 years after the flood, with thousands of homeless people living in the city's abandoned buildings. Fully 75 percent of these individuals were Katrina survivors, and alarmingly, most had been stably housed prior to the storm (UNITY, 2010).

Special efforts are needed to address the particular challenges facing homeless populations during disasters and to combat systemic issues that cause the most vulnerable victims of a disaster to fall into homelessness. Strategies proposed on the basis of experience with past disasters include

- a communication plan to relay timely and accurate information to health and human service agencies, and a platform for reporting operational status and needs;
- a homeless-specific sheltering and evacuation plan (National Coalition for the Homeless, 2014);
- the conversion of abandoned buildings into permanent supportive housing, where on-site case management services are available to help homeless individuals with disabilities remain stably housed after a disaster;
- the formation of outreach and housing search teams to identify homeless individuals and families and connect them with temporary and permanent housing; and
- continued investment in addressing affordable housing shortages to help low-income homeowners and renters finds new homes (UNITY, 2010).

These strategies require concerted collaboration among governmental and nongovernmental stakeholders from the social services and housing sectors.

INTERMEDIATE- TO LONG-TERM RECOVERY: OPPORTUNITIES TO ADVANCE HEALTHIER AND MORE RESILIENT AND SUSTAINABLE COMMUNITIES

A central theme of this report, cutting across all sectors involved in disaster recovery, is that rebuilding homes, buildings, and neighborhoods after a disaster creates an opportunity to rebuild in a way that supports residents' health, is more resilient to the next disaster, and is more sustainable. The Urban Land Institute (2014) suggests five elements that should be considered when creating such communities (see Box 10-3 for details on how Greensburg, Kansas, incorporated these elements after a tornado):

- Compact, walkable, and mixed-use—Communities that are pedestrian friendly and provide easy access to services are more resilient to extreme weather, contribute to the health of their residents, reduce environmental impacts, and encourage social networks.
- Equity—Encouraging equity and the participation of vulnerable groups in community planning, housing and land use decisions, and disaster preparedness can reduce disproportionate health impacts in both steady-state and disaster times and improve the resilience of the entire community.
- Social capital—A strong and interconnected community—including partnerships among residents, organizations, and government—is a "prerequisite for recovery following catastrophic events" (ULI, 2014, p. 9) and it also has a positive impact on health generally.

- Efficient and durable housing—Housing that is designed to reduce the use of resources and to withstand extreme weather events can improve residents' health and minimize damage during a disaster.
- Continuous adaptation—Community resilience is an iterative process, in which plans and designs must continually be reassessed after disasters and in the face of a changing climate (ULI, 2014).

It is important that multifamily residences be rebuilt in accordance with principles of resiliency and healthy living since the design of such a building can affect the health and well-being of a large number of individuals. In other words, economies of scale may be realized. With multifamily housing, steps to promote recovery and improve overall health can impact all building residents. Greater efficiencies of operation are possible in multifamily buildings, as well as different kinds of educational programs and training compared with those possible with single-family housing.

Efforts to reduce the vulnerability of residents of multifamily buildings to the effects of disasters are an important consideration. After Hurricane Sandy, tens of thousands of residents of such buildings, including those in public housing, were left without heat or power because of flooding in the basements where heating and electrical systems were located (Furman Center, 2013). Hazard mitigation measures, including the presence of generators, emergency boilers, and pumps, could have prevented widespread hardship (Hurricane Sandy Rebuilding Task Force, 2013), and such measures need to be incorporated into more resilient multifamily unit designs. In contrast to past recovery efforts, recovery from Hurricane

---

BOX 10-3
Rebuilding in Greensburg, Kansas

In 2007, the small town of Greensburg, Kansas, was struck by the strongest class of tornado. The rural town, with a population of only 1,500, was nearly wiped out. The tornado destroyed or severely damaged 90 percent of the structures in the town, including 600 homes. Despite the scope of the damage and the crippling costs to the community of more than $500 million, Greensburg residents used the disaster as an opportunity to build back in a healthier and more resilient and sustainable way, demonstrating that such approaches are not applicable only to metropolitan areas.

The town set out to craft a new standard for resiliency and energy efficiency in rural communities, an approach rooted in Kansan values, such as respect for the earth and a commitment to future generations. Under Greensburg's Long-Term Community Recovery Plan, the town built on the preexisting compact size of the rural community to create its new downtown, a mixed-use area with walkable streets, and added green space and recreational facilities. Affordable housing was built within walking distance of stores, parks, the school, the hospital, and the city hall. Many of the homes that were destroyed were rebuilt using green building standards, as well as hazard mitigation features such as storm shelters and bolting of the structure to concrete. Some homes incorporated a wall system capable of withstanding winds up to 195 miles per hour. Publically funded buildings of more than 4,000 square feet were required to be built to Leadership in Energy & Environmental Design (LEED) Platinum Certification standards, and the town is now home to the most LEED-certified buildings per capita in the world.

The Greensburg Sustainable Comprehensive Plan, designed and adopted by the community, provides a vision for the town and will continue to guide the rebuilding and redevelopment efforts. For rural communities such as Greensburg, collective community action is crucial to the overall healing process. Furthermore, the social cohesion common to rural communities drives efforts to rebuild in a more resilient and sustainable manner, addressing preexisting challenges and working to ensure that the community is not only more prepared for future disasters but stronger and healthier overall.

SOURCE: ULI, 2014.

Sandy has included focusing recovery funds on public and multifamily housing. The CDBG-DR notice discussed earlier included a provision designed to encourage grantees to emphasize public and multifamily housing. HUD required grantees to specify how they would meet the rehabilitation, mitigation, and new construction needs of all affected public housing agencies and the multifamily assisted housing within these agencies' jurisdictions.[6]

In addition to taking steps to better shield residents from the effects of disasters, there may be special opportunities in a multifamily residence to incorporate features that contribute to residents' health on a daily basis. For example, buildings can include health centers. An example is the Brandywine Center in Pennsylvania, which has affordable housing for seniors on the upper floors and a federally qualified health center on the first floor that offers health care, mental health, and dental services (Brandywine Center, 2009).

Incentivizing the Use of Green and Healthy Housing Standards

HUD recently required compliance with an industry-recognized "green" standard for construction and rehabilitation of housing damaged by Hurricane Sandy that is supported by CDBG-DR funds[7] (see Box 10-4). This important development shows that using green healthy housing standards in the context of disaster recovery is feasible and can be accomplished at the programmatic level. Although there may be some increased upfront costs associated with building in accordance with these standards, testimony provided to the committee suggested there was little resistance to complying with such standards (Smith Parker, 2014). Based on the demonstrated positive impacts of green building standards to health (discussed earlier in this chapter), the committee believes that HUD's requirement should be extended to all recovery efforts.

Housing regulations and standards typically are triggered during the course of specific building stages (e.g., obtaining permits for new construction projects) and housing transactions (e.g., sales, rentals, subsidies, financing), as well as in response to public health concerns (e.g., noise complaints, vermin, surveillance of lead poisoning in children due to lead-based paint). Little clarity exists, however, as to how housing—either temporary or rebuilt after a disaster—should comply with such standards. HUD's requirement to rebuild housing in the wake of Hurricane Sandy in compliance with green healthy housing standards is commendable (HUD, 2013). Given the proliferation of such green standards, however, additional guidance is needed to help communities understand the specific standards that should be applied.

Establishing Permitting and Code Enforcement Policies That Promote and Protect Health

Following a disaster, a community may wish to establish temporary permitting processes to speed rebuilding. There may be pressure to waive existing land use, zoning, and building codes in the interest of facilitating rapid reconstruction. However, it is important that such temporary measures be carefully considered and only taken when truly necessary. Such waivers may in fact compromise public safety and a community's resilience to withstand future disasters and thus are generally not recommended.

Single-family and multifamily housing can pose different health issues in the context of disaster recovery. Multifamily units, for example, can have more complex heating, ventilation, and air-conditioning systems that require different levels of expertise and standards. Electrical and fire protection systems also differ between the two types of housing. These distinctions, however, offer an opportunity to incorporate health into long-term recovery. If, for instance, a multifamily building does not comply with safety and building standards, such as the American Society of Heating, Refrigerating, and Air-Conditioning Engineers (ASHRAE) standard, before a disaster, the rebuilding effort can be used to promote compliance with healthier standards overall.

---

[6] 78 F.R. 69104-69113.
[7] 78 F.R. 14329-14349.

BOX 10-4
Post-Hurricane Sandy Requirements for "Green" Rebuilding

In specifying how Community Development Block Grant for Disaster Recovery (CDBG-DR) funds can be used in Hurricane Sandy rebuilding efforts, the U.S. Department of Housing and Urban Development (HUD) issued a notice stating that such funds may be used only for housing that complies with green standards. (A notice is for all practical purposes legally enforceable.) That notice requires (in part) that local jurisdictions receiving HUD CDBG-DR funds provide:

"(5) A description of how the grantee's programs or activities will attempt to protect people and property from harm, and how the grantee will encourage construction methods that emphasize high quality, durability, energy efficiency, a healthy indoor environment, sustainability, and water or mold resistance, including how it will support adoption and enforcement of modern building codes and mitigation of hazard risk, including possible sea level rise, storm surge, and flooding, where appropriate. All rehabilitation, reconstruction, and new construction should be designed to incorporate principles of sustainability, including water and energy efficiency, resilience and mitigating the impact of future disasters. Whenever feasible, grantees should follow best practices such as those provided by the U.S. Department of Energy Home Energy Professionals: Professional Certifications and Standard Work Specifications.

"To foster the rebuilding of more resilient neighborhoods and communities, HUD strongly encourages grantees to consider sustainable rebuilding scenarios such as the use of different development patterns, infill development and its reuse, alternative neighborhood designs, and the use of green infrastructure. The Partnership for Sustainable Communities is an interagency partnership between HUD, the Department of Transportation, and the Environmental Protection Agency. The Partnership for Sustainable Communities' six Livability Principles should serve as a guide to grantees working in areas that were substantially destroyed. When grantees seek to rebuild such areas, grantees should describe how they will consider sustainable urban design and construction in their redevelopment planning process. The Livability Principles can be found at the Partnership for Sustainable Communities' Web site www.sustainablecommunities.gov.

"At a minimum, HUD is requiring the following construction standards [emphasis added]:

"(a) Green Building Standard for Replacement and New Construction of Residential Housing. Grantees must meet the Green Building Standard in this subparagraph for: (i) all new construction of residential buildings; and (ii) all replacement of substantially-damaged residential buildings. Replacement of residential buildings may include reconstruction (i.e., demolishing and re-building a housing unit on the same lot in substantially the same manner) and may include changes to structural elements such as flooring systems, columns or load bearing interior or exterior walls.

"(b) For purposes of this Notice, the Green Building Standard means the grantee will require that all construction covered by subparagraph (a), above, meet an industry-recognized standard that has achieved certification under at least one of the following programs: (i) ENERGY STAR (Certified Homes or Multi-family High Rise); (ii) Enterprise Green Communities; (iii) LEED (NC, Homes, Midrise, Existing Buildings O&M, or Neighborhood Development); (iv) ICC-700 National Green Building Standard; (v) EPA Indoor AirPlus (ENERGY STAR a prerequisite); or (vi) any other equivalent comprehensive green building program, including regional programs such as those operated by the New York State Energy Research and Development Authority or the New Jersey Clean Energy Program."

SOURCE: 78 F.R. 14329-14349.

A community also may need to be strategic in the way permits are provided so that rebuilding is not piecemeal but synchronized with the availability of other services. For example, permits may not be issued for areas where commercial power has not yet been restored. In some cases, a moratorium on issuing permits may provide needed time to consider mitigation measures prior to reconstruction. Permitting processes can also be used as incentives to encourage green building by giving priority to developers that use green and healthy housing standards (Hillsborough County Government, 2010).

Strengthening the Resiliency of Housing

Rebuilding in a way that mitigates against future disasters helps "break the cycle of disaster damage, reconstruction, and repeated damage" (FEMA, 2014). Mitigation protects against damage and loss of life, enables a community to recover more quickly, and reduces the financial impact of a disaster. Mitigation can be performed on individual homes, neighborhoods, or entire communities. Mitigation methods include floodproofing; elevating structures; reinforcing roofs, windows, walls, and doors; using fire-resistant materials (excluding those containing asbestos); planting vegetation to control stormwater; building levees and dams; and moving homes away from disaster-prone areas.

Funds are available to both individuals and communities for mitigation activities. Individuals may apply for home disaster loans through the SBA, and additional funding is available specifically for mitigation activities—up to 20 percent of the total amount of disaster damage. The SBA's low-interest disaster loans are available to businesses, nonprofits, homeowners, and those with rental properties for purposes of repairing or replacing real estate, personal property, and business assets (SBA, 2014). In addition, CDBG-DR and FEMA's Hazard Mitigation Grant Program funds can be used by states and communities for such purposes as purchase of hazard-prone homes and conversion of the land to green spaces, recreational areas, or wetlands; stormwater management; structure elevation; floodproofing; and retrofitting of existing buildings. Special considerations related to buyouts are discussed in Chapter 9.

Ensuring Adequate Affordable Healthy Housing

Affordability is a key component of healthy housing and healthy neighborhoods. If housing improvements following a disaster are not affordable, families may be forced to leave the area or to choose between paying rent and taking care of their health (as described in the "Heat or Eat" study reviewed above). According to the Homeless Coalition of Hillsborough County, "the biggest contributing factor to the rising number of homeless people is the shortage of affordable housing for people with limited incomes," a shortage that is only likely to increase following a disaster (Hillsborough County, 2010).

Beyond the disaster recovery context, housing affordability is related to health outcomes generally. For example, renters who receive financial assistance for housing under HUD's Housing Choice Vouchers (Section 8) are less likely to suffer housing-related health issues than non-voucher holders (Lindberg et al., 2010). Voucher holders are less likely to experience

- overcrowding,
- malnutrition due to food insecurity,
- concentrated neighborhood poverty (Lindberg et al., 2010),
- higher rent burdens (Van Ryzin and Kamber, 2002), and
- low age-standardized weight for children (Meyers et al., 2005).

At the neighborhood level, those with high poverty rates also have many poor health outcomes, including mortality, poor child and adult physical and mental health, and negative health behaviors (Diez-Roux et al., 1997; Ellen and Turner, 2003; Ellen et al., 2001; Kawachi and Berkman, 2003; Macintyre and Ellaway, 2000, 2003; Macintyre et al., 2002; Pickett and Pearl, 2001; Waitzman and Smith, 1998). Living in such neighborhoods can limit residents' access to education and employment, which in turn can contribute to housing instability or homelessness (Lindberg et al., 2010), both of which are exacerbated by disasters.

Many communities already lack adequate affordable housing before a disaster, so a disaster can present an opportunity to increase the supply of such housing. Funding for disaster recovery far outpaces funding for community development generally—the funding request for traditional CDBGs in 2013 was about $3 billion, while $16 billion was allocated in CDBG-DR funds for post–Hurricane Sandy recovery (Gilmore and Standaert, 2013). In addition to the use of federal funding, a community can increase affordable housing by requiring or incentivizing developers to build certain types of housing. A program in Cedar Rapids, Iowa, for example, allows developers to build homes on city-owned lots provided that the homes' final sale price does not exceed $150,000 (Cedar Rapids, 2014a).

Some communities have sought to develop mixed-income housing, which includes housing for low-, middle-, and high-income individuals within a defined area, usually a building or neighborhood (Levy et al., 2010). Yet while the evidence that segregated neighborhoods and housing are associated with poor health outcomes is clear (Jacobs, 2011), the evidence that mixed-income neighborhoods are associated with positive health outcomes is mixed. Because no studies qualified for review, the Community Preventive Services Task Force was unable to find sufficient evidence to determine the effectiveness of creating mixed-income housing developments as an approach to reversing neighborhood deterioration, improving physical or mental health status, or increasing community cohesion and civic engagement (TFCPS, 2003). There is some evidence that moving into mixed-income communities leads to improvements in obesity in adults and mental health improvements in girls aged 12-19 (Orr et al., 2003), but the evidence for potential mental health improvements is mixed. One recent study, for example, found an increased prevalence of mental health disorders in boys aged 10-15 who had moved into a mixed-income community compared with those who had not moved into such a community (Kessler et al., 2014). While a disaster may present the opportunity to develop mixed-income housing, further research is needed on the associated health outcomes. In addition, turning formerly low-income areas into mixed-income housing may decrease the concentration of poverty, but it also may decrease the supply of affordable housing and leave some residents without realistic housing options (Ross, 2013).

Providing Financial Incentives

Financial incentives can be used to encourage rebuilding in a healthier and more resilient and sustainable way, including the use of green or healthy standards, the building of affordable housing, or rebuilding on land that is not disaster-prone. In Cedar Rapids, Iowa, for example, the city used a combination of incentives and disincentives for rebuilding after a flood. The city purchased approximately 1,400 properties that were in flood-prone areas or had been severely damaged, which helped homeowners move on financially. CDBG-DR funds were used to create mixed-income housing, and state and local tax credits were offered to developers for building in a downtown core area, which improved the availability of dense, multifamily, affordable housing in mixed-use neighborhoods. The city council distributed public funding for rebuilding only in areas that were not in the 100-year flood plain or in the path of the city's new flood control system. Moreover, a city program designed to "fill in" vacant properties provides free lots to builders when they agree to use build affordable homes using green standards, among other requirements (Cedar Rapids, 2014a,b). Other methods can include

- expedited building permits or reduced fees for homeowners that include mitigation and sustainability measures in their repairs;
- expedited permitting for rebuilding in an area that has been designated as a priority for redevelopment (Hillsborough County Government, 2010); and
- using green or healthy building standards as additional "points" in a competitive bidding program for developers seeking to build.

One consideration, however, is that there must be a need for the type of housing that is incentivized; otherwise, there will be an imbalance in housing stock supply and demand. In Hancock County, Mississippi, for example, the supply of multifamily rental units was increased because of post-hurricane incentives; however, there is little demand for this type of housing in the community (Hillsborough County Government, 2010).

Federal requirements tied to grants are also important drivers of forward-looking approaches to redevelopment and consideration of vulnerable populations. Communities using CDBG-DR funds after a disaster, for example, are required by HUD to use at least 50 percent of the funds to benefit low- or moderate-income people (HUD, 2014b), and post-Sandy rebuilding using CDBG was required to conform to green building standards (see Box 10-4).

RESEARCH NEEDS

Although there is a fair amount of evidence on the link between health and housing, more research is needed in the post-disaster context, particularly to produce

- evidence of improved outcomes resulting from a collaborative approach to housing recovery that integrates design, social/behavioral, and health perspectives;
- temporary housing strategies that improve social connectedness and associated impacts on health;
- evidence of the link between health outcomes and post-disaster housing reconstruction that complies with green healthy housing building standards; and
- knowledge of the key barriers to adoption of green building standards for post-disaster housing reconstruction.

SUMMARY OF FINDINGS AND RECOMMENDATION

Housing meets some of people's most basic needs (shelter from the elements, privacy, a place of respite and socialization), and healthy, affordable housing is fundamental to healthy communities. After a disaster, providing housing rapidly and appropriately is essential to health and well-being. However, it is also critical to ensure that the urgency of post-disaster housing reconstruction does not result in practices that compromise health and preclude opportunities to promote long-term the affordability, resiliency, and sustainability of housing. Experience with past disasters has shown that the ways in which housing can either support or compromise health during and after recovery often are not adequately understood, resulting in unintended health impacts. Adoption of housing standards that are known to support and promote health, such as those for green and healthy housing, provides a mechanism for ensuring that health considerations are integrated into housing recovery efforts.

Recommendation 12: *Ensure Healthy and Affordable Post-Disaster Housing.*

To reduce housing-related health risks, federal, state, and local governmental housing agencies should require that new residential construction and substantial rehabilitation of existing residences financed with public funds after disasters comply fully with Enterprise Green Communities standards or their equivalent and with the minimum requirements set forth in the National Healthy Housing Standard. Federal and state funding agencies should tie these requirements to recovery funds, and private funders should consider incentivizing compliance with these standards. Additionally, multiple affordable housing options should be considered during redevelopment to ensure that people of all income levels can remain in the community.

HOUSING SECTOR RECOVERY CHECKLIST

The committee has identified three pre-event and seven post-disaster critical recovery priorities for the housing sector that are inextricably linked to strengthening the health, resilience, and sustainability of a community. Action steps for each of these priorities are provided in the following checklist. Although housing sector leaders will need to adapt these actions to the local context, this guidance provides an indicative set of concerns to be considered during recovery. The checklist illustrates how the following five key recovery strategies, identified as recurring themes at the beginning of this chapter, apply to individual priority areas:

- Protect survivors and recovery workers from health hazards associated with unhealthy or unsafe housing.
- Preserve and promote social connectedness in plans for immediate response, short-term housing, and long-term rebuilding.
- Consider needs for access to health and social services during all phases of housing recovery.
- Incentivize the use of healthy and/or green criteria for the rebuilding of homes, buildings, and neighborhoods.
- Engage community members, including representatives of and advocates for vulnerable populations, in the development of post-disaster housing plans to ensure that the needs of all community members are met.

Pre-Event

Priority: Establish a Disaster Housing Task Force and Integrate It into Community Recovery Organizational Structures under the National Disaster Recovery Framework (NDRF)

Primary Actors[1]: Housing Agencies
Key Partners: State/Local Health Departments,[2] Social Services Agencies, Emergency Management Agencies, Environmental Health Agencies, Health and Medical System Partners (including Nursing Homes and Other Long-Term Care Institutions), Community Development Organizations, Public Works and Utilities, Disaster Relief Organizations (including the American Red Cross and Long-Term Recovery Committees), Federal Agencies (including the U.S. Department of Housing and Urban Development [HUD] and Federal Emergency Management Agency [FEMA]), Private Sector (including Housing Finance Entities and Developers)

Key Recovery Strategy:
- Engage community members, including representatives of and advocates for vulnerable populations, in the development of post-disaster housing plans to ensure that the needs of all community members are met.

Activities include but are not limited to:
- ☐ Bring together a wide variety of governmental and nongovernmental organizations under the umbrella of a disaster housing task force to establish plans and identify resources for recovery.
- ☐ Ensure that key health and social services organizations are represented on the disaster housing task force.

- -

Priority: Conduct Vulnerability and Capacity Assessments, Including an Inventory of Existing Plans and Housing Stock

Primary Actor: Disaster Housing Task Force
Key Partners: Housing Agencies, Urban and Regional Planning Agencies, Community Development Organizations, Emergency Management Agencies, State/Local Health Departments, Social Services Agencies, Private Sector (including Housing Manufacturers, Providers, and Developers)

Key Recovery Strategy:
- Engage community members, including representatives of and advocates for vulnerable populations, in the development of post-disaster housing plans to ensure that the needs of all community members are met.

---

[1] See Appendix F for further description of terms used to describe Primary Actors and Key Partners in this checklist.
[2] Throughout this checklist, "State/Local" is used for the purposes of brevity but should be inferred to include tribal and territorial as well.

Pre-Event

Activities include but are not limited to:
- ☐ Assess the current housing stock, including vacancy rates and the suitability of vacant properties for post-disaster housing.
- ☐ Assess the vulnerabilities of the local housing stock according to the risks that the community faces.
- ☐ Consider current community health and social welfare problems during the identification of priority redevelopment areas (e.g., locations already suffering from blight and associated with significant health disparities).
- ☐ Assess institutional capacity for housing recovery: What organizations exist, what are their roles and expertise, and how can they collaborate during recovery?
- ☐ Identify manufactured housing vendors and determine which are capable of providing temporary housing units. Establish preliminary but flexible relationships with vendors.
- ☐ Inventory the local plans, programs, or procedures that are relevant to housing during long-term recovery to identify opportunities to leverage existing programs, including those already serving vulnerable populations.

- -

Priority: Plan for Siting of Temporary Housing

Primary Actor: Disaster Housing Task Force
Key Partners: Urban and Regional Planning Agencies, Community Development Organizations, State/Local Health Departments, Transportation Agencies, Social Services Agencies, Public Works and Utilities, Private Sector, Federal Agencies (including FEMA), Community Members

Key Recovery Strategies:
- Protect survivors and recovery workers from health hazards associated with unhealthy or unsafe housing.
- Preserve and promote social connectedness in plans for immediate response, short-term housing, and long-term rebuilding.
- Consider needs for access to health and social services during all phases of housing recovery.
- Engage community members, including representatives of and advocates for vulnerable populations, in the development of post-disaster housing plans to ensure that the needs of all community members are met.

Activities include but are not limited to:
- ☐ Identify potential sites for temporary housing and develop criteria for housing sites to be applied after a disaster.
- ☐ Ensure that sites are free of health hazards and not subject to further damage or disaster-related risks.
- ☐ If possible, locate temporary housing sites near essential community services and public transportation to facilitate access to goods, services, and employment.
- ☐ For long-term temporary housing, consider a site that could be converted to permanent housing units, thus capitalizing on necessary investments in infrastructure.
- ☐ Collaborate with the community and urban and regional planning agencies to identify appropriate locations.

Short-Term Recovery

Priority: Assess Housing Needs

Primary Actor: Disaster Housing Task Force
Key Partners: Federal Agencies (including HUD and FEMA)

Key Recovery Strategies:
- Protect survivors and recovery workers from health hazards associated with unhealthy or unsafe housing.
- Consider needs for access to health and social services during all phases of housing recovery.
- Engage community members, including representatives of and advocates for vulnerable populations, in the development of post-disaster housing plans to ensure that the needs of all community members are met.

Activities include but are not limited to:
- ☐ Quantify available housing stock in and near the community, including HUD-assisted and HUD-owned housing.
- ☐ Assess the extent of damage to the housing stock and its suitability (health/safety) for temporary housing.
- ☐ Determine the need for temporary housing and whether the existing housing stock can fulfill that need.

- -

Priority: Prevent Unnecessary Displacement

Primary Actor: Disaster Housing Task Force
Key Partners: Private Sector (including Mortgage Servicers), Federal Agencies (including HUD's Federal Housing Administration [FHA], and FEMA)

Key Recovery Strategies:
- Protect survivors and recovery workers from health hazards associated with unhealthy or unsafe housing.
- Preserve and promote social connectedness in plans for immediate response, short-term housing, and long-term rebuilding.
- Consider needs for access to health and social services during all phases of housing recovery.
- Engage community members, including representatives of and advocates for vulnerable populations, in the development of post-disaster housing plans to ensure that the needs of all community members are met.

Activities include but are not limited to:
- ☐ Consider implementing a "rapid repair" program for housing requiring relatively simple repairs so people can remain in their homes.

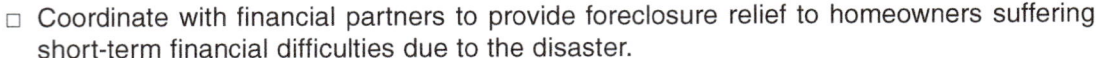

Short-Term Recovery

☐ Coordinate with financial partners to provide foreclosure relief to homeowners suffering short-term financial difficulties due to the disaster.
☐ Provide assistance to homeowners, particularly the most vulnerable, who lack adequate insurance or means of repairing their own homes.

- -

Priority: Protect Homeowners and Recovery Workers Against Health Risks

Primary Actors: State/Local Health Departments
Key Partners: Housing Agencies, Environmental Health Agencies, Health and Medical System Partners, Federal Agencies (including the National Institute of Environmental Health Sciences [NIEHS])

Key Recovery Strategy:
- Protect survivors and recovery workers from health hazards associated with unhealthy or unsafe housing.

Activities include but are not limited to:
☐ Train recovery and repair workers and volunteers in identifying hazards (e.g., mold, asbestos), protecting themselves, and mitigating the hazards.
☐ Provide information to homeowners, occupants, volunteers, and contractors regarding hazard identification, protective measures, and mitigation (e.g., by disseminating pamphlets at disaster recovery centers and home repair retail stores).
☐ Provide personal protective equipment (e.g., respirators, goggles, clothing) as needed.

- -

Priority: Provide Short- and Long-Term Temporary Housing That Meets Health and Human Service Needs

Primary Actors: Housing Agencies, Federal Agencies (including FEMA and HUD)
Key Partners: Private Sector (including Land and Housing Owners), State/Local Health Departments, Social Services Agencies, Transportation Agencies

Key Recovery Strategies:
- Protect survivors and recovery workers from health hazards associated with unhealthy or unsafe housing.
- Preserve and promote social connectedness in plans for immediate response, short-term housing, and long-term rebuilding.
- Consider needs for access to health and social services during all phases of housing recovery.
- Engage community members, including representatives of and advocates for vulnerable

Short-Term Recovery

populations, in the development of post-disaster housing plans to ensure that the needs of all community members are met.

Activities include but are not limited to:
- Provide housing by leveraging existing buildings and/or purchasing temporary housing units.
- Utilize FEMA's Rental Repair Program to repair rental housing and make it available to disaster victims.
- Make sure new or repaired units comply with the National Healthy Housing Standard and applicable housing codes.
- Conduct advance planning to ensure adequate personnel and training for special-needs and medical shelters and appropriate temporary housing for special-needs populations.
- Ensure that shelters and temporary housing are compliant with the Americans with Disabilities Act.
- Consider placing housing units on homeowners' property to minimize disruption and maintain neighborhood cohesion, social connectedness, and access to services.
- If housing units are placed on group sites,
    - arrange the site in a configuration that encourages social connectedness; and
    - if possible, locate the site near or with "wraparound" services such as health care, schools, daycare, social services, public transportation, and employment counseling.

Intermediate- to Long-Term Recovery

Priority: Incentivize the Use of Green and Healthy Housing Standards

Primary Actors: Elected Officials and Community Leaders, Federal Agencies (including HUD)
Key Partners: Housing Agencies, Urban and Regional Planning Agencies, Community Development Organizations, State/Local Health Departments, Environmental Health Agencies, Private Sector (including Developers)

Key Recovery Strategies:
- Protect survivors and recovery workers from health hazards associated with unhealthy or unsafe housing.
- Consider needs for access to health and social services during all phases of housing recovery.
- Incentivize the use of healthy and/or green criteria for the rebuilding of homes, buildings, and neighborhoods.

Activities include but are not limited to:
- ☐ Ensure that long-term housing is built in compliance with current housing codes (even if compliance was waived during short-term recovery).
- ☐ Use permitting processes strategically to ensure that houses are rebuilt in concert with the availability of necessary services and infrastructure.
- ☐ Give expedited permitting or financial incentives (e.g., tax credits) to builders using healthy and green housing standards.
- ☐ If the local government is allocating funding for the building or repair of properties, require the use of healthy housing and green standards.

- -

Priority: Strengthen the Resiliency of Housing

Primary Actors: Elected Officials and Community Leaders, Housing Agencies
Key Partners: Federal Agencies (including HUD), Environmental Health Agencies, Emergency Management Agencies, Urban and Regional Planning Agencies, Community Development Organizations

Key Recovery Strategies:
- Protect survivors and recovery workers from health hazards associated with unhealthy or unsafe housing.
- Preserve and promote social connectedness in plans for immediate response, short-term housing, and long-term rebuilding.
- Consider needs for access to health and social services during all phases of housing recovery.
- Incentivize the use of healthy and/or green criteria for the rebuilding of homes, buildings, and neighborhoods.
- Engage community members, including representatives of and advocates for vulnerable populations, in the development of post-disaster housing plans to ensure that the needs of all community members are met.

Intermediate- to Long-Term Recovery

Activities include but are not limited to:
- □ Rebuild homes, neighborhoods, and communities using principles of resiliency:
  - – Neighborhoods are compact, walkable, and mixed-use.
  - – All members of the community participate in planning and decisions with an eye toward making the community more equitable.
  - – Connections and partnerships in the community are preserved and strengthened.
  - – Housing is efficient and durable.
  - – Preparedness and recovery plans are continually reassessed.
- □ Consider disaster-resistant building strategies, such as installing elevated mechanical systems and locating living space above the ground floor.
- □ Consider opportunities to mitigate against future disaster damage by buying out disaster-prone properties and converting them to green or community space.
- □ Give financial incentives to builders or homeowners that incorporate mitigation in their repairs or rebuilding.

- -

Priority: Ensure Adequate Affordable Healthy Housing

Primary Actors: Elected Officials and Community Leaders, Housing Agencies
Key Partners: Community- and Faith-Based Organizations, Federal Agencies (including HUD), Community Development Organizations, Private Sector (including Developers)

Key Recovery Strategy:
- Engage community members, including representatives of and advocates for vulnerable populations, in the development of post-disaster housing plans to ensure that the needs of all community members are met.

Activities include but are not limited to:
- □ Use federally assisted housing programs, such as Housing Choice Vouchers and others, to help low-income residents afford housing that is regulated for health and safety.
- □ Use financial incentives or expedited permitting to encourage the building of affordable housing or mixed-income neighborhoods.

REFERENCES

ADA (Americans with Disabilities Act). 2007. The ADA and emergency shelters: Access for all in emergencies and disasters. In *ADA best practices tool kit for state and local governments*, Ch.7, addendum 2. Washington, DC: ADA.

AlJazeera America. 2013. Eight years after Hurricane Katrina, many evacuees yet to return. *AlJazeera America*, http://america.aljazeera.com/articles/2013/8/29/eight-years-afterkatrinalowincomeevacueeshaveyettoreturn.html (accessed December 4, 2014).

APA (American Planning Association). 1998. *Planning for post-disaster recovery and reconstruction*. PAS Report No. 484/484. Chicago, IL: APA.

APHA (American Public Health Association), and NCHH (National Center for Healthy Housing). 2014. *National healthy housing standard*. http://www.nchh.org/Portals/0/Contents/NHHS_Full_Doc.pdf (accessed October 31, 2014).

ARC (American Red Cross). 1998. *Building community partnerships in disaster recovery: The rental housing replacement revolving fund final report*. Washington, DC: ARC.

Association of Bay Area Governments. 2014. *Housing and community risk key issue statements*. http://resilience.abag.ca.gov/wp-content/documents/housing/8.26.14%20Handouts.pdf (accessed October 31, 2014).

Brandywine Center. 2009. *About the Brandywine Center*. http://www.brandywinecenter.org/about.html (accessed December 4, 2014).

Burstrom, B., and P. Fredlund. 2001. Self rated health: Is it as good a predictor of subsequent mortality among adults in lower as well as in higher social classes? *Journal of Epidemiology and Community Health* 55(11):836-840.

CA Department of Conservation. 2013. *Facts about the Loma Prieta earthquake*. http://www.conservation.ca.gov/cgs/News/Pages/loma_prieta.aspx (accessed December 4, 2014).

CDC (Centers for Disease Control and Prevention). 2010. *Final report on formaldehyde levels in FEMA-supplied travel trailers, park models, and mobile homes*. Atlanta, GA: CDC.

CDC. 2014. *Falls among older adults: An overview*. http://www.cdc.gov/homeandrecreationalsafety/falls/adultfalls.html (accessed December 4, 2014).

Cedar Rapids. 2014a. *Single family new construction program 4th round: Mandatory and optional green building guidelines*. Cedar Rapids, IA: Cedar Rapids.

Cedar Rapids. 2014b. *Roots properties*. http://www.cedar-rapids.org/government/departments/community-development/housing/ROOTs/Pages/Properties.aspx (accessed December 4, 2014).

Chew, G. L., J. Wilson, F. A. Rabito, F. Grimsley, S. Iqbal, T. Reponen, M. L. Muilenberg, P. S. Thorne, D. G. Dearborn, and R. L. Morley. 2006. Mold and endotoxin levels in the aftermath of Hurricane Katrina: A pilot project of homes in New Orleans undergoing renovation. *Environmental Health Perspectives* 114(12):1883-1889.

Crocker, D. D., S. Kinyota, G. G. Dumitru, C. B. Ligon, E. J. Herman, J. M. Ferdinands, D. P. Hopkins, B. M. Lawrence, and T. A. Sipe. 2011. Effectiveness of home-based, multi-trigger, multicomponent interventions with an environmental focus for reducing asthma morbidity: A community guide systematic review. *American Journal of Preventive Medicine* 41(2, Suppl. 1):S5-S32.

Diez-Roux, A. V., F. J. Nieto, C. Muntaner, H. A. Tyroler, G. W. Comstock, E. Shahar, L. S. Cooper, R. L. Watson, and M. Szklo. 1997. Neighborhood environments and coronary heart disease: A multilevel analysis. *American Journal of Epidemiology* 146(1):48-63.

DiGuiseppi, C., D. E. Jacobs, K. J. Phelan, A. D. Mickalide, and D. Ormandy. 2010. Housing interventions and control of injury-related structural deficiencies: A review of the evidence. *Journal of Public Health Management and Practice* 16(5 Suppl.):S34-S43.

Duvall, D., and A. Booth. 1978. The housing environment and women's health. *Journal of Health and Social Behavior* 19(4):410-417.

Ellen, I. G., and M. A. Turner. 2003. Do neighborhoods matter and why? In *Choosing a better life? Evaluating the moving to opportunity social experiment*, edited by J. Goering and J. D. Feins. Washington, DC: The Urban Institute Press. Pp. 313-338.

Ellen, I. G., T. Mijanovich, and K.-N. Dillman. 2001. Neighborhood effects on health: Exploring the links and assessing the evidence. *Journal of Urban Affairs* 23(3-4):391-408.

Elton, P. J., and J. M. Packer. 1986. A prospective randomised trial of the value of rehousing on the grounds of mental ill-health. *Journal of Chronic Diseases* 39(3):221-227.

Enterprise. 2011. *Enterprise green communities criteria checklist*. http://www.enterprisecommunity.com/servlet/servlet.FileDownload?file=00P30000008rMSlEAM (accessed December 4, 2014).

EPA (U.S. Environmental Protection Agency). 2010. *A brief guide to mold, moisture, and your home.* www.epa.gov/mold/moldguide.html (accessed December 4, 2014).

EPA. 2012. *A citizen's guide to radon: The guide to protecting yourself and your family from radon.* http://www.epa.gov/radon/pubs/citguide.html (accessed December 4, 2014).

EPA. 2014. *Green building: Basic information.* http://www.epa.gov/greenbuilding/pubs/about.htm (accessed December 4, 2014).

Evans, G. W., N. M. Wells, H.-Y. E. Chan, and H. Saltzman. 2000. Housing quality and mental health. *Journal of Consulting and Clinical Psychology* 68(3):526-530.

Evans, G. W., N. M. Wells, and A. Moch. 2003. Housing and mental health: A review of the evidence and a methodological and conceptual critique. *Journal of Social Issues* 59(3):475-500.

FEMA (Federal Emergency Management Agency). 2009a. *National disaster housing strategy.* Washington, DC: FEMA.

FEMA. 2009b. *National disaster housing strategy: Annexes.* Washington, DC: FEMA.

FEMA. 2013a. *Hazard mitigation assistance unified guidance.* Washington, DC: FEMA.

FEMA. 2013b. *Recovery policy: Multi-family lease and repair program—direct temporary housing assistance.* http://www.fema.gov/media-library-data/1384452357718-95f11f1ef06e063e305edd22bee70964/MLRP%20Policy.pdf (accessed February 12, 2015).

FEMA. 2014. *Multi-hazard mitigation planning.* https://www.fema.gov/multi-hazard-mitigation-planning (accessed November 25, 2014).

FEMA. 2015. *Interim housing resources.* https://www.fema.gov/interim-housing-resources (accessed March 9, 2015).

Florida Department of Community Affairs. 2010. *Post-disaster redevelopment planning: A guide for Florida communities.* http://www.floridadisaster.org/recovery/documents/Post%20Disaster%20Redevelopment%20Planning%20Guidebook%20Lo.pdf (accessed October 21, 2014).

Frank, D. A., N. B. Neault, A. Skalicky, J. T. Cook, J. D. Wilson, S. Levenson, A. F. Meyers, T. Heeren, D. B. Cutts, P. H. Casey, M. M. Black, and C. Berkowitz. 2006. Heat or eat: The low income home energy assistance program and nutritional and health risks among children less than 3 years of age. *Pediatrics* 118(5):e1293-e1302.

Freedy, J. R., and W. M. Simpson. 2007. Disaster-related physical and mental health: A role for the family physician. *American Family Physician* 75(6):841-846.

Furman Center. 2013. *Sandy's effects on housing in New York City.* New York: Furman Center, Moelis Institute.

Geaghan, K. A. 2011. *Forced to move: An analysis of Hurricane Katrina movers.* Washington, DC: U.S. Census Bureau.

Gifford, R., and C. Lacombe. 2006. Housing quality and children's socioemotional health. *Journal of Housing and the Built Environment* 21(2):177-189.

Gilmore, D. R., and D. M. Standaert. 2013. Introduction and table of contents. In *Building community resilience post-disaster: A guide for affordable housing and community economic development practitioners*, edited by D. R. Gilmore and D. M. Standaert. Chicago, IL: American Bar Association.

Halford, C., T. Wallman, L. Welin, A. Rosengren, A. Bardel, S. Johansson, H. Eriksson, E. Palmer, L. Wilhelmsen, and K. Svardsudd. 2012. Effects of self-rated health on sick leave, disability pension, hospital admissions and mortality. A population-based longitudinal study of nearly 15,000 observations among Swedish women and men. *BMC Public Health* 12:1103.

Halpern, D. 1995. *Mental health and the built environment.* London: Taylor & Francis.

HHS (U.S. Department of Health and Human Services). 2009. *The surgeon general's call to action to promote healthy homes.* Rockville, MD: HHS, Office of the Surgeon General.

HHS. 2012. *Gaps continue to exist in nursing home emergency preparedness and response during disasters: 2007-2010.* Washington, DC: HHS.

HHS and HUD (U.S. Department of Housing and Urban Development). 2006. *Healthy housing reference manual.* Washington, DC: HHS and HUD.

Hillsborough County Government. 2010. *Post-disaster redevelopment plan* http://www.hillsboroughcounty.org/index.aspx?nid=1795 (accessed November 3, 2014).

Howden-Chapman, P., A. Matheson, J. Crane, H. Viggers, M. Cunningham, T. Blakely, C. Cunningham, A. Woodward, K. Saville-Smith, D. O'Dea, M. Kennedy, M. Baker, N. Waipara, R. Chapman, and G. Davie. 2007. Effect of insulating existing houses on health inequality: Cluster randomised study in the community. *British Medical Journal* 334(7591):460.

HUD. 1994. *4330.1 rev-5: Chapter 8. HUD-approved relief provisions.* http://portal.hud.gov/hudportal/documents/huddoc?id=43301c8HSGH.pdf (accessed December 4, 2014).

HUD. 2000. *Mortgagee letter 00-05: Loss mitigation program-comprehensive clarification of policy and notice of procedural changes*. Washington, DC: HUD.

HUD. 2002. *Mortgagee letter 2002-17: Special forbearance: Program changes and updates*. Washington, DC: HUD.

HUD. 2007. *2007 metropolitan disaster planning: Analytical support of the American Housing Survey*. Washington, DC: HUD.

HUD. 2009a. *Housing habitability standards inspection checklist*. http://portal.hud.gov/hudportal/documents/huddoc?id=dhapsandyhabitchklist.pdf (accessed December 4, 2014).

HUD. 2009b. *HUD to assist homeowners facing problem drywall: Temporary relief available to make home repairs affordable for at-risk borrowers*. http://portal.hud.gov/hudportal/HUD?src=/press/press_releases_media_advisories/2009/HUDNo.09-237 (accessed December 4, 2014).

HUD. 2013. *Second allocation, waivers, and alternative requirements for grantees receiving Community Development Block Grant (CDBG) Disaster Recovery funds in response to Hurricane Sandy*. https://www.hudexchange.info/resource/3301/second-notice-cdbg-dr-funds-hurricane-sandy (accessed December 4, 2014).

HUD. 2014a. *Administration of insured home mortgages (4330.1)*. http://portal.hud.gov/hudportal/HUD?src=/program_offices/administration/hudclips/handbooks/hsgh/4330.1 (accessed December 4, 2014).

HUD. 2014b. *CDBG-DR eligibility requirements*. https://www.hudexchange.info/cdbg-dr/cdbg-dr-eligibility-requirements (accessed December 4, 2014).

HUD. 2014c. *Disaster Housing Assistance Program—Sandy (DHAP-Sandy)*. http://portal.hud.gov/hudportal/HUD?src=/program_offices/public_indian_housing/programs/ph/sandy (accessed December 4, 2014).

HUD. 2014d. *Disaster recovery*. http://portal.hud.gov/hudportal/HUD?src=/program_offices/healthy_homes/disaster recovery (accessed December 4, 2014).

HUD. 2014e. *HUD disaster resources*. http://portal.hud.gov/hudportal/HUD?src=/info/disasterresources (accessed December 4, 2014).

Hurricane Sandy Rebuilding Task Force. 2013. *Hurricane strategy rebuilding strategy: Stronger communities, a resilient region*. Washington, DC: HUD.

Idler, E. L., L. B. Russell, and D. Davis. 2000. Survival, functional limitations, and self-rated health in the NHANES I Epidemiologic Follow-up Study, 1992. First National Health and Nutrition Examination Survey. *American Journal of Epidemiology* 152(9):874-883.

Insurance Institute for Business & Home Safety. 2012. *Fortified home: Hurricane standards*. Tampa, FL: Insurance Institute for Business & Home Safety.

IOM (Institute of Medicine). 2004. *Damp indoor spaces and health*. Washington, DC: The National Academies Press.

Jacobs, D. E. 1995. Lead-based paint as a major source of childhood lead poisoning: A review of the evidence. In *Lead in paint, soil and dust: Health risks, exposure studies, control measures and quality assurance*, edited by M. E. Beard and S. D. Allen Iske. Philadelphia, PA: American Society for Testing and Materials. Pp. 175-187.

Jacobs, D. E. 2011. Environmental health disparities in housing. *American Journal of Public Health* 101(Suppl. 1):S115-S122.

Jacobs, D. E., R. P. Clickner, J. Y. Zhou, S. M. Viet, D. A. Marker, J. W. Rogers, D. C. Zeldin, P. Broene, and W. Friedman. 2002. The prevalence of lead-based paint hazards in U.S. housing. *Environmental Health Perspectives* 110(10):A599-A606.

Jacobs, D. E., M. J. Brown, A. Baeder, M. S. Sucosky, S. Margolis, J. Hershovitz, L. Kolb, and R. L. Morley. 2010. A systematic review of housing interventions and health: Introduction, methods, and summary findings. *Journal of Public Health Management and Practice* 16(5 Suppl.):S5-S10.

Jacobs, D. E., E. Ahonen, S. L. Dixon, S. Dorevitch, J. Breysse, J. Smith, A. Evens, D. Dobrez, M. Isaacson, C. Murphy, L. Conroy, and P. Levavi. 2014a. Moving into green healthy housing. *Journal of Public Health Management and Practice* 21(4):345-354.

Jacobs, D. E., J. Breysse, S. L. Dixon, S. Aceti, C. Kawecki, M. James, and J. Wilson. 2014b. Health and housing outcomes from green renovation of low-income housing in Washington, DC. *Journal of Environmental Health* 76(7):8-16; quiz 60.

Kawachi, I., and L. F. Berkman, editors. 2003. *Neighborhoods and health*. New York: Oxford University Press.

Kessler, R. C., G. J. Duncan, L. A. Gennetian, L. F. Katz, J. R. Kling, N. A. Sampson, L. Sanbonmatsu, A. M. Zaslavsky, and J. Ludwig. 2014. Associations of housing mobility interventions for children in high-poverty neighborhoods with subsequent mental disorders during adolescence. *Journal of the American Medical Association* 311(9):937-948.

Krieger, J. 2010. Home is where the triggers are: Increasing asthma control by improving the home environment. *Pediatric Allergy, Immunology, and Pulmonology* 23(2):139-145.

Krieger, J., and D. L. Higgins. 2002. Housing and health: Time again for public health action. *American Journal of Public Health* 92(5):758-768.

Krieger, J., D. E. Jacobs, P. J. Ashley, A. Baeder, G. L. Chew, D. Dearborn, H. P. Hynes, J. D. Miller, R. Morley, F. Rabito, and D. C. Zeldin. 2010. Housing interventions and control of asthma-related indoor biologic agents: A review of the evidence. *Journal of Public Health Management and Practice* 16(5 Suppl.):S11-S20.

Krokstad, S., R. Johnsen, and S. Westin. 2002. Social determinants of disability pension: A 10-year follow-up of 62,000 people in a Norwegian county population. *International Journal of Epidemiology* 31(6):1183-1191.

Landrigan, P. J. 1998. Asbestos—still a carcinogen. *New England Journal of Medicine* 338(22):1618-1619.

Leech, J. A., M. Raizenne, and J. Gusdorf. 2004. Health in occupants of energy efficient new homes. *Indoor Air* 14(3):169-173.

Levy, D. K., Z. McDade, and K. Dumlao. 2010. *Effects from living in mixed-income communities for low-income families: A review of the literature*. Washington, DC: The Urban Institute.

Lew, H. S. 1990. *Performance of structures during the Loma Prieta earthquake of October 17, 1989*. Vol. 778. Washington, DC: U.S. Department of Commerce, National Institute of Standards and Technology.

Li, C. L., H. Y. Chang, H. H. Wang, and Y. B. Bai. 2011. Diabetes, functional ability, and self-rated health independently predict hospital admission within one year among older adults: A population based cohort study. *Archives of Gerontology and Geriatrics* 52(2):147-152.

Lindberg, R. A., E. D. Shenassa, D. Acevedo-Garcia, S. J. Popkin, A. Villaveces, and R. L. Morley. 2010. Housing interventions at the neighborhood level and health: A review of the evidence. *Journal of Public Health Management and Practice* 16(5 Suppl.):S44-S52.

Lonigan, C. J., M. P. Shannon, C. M. Taylor, A. J. Finch, Jr., and F. R. Sallee. 1994. Children exposed to disaster: II. Risk factors for the development of post-traumatic symptomatology. *Journal of the American Academy of Child and Adolescent Psychiatry* 33(1):94-105.

Lowry, S. 1991. Housing and health. *British Medical Journal*. London.

Lubin, J. H., and J. D. Boice, Jr. 1997. Lung cancer risk from residential radon: Meta-analysis of eight epidemiologic studies. *Journal of the National Cancer Institute* 89(1):49-57.

Macintyre, S., and A. Ellaway. 2000. Ecological approaches: Rediscovering the role of the physical and social environment. In *Social epidemiology*, edited by L. F. Berkman and I. Kawachi. New York: Oxford University Press.

Macintyre, S., and A. Ellaway. 2003. Neighborhoods and health: An overview. In *Neighborhoods and health*, edited by I. Kawachi and L. F. Berkman. New York: Oxford University Press. Pp. 20-42.

Macintyre, S., A. Ellaway, and S. Cummins. 2002. Place effects on health: How can we conceptualise, operationalise and measure them? *Social Science & Medicine* 55(1):125-139.

Mansson, N. O., and L. Rastam. 2001. Self-rated health as a predictor of disability pension and death—a prospective study of middle-aged men. *Scandinavian Journal of Public Health* 29(2):151-158.

Marin County Sheriff. 2003. *Post-disaster housing annex: Marin operational area emergency operations plan*. http://marinsheriff.org/uploads/documents/Post-Disaster%20Housing%20Annex.pdf (accessed October 31, 2014).

Marmot, M., A. Feeney, M. Shipley, F. North, and S. L. Syme. 1995. Sickness absence as a measure of health status and functioning: From the UK Whitehall II Study. *Journal of Epidemiology and Community Health* 49(2):124-130.

McIntosh, J. 2013. The implications of post disaster recovery for affordable housing. In *Approaches to disaster management—examining the implications of hazards, emergencies and disasters*, edited by J. Tiefenbacher. Rijeka, Croatia: InTech. Pp. 205-217.

Meeds, D. 2013. *Joplin pays it forward*. http://joplincc.com/Joplin%20Pays%20It%20Forward%20-%20Community%20Leaders%20Share%20Our%20Recovery%20Lessons.pdf (accessed February 26, 2015).

Meyers, A., D. Cutts, D. A. Frank, S. Levenson, A. Skalicky, T. Heeren, J. Cook, C. Berkowitz, M. Black, P. Casey, and N. Zaldivar. 2005. Subsidized housing and children's nutritional status: Data from a multisite surveillance study. *Archives of Pediatrics and Adolescent Medicine* 159(6):551-556.

Miilunpalo, S., I. Vuori, P. Oja, M. Pasanen, and H. Urponen. 1997. Self-rated health status as a health measure: The predictive value of self-reported health status on the use of physician services and on mortality in the working-age population. *Journal of Clinical Epidemiology* 50(5):517-528.

Morgan, W. J., E. F. Crain, R. S. Gruchalla, G. T. O'Connor, M. Kattan, R. Evans, III, J. Stout, G. Malindzak, E. Smartt, M. Plaut, M. Walter, B. Vaughn, and H. Mitchell. 2004. Results of a home-based environmental intervention among urban children with asthma. *New England Journal of Medicine* 351(11):1068-1080.

Murphy, M. W., J. F. Lando, S. M. Kieszak, M. E. Sutter, G. P. Noonan, J. M. Brunkard, and M. A. McGeehin. 2013. Formaldehyde levels in FEMA-supplied travel trailers, park models, and mobile homes in Louisiana and Mississippi. *Indoor Air* 23(2):134-141.

Nagaraja, J., J. Menkedick, K. J. Phelan, P. Ashley, X. Zhang, and B. P. Lanphear. 2005. Deaths from residential injuries in US children and adolescents, 1985-1997. *Pediatrics* 116(2):454-461.

National Center for Healthy Housing. 2008. *Creating a healthy home: A field guide for clean-up of flooded homes.* Columbia, MD: Enterprise Community Partners, National Center for Healthy Housing.

National Coalition for the Homeless. 2009. *Mental illness and homelessness.* http://www.nationalhomeless.org/factsheets/Mental_Illness.pdf (accessed March 10, 2015).

National Coalition for the Homeless. 2014. *Integrating homeless service providers and clients in disaster preparedness, response, and recovery.* http://www.nhchc.org/wp-content/uploads/2014/09/disasterbrief092014.pdf (accessed March 10, 2015).

New York State Governor. 2013. *Governor Cuomo announces federal reimbursement to New York City for Superstorm Sandy costs.* http://www.governor.ny.gov/news/governor-cuomo-announces-federal-reimbursement-new-york-city-superstorm-sandy-costs (accessed December 4, 2014).

NIEHS (National Institute of Environmental Health Sciences). 2013. *NIEHS Hurricane Sandy response report.* Washington, DC. NIEHS. http://tools.niehs.nih.gov/wetp/public/hasl_get_blob.cfm?ID=9939#sthash.GPOGbMG4.dpuf (accessed March 26, 2015).

Nolen, A. 2014. *A Health in All Policies approach to disaster recovery: Lessons from Galveston.* Paper presented at IOM Committee on Post-Disaster Recovery of a Community's Public Health, Medical, and Social Services: Meeting Four, June 13, Washington, DC.

NTP (National Toxicology Program). 2012. *NTP monograph: Health effects of low-level lead.* Research Triangle Park, NC: HHS.

NYC (New York City). 2013. *Mayor Bloomberg announces first-of-its-kind NYC rapid repairs program completes work on more than 20,000 homes damaged by Hurricane Sandy.* http://www1.nyc.gov/office-of-the-mayor/news/109-13/mayor-bloomberg-first-of-its-kind-nyc-rapid-repairs-program-completes-work-more-than (accessed December 4, 2014).

Orr, L., J. D. Feins, R. Jacob, and E. Beecroft. 2003. *Moving to opportunity interim impacts evaluation. Final report.* Washington, DC: HUD, Office of Policy Development and Research.

Osofsky, H. J., J. D. Osofsky, M. Kronenberg, A. Brennan, and T. C. Hansel. 2009. Posttraumatic stress symptoms in children after Hurricane Katrina: Predicting the need for mental health services. *American Journal of Orthopsychiatry* 79(2):212-220.

Pickett, K. E., and M. Pearl. 2001. Multilevel analyses of neighbourhood socioeconomic context and health outcomes: A critical review. *Journal of Epidemiology and Community Health* 55(2):111-122.

Pietilainen, O., M. Laaksonen, O. Rahkonen, and E. Lahelma. 2011. Self-rated health as a predictor of disability retirement—the contribution of ill-health and working conditions. *PLoS ONE* 6(9):e25004.

Rezaeian, M. 2013. The association between natural disasters and violence: A systematic review of the literature and a call for more epidemiological studies. *Journal of Research in Medical Sciences: The Official Journal of Isfahan University of Medical Sciences* 18(12):1103-1107.

Rodier, P. M. 1995. Developing brain as a target of toxicity. *Environmental Health Perspectives* 103(Suppl. 6):73-76.

Ross, T. 2013. *A disaster in the making: Addressing the vulnerability of low-income communities to extreme weather.* Washington, DC: Center for American Progress.

Rudge, J. 2011. Indoor cold and mortality. In *Environmental burden of disease associated with inadequate housing: A method guide to the quantification of health impacts of selected housing risks in the WHO European Region,* edited by M. Braubach, D. E. Jacobs, and D. Ormandy. Geneva, Switzerland: WHO.

Runkle, J. D., A. Brock-Martin, W. Karmaus, and E. R. Svendsen. 2012. Secondary surge capacity: A framework for understanding long-term access to primary care for medically vulnerable populations in disaster recovery. *American Journal of Public Health* 102(12):e24-e32.

Sandel, M., A. Baeder, A. Bradman, J. Hughes, C. Mitchell, R. Shaughnessy, T. K. Takaro, and D. E. Jacobs. 2010. Housing interventions and control of health-related chemical agents: A review of the evidence. *Journal of Public Health Management and Practice* 16(5 Suppl.):S24-S33.

Sattler, D., J. Sattler, C. Kaiser, B. Hamby, M. Adams, L. Love, J. Winkler, C. Abu-Ukkaz, B. Watts, and A. Beatty. 1995. Hurricane Andrew: Psychological distress among shelter victims. *International Journal of Stress Management* 2(3):133-143.

SBA (U.S. Small Business Administration). 2014. *Disaster loans.* https://www.sba.gov/category/navigation-structure/loans-grants/small-business-loans/disaster-loans (accessed November 25, 2014).

Singh-Manoux, A., A. Gueguen, P. Martikainen, J. Ferrie, M. Marmot, and M. Shipley. 2007. Self-rated health and mortality: Short- and long-term associations in the Whitehall II Study. *Psychosomatic Medicine* 69(2):138-143.

Smith Parker, T. 2014. *CDBG Disaster Recovery overview.* Paper presented at IOM Committee on Post-Disaster Recovery of a Community's Public Health, Medical, and Social Services: Meeting Two, February 3, Washington, DC.

Spokane, A. R., Y. Mori, and F. Martinez. 2012. Housing arrays following disasters: Social vulnerability considerations in designing transitional communities. *Environment and Behavior* 1-25.

Takaro, T. K., J. Krieger, L. Song, D. Sharify, and N. Beaudet. 2011. The breathe-easy home: The impact of asthma-friendly home construction on clinical outcomes and trigger exposure. *American Journal of Public Health* 101(1):55-62.

TFCPS (Task Force on Community Preventive Services). 2003. Recommendations to promote healthy social environments. *American Journal of Preventive Medicine* 24(3):21-24.

ULI (Urban Land Institute). 2014. *Housing in America: Integrating housing, health, and resilience in a changing environment.* Washington, DC: ULI.

UNITY. 2010. *Search and rescue five years later: Saving people still trapped in Katrina's ruins.* http://unitygno.org/wp-content/uploads/2010/08/UNITY_AB-Report_August2010.pdf (accessed March 10, 2015).

Uscher-Pines, L. 2009. Health effects of relocation following disaster: A systematic review of the literature. *Disasters* 33(1):1-22.

USGBC (U.S. Green Building Council). 2009. *LEED for new construction & major renovations.* Washington, DC: USGBC.

Van Ryzin, G. G., and T. Kamber. 2002. Subtenures and housing outcomes for low income renters in New York City. *Journal of Urban Affairs* 24(2):197-218.

Waitzman, N. J., and K. R. Smith. 1998. Phantom of the area: Poverty-area residence and mortality in the United States. *American Journal of Public Health* 88(6):973-976.

Weich, S., and G. Lewis. 1998. Material standard of living, social class, and the prevalence of the common mental disorders in Great Britain. *Journal of Epidemiology and Community Health* 52(1):8-14.

WHO (World Health Organization). 2011. *Environmental burden of disease associated with inadequate housing: A method guide to the quantification of health effects of selected housing risks in the WHO European region.* Edited by M. Braubach, D. E. Jacobs, and D. Ormandy. Geneva, Switzerland: WHO.

Wilner, D. M., R. P. Walkley, T. C. Pinkerton, and M. Tayback. 1962. *The housing environment and family life a longitudinal study of the effects of housing on morbidity and mental health.* http://catalog.hathitrust.org/api/volumes/oclc/233806.html (accessed March 30, 2015).

Wilson, J., S. L. Dixon, P. Breysse, D. Jacobs, G. Adamkiewicz, G. L. Chew, D. Dearborn, J. Krieger, M. Sandel, and A. Spanier. 2010. Housing and allergens: A pooled analysis of nine US studies. *Environmental Research* 110(2):189-198.

Wilson, J., S. Dixon, D. Jacobs, J. Breysse, J. Akoto, E. Tohn, M. Isaacson, A. Evens, and Y. Hernandez. 2014. Watts-to-wellbeing: Does residential energy conservation improve health? *Energy Efficiency* 7(1):151-160.

Zock, J.-P., D. Jarvis, C. Luczynska, J. Sunyer, and P. Burney. 2002. Housing characteristics, reported mold exposure, and asthma in the European Community Respiratory Health Survey. *Journal of Allergy and Clinical Immunology* 110(2):285-292.

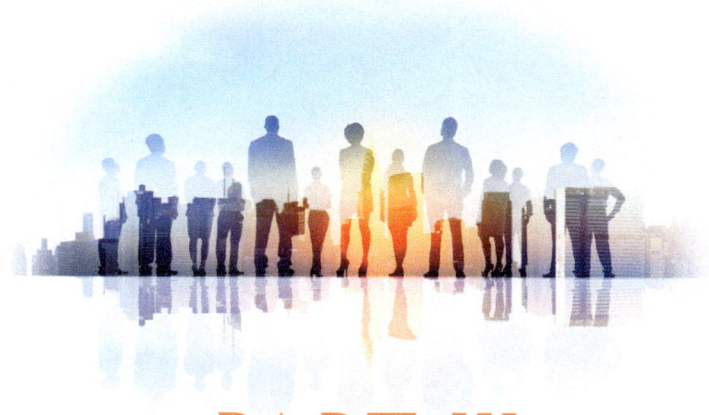

PART III

APPENDIXES

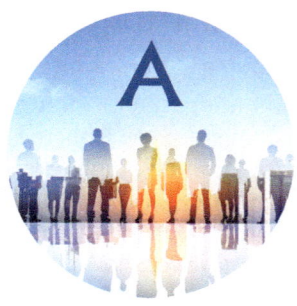

The Federal Policy Environment
Influencing Disaster Recovery

Over the last decades, a number of pieces of legislation and policy directives have included to varying degrees a focus on recovery as an intrinsic element of the national approach to managing disasters: the Robert T. Stafford Disaster Relief and Emergency Assistance Act, the Disaster Mitigation Act of 2000, the Homeland Security Act of 2002, the Post-Katrina Emergency Reform Act of 2006, the Pandemic and All-Hazards Preparedness Act of 2006 and its reauthorization in 2013, Presidential Policy Directive 8: National Preparedness, and the Hurricane Sandy Rebuilding Strategy. Each of these policies is discussed below in the context of disaster recovery.

ROBERT T. STAFFORD DISASTER RELIEF AND EMERGENCY ASSISTANCE ACT,[1] MOST RECENTLY AMENDED BY THE SANDY RECOVERY IMPROVEMENT ACT OF 2013[2]

The Stafford Act (Public Law 93-288) is the main source of authorities for the Federal Emergency Management Agency's (FEMA's) disaster assistance programs. Under this act, the President is authorized to issue major disaster or emergency declarations, resulting in the distribution of wide-ranging federal aid to individuals and families, certain nonprofit organizations, and public agencies. The Sandy Recovery Improvement Act of 2013 amended the Stafford Act to establish new procedures designed to improve the efficiency and quality of disaster assistance; it created a set of alternative procedures for FEMA's administration of its Public Assistance program, which offers funding for the removal of debris and the repair and restoration of eligible facilities. Among the other provisions of the Sandy Recovery Improvement Act is the authorization for a chief executive of an Indian tribal nation to request a major disaster or emergency declaration, separately from the state. The act also authorizes FEMA to pay for child care expenses as disaster assistance under the Other Needs Assistance provision of the Individuals and Households Program. This provision for child care is critical to protecting a vulnerable population. Finally, the Sandy Recovery Improvement Act also makes changes to streamline the Hazard Mitigation Grant Program process, and it allows FEMA to provide up to 25 percent of the estimated costs of hazard mitigation to a grantee in advance of the costs being incurred (Brown et al., 2013).

---

[1] 42 U.S.C. § 5121 et seq.
[2] Sandy Recovery Improvement Act of 2013, Public Law 113-2, 113th Cong., H.R.152 (January 29, 2014).

DISASTER MITIGATION ACT OF 2000[3]

The Disaster Mitigation Act of 2000 (Public Law 106-390) authorizes FEMA's requirement that state, local, and Indian tribal governments carry out mitigation planning as a condition for receiving post-disaster mitigation grant assistance. The DMA also "amended the Robert T. Stafford Disaster Relief and Emergency Assistance Act by repealing the previous mitigation planning provisions and replacing them with a new set of requirements that emphasize the need for state, local, and Indian Tribal entities to closely coordinate mitigation planning and implementation efforts" (FEMA, 2013). The act added incentives, authorizing increased funding for states demonstrating improved coordination and integration of mitigation planning and implementation. Finally, the act established a new requirement for local mitigation plans and authorizes the use of up to 7 percent of Hazard Mitigation Grant Program funds available to a state for the development of state, local, and Indian tribal mitigation plans (FEMA, 2013). Mitigation, conceived of as a cornerstone of emergency management, refers to activities that reduce a disaster's impact on lives and property through, for example, damage prevention and flood insurance.

HOMELAND SECURITY ACT OF 2002[4]

The Homeland Security Act of 2002 created the U.S. Department of Homeland Security (DHS) and placed FEMA, which had been an independent agency created in 1979, within this new department. It also called for the consolidation of existing federal emergency response plans into a National Response Plan (NRP), which was to establish a single, comprehensive approach to domestic incident management. The NRP was completed in December 2004, and subsequently superseded by the National Response Framework (NRF), first published in January 2008 and updated in May 2013. The NRP and NRF were designed to be used in efforts to prevent, prepare for, respond to, and recover from emergencies, including terrorist attacks and disasters (FEMA, 2015c). The NRP and the first version of the NRF included a special focus on long-term community recovery through a specific Emergency Support Function (ESF) #14.[5] The Homeland Security Act also called for the establishment of a National Incident Management System, which specifies a systematic approach for how to manage emergencies involving all threats and hazards, regardless of the cause, size, location, or complexity of the incident (FEMA, 2015b). Relatedly, a presidential directive—Homeland Security Presidential Directive (HSPD)-5: Management of Domestic Incidents—was issued.[6] It directed the development and administration of a National Incident Management System (NIMS), first released on March 1, 2004, by DHS (DHS, 2008). The NIMS is a comprehensive, scalable, and systematic approach to incident management that specifies core doctrine, concepts, and organizational processes for all hazards.

THE POST-KATRINA EMERGENCY REFORM ACT OF 2006[7] AND THE NATIONAL DISASTER RECOVERY FRAMEWORK

Spurred by the highly visible failures surrounding the response to Hurricane Katrina, one of the main goals of the Post-Katrina Emergency Reform Act of 2006 was to reconfigure FEMA. It established 10 regional FEMA offices, each with a regional administrator, and it conferred on FEMA more organizational autonomy. Among its other provisions, especially relevant to recovery, was adding to the Stafford Act mission a focus on reunification of families through the development of a National Emergency Family Registry and Locator System and a Child Locator Center. The act also established a National Advisory Council, and it called for the appointment of a FEMA disability coordinator and a small state and rural

---

[3] Disaster Mitigation Act of 2000, Public Law 106-390, 106th Cong., H.R.707 (October 30, 2000).

[4] Homeland Security Act of 2002, Public Law 107-296, 107th Cong., H.R.5005 (November 25, 2002).

[5] ESF #14 was subsequently replaced by Recovery Support Functions under the National Disaster Recovery Framework.

[6] Homeland Security Presidential Directive (HSPD)-5, *Management of Domestic Incidents* (February 28, 2003).

[7] Post-Katrina Emergency Management Reform Act of 2006, 109th Cong., S.3721 (October 4, 2006).

advocate. These last two provisions in particular are key to protecting vulnerable populations during response and recovery (Bea et al., 2006).

The act also called for the establishment of the National Disaster Housing Strategy, released January 16, 2009, which addresses temporary housing needs and the rebuilding of permanent housing—including rental housing—and includes a focus on the housing needs of disabled persons (FEMA, 2009). The act also amended the Stafford Act regarding disaster assistance, transportation assistance, and case management services, all of which are important in the early phases of recovery.

The act also called on FEMA to assemble a group of federal and nongovernmental organizations to develop a National Disaster Recovery Strategy, summarizing existing programs and evaluating their utility following a disaster (Bea et al., 2006). In 2009, the President created the White House Long-Term Disaster Recovery Working Group to develop this strategy, which was accomplished by sponsoring outreach sessions and creating a Web portal enabling more than 600 stakeholders to provide thousands of comments. The National Disaster Recovery Strategy was renamed the National Disaster Recovery Framework (NDRF) and released in September 2011. The NDRF grew out of recognition of the failure to plan for recovery after Hurricane Katrina, the failure to relate local needs to available resources, and the failure to plan for the actions of multiple parties to address disagreements about resource allocation (Smith, 2011). It specifies "core recovery principles; roles and responsibilities of recovery coordinators and other stakeholders; a coordinating structure that facilitates communication and collaboration among all stakeholders; guidance for pre- and post-disaster recovery planning; and the overall process by which communities can capitalize on opportunities to rebuild" what the NDRF asserts will be "stronger, smarter, and safer" communities (FEMA, 2011, p. 1).

The NDRF provides a guide for the federal government to facilitate effective recovery at the community level (FEMA, 2011). Spearheaded by FEMA and its federal partners, the NDRF is not an explicit plan but is, rather, a document that defines how federal agencies organize and operate during recovery to support states, tribes, and localities. The NDRF is intended for a wide audience of governmental, private sector, and nongovernmental stakeholders. A companion document, the Recovery Federal Interagency Operational Plan, was released in 2014. That document operationalizes the NDRF and is far more specific about federal tasks and responsibilities, as well as detailed resource, personnel, and sourcing requirements (FEMA, 2014).

PANDEMIC AND ALL-HAZARDS PREPAREDNESS ACT,[8] PANDEMIC AND ALL-HAZARDS PREPAREDNESS REAUTHORIZATION ACT OF 2013[9] AND NATIONAL HEALTH SECURITY STRATEGY

The Pandemic and All-Hazards Preparedness Act (PAHPA) of December 2006 amended the Public Health Service Act to establish the position of the Assistant Secretary for Preparedness and Response (ASPR) within the U.S. Department of Health and Human Services. It then gave ASPR authority over and responsibility for the National Disaster Medical System and the Hospital Preparedness Program (HPP) Cooperative Agreement. Relatedly, it formally established in law the Medical Reserve Corps (MRC) and reassigned responsibility for the Emergency System for Advance Registration of Volunteer Health Professionals (ESAR-VHP) to ASPR. These two programs establish guidelines and standards for registration, credentialing, and deployment of medical professionals in a national emergency.

The PAHPA also called for establishment of the National Health Security Strategy (NHSS) (HHS, 2009). The original NHSS, released in December 2009, presented a vision of national health security—a secure and resilient nation "in the face of diverse incidents with health consequences"—and identified priorities to direct this effort. Progress toward achieving the stated goal to "strengthen and sustain com-

---

[8] Pandemic and All-Hazards Preparedness Act, Public Law 109-417, 109th Cong., S.3678 (December 19, 2006).

[9] Pandemic and All-Hazards Preparedness Reauthorization Act of 2013, Public Law 113-5, 113th Cong., H.R.307 (March 13, 2013).

munities' abilities to prevent, protect against, mitigate the effects of, respond to, and recover from incidents with negative health consequences" is assessed and reported every four years (HHS, 2015, p. 6). Following the release of the National Health Security Review 2010-2014, an updated National Health Security Strategy Implementation Plan (NHSS/IP) 2015-2018 was released in February 2015. The NHSS/IP offers five strategic objectives, the first of which is to "build and sustain healthy, resilient communities" (HHS, 2015, p. 9). This objective calls for efforts to build social connectedness, to improve the coordination of health and human services through community partnerships, and to foster a culture of resilience throughout the nation (HHS, 2015). Remaining objectives include enhancing the national capability to produce and effectively use both medical countermeasures and non-pharmaceutical interventions; ensuring comprehensive health situational awareness to support decision making before incidents and during response and recovery operations; enhancing the integration and effectiveness of the public health, health care, and emergency management systems; and strengthening global health security (HHS, 2015).

The NHSS is supported by the HPP Cooperative Agreement, which is administered by ASPR, and the Public Health Emergency Preparedness (PHEP) Cooperative Agreement, which is administered by the Centers for Disease Control and Prevention. These Cooperative Agreements are authorized by sections 319C-1 and 319C-2 of the Public Health Service Act, as amended by the PAHPA.[10]

Defined sets of public health and health care preparedness capabilities have been developed by CDC and ASPR, respectively, to help public health and health care organizations with strategic planning for preparedness and response. These capabilities form the basis of the program measures and evaluations required by the PHEP and HPP Cooperative Agreements.

Recovery is one of 15 capabilities specified in Public Health Preparedness Capabilities: National Standards for State and Local Planning (CDC, 2011) and one of eight capabilities specified in Healthcare Preparedness Capabilities: National Guidance for Healthcare System Preparedness (ASPR, 2012). For public health, the capability for community recovery is designed to help community partners "plan and advocate for the rebuilding of public health, medical, and mental/behavioral health systems to at least a level functioning comparable to pre-incident levels, and improved levels where possible" (CDC, 2011, p. 10). For health care, the capability for health care system recovery relates to the development of efficient processes for achieving continuity of operations and the return to normalcy in the delivery of health care to a community.

PRESIDENTIAL POLICY DIRECTIVE 8: NATIONAL PREPAREDNESS

Presidential Policy Directive 8, which was signed on March 30, 2011, directed the development of a National Preparedness Goal and a National Preparedness System, among other provisions (Brown, 2011).[11] The National Preparedness Goal (released September 2011) established what it means for the whole community[12] to be prepared for disasters of all types. The National Preparedness Goal, which was issued subsequently, is "a secure and resilient nation with the capabilities required across the whole community to prevent, protect against, mitigate, respond to, and recover from the threats and hazards that pose the greatest risk." The National Preparedness Goal then defines 31 core capabilities that address the greatest risks to the nation. The core capabilities are organized into five mission areas: prevention, protection, mitigation, response, and recovery (FEMA, 2015d). The presidential directive defines "recovery" as "rebuilding infrastructure systems; providing adequate interim and long-term housing for survivors;

---

[10] Public Health Service Act § 319(C)(1-2), as amended by the Pandemic and All-Hazards Preparedness Act, Public Law 109-417, 109th Cong., S.3678 (December 19, 2006).

[11] This directive replaces Homeland Security Presidential Directive (HSPD)-8: National Preparedness, issued December 17, 2003, and HSPD-8 Annex I: National Planning, issued December 4, 2007, both by President Bush.

[12] The whole-community approach to preparedness "recognizes that everyone can contribute to and benefit from national preparedness efforts. This includes individuals and families (including those with disabilities and others with access and functional needs), businesses, community and faith-based groups, nonprofit organizations, and all levels of government" (FEMA, 2015c).

restoring health, social, and community services; promoting economic development; and restoring natural and cultural resources" (DHS, 2011).

The National Preparedness System is an integrated set of guidance, programs, and processes designed for all levels of government, private and nonprofit sectors, and the public to guide the United States toward meeting the National Preparedness Goal. The National Preparedness System includes a series of integrated national planning frameworks covering each of the five preparedness mission areas: prevention (the National Prevention Framework, released in May 2013); protection (the National Protection Framework, released in June 2014); mitigation (the National Mitigation Framework, released in May 2013); response (the NRF, first edition released in 2008 and second edition in May 2013); and recovery (NDRF, released in September 2011) (FEMA, 2015c).

Each framework explains its purpose, including guiding principles and scope of mission area; provides an overview of the roles and responsibilities of each part of the community; identifies the mission area's core capabilities, providing key examples of crucial tasks; and defines coordinating structures, whether new or existing, that can enable the whole community to work collaboratively to deliver the core capabilities. Each framework also provides information that state, local, tribal, and territorial governments can utilize to revise their own operational plans (FEMA, 2015a).

Each of the frameworks also is associated with a Federal Interagency Operational Plan that is designed to enable the federal government to implement the framework. Each operational plan describes how federal activities can integrate with and support state and local recovery efforts. Each operational plan also describes critical federal tasks and responsibilities, including resource, personnel, and sourcing requirements and offers guidelines for integrating resources and staff quickly and efficiently. These plans are intended to serve as the federal government's concept of operations for each of the five preparedness mission areas (FEMA, 2015a). Finally, Presidential Directive 8 requires an annual report, the National Preparedness Report, which summarizes progress toward core capabilities in the National Preparedness Goal. Such reports were released on March 30, 2012; March 30, 2013; and March 30, 2014 (see FEMA, 2015e).

HURRICANE SANDY REBUILDING STRATEGY

On December 7, 2012, President Obama signed an executive order establishing the Hurricane Sandy Rebuilding Task Force. That task force was responsible for writing the Hurricane Sandy Rebuilding Strategy, a comprehensive plan, released in August 2013, that is designed to guide the expenditure of the $50 billion appropriated under the Disaster Relief Appropriations Act of 2013, which supports recovery from Hurricane Sandy (Hurricane Sandy Rebuilding Task Force, 2013). From the outset, the strategy envisioned rebuilding the affected region in a way that is stronger and smarter, including more resilient—that is, better able to withstand future storms. The strategy sets forth 69 recommendations designed to achieve the following goals: "promoting resilient rebuilding through innovative ideas and a thorough understanding of current and future risk; ensuring a regionally coordinated, resilient approach to infrastructure investment; restoring and strengthening homes and providing families with safe, affordable housing options; supporting small businesses and revitalizing local economies; addressing insurance challenges, understanding, and affordability; building state and local capacity to plan for and implement long-term recovery and rebuilding; [and] improving data sharing between federal, state and local officials" (Hurricane Sandy Rebuilding Task Force, 2013, p. 39). Some of the specific recommendations are to make the electrical grid smarter and more flexible and to protect the liquid fuel supply chain so that it can better withstand future disasters. Another recommendation is to make housing units—both individual and multifamily—more sustainable and resilient through recovery steps such as elevating units well above flood risk levels and increasing energy efficiency. Still another is to fund local disaster recovery manager positions in communities in the Sandy-affected region (Hurricane Sandy Rebuilding Task Force, 2013).

REFERENCES

ASPR (Office of the Assistant Secretary for Preparedness and Response). 2012. *Healthcare preparedness capabilities: National guidance for healthcare system preparedness*. Washington, DC: HHS.

Bea, K., E. Halchin, H. Hogue, F. Kaiser, N. Love, F. X. McCarthy, S. Reese, and B. Schwemle. 2006. *Federal emergency management policy changes after Hurricane Katrina: A summary of statutory provisions*. CRS Report RL33729. Washington, DC: CRS, Library of Congress.

Brown, J. T. 2011. *Presidential Policy Directive 8 and the National Preparedness System: Background and issues for Congress*. CRS Report R42073. Washington, DC: CRS, Library of Congress.

Brown, J. T., F. X. McCarthy, and E. C. Liu. 2013. *Analysis of the Sandy Recovery Improvement Act of 2013*. CRS Report R42991. Washington, DC: CRS, Library of Congress.

CDC (Centers for Disease Control and Prevention). 2011. *Public health preparedness capabilities: National standards for state and local planning*. Atlanta, GA: CDC.

DHS (U.S. Department of Homeland Security). 2008. *National Incident Management System*. Washington, DC: DHS.

DHS. 2011. *Presidential Policy Directive/PPD-8: National preparedness*. http://www.dhs.gov/presidential-policy-directive-8-national-preparedness (accessed December 2, 2014).

FEMA (Federal Emergency Management Agency). 2009. *National disaster housing strategy*. Washington, DC: FEMA.

FEMA. 2011. *National disaster recovery framework*. Washington, DC: FEMA.

FEMA. 2013. *Disaster Mitigation Act of 2000*. https://www.fema.gov/media-library/assets/documents/4596 (accessed March 26, 2015).

FEMA. 2014. *Recovery federal interagency operational plan*. Washington, DC: FEMA.

FEMA. 2015a. *Federal interagency operational plans*. https://www.fema.gov/federal-interagency-operational-plans (accessed March 26, 2015).

FEMA. 2015b. *National Incident Management System*. https://www.fema.gov/national-incident-management-system (accessed March 26, 2015).

FEMA. 2015c. *National planning frameworks*. https://www.fema.gov/national-planning-frameworks (accessed April 13, 2015).

FEMA. 2015d. *National preparedness goal*. https://www.fema.gov/national-preparedness-goal (accessed April 13, 2015).

FEMA. 2015e. *National preparedness report*. https://www.fema.gov/national-preparedness-report (accessed March 20, 2015).

HHS (U.S. Department of Health and Human Services). 2009. *National health security strategy of the United States of America*. Washington, DC: HHS.

HHS. 2015. *National Health Security Strategy and Implementation Plan 2015-2018*. http://www.phe.gov/Preparedness/planning/authority/nhss/Pages/strategy.aspx (accessed April 13, 2015).

Hurricane Sandy Rebuilding Task Force. 2013. *Hurricane Sandy rebuilding strategy*. Washington, DC: Hurricane Sandy Rebuilding Task Force.

Smith, G. 2011. *Planning for post-disaster recovery: A review of the United States disaster assistance framework*. Fairfax, VA: Public Entity Risk Institute.

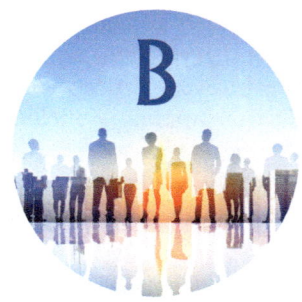

Disaster Recovery Funding: Achieving a Resilient Future?[1]

June 21, 2014

Gavin Smith, Ph.D., AICP
Executive Director, Department of Homeland Security Coastal Hazards Center of Excellence
Associate Professor
Department of City and Regional Planning
University of North Carolina at Chapel Hill

PURPOSE OF REPORT

The Institute of Medicine (IOM) Committee on Post-Disaster Recovery of a Community's Public Health, Medical, and Social Services has been tasked with providing practical guidance on recovery practices that, if implemented, can improve short-, intermediate- and long-term health outcomes in a disaster-affected community. The committee has commissioned this paper to inform its deliberations regarding opportunities to leverage resources that become available in the post-disaster environment to improve the health and social welfare of community members by meeting short- and long-term public health, medical, and social service needs. Specifically, this paper seeks to describe the major governmental and nongovernmental funding sources for disaster recovery, delineate the complex pathways by which those funds reach affected communities and are allocated for recovery activities, and identify key decision makers at state and local levels responsible for directing the dissemination of recovery funds.

INTRODUCTION

Disaster recovery can be defined as "the differential process of restoring, rebuilding, and reshaping the physical, social, economic, and natural environment through pre-event planning and post-event actions"

---

[1] A white paper prepared for the National Academy of Sciences, Institute of Medicine Committee on Post-Disaster Recovery of a Community's Public Health, Medical, and Social Services. The author is responsible for the content of this article, which does not necessarily represent the views of the Institute of Medicine.

(Smith and Wenger, 2006, p. 237). Disaster recovery is a complex process comprised of many interrelated elements and the means by which it is achieved varies across individuals, organizations, institutions, and communities based on a series of pre- and post-event actions. Disaster recovery is shaped by a combination of pre-disaster investments and post-disaster funding, policies, and technical assistance strategies. The overemphasis on post-event aid versus investing in pre-event capacity building and collaborative decision making can hinder recovery outcomes. Similarly, a focus on what amount to narrowly defined federal post-disaster funding streams disproportionately drives the trajectory of recovery, thereby hindering a community's ability to achieve a more resilient and sustainable future.

Sustainable development, and more recently, the concept of resilience have been used to help frame disaster recovery (Berke and Beatley, 1997; Berke and Campanella, 2006; Berke et al., 1993; Campanella, 2006; NRC, 2012). Both have important practical applications and can be used to help guide improved policies and funding strategies, if they are effectively operationalized (Smith and Wenger, 2006). Significant challenges remain as both concepts are elusive in practice, as evidenced by the lack of tangible, coordinated policies and funding mechanisms focused on these aims that are guided by a national resilience strategy. Researchers suggest that a locally-focused capacity-building effort, supported by a broad governance network is needed (NRC, 2012, pp. 3-9). While many federal, state, and local units of government suggest that their organizations rely on sustainability and resilience-based concepts to help drive disaster recovery funding programs, these endeavors are often undertaken in isolation, which undermines resilience (Smith, 2011).

Disaster Recovery Assistance Network

Accessing post-disaster funding is a critical part of recovery (Bates and Peacock, 1987; Friesema, 1979; Olshansky and Johnson, 2010, pp. 227-230; Platt, 1999). Additional resources include policy and technical assistance in the form of education, outreach, and training initiatives. Each of these interconnected resources are delivered by a host of actors collectively defined as the disaster recovery assistance network (see Figure B-1). The network is characterized as a loosely coupled set of organizations whose

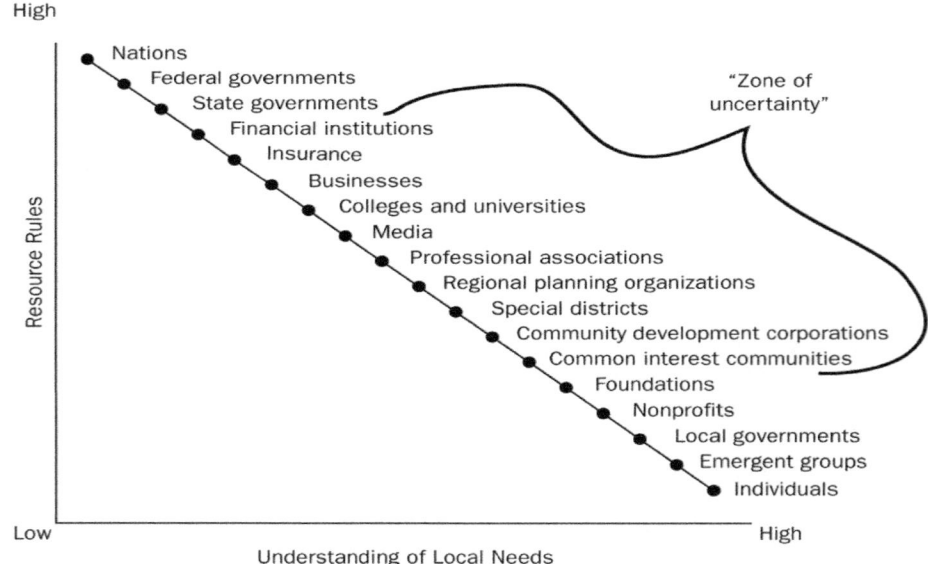

FIGURE B-1 Disaster recovery assistance network.
SOURCE: Smith, 2011, p. 14.

level of interaction varies over time and space and the degree to which the resources delivered by these organizations is coordinated temporally or meets local needs is also highly variable.

The three resources (funding, policy, and technical assistance) and the rules associated with their distribution differ across the network as Figure B-1 indicates. While the graphic represents a hypothetical assistance network that is subject to change over time, the notion that the rules used to manage the resources can range from highly prescriptive (e.g., those administered by nations and federal agencies) to highly flexible (e.g., emergent groups and individuals) has important implications. For instance, the highly prescriptive rules delivered by federal agencies post-disaster have been found to disproportionately drive recovery outcomes, as substantial attention is placed on the management of these resources even though they may not reflect local needs at the community or individual level (Smith, 2011, pp. 35-36). Conversely, those who may possess a deep understanding of local needs are often excluded from participating in the development of national recovery policy, including those shaping the distribution of funding. Further exacerbating the ability to develop a coherent recovery strategy driven by collaboration and the coordinated distribution of assistance is the large number of actors who fall within what can be called "the zone of uncertainty" as both practitioners often fail to involve them in pre-event planning for post-disaster recovery and researchers know less about their roles in recovery (Smith, 2011, p. 15).

TIMING OF ASSISTANCE

The timing of disaster recovery assistance includes pre- and post-event activities. As noted in the definition of disaster recovery, pre-event planning and post-event actions assume an ideal condition as the United States does not have in place a robust pre-event planning policy nor do most states or local governments maintain pre-disaster recovery plans that address the coordinated timing of assistance. For example, the National Disaster Recovery Framework, developed due to a congressional mandate established following Hurricane Katrina, has not been fully codified nor is there sufficient attention tied to pre-event planning.[2] Even with the advent of the NDRF, the vast majority of attention remains placed on the administration of the often substantial influx of post-disaster funding rather than a meaningful commitment to pre-event investments in capacity building and the modification of policies dominated by a response or post-disaster orientation.[3] A focus on response and post-disaster funding has limited the development of a thoughtful set of procedures, put in place before a disaster and agreed to by stakeholders, to coordinate the timing of that assistance across members of the assistance network.

The lack of investments in pre-event planning is particularly troubling given the strong post-disaster forces at work, namely, the post-disaster problems that Olshansky (2006) refers to as speed versus deliberation and time compression (Olshansky and Johnson, 2010, pp. 225-226). Following disasters there is an intense pressure to return to a sense of normalcy, even if pre-event conditions include inequitable housing, poor public health, sprawling development and high hazard vulnerability (Smith, 2011). Attempts to alter pre-event conditions through post-disaster deliberation followed by a thoughtful implementation strategy is hard to achieve in practice (Campanella, 2006; Vale and Campanella, 2005). Taking the time needed to contemplate changes in long-standing human settlement patterns or identifying those who can assist the disenfranchised when traditional aid programs like loans cannot achieve this end requires a long-term commitment that can run headlong into public pressures to rebuild as quickly as possible and make policy choices that do not necessarily represent the public good, including those that are shaped by

---

[2] Prior to Hurricane Katrina, the U.S. government did not have in place a national disaster recovery strategy. Rather, guidance on recovery activities, which focused entirely on the distribution of post-disaster federal grant programs, was located in an appendix of the National Response Framework. This condition provides a powerful indicator of the strong response orientation of Federal Emergency Management Agency (FEMA) and the emergency management profession across the United States.

[3] A common refrain among local government officials who have experienced a major disaster is the difficulty of financially managing the large sums of money that flow into their community, which can dramatically exceed annual operating budgets and the ability of existing staff to administer new and unfamiliar programs in addition to their day-to-day responsibilities associated with typical government operations.

development interests (Freudenburg et al., 2009) or those that influence the distribution of post-disaster aid. Promises of "building back better" often ring hollow for those who were among the most vulnerable and least powerful in a community.

Understood relative to the disaster recovery assistance network, the timing of assistance varies across each member of the network, in part, because of the lack of good pre-event planning and collaborative problem solving (Smith, 2011, pp. 18-22). The resources delivered by most actors (disproportionately in the post-disaster timeframe) remain uncoordinated, duplicative, and in many cases counterproductive. If one assumes that each member of the assistance network is delivering funding; creating, influencing, or implementing policies; and delivering technical assistance across a temporally defined disaster recovery continuum, the complexities of disaster recovery become more apparent.

Take, for instance, two sets of actors (e.g., nonprofits and local governments), both of whom implement post-disaster housing-related policies. Following disasters, nonprofit organizations often offer assistance to low-income homeowners through the repair or reconstruction of damaged housing. If done before local governments have considered strengthening building codes and standards, or re-mapped hazardous locations in accordance with the latest technology or tools used to assess risk, homes may be built back to standards that were in place at the time of the event, rather than in accordance with the best available information. The rapid repair or rebuilding of housing can also precede access to federal funding that could be used to incorporate a range of risk reduction measures such as the relocation or elevation of flood and storm-surge prone housing, the use of fire resistant building materials, and the retrofitting of homes to better withstand earthquake-induced ground motion. The failure to incorporate these measures into recovery has the effect of perpetuating social vulnerability. The lack of coordination horizontally (e.g., between local government and nonprofits) and vertically (between federal, state, and local government actors) is another problematic characteristic of the disaster assistance framework.

HORIZONTAL AND VERTICAL INTEGRATION

The concept of horizontal and vertical integration is a useful way to help to understand the interaction of governmental and non-governmental actors and has been applied to disaster recovery as a way to help explain the benefits of inter-organizational cooperation and the implications of failing to do so (Berke and Beatley, 1997; Berke et al., 1993; Smith, 2011) (see Figure B-2).

A Type 1 community, which is characterized by strong horizontal and vertical connectivity, is able to recover more quickly and in a manner that addresses local needs, controlling for other factors such as size of the disaster and its impacts, wealth, and disaster experience. A Type 1 community has strong ties among locally-based organizations as well as established relationships with state and federal organizations involved in disaster recovery. This condition fosters a good understanding of local needs and external sources of assistance, including the degree to which state and federal resources meet identified needs.

Type 2 communities possess strong horizontal but weak vertical integration. Rural locales often possess the characteristics of a Type 2 community as they tend to be tight-knit and yet may not maintain strong relationships with state and federal organizations. This means that while they may have a good understanding of local conditions and needs, their ability to assess the types of external assistance available, including the degree to which it will meet local needs, may be limited.

Type 3 communities have weak horizontal but strong vertical integration. Since these communities have a good understanding of federal and state assistance programs and their associated funding mechanisms, but weak horizontal connectivity, recovery is strongly influenced by narrowly defined federal and state programs rather than a locally-developed and grounded vision for recovery.

Type 4 communities are characterized by weak horizontal and vertical integration. As such, they are likely to be the most ill-equipped to deal with the complexities of disaster recovery. Their ability to seek external assistance or coordinate locally available resources is limited.

Vertical / Horizontal	Strong	Weak
Strong	Type 1	Type 2
Weak	Type 3	Type 4

FIGURE B-2 Horizontal and vertical integration typology.
SOURCE: Smith, 2011, p. 25.

PRE- AND POST-DISASTER RECOVERY FUNDING ACROSS THE DISASTER RECOVERY ASSISTANCE NETWORK

The remainder of this paper will focus on the role of disaster recovery funding, including how it affects the three dimensions of the assistance framework (resources and local needs, timing of assistance and horizontal and vertical integration). The pre- and post-disaster funding mechanisms in place in the United States have a strong effect on the use of available resources and the degree to which they meet local needs. This is most evident among federal assistance as many of these programs are delivered in the aftermath of a disaster, rather than pre-event; they are narrow in scope and highly prescriptive in nature; and local governments struggle to implement these federal programs, and may not be able to muster the additional resources needed to effectively address larger policy and planning issues such as developing a broader vision of what they want their community to be in the aftermath of an extreme event.

The lack of pre-disaster funding investments in capacity building efforts like training and the hiring of on-call local staff (either contractors or temporary government officials) to support the effective management of post-disaster grant programs often results in overwhelmed local government staff, whose day-to-day roles may become consumed by the search for or implementation of grants rather than addressing other key issues like case management, building code enforcement, public health concerns, and the implementation of pre-existing plans and policies that were in place at the local level before the disaster struck.

The timing of funding delivery across the network of aid providers also has a significant effect on recovery outcomes. Ill-timed and/or uncoordinated funding strategies can lead to suboptimal results among members of the assistance network, as the housing example suggests. The failure to coordinate the timing of funding disbursements across all members of the disaster recovery assistance network is exceedingly difficult and requires a commitment to build a robust and sustained pledge to pre-event planning and post-event actions that are maintained over the life of the often lengthy recovery process. The lack of commitment to this effort, while troubling, is not surprising given the episodic nature of extreme events.

The ability to build on established relationships and strengthen those that remain nascent, non-existent or emergent in the aftermath of a disaster can be expressed through the horizontal and vertical integration typology. While varied organizations provide recovery-related funding before and after disasters, their effective coordination remains elusive. Further, the use of these funds once received by communities of differing types can vary significantly. In both cases, the level of horizontal and vertical integration can help to understand these relationships. For instance, the ability of local governments to effectively manage the receipt of government-based funding that is provided by external state and federal agencies is often incumbent on their awareness and understanding of varied eligibility requirements and the timing of their distribution. It is also shaped by relationships established over time, often in the throes of the disaster recovery process. Thus local governments that have experienced past disasters can learn the myriad sources of funding and how they can be stitched together to address local conditions and available local assets. Inexperienced communities must rapidly assimilate substantial amounts of information regarding grant and loan eligibility criteria while they struggle to address a range of new duties that many local officials are unprepared to address in a comprehensive, integrated manner. Strong inter-organizational relationships at the community level are also critically important. The ability to effectively manage limited resources that will rapidly become overtaxed while assessing local post-disaster needs benefits from a cohesive set of local actors.

Types of Funding and Eligibility

Pre- and post-disaster recovery funding is comprised of several types, including direct assistance in the form of grants and loans and assistance targeting capacity building initiatives like planning. Direct assistance may be provided to individuals, institutions, and organizations as well as communities to fund a range of activities, many of which focus on projects tied to the physical reconstruction or repair of housing, damaged infrastructure, and public facilities like hospitals, police, and fire stations. The nature of assistance received by individuals, including insurance payouts, grants or loans can influence not only individuals and family outcomes, but also community-level recovery. Likewise, the type of funds received by communities can shape options and associated outcomes among individuals and families. The nature of housing assistance is a powerful case in point as the majority of federal funding targets homeowners and not renters, who are disproportionately low income. For instance, insurance payments or post-disaster grants that pay for housing repairs increase the likelihood that these residents will stay in a given area, even if it is subject to repeated hazard events, whereas the limited funding available for renters post-disaster may exacerbate the loss of affordable housing, sometimes resulting in the "disaster gentrification" of low-income areas hit by disaster (Smith, 2014).[4]

Another problematic issue involves the rebuilding of communities to their pre-event condition rather than the systematic incorporation of risk reduction measures into the repair of damaged housing, infrastructure, and public facilities. The Hazard Mitigation Grant Program (HMGP) can be used to fund a series of risk reduction measures such as the acquisition or elevation of flood-prone housing and the strengthening of homes and buildings to withstand the forces of nature (e.g., ground motion associated with earthquakes, high wind tied to hurricanes or tornadoes, or storm surge tied to coastal storms).

The amount of HMGP available following a federally declared disaster is predicated on 15 percent of

---

[4] While post-disaster assistance following federally declared disasters tends to receive the most attention from researchers and practitioners, the cumulative amount of damages sustained from non-declared events exceeds that recorded for large scale disasters (National Emergency Management Association and the Council on State Governments, 1998). This has important implications for state and local officials tasked with the provision of assistance following localized emergencies when federal assets are not available and the value of proactively applying existing, locally-based resources, tools, and techniques—such as long-standing partnerships, an in-depth knowledge of local conditions and capabilities, and land use measures—are often unrecognized. The preponderance of smaller localized events also highlights the important role insurance plays in recovery as access to insurance proceeds are not tied to a disaster declaration, per se, but rather to incurring damages that are covered by the policy. Significant challenges remain, however, on both counts. The failure to involve key stakeholders at the local level, like land use planners in pre-event recovery planning, has been shown to limit the use of readily available tools and techniques, while disaster-based insurance (e.g., flood and earthquake) is less likely to be maintained by low-income individuals and families, nor is it likely to be maintained over time when it is a required criterion for accessing post-disaster housing assistance grant programs.

total disaster costs, and as such, is still a modest amount of funding committed to risk reduction.[5] Further, since the funds are made available after a disaster, they are typically used to address at-risk properties that have been damaged by the event in question. Conversely, the Pre-Disaster Mitigation (PDM) grant program, which is a component of the Disaster Mitigation Act of 2000, recognizes that hazard mitigation is best initiated prior to a disaster and therefore represents an important advancement in the larger policy dialogue surrounding disaster resilience. In order to remain eligible for PDM funding, states and local governments are required to develop pre-disaster hazard mitigation plans. Linking pre- and post-disaster assistance to engaging in pre-disaster hazard mitigation planning is a step in the right direction. However, a 6-year study of the quality of state and local hazard mitigation plans uncovers several key problems. First, plans did not do a good job linking the results of the risk assessment and the development of risk reduction policies and projects. Second, many plans did not address land use as a key aspect of a larger risk reduction strategy. Third, very few plans made the link between hazard risk reduction and climate change adaptation (Lyles et al., 2014).

The Public Assistance (PA) program typically represents the largest allocation of funding following federally-declared disasters. PA funds are used to pay for post-disaster debris removal, the funding of the additional time required of local and state officials to address recovery-related tasks, and the repair or reconstruction of damaged public facilities. The PA 406 program represents an important, albeit unde-rutilized, means to incorporate hazard mitigation into the repair of damaged infrastructure. Eligibility determinants of the 406 program, namely, cost effectiveness, requires collecting additional data and con-ducting benefit cost analyses. The additional time required to perform the analysis can deter the pursuit of the funds used to repair damaged infrastructure, like hospitals, fire and police stations, and roads in a manner that makes them less susceptible to future damages. As noted earlier, local elected officials are under intense pressure to return communities to "normal" as quickly as possible and the additional time needed to rebuild the community in a safer manner may be met with heated opposition. Similarly, FEMA PA staff are trained in disaster-based cost containment procedures and the expenditure of additional post-disaster funding (even if it is cost-effective in the long run) can sometimes manifest itself in a general reluctance to aggressively pursue hazard mitigation measures (Smith, 2011, pp. 61-62).

Following major federally-declared disasters, Congress may deem it necessary to provide additional assistance beyond that offered under the Robert T. Stafford Disaster Relief and Emergency Assistance Act (Stafford Act), which is the traditional federal vehicle through which post-disaster assistance is delivered. Among the largest single sources of "supplemental assistance" is the Community Development Block Grant for Disaster Recovery (CDBG-DR). Administered by the U.S. Department of Housing and Urban Development (HUD), the CDBG-DR can be used to fund a variety of disaster recovery activities, includ-ing (1) the acquisition and relocation of flood-damaged housing; (2) relocation payments for people and businesses displaced by a disaster; (3) debris removal not covered by FEMA; (4) rehabilitation of homes and buildings damaged by a disaster; (5) buying, constructing, or rehabilitating public facilities such as streets, neighborhood centers, and water, sewer, and drainage systems; (6) code enforcement; (7) home-ownership activities such as down payment assistance, interest rate subsidies, and loan guarantees; (8) public services; (9) helping businesses retain or create jobs in disaster impacted areas; and (10) planning and administration costs (HUD, 2015]).

The CDBG-DR funds target those communities that have demonstrated significant unmet needs not addressed by other grant programs. At least half of CDBG-DR funds must be used to assist low and moderate income persons. The HUD criteria help to address three important shortfalls described in the larger disaster recovery assistance network: grant flexibility, the ability to address unmet needs, and assistance provided to socially vulnerable populations. The effective delivery of post-disaster assistance

---

[5] States that develop an enhanced hazard mitigation plan are allotted HMGP funds that represent 20 percent of total federal disaster costs. Enhanced state hazard mitigation plan status is based on a state's demonstrated ability to manage HMGP funds, not necessarily an enhanced ability to build local capacity or commitment to reduce hazard risk. The enhanced status criteria further demonstrates the federal emphasis on grants management and the processing of grant funds rather than a more comprehensive ap-proach to state-wide risk reduction.

also benefits from a high level of engagement with local governments tasked with the implementation of disaster recovery funding. Historically, HUD staff charged with CDBG-DR program administration have not provided the same level of daily face-to-face interaction and dialogue with local governments and individual post-disaster aid recipients as other FEMA and state grant program managers typically do. The ability to draw lessons from the more flexible CDBG program and apply them to other more narrowly defined post-disaster recovery grant programs described in this paper while developing an enhanced and enduring CDBG-DR engagement strategy with future grant recipients (to include pre- and post-disaster training and capacity building initiatives) could conceivable improve both approaches.[6]

Direct assistance to local governments can take many forms, including grants, loans, and insurance proceeds. Funds may include federal grants to provide the financial capital needed to continue governmental operations and services, loans obtained through lending companies to finance reconstruction activities not covered by public sector programs, insurance payouts for insured facilities, and the incorporation of risk reduction measures into the recovery and reconstruction process. At the individual and family level, funds may include federal funding to make temporary repairs to damaged housing; individual loans procured through local banks, lending institutions, relatives, or the Small Business Administration; and insurance proceeds.[7] Challenges remain, particularly for poor families that may not qualify for a grant or loan.

The financial investment in pre- and post-event disaster recovery capacity building efforts in the United States remains woefully inadequate, particularly when compared to the massive, albeit episodic expenditures made after a federally-declared disaster occurs. The overemphasis on post-disaster assistance has had several negative effects. One, because communities do not receive significant assistance unless they have been impacted by a major disaster, their capacity to recover from an extreme event when it does occur remains low. Thus, it should not be surprising that recovery outcomes are often suboptimal, lengthy processes that may leave the community in worse shape than it was before the disaster. Two, there is little incentive for communities to be proactive and adopt forward-looking strategies that embrace hazard mitigation measures, for instance, when they believe that sufficient post-disaster aid is available regardless of the pre-disaster choices made by them.[8]

Pre- and post-disaster planning grants have the potential to positively influence disaster recovery outcomes if specific changes to existing guidance and requirements are made. Grants that are most relevant to disaster recovery include comprehensive local planning grants, hazard mitigation planning grants, and post-disaster recovery planning grants. In many states, funds are provided to local governments to develop comprehensive land use plans. These plans are intended to serve as a means to develop a common vision of the future and the steps needed to achieve it. Given that these plans should be developed through an extensive participatory process and possess regulatory and legal standing they should provide a good way to help chart the recovery process should a disaster strike. However, many communities have not incorpo-

---

[6] Options to improve the delivery of CDBG-DR include the hiring of additional HUD field staff that are committed to work more closely (and for an extended period of time in the field) with states, communities, and individual grant recipients on a pre- and post-disaster basis and enhancing the existing working relationship with FEMA's Community Planning and Capacity Building (CPCB) teams. Each FEMA regional office now includes CPCB officials tasked with assisting states and communities develop disaster recovery plans and build local recovery capacity. Addressing the initial option will require an organizational change at HUD to become more committed to placing staff in the field for long periods of time after disasters rather than simply releasing funds and expecting states and local governments to possess the capacity to implement them with little support. The ability to more effectively use the latter approach to disseminate HUD CDBG-DR information through the CPCB will require the development of clear messaging agreed to by both HUD and FEMA as grant administrators may be reticent to have "non-experts" deliver what amounts to highly technical and nuanced information to potential grant recipients.

[7] Insurance coverage varies by income and race. Low-income minorities are less likely to obtain and maintain insurance than middle income non-minority populations. Similarly, renters, which are disproportionately comprised of lower-income tenants, are less likely to maintain insurance relative to homeowners, in part because of mortgage-based requirements. Of those that live in and adjacent to flood-prone areas, low-income residents are less likely to maintain flood insurance and may be unaware that homeowners insurance does not cover flood-related losses.

[8] Hazard mitigation planning research has shown that many local governments have developed plans that meet minimal requirements in order to remain eligible for pre- and post-disaster funding rather than as a means to reduce hazard risk (Smith, 2009).

rated recovery actions in the comprehensive plan. In most cases, if disaster recovery has been addressed at all, it is located in an annex to their local emergency management plan, which like the National Response Framework, places a strong emphasis on response, not disaster recovery goals. While there are federal funds that can be used to pay for the development of pre-disaster recovery plans, like Hazard Mitigation Assistance (HMA) program, Emergency Management Performance Grants (EMPG), and the Homeland Security Grant Program (HSGP), local governments have to make the development of recovery plans a priority as the noted grant programs have historically been used to fund hazard mitigation projects (HMA) and response-related activities (EMPG and HSGP).[9]

The disconnect between plans developed by land use planners and emergency managers is a real problem. The disaster recovery process involves a myriad set of challenges tied to grants administration, building code regulations and permitting, the reconstruction of damaged infrastructure and housing, environmental restoration, economic development, and the reconstitution of social networks. In many ways, these issues are the purview of the land use planner. Yet many of the major funding streams that flow from federal and state agencies are associated with the Stafford Act, the federal legislation that governs FEMA's roles and responsibilities in the aftermath of a disaster. The more recent passage of the Disaster Mitigation Act of 2000 and the Post-Katrina Emergency Management Reform Act also serve to clarify and expand these roles. Thus, much of post-disaster federal funding assistance flows through FEMA and is managed by state and local emergency management offices. Yet, the development of a community's future-oriented vision is largely the responsibility of land use planners. The ability to link post-disaster funding, which serves as a key implementation vehicle for recovery and the community's vision of *recovery* is not always clear as few communities have actually developed a recovery plan in advance of a disaster (Smith, 2010).

The Disaster Mitigation Act of 2000 has the potential to play an important role in shaping post-disaster recovery outcomes that are more resilient. These plans are intended to identify ways to reduce future risk through specific projects (e.g., relocation of flood-prone homes out of the flood plain, the strengthening of infrastructure to better withstand the forces of earthquakes) and policies (e.g., the adoption of more stringent building codes and the disinvestment of capital improvements in high hazard areas) based on their assessment of risk. The plans also provide a means to implement identified projects post-disaster as a federally-declared disaster triggers the release of Hazard Mitigation Grant Program funding. A 6-year study assessing the quality of state and local hazard mitigation plans has found, however, that many of the plans represent a means to an end, namely, ensuring access to post-disaster hazard mitigation funds rather than serving as a future-oriented vehicle to help guide future development away from known hazard areas (Berke and Smith, 2009, p. 7; Lyles et al., 2014; Smith, 2010).

The passage of the Post-Katrina Emergency Management Reform Act has sought to place greater emphasis on disaster recovery, to include planning. While several congressional investigations following Hurricane Katrina have led to the development of the National Disaster Recovery Framework (NDRF),[10] the NDRF is still being operationalized almost 10 years after Katrina struck. Specific tasks currently underway include the development of state and local recovery planning guidance, the hiring of federal recovery coordinators in each FEMA region, and the provision of post-disaster planning assistance through the

---

[9] A number of programs that have a distinct response orientation could be modified to address pre-disaster recovery needs, including local planning and other key capacity building initiatives. Examples of specific actions include: (1) a shift in FEMA's Community Planning and Capacity Building group to include a greater commitment to pre-event disaster recovery planning; (2) the modification of the Emergency Management Assistance Compact to include a greater emphasis on the sharing of resources that are focused on disaster recovery (rather than just response); (3) the modification of emergency management accreditation programs to include a greater emphasis on recovery; (4) the expansion of the roles associated with the members of National Volunteer Organizations Active in Disasters; and (5) the expansion of the Community Emergency Response Teams to include preparing for disaster recovery (see Smith, 2011, pp. 345-361). Similar challenges remain in the health profession as the Hospital Preparedness Program (HPP), Public Health Emergency Preparedness (PHEP) performance measures focus on disaster preparedness and not disaster recovery.

[10] FEMA has developed a series of frameworks addressing response, hazard mitigation, and disaster recovery. The reluctance to refer to these documents as plans stems, in part, because of their general reluctance to be overly prescriptive regarding the guidance provided to states and local governments. However, the frameworks can be vague and offer limited direction for states and local governments.

Community Planning and Capacity Building team. While planning guidance encourages states and local governments to develop pre-disaster recovery plans, they are not required. Nor is significant pre-event assistance (e.g., capacity building) provided. Rather, emphasis remains on the provision of assistance following a federally-declared disaster where CPCB staff assist communities develop post-disaster recovery plans.

The Sandy Recovery Improvement Act of 2013 represents another piece of legislation crafted after a major disaster that strives to address long-standing problems associated with disaster recovery.[11] Broad aims include efforts to improve the quality and efficiency of recovery through a number of amendments to the Stafford Act. More specific provisions include: (1) streamlining HMGP and PA grant procedures and emphasizing greater flexibility in order to speed the disbursement of funds; (2) expanding rental housing assistance options; (3) expanding the use of Alternative Dispute Resolution techniques to resolve grant disputes; and (4) creating a national strategy for reducing future risk (Brown et al., 2013). The improvements in funding, to include specific changes in grant rules that enhance flexibility and streamline procedural requirements (which have the potential to better address local needs and enhance the speed of disaster assistance) represent important advances in federal grant programs. The overriding emphasis on grants administration in the Sandy Recovery Act of 2013 provides another example of a government-centric approach focused on the post-disaster release of funding, without a similar commitment to pre-event planning, to include how good pre-event plans engage the larger network of resource providers in the collaborative development of coordinated funding strategies that better meet local needs and are appropriately timed.

The last proposed measure in the Sandy Recovery Improvement Act (creating a national strategy for reducing risk) is also significant in that it points out a gap in the capacity of federal agencies to craft national policy in a timely, yet thoughtful manner. The action proposed in the Sandy Recovery Improvement Act, for instance, is very similar to the existing National Mitigation Framework, which at the time the post-Sandy legislation was written, was more than a year overdue (Brown et al., 2013, p. 22). The National Mitigation Framework has since been approved as part of Presidential Policy Directive 8: National Preparedness (PPD-8). As evidenced by PKEMRA and the Sandy Recovery Improvement Act of 2013, much of our national disaster policymaking remains reactionary, piecemeal, and slow to implement. Further evidence of this problem is the fact that much of the Sandy Improvement Act of 2013 was proposed several years ago as part of the Disaster Recovery Act (Brown et al., 2013, pp. 25-26).[12] While we often associate capacity building initiatives with states and local governments, it is evident that additional resources (perhaps drawn from the more active engagement of the larger network) are needed to build the capacity of federal agencies to craft and implement sound national policy, including those policies that link planning and the provision of disaster recovery funding.

DISASTER RECOVERY FUNDING PROVIDERS AND RECIPIENTS

There are a number of entities that provide and receive pre- and post-disaster recovery funding across the disaster recovery assistance network as shown in Figure B-1. One of the great challenges in disaster recovery is to effectively coordinate the distribution and timing of these funds. Members of the public sector, including federal, state, and local government agencies disburse, manage, and receive monetary

[11] The history of national disaster policymaking in the United States is highly reactionary, as policy shifts tend to occur following major disasters (Rubin and Renda-Tanali, 2001).

[12] Many of the proposed changes to disaster recovery approved following Hurricane Sandy were initially part of the Disaster Recovery Act of 2012 which was passed by the Senate in the 112th Congress (H.R. 1) but never ratified. The Disaster Recovery Act of 2012 was part of the Senate-passed Disaster Relief Appropriations Act, 2013 that was not taken up for a vote in the 112th House. Key provisions of the proposed Disaster Recovery Act were drawn from Smith (2011, pp. 321-376). Broad actions proposed by Smith include (1) Conduct an audit of state and local disaster recovery plans; (2) Mandate state and local recovery planning; (3) Mandate the use of Alternative Dispute Resolution to address pre- and post-disaster recovery conflicts; (4) Establish collaborative leadership initiatives; (5) Develop an education, training, and outreach agenda; (6) Establish a national recovery coalition through improved planning practices; (7) Assess and modify emergency management programs and the scope of plans; and (8) Enhance local self-reliance and accountability: Create a culture of planning for recovery.

assistance in the form of grants and loans. The distribution of federal post-disaster funds following a presidentially declared disaster tends to overwhelm state and local governments who are often ill-prepared to manage budgets of this size. Focusing on the administration of these funds at the state and local level tends to shift attention away from a thoughtful discourse surrounding other issues such as achieving pre-existing state and community goals, coordinating federal assistance with other types of aid that comes from the larger assistance network, and ensuring that socially vulnerable populations are receiving the help they need (Smith, 2011).

The manner in which post-disaster federal assistance flows to states, local governments, and individuals necessitates close attention by recipients and further complicates the recovery process, including the ability to "plan" in the aftermath of a disaster. Among the most difficult issues for local governments to address is the uncertainty associated with when they will receive varied grant program funding to implement recovery and reconstruction efforts. Considering the interconnected elements of recovery, such as the clearing of debris, the repair of damaged infrastructure, and the reconstitution of affected neighborhoods, the inability to easily determine when differing funds will be available to implement identified projects in a logical manner often results in recovery outcomes being driven by these ambiguous timelines rather than a more coherent, integrative approach.

Each governmental layer involved in this process adds complexity and uncertainty. Federal programs have varied rules that affect the timing of its delivery. For instance, HMGP funds are extremely difficult to administer. It is not uncommon for an individual grant recipient like a homeowner who is slated to have their home acquired to wait for more than a year to receive these funds.[13] Federal programs, which are administered through a number of agencies in regional offices located across the United States, possess widely differing levels of capacity to manage these programs due to staffing levels and post-disaster experience.

States, which often serve as "pass through" organizations responsible for administering federal grants like HMGP, PA, and CDBG, in coordination with local governments, have differing levels of disaster experience and staffing capacity, which can dramatically affect the speed with which federal funds ultimately reach local governments and individuals (Smith, 2011; Smith et al., 2013). State officials in various agencies work with federal agency representatives and local government officials to assess post-disaster needs and determine if damages sustained to infrastructure, critical facilities, and housing are eligible for assistance. State responsibilities also include creating prioritization plans for certain grants like HMGP and CDBG, whereby the state establishes the types of projects that can be funded, recognizing broader federal guidelines such as "cost-effectiveness" in the case of HMGP and assisting a determined percentage of low-income disaster recipients as prescribed under HUD CDBG guidelines. Additional restrictions can be placed on the receipt of federal assistance, although this is uncommon. Evidence suggests that this is due to concerns about further slowing down a process that is already mired in bureaucracy (Smith et al., 2013). State restrictions on federal grant programs may require receiving jurisdictions to adopt higher codes and standards than currently exist or requiring the development of plans or policies as a precursor to the release of funds.[14]

Some states create disaster recovery programs tied to ongoing revenue sources or "rainy day" funds. State programs are developed to address needs that are unmet by federal assistance. In the case of state

---

[13] The development of a pre-disaster hazard mitigation project, linked to a disaster recovery plan which establishes a framework for post-disaster decision making, can significantly speed up this process. A comparison between two disasters that struck the same community provides a powerful case in point. Following Hurricane Fran, which struck North Carolina in 1996, it took 1 year to develop and approve the acquisition of approximately 360 flood-damaged homes using HMGP funds. After all of the available HMGP funds were expended, Kinston, North Carolina, developed a HMGP application in anticipation of a future disaster and the release of additional funding. The grant was developed in close coordination with state and federal officials, all of whom had gained valuable knowledge in the development of an eligible grant application following Hurricane Fran. Three years later, Hurricane Floyd struck, devastating the town again. This time, it took approximately 1 week to have a grant approved for the acquisition of more than 300 homes and funds began to flow into the community shortly thereafter (Smith, 2011, p. 65).

[14] In North Carolina following Hurricane Fran, the state required communities receiving HMGP funds to develop hazard mitigation plans. This requirement pre-dated the similar stipulation adopted by FEMA under the Disaster Mitigation Act of 2000.

funds, local governments apply for these resources through a grant application process created by the administering agency. State agencies responsible for the administration of these funds tend to align with the nature of the grant and may include state emergency management, community development, environmental management, and social services.

Local government departments often represent the recipients of post-disaster federal and state assistance. For instance, public works departments, working closely with the jurisdictions financial management department, may be responsible for the administration of Public Assistance funds used to repair damaged infrastructure, whereas the housing and economic development department may assume responsibility for the management of an HMGP grant to acquire flood-prone properties. In many cases, local governments contract with consultants to assist in the writing of grant proposals as well as their implementation once approved.

While nonprofits, volunteer organizations, and foundations often seek to assist those whose needs are not met by federal and state assistance programs, and their ability to act is not as constrained by bureaucratic rules that slow monetary assistance, the very organizational culture that makes them more nimble can hinder overall recovery efforts. Nonprofits can grow impatient with more bureaucratic organizations and provide assistance without coordinating with government agencies. It is also important to recognize that nonprofits and foundations vary in terms of the speed with which they can assist others. For instance, the Salvation Army has proven more adept at identifying local needs and delivering targeted assistance more rapidly than the Red Cross, which has proven less organizationally responsive (GAO, 2006; Smith, 2011, pp. 131-132).[15] Foundations, which may assume public or private characteristics, provide grants directly to individuals or local organizations tasked with recovery-related activities. The actions of foundations can prove critically important as local nonprofits are often over taxed after disasters and benefit from post-disaster funding which can be used to augment their capacity to assist their constituents or serve as a pass through for targeted disaster assistance funding.[16]

Quasi-governmental organizations, which include regional planning organizations, community development corporations, and homeowners associations perform many of the duties assumed by governments, including those following disasters. Examples include land use plan-making, code development and enforcement, grants management, and other contracted services as assigned. Regional planning organizations, for instance, are often contracted by local governments to write pre- and post-disaster recovery plans as well as write and administer post-disaster grants received by communities. Community development corporations may seek funds to repair or reconstruct damaged affordable housing as private sector developers may not view this as a profitable venture.

A host of private-sector organizations strongly influence recovery outcomes, including corporations, businesses, insurance companies, investment firms, and consultants. Corporations may provide financial assistance to communities or employees that reside in an affected area. In other cases, corporation may provide donations to a foundation or non-profit to distribute as they see fit. The return of businesses to an area affected by disaster can signal an important part of the overall recovery process as they can begin to provide needed goods and services needed by those who seek to return to their communities. Examples include home improvement retailers who provide building materials and white goods that are needed to repair damaged housing as well as small businesses who offer specialized services unique to the area. The distribution of insurance claims are vital to community and household recovery and provide an economic stimulus as these funds are re-injected into the community. Investment firms, developers, and construction

---

[15] The Red Cross has a congressional mandate to provide assistance and is thus encumbered by rules established in Washington, DC. The Salvation Army is a more decentralized organization that allows for more local autonomy and improvisation (Smith, 2011, p. 138).

[16] Foundation-based funding is driven by the makeup and orientation of board members who ultimately shape the distribution of monetary aid. In some cases this may not match local needs. Foundations, like other organizations that provide funding, want to be able to demonstrate their relevance and this can manifest itself in the quick rather than thoughtful distribution of funding or the release of funds to address an issue highlighted by the media rather than one explicitly needed by underrepresented groups (Smith, 2011, pp. 140-141, 171).

firms provide the capital, plans, and manpower to physically rebuild damaged housing, businesses, public facilities, and infrastructure. Consultants, many of whom specialize in post-disaster recovery activities, assist local governments in writing and implementing grants, picking up disaster-generated debris, and writing plans. The practice of post-disaster recovery, like emergency management as a whole, is becoming increasingly privatized which has important implications. Some research suggests that private sector firms are more nimble and able to specialize in post-disaster recovery whereas other research suggests that private contractors may not have the best interests of a community in mind and are influenced by profit motive, leading to shoddy construction, price gouging, and unscrupulous business practices.

Following major disasters like Hurricane Katrina, international aid organizations and nations attempted to provide a range of resources, including monetary donations to U.S. based foundations and technical assistance (e.g., search and rescue crews, medical teams, and engineering-based assistance tied to the repair of damaged levee infrastructure). Much of the assistance was not accepted as the United States did not have in place clear international protocols to accept disaster aid from other nations or the aid was offered by nations in which the United States does not maintain positive diplomatic relationships. In the case of the former, the concept of "absorptive capacity," which is typically applied to developing nations (Harrell-Bond, 1986) can be applied to the United States which did not have in place the means to accept and use the external assistance offered (Smith, 2011, pp. 198-199). In the case of the later example, the establishment of conditions under which the assistance will be accepted is referred to as "conditionality," (Susskind, 1994, pp. 18-24) and can hinder the likelihood that a receiving nation will accept that assistance. In the case of the United States, President Bush was reticent to accept offers from other nations, stating the United States had the capacity to address recovery needs.

In Ilan Kelman's concept of disaster diplomacy, nations that view themselves as "enemies," can in fact work together collaboratively after disaster through the sending and willing receipt of assistance. Following Katrina several examples exist in which disaster diplomacy failed. For instance, the offer of Cuban physicians was met by a response from the White House that effectively said the United States would not accept this aid until Fidel Castro was no longer in power (Smith, 2011, p. 201). Additional examples include Argentina's offer of physicians, the willingness of the British to deliver meals ready to eat (which were destroyed due to fears of mad cow disease), and the use of Greek cruise ships for use as hotels or hospitals (which were ultimately turned down once it was realized that it would take over a month to process the needed paperwork) (Smith, 2011, p. 203).

The difficulties experienced by the United States in accepting international assistance is troubling considering that international aid is routinely delivered to other nations as part of the missions of several U.S. organizations like the United States Agency for International Development (USAID) and the Office of Foreign Disaster Assistance (OFDA). The ability to draw lessons from these experiences, including concepts like absorptive capacity, conditionality, and disaster diplomacy, was seemingly ignored, nor was it used to critically assess our own ability to accept aid from other nations and make necessary changes in international relief protocols. Hurricane Katrina has led to a further examination of this issue, which merits increased attention, particularly in light of the global ramifications of a changing climate and how this affects weather patterns both in the United States and abroad. Significant concerns remain as the United States has largely failed to effectively incorporate lessons from developing nations regarding post-disaster recovery, including the value of investing in pre-event capacity building measures (which is a long-standing approach used in international development strategies) and the importance of drawing on deeply held indigenous knowledge as a means to better understand local needs.

The creation of emergent groups after disasters is well documented in the response literature, as groups form in reaction to an issue that is perceived to merit increased attention and such group tends to dissolve once the problem is addressed. Much less attention has been placed on emergent groups in disaster recovery as evidenced both in the existing academic literature on recovery as well as in practice. Members of emergent groups are lacking in most pre-disaster recovery plans (in part because they do not exist prior to a disaster), nor do emergent groups tend to be adequately involved in post-disaster decision making, even though they play important roles in filling gaps in disaster recovery assistance networks (Smith,

2011, pp. 244-245). The involvement of these groups in recovery can be planned for and incorporated into policy making and resource distribution processes when a disaster occurs. The rapid identification of these groups post-disaster and their meaningful involvement in recovery operations provides another example of the value of pre-disaster planning and adaptive post-disaster actions. Examples of emergent group actions include assisting non-English speaking individuals [to] apply for assistance, advocating for limited post-disaster redevelopment in flood-prone areas, promoting the construction of low-income post-disaster housing and providing free bicycles for those without an automobile following Hurricane Katrina (Smith, 2011, p. 243).

Individuals, including their social networks, possess a vital awareness of local conditions in a community, yet these resources are often underutilized by larger disaster recovery assistance networks. In some ways this is manifest in the labeling of individuals as "disaster victims," implying a helplessness and an inability to act to confront the challenges following a disaster. The discounting of their importance in recovery can be seen in limited engagement and empowerment strategies in which individuals are actively involved in conveying needs and developing or modifying existing policies and funding strategies provided by others. In the immediate aftermath of a disaster, individuals are typically the first providers of assistance through search and rescue activities, sheltering, and provision of food. In long-term recovery, individuals, who may experience an initial psychological shock, often feel a higher purpose which drives more self-directed actions (Hoffman, 1999; Smith, 2011, p. 241). Research has shown that individuals and households recovering from a disaster rely on a mix of autonomous, kinship, and institutional resources. Autonomous resources include personally held financial, material, and individual skills. Kinship resources include those delivered by family, friends, and associates which vary according to the level of damage sustained to the provider's property, distance from one another, and the potential harm faced during the delivery process. Institutional resources include that delivered by others in the larger disaster assistance network. The ability to make sense of the myriad funding programs and their confusing rules can prove overwhelming and the ability to decipher them benefits from past disaster experience as well as boundary-spanning organizations like nonprofit organizations who may serve as case managers.

A TEMPORAL REVIEW OF DISASTER RECOVERY FUNDING

Next, we discuss the timing of funding across the disaster recovery assistance network, emphasizing pre- and post-disaster timeframes. Pre-event recovery activities that influence the access to funding involve preparedness, planning, and capacity-building initiatives. An important reality remains in that many local and state governments invest little funding in disaster recovery preparedness, planning, and capacity-building initiatives, often resulting in significant hardships when, in fact, they must confront the many challenges of disaster recovery after an extreme event. Pre-event preparedness activities may include the identification of members of their disaster recovery assistance network, including those that are local as well as external providers of assistance (e.g., state, federal, and international). Planning efforts include developing, exercising, monitoring, implementing, and updating disaster recovery plan over time. It is critically important to involve members of the disaster recovery assistance network (identified as part of preparedness activities) to include the development of mutually agreeable goals, objectives, and policies that drive the temporally coordinated use of the resources they possess. Capacity-building actions, ideally delivered prior to a disaster, involve education, training, and outreach efforts, of which planning can play an important role. The act of planning serves as a capacity building process achieved through learning about one another's roles and capabilities and enhancing the collective capacity of the group through the optimization of resources (e.g., limiting duplicative or contradictory funding strategies) that are undergirded by a common set of goals identified in the recovery plan. Another approach used to optimize resources could involve the reprogramming of existing funds already awarded to communities. Reprogramming already distributed funding may prove difficult to achieve in practice due to rules governing their use after being awarded. An alternative involves the creation of a pre-disaster collaborative process spanning funding providers to establish a funding eligibility matrix tied to agreeable goals. For instance, CDBG funds can be used to assist with the repair of low-income housing. The degree to which these funds also increase disaster resilience varies because federal rules do not require it and state agencies responsible for crafting eligibility rules in their respective states may not have considered it an important criterion. Good pre-disaster recovery planning, including the creation of committees tasked with addressing the coordination of pre- and post-disaster funding streams, should embrace this responsibility.

Post-disaster recovery activities are described in three temporally-defined phases: (1) response and the transition to short-term recovery, (2) mid-term, and (3) long-term recovery. It is important to note that the characterization of the recovery process as a simple linear process discounts the reality that recovery is achieved at different speeds and through differing pathways at the community and individual level (Smith, 2011, pp. 19-22). While there is not a clear line of demarcation separating the initial response and short-term recovery, the actions taken immediately after a disaster can shape what follows.

Response and short-term recovery activities include the provision of feeding operations (e.g., feeding stations provided by the Salvation Army, Red Cross, and other nonprofit and emergent groups); sheltering (e.g., evacuation shelters like those provided by the Red Cross, hotels, or staying with family and friends); preliminary mental health interventions (e.g., psychological first aid); non-emergency medical care and prescription access; early debris clearing efforts (e.g., clearing roadways for emergency access to hospitals and other critical facilities); and the provision of generators and early restoration of power. The funding of these emergency services are typically reimbursable by state and federal emergency management agencies if a state or federal disaster declaration has occurred. Depending on the scale (breadth of impact) and type (e.g., Tohoku earthquake and tsunami and resulting damages to the Fukushima Daiichi nuclear plant) of disaster and the capacity of local, state, and federal agencies (and the larger disaster recovery assistance network), this phase of the disaster can take days or even months to achieve. These characteristics can also differentially shape the temporal distribution of recovery as those communities and networks with fewer resources may be much slower to recover than others and these variations occur at multiple scales, including neighborhoods, households, and individuals. Further, response-related funds often carry over into the intermediate phase of recovery.

Specific actions undertaken during the intermediate phase of recovery include the provision of transitional housing (e.g., FEMA-provided trailers and rental assistance), temporary education and public services facilities; provision of monetary aid to allow for normal governmental operations (e.g., meeting payroll, hiring of additional staff, meeting existing and new financial obligations); continued mental health interventions; access to medical and social services, the restoration of public infrastructure (e.g., the complete restoration of power, water, and sewer services); the repair and reconstruction of damaged public infrastructure; the provision of economic redevelopment assistance (e.g., post-disaster employment, delivery of economic development grants and loans); and post-disaster planning for long-term recovery.[17]

During the long-term phase of disaster recovery, communities must confront a number of complex issues tied to rebuilding and reconstruction, including decisions surrounding the degree to which hazard mitigation is incorporated into recovery; the restoration of environmental systems; economic redevelopment; and the reconstitution of social networks. Hazard mitigation, or the adoption of policies and projects intended to reduce future hazard risk and exposure, is often achieved in the aftermath of a disaster when funds are available for this purpose. Specific measures may include the relocation or elevation of flood-prone housing, the strengthening (retrofit) of public facilities and infrastructure, the adoption of new or modified codes and standards, the use of hazards-based insurance (e.g., flood, wind, fire or earthquake), and the proactive application of land use tools and techniques (e.g., capital improvements planning, cluster development, open space preservation, transfer of development rights). During the recovery process this may include the disinvestment of public and private assets (e.g., infrastructure, housing, public facilities)

---

[17] While the development of disaster recovery plans are ideally developed before a disaster occurs, thereby providing the time needed for disaster recovery committees and the larger public to discuss the complexities of recovery and develop coordinative strategies to address them, recovery plans are often developed in the aftermath of a disaster. The development of these plans often begins as communities transition out of the immediate response and into the early phase of recovery as a number of pressing issues limit the time that can be devoted to a thoughtful planning process.

in high hazard areas and the resettlement in less vulnerable locations. The application of hazard mitigation techniques to housing-related issues, including relocation provides an interesting case in point. The choices made by federal, state, and local governments regarding the use of post-disaster mitigation funds can powerfully influence the choices made by individuals. For instance, hazard mitigation funds are disproportionately used for owner-occupied housing versus rental properties. This can have the effect of assisting homeowners who may be more wealthy (on average) than renters.

The adoption of new or strengthened codes and standards can play an important role in reducing future losses. The adoption of new standards may be influenced by the real or perceived additional costs and the ability of proponents to adequately convey their benefits. Developing higher standards post-disaster may be opposed by some who see these additional requirements as restraining the pace of reconstruction or adding to the costs of repairs and new development in the affected area.

Additional factors shaping the adoption of new standards include the ability to collect and analyze the data required to select "appropriate" code standards. The analysis and re-mapping of such areas takes time and may result in the development of initial maps that depict an assessment that may need to be refined over time but can be used to help inform post-disaster reconstruction. Challenges remain when using this approach as communities must decide whether to adopt these new standards and associated maps in lieu of existing codes. In addition, new temporary standards require the vigilant enforcement of these advisory maps during a time when building code officials are overtaxed reviewing the influx of permits that invariably follow a major disaster.

The determination of appropriate codes and standards can be problematic as they are designed to withstand the hazard forces (e.g., high water, storm surge, ground motion, wind speed) associated a given "return period" event (e.g., 100-year flood or 1-percent annual chance event). The development of standards to a set return period event does not effectively account for the dynamism of hazards and the effects of growth in hazardous areas and adjacent locales. For instance, barrier islands are inexorably moving toward the mainland as part of a natural process. The construction of homes, infrastructure, and businesses, which are placed in a fixed location, must regularly confront this dynamism. Options include building protective measures like levees and seawalls, implementing beach re-nourishment and dune restoration projects, elevating structures, or limiting development in vulnerable locations. Researchers have coined the term "safe development paradox" to describe the false sense of security that protective measures can provide. The funding of these types of measures has the effect of encouraging development in these areas, leading to even larger disasters when the design parameters of levees and seawalls are exceeded, leading to increasing post-disaster payouts (Burby and French, 1981; Burby et al., 2006).

Growth in and adjacent to hazardous areas can also exacerbate risk as new development in floodplains, for instance, results in an increase in impervious surface, which speeds rainfall runoff, leading to increased flood elevations relative to what may be reflected on Flood Insurance Rate Maps developed in the past. Structures built to what amount to outdated codes and standards suffer the consequences. Upstream development and development adjacent to the floodplain can also increase flood hazard vulnerability as the cumulative effects are realized.

The adroit use of pre- and post-disaster funding can be used to address may of the shortfalls addressed in this paper, including the development and implementation of a strategy emphasizing sustainability and disaster resilience (Burby and Dalton, 1994; Burby, 1998). Ideally this involves drawing on pre-existing goals and incorporating them into post-disaster "opportunities" identified through a robust community engagement effort. The integration of physical, social, economic, and environmental dimensions, achieved through the implementation of complementary policies and projects, requires gaining access to the funds needed to realize these aspirations.

A Hypothetical Disaster Recovery Scenario

While drawing on the myriad resources of the disaster recovery assistance network is critically important, it is equally important to develop a strategy or plan to help shape the integration and temporal distribution of these assets. The development and implementation of an agreed upon plan greatly increases a community's chances of successfully achieving this aim. The following hypothetical example provides a simplified explanation of this process. Following a major flood, a community begins to assess the effects of the event. Based on the assessment, the disaster merits a presidential disaster declaration, which triggers the release of federal aid as well as the assistance of the larger disaster recovery assistance network. As part of the recovery process, the community assesses its needs and forms a disaster recovery committee.

The committee identifies existing local policies and plans that pre-date the disaster and assesses how these documents can inform the development of a disaster recovery plan. As part of this assessment, those policies that contradict the aims of the recovery plan's goals (as developed by the committee and citizen involvement) may be modified to reflect the recovery plan's vision. One of the plans that should be assessed is their hazard mitigation plan, which should identify the hazards prevalent in their community as well as the vulnerability of their assets (e.g., housing, infrastructure, critical public facilities) to these hazards. The policy and plan review, commonly referred to as a capability assessment, and the risk assessment form the fact base upon which recovery policies are developed.

If we assume a primary vision of the recovery plan is to achieve a more resilient future, a set of goals are developed that address physical, economic, social, and environmental themes. Each of these goals are supported by policies and projects that include established implementation timelines. Careful attention should be placed on the development of policies and projects that are complimentary in nature to both individual goals as well as the larger plan's vision.

For instance, let's assume the community and its citizens decide to relocate a flood damaged community out of the flood plain. Once the land is acquired and the properties removed, the area might become a greenway, thereby reducing future flood-related damages, improving water quality, and enhancing public health and recreational opportunities. In addition, the property adjacent to the greenway may increase in value. Thus this one measure achieves multiple, integrated benefits for the community. If we assume the area was comprised of low-income residents, care must be taken to identify the means to relocate these residents to safe and decent housing. In addition, thoughtful consideration should be given to relocating the entire neighborhood to another area, thereby maintaining social networks, or identifying scattered housing sites throughout the community to avoid the aggregation of low-income housing.

Achieving a resilient future means more than taking steps to make a community less vulnerable to future disasters, as this brief hypothetical scenario suggests. As descried earlier in this paper, recovery also involves the clearing of debris; the restoration of damaged infrastructure; the provision of temporary and permanent housing solutions; the reconstruction of damaged public facilities, businesses, and housing; the repair of damaged ecosystems; and the reconstitution of disrupted social networks. It also means drawing on the resources held by members of the assistance network to achieve these aims. It also means collectively learning from past events and developing a sustained approach that is incorporated into the day-to-day activities of all members of the disaster assistance network.

KEY CHALLENGES AND OPPORTUNITIES TO ACHIEVING DISASTER RESILIENT OUTCOMES

Achieving disaster resilient outcomes following disasters is challenging, and is closely tied to the way in which funding assistance is provided across a network of stakeholders. Among the most problematic issues are the delivery of funding in isolation, narrowly defined programs that do not address local needs, creating and maintaining issue salience surrounding disaster recovery, and the timing of assistance. Most members of the assistance network provide funding in a way that is not coordinated with others, leading to duplication, contradicting results, and ill-timed aid that often hinders the ability of communities to achieve disaster resilient outcomes. Addressing the issues common to disaster recovery remains difficult as pre-disaster recovery planning is less salient to local officials, particularly when compared to pressing day-to-day activities.

In the aftermath of a disaster there is an intense pressure to return to a sense of normalcy, even though it may take more time in the short run to inject resilience measures into recovery. The common refrain among locally elected as well as state and federal government officials denote a disaster as "an opportunity" to address long-standing pre-event conditions and human settlement patterns should be carefully evaluated and questioned. Critically reflecting on this statement requires asking the question: opportunities for whom and at what cost? Disasters provide a powerful means to expose pre-event conditions, including inequity, high risk, and the existence (or not) of a collaborative planning culture.

Improving resilience across physical, social, economic, and environmental domains means adopting an integrative, long-term strategy. In today's era of climate change, this means expanding our assistance network and a suite of temporally-defined strategies to include those that are engaged in understanding the linkage between our changing climate and its effects on natural hazards and disasters as well as the rapidly emerging collection of social scientists, planners, activists, engineers, and medical professionals who are developing adaptive strategies to our still emerging understanding of these episodic and long-term threats. Developing clear linkages between pre- and post-disaster recovery funding allocations and the incorporation of adaptation measures during the recovery process provide a unique "opportunity" that merits increased attention.

RECOMMENDATIONS

The following recommendations result from a distillation of the disaster recovery research and a critical assessment of existing national policy. The proposed changes, which are significant and require changes in national policy, represent a set of actions that are much needed and could be incorporated into the still emerging national dialogue surrounding disaster recovery and resilience. Two important venues provide a means through which to inject the recommendations that follow: the National Disaster Recovery Framework and Hurricane Sandy-related initiatives.

Increase the Pre-Event Investments in Capacity Building and Planning. The reluctance of federal, state, and local governments to invest the resources in pre-event capacity building and the closely associated means by which this can be achieved and ultimately acted upon through the policies and public investments identified in plans, is perhaps the single greatest problem facing those who seek to systematically address disaster resilience in a meaningful way. Today's disaster recovery policy milieu is dominated by a post-disaster orientation as evidenced by the large-scale investments in monetary assistance after a disaster strikes with a proportionately low expenditure of funds, pre-emptive policies, or training before an event occurs. Nor is there meaningful attention paid to pre-event planning for post-disaster recovery. In a recent study of local disaster recovery plans in the southeastern United States (an area highly prone to disasters) researchers found that using a liberal definition of recovery plans, less than one-third of communities had a disaster recovery plan in place and among those that did, the plans were of poor quality (Berke et al., 2014). While this is slowly changing per the National Disaster Recovery Framework, state and local pre-event recovery plans are not required in order to gain access to post-disaster assistance. Smith has suggested that while the development of recovery plans should be required, an incremental policy approach should be undertaken in tandem with an increased investment in pre-event capacity building that targets measureable improvements in the quality of those plans over time. The ultimate aim of this strategy would be to hold communities more accountable by linking the creation of high quality plans to post-disaster funding access (Smith, 2011).

Improve the Coordinated Management of Pre- and Post-Disaster Funding. Planning provides one way to improve the coordination of funding across the disaster recovery assistance network. This holds true, however, only if all members participate in a meaningful process that fosters collective action over time. Current federal initiatives to further improve governance strategies, namely the "whole of community" concept, have yet to be effectively realized through clear and actionable policies. In its current state, it is more reflective of a desired end state without guidance, rules, and a mix of incentives and sanctions furthering compliance with what still remains a broad and elusive term. Further complicating matters is the varied funding sources provided from non-governmental actors (e.g., nonprofits, businesses, quasi-governmental organizations, emergent groups, and individuals), whose compliance with governmental mandates is highly variable. Facilitating the coordinated expenditure of pre- and post-disaster funding across the assistance network, first requires gaining a depth of understanding among all providers of assistance as to the resources each provides and when they provide it. It also means identifying the underlying interests of each provider of assistance and how this is manifest in specific funding strategies. Gaining an understanding of underlying interests provides an opportunity to seek mutually compatible policies that can guide resource distribution in a cooperative manner while also identifying and modifying duplicative or counterproductive actions. One indicator of the degree to which this has occurred may be the willingness of organizations to reprogram pre-disaster funding criteria to include key disaster recovery goals such as disaster resilience.

Hold States and Local Governments More Accountable. It is incumbent on governmental actors to lead the development of clear policies that encourage—and, in some cases, require—compliance with disaster recovery program goals like achieving a more disaster resilient future if in fact post-disaster aid is an expectation following extreme events. Any shift in policy that increases accountability should be balanced with a concerted effort to build capacity both within organizations and across the larger network. Otherwise, increasing standards will likely lead to the creation of non-compliant plans or the abandonment of the process altogether.

Examples of this approach could include requiring communities and states to develop pre-disaster recovery plans that meet increasingly higher standards of practice over time, while investing in training, education, outreach, as well as providing the financial resources needed to develop these plans. Good recovery plans include strong inter-organizational coordination and implementation mechanisms, among other principles.[18]

Operationalize Broad Concepts Found in National Disaster Recovery Framework Through Coordinated Actions Implemented by Identified Members of the Disaster Recovery Assistance Network and the Passage of the Disaster Recovery Act. The good news is that attention has been placed on operationalizing the elements found in the NDRF. Examples include the national roll out of the NDRF through public meetings and conference calls, hiring of regional FEMA recovery coordinators, designation of state counterparts (state recovery coordinators), and development of FEMA committees comprised of state and local officials tasked with the development of training materials and guidance documents. However, the CPCB team has not begun a sincere effort to engage in a robust pre-disaster capacity building initiative to assist states and communities in developing and exercising recovery plans in advance of extreme events. Several factors are contributing to this still somewhat reactive approach: (1) limited federal resources and agency support to advance the aims of the NDRF, (2) the lack of a clear mandate to require the development of state and local pre-disaster recovery plans, and (3) insufficient authority to act in pre- and post-disaster plan-making settings (GAO, 2010; Smith 2011, pp. 321-323).

Following Hurricane Sandy, the CPCB team offered assistance after the disaster occurred. This has become the standard approach to recovery planning. It is incumbent on FEMA and the larger disaster recovery assistance network to engage in a more concerted pre-disaster recovery planning process, applying the tenets of good recovery planning, including in particular an emphasis on pre-event planning for post-disaster recovery. States like Florida have begun developing pre-disaster disaster recovery plans and lessons should be drawn from this process.

The adoption and more focused operationalization of the NDRF can provide the venue through which many of the problems noted in this paper can be addressed. In order for this to occur, a greater empha-

---

[18] A discussion of disaster recovery planning principles can be found in *Planning for Post-Disaster Recovery: A Review of the United States Disaster Assistance Framework* (Smith, 2011, pp. 275-292). See Sandler and Smith (2013) for a discussion of plan quality principles applied to state disaster recovery plans.

sis needs to be placed on the three previous policy recommendations, including (1) increasing pre-event investments in capacity building and planning; (2) improving the coordinated management of pre- and post-disaster funding; and (3) holding states and local governmental more accountable for their actions (and lack thereof). Any serious policy discussion should discuss the realities of funding as a motivator for action, including the need to invest substantial pre-disaster resources in planning and capacity building while gradually withholding funding from those states and local governments that do not agree to develop, adopt, exercise, and implement robust, inclusively created recovery plans. Federal legislation like the proposed Disaster Recovery Act should be passed to provide the federal government the resources they need to carry out the intent of the NDRF.

ENHANCE THE INTEGRATION OF HEALTH CARE ORGANIZATIONS AND PROVIDERS IN THE DISASTER RECOVERY ASSISTANCE NETWORK

A review of the NDRF suggests that it focuses primarily on the repair of infrastructure and places inadequate attention on "human recovery," including the psychological effects of disasters as well as acute and chronic health issues faced during recovery (Chandra and Acosta, 2010). Chandra and Acosta suggest that in order to achieve more resilient health outcomes, a clear definition of health and human recovery should be developed, benchmarks established, and a vulnerability index created to help identify pre-disaster health and social service needs in order to identify and evaluate the resources required to address them, manage expectations, and track outcomes (Chandra and Acosta, 2010, p. 1609). The broader issues (e.g., social vulnerability, resilience, and recovery metrics/indicators and outcomes) have been discussed by a number of researchers and practitioners in other disciplines, including geography, psychology, planning, emergency management, and sociology, and a growing number have begun to develop, apply, and track indices of social vulnerability, recovery, and resilience. In fact, "wellness" has been used to as an indicator of resilience and a measure by which adaptation to a stressor (e.g., disaster) has occurred (Norris et al., 2008). Yet, like many such efforts, the degree to which health-related measures are integrated into a holistic system remains unattained (NRC, 2012, p. 5). Rather, like a central challenge in recovery, medical and public health groups have tended to act in isolation, rather than as part of a larger multidisciplinary group (Shoaf and Rottman, 2000). There are existing post-disaster grant programs focused on social, health, and mental health services. For instance, the Social Services Block Grant (SSBG) program targets health care and other human service providers, including community-based organizations. Eligible costs include paying for the provision of social, health, and mental health services and the repair and reconstruction of health care facilities, child care facilities, and other social services buildings and associated infrastructure. The degree to which these programs are connected with other post-disaster grant programs varies significantly across states and local governments.

Not surprisingly, the development of indicators do not necessarily span the broad network of aid providers and recipients to include medical and public health care providers. Additional research has shown, for instance, the valued, but underutilized or misunderstood, roles in recovery of several stakeholders in health-related fields, including nongovernmental organizations (Acosta et al., 2013) and local and regional public health providers (Koh et al., 2008). The ability to include them in the disaster recovery assistance network is increasingly prescient given the additional public health threats associated with increased disasters and the inexorable shift in climate-borne health impacts, including those tied to ecological, social, and physical disruption (Greenough et al., 2001).

DISASTER RECOVERY IN THE AGE OF CLIMATE CHANGE

Disaster recovery is a complex process, affected by a number of pre- and post-disaster conditions. The effects of a changing climate and adapting to these emerging conditions represents another issue that must be addressed in a thoughtful manner, recognizing that it adds an additional layer of complexity to disaster recovery. Like disaster recovery, adaptation has been framed in the context of sustainability and resilience (Godschalk, 2003; Peacock et al., 2008). Disaster recovery in the age of climate change means planning for uncertainty. One way to confront this challenge is through the development of a flexible suite of robust and contingent adaptation strategies (Berke, 2014, p. 187). Robust strategies are often referred to as "no-regrets" actions that address a range of scenarios. Contingent strategies are designed to address specific scenarios, including worst case conditions. In some ways, disaster recovery in this new era provides an opportunity for positive change, expanded networks, and complimentary aims linking risk reduction and adaptation, both of which can be framed and acted upon in a way that advances resilience. The future sustainability and resilience of our communities depend on it.

REFERENCES

Acosta, J. D., A. Chandra, and J. S. Ringel. 2013. Nongovernmental resources to support disaster preparedness, response and recovery. *Disaster Medicine and Public Health Preparedness* 7(4):348-353.

Bates, F. L., and W. G. Peacock. 1987. Disasters and social change. In *The sociology and disasters*, edited by R. R. Dynes, B. Demarchi, and Pelanda. Milan, Italy: Franco Angeli Press. Pp. 291-330.

Berke, P. 2014. Rising to the challenge: Planning for adaptation in the age of climate change. In *Adapting to Climate Change: Lessons from Natural Hazards Planning*, Ch. 8, edited by B. Glavovic and G. Smith. New York: Springer. Pp. 171-190.

Berke, P., and T. Beatley. 1997. *After the hurricane: Linking recovery to sustainable development in the Caribbean.* Baltimore, MD: Johns Hopkins University Press.

Berke, P., and T. J. Campanella. 2006. Planning for postdisaster resiliency. *The Annals of the American Academy of Political and Social Science* 604(1):192-207.

Berke, P., and G. Smith. 2009. Hazard mitigation, planning and disaster resiliency: Challenges and strategic choices for the 21st century. In *Building safer communities: Risk, governance, spatial planning and responses to natural hazards*, Ch. 1, Vol. 58, edited by U. Fra Paleo. Amsterdam: ISO Press. Pp. 1-20.

Berke, P. R., J. Kartez, and D. Wenger. 1993. Recovery after disasters: Achieving sustainable development, mitigation and equity. *Disasters* 17(2):93-109.

Berke, P., J. Cooper, M. Aminto, J. Horney, and S. Grabich. 2014. Adaptive planning for disaster recovery and resiliency: An evaluation of 87 local recovery plans in eight states. *Journal of the American Planning Association* 80(4):310-323.

Brown, J. T., F. X. McCarthy, and E. C. Liu. 2013. *Analysis of the Sandy Recovery Improvement Act of 2013.* CRS Report 42991. Washington, DC: Congressional Research Service.

Burby, R. 1998. *Cooperating with nature: Confronting natural hazards with land-use planning for sustainable communities.* Washington, DC: Joseph Henry Press.

Burby, R. J., and L. Dalton. 1994. Plans can matter! The role of land use and state planning mandates on limiting development in hazardous areas. *Public Administration Review* 54(3):229-238.

Burby, R., and S. French. 1981. Coping with floods: The land use management paradox. *Journal of the American Planning Association* 47:289-300.

Burby, R. J., A. C. Nelson, and T. W. Sanchez. 2006. The problems containment and the promise of planning. In *Rebuilding urban places after disasters: Lessons from Hurricane Katrina*, edited by E. L. Birch and S. M. Wachter. Philadelphia: University of Pennsylvania Press.

Campanella, T. J. 2006. Urban resilience and the recovery of New Orleans. *Journal of the American Planning Association* 72(2):141-146.

Chandra, A., and J. Acosta. 2010. Disaster recovery also involves human recovery. *Journal of the American Medical Association* 304(14):1608-1609.

Freudenberg, W., R. Gramling, S. Laska, and K. Erickson. 2009. *Catastrophe in the making: The engineering of Katrina and the disasters of tomorrow.* Washington, DC: Island Press.

Friesema, P. 1979. *Aftermath: Communities after natural disasters.* Beverly Hills, CA: Sage Publications.

GAO (U.S. Government Accountability Office). 2006. *Hurricanes Katrina and Rita. Coordination between FEMA and the Red Cross should be improved for the 2006 hurricane season.* GAO-06-712. Washington, DC: GAO.

GAO. 2010. *Report to Congressional requesters. Disaster recovery: FEMA's long-term assistance was helpful to state and local governments but had some limitations.* GAO-10-404. Washington, DC: GAO.

Godschalk, D. R. 2003. Urban hazard mitigation: Creating resilient cities. *Natural Hazards Review* 4(3):136-142.

Greenough, G., M. McGeehin, S. M. Bernard, J. Trtanj, J. Riad, and D. Engelberg. 2001. The potential impacts of climate variability and change on health impacts of extreme weather events in the United States. *Environmental Health Perspectives* 109(Suppl. 2):191-198.

Harrell-Bond, E. 1986. *Imposing aid: Emergency assistance to refugees.* Oxford: Oxford University Press.

Hoffman, S. 1999. The worst of times, the best of times: Toward a model of cultural response to disaster. In *Catastrophe and culture: The anthropology of disaster,* edited by S. M. Hoffman and A. Oliver-Smith. Santa Fe, NM: School of American Research Press. Pp. 135-155.

HUD (U.S. Department of Housing and Urban Development). 2015. *CDBG-DR eligibility requirements.* https://www.hudexchange.info/cdbg-dr/cdbg-dr-eligibility-requirements (accessed June 17, 2015).

Koh, H. K., L. J. Elqura, C. M. Judge, and M. A. Soto. 2008. Regionalization of local public health systems in the era of preparedness. *Annual Review of Public Health* 29:205-218.

Lyles, W., P. Berke, and G. Smith. 2014. A comparison of local hazard mitigation plan quality in six states, USA. *Landscape and Urban Planning* 122:89-99.

NRC (National Research Council). 2012. *Disaster resilience: A national imperative.* Washington, DC: The National Academies Press.

National Emergency Management Association and the Council on State Governments. 1998. *Report on state emergency management funding and structures.* Lexington, KY: Council on State Governments.

Norris, F. H., S. P. Stevens, B. Pfefferbaum, K. F. Wyche, and R. L. Pfefferbaum. 2008. Community resilience as a metaphor, theory, set of capacities, and strategy for disaster readiness. *American Journal of Community Psychology* 41(1-2):127-150.

Olshansky, R. B. 2006. Planning after Hurricane Katrina. *Journal of the American Planning Association* 72(2):147-153.

Olshansky, R. B., and L. A. Johnson. 2010. *Clear as mud: Planning for the rebuilding of New Orleans.* Chicago, IL: American Planning Association.

Peacock, W. G., H. Kunreuther, W. H. Hooke, S. L.Cutter, S. E. Chang, and P. R. Berke. 2008. Toward a Resiliency and Vulnerability Observatory Network: RAVON. HRRC reports 08-02R. http://hrrc.arch.tamu.edu/publications/reports (accessed June 17, 2015).

Platt, R. 1999. *Disasters and democracy: The politics of extreme natural events.* Washington, DC: Island Press.

Rubin, C. B., and I. Renda-Tanali. 2001. *Disaster timeline.* Arlington, VA: Claire Rubin and Associates.

Sandler, D., and G. Smith. 2013. Assessing the quality of state disaster recovery plans: Implications for policy and practice. *Journal of Emergency Management* 11(4):281-291.

Shoaf, K. I., and S. J. Rottman. 2000. The role of public health in disaster preparedness, mitigation, response and recovery. *Prehospital and Disaster Medicine* 15(4):144-146.

Smith, G. 2009. Planning for sustainable and disaster resilient communities. In *Natural hazards analysis: Reducing the impact of disasters,* Ch. 9, edited by J. Pine. Boca Raton, FL: CRC Press. Pp. 221-247.

Smith, G. 2010. Disaster recovery planning in the United States: Lessons for the Australasian audience. Special Issue of the *Australasian Journal of Disaster and Trauma Studies. Natural Hazards Planning in Australasia,* ISSN:1174-4707, Vol. 2010-1.

Smith, G. 2011. *Planning for post-disaster recovery: A review of the United States Disaster Assistance Framework.* Washington, DC: Island Press.

Smith, G. 2014. Disaster recovery in Coastal Mississippi (USA): Lesson drawing from Hurricanes Camille and Katrina. In *Adapting to climate change: Lessons from natural hazards planning,* Ch.14, edited by B. Glavovic and G. Smith. New York: Springer. Pp. 339-368.

Smith, G., and D. Wenger. 2006. Sustainable disaster recovery: Operationalizing an existing framework. In *Handbook of Disaster Research,* edited by H. Rodriguez, E. Quarantelli, and R. Dynes. New York: Springer. Pp. 234-257.

Smith, G., W. Lyles, and P. Berke. 2013. The role of the state in building local capacity and commitment for hazard mitigation planning. *International Journal of Mass Emergencies and Disasters* 31(2):178-203.

Susskind, L. 1994. *Environmental diplomacy: Negotiating more effective global agreements.* New York: Oxford Press.

Vale, L., and T. Campanella. 2005. *The resilient city: How modern cities recover from disasters.* New York: Oxford University Press.

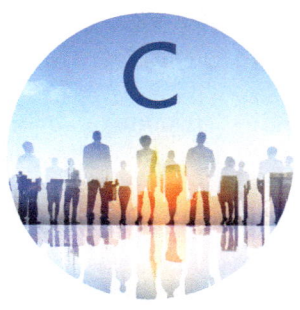

Additional Resources[1]

BUILDING SOCIAL COHESION

- Lyttelton Harbour Timebank, a program in which community members trade skills to develop local cohesion and build better trust among residents, available at http://www.lyttelton.net.nz/timebank
- SF72, an emergency preparedness program developed by the San Francisco Department of Emergency Management that emphasizes increasing social connectedness, available at http://www.sf72.org/home

DISASTER BEHAVIORAL HEALTH, EMOTIONAL, AND SPIRITUAL CARE

- Substance Abuse and Mental Health Services Administration's (SAMHSA's) *Disaster Planning Handbook for Behavioral Health Treatment Programs*, available at http://store.samhsa.gov/shin/content/SMA13-4779/SMA13-4779.pdf
- SAMHSA and the National Institute of Environmental Health Science's efforts to provide worker resiliency training before or after disasters, available at http://tools.niehs.nih.gov/wetp/index.cfm?id=2528
- SAMHSA's *Tips for Talking with and Helping Children and Youth Cope After a Disaster or Traumatic Event*, available at http://store.samhsa.gov/shin/content/SMA12-4732/SMA12-4732.pdf
- The National Center for Trauma Informed Care (NCTIC), funded by SAMHSA, provides training and technical assistance, available at http://www.samhsa.gov/nctic/training-technical-assistance
- National Child Traumatic Stress Network's *Parent Guidelines for Helping Children after a Hurricane,* available at http://www.nctsn.org/sites/default/files/assets/pdfs/parents_guidelines_talk_children_hurricanes.pdf
- National Child Traumatic Stress Network's *Helping Young Children and Families Cope with Trauma*, available at http://nctsn.org/sites/default/files/assets/pdfs/Helping_Young_Children_and_Families_Cope_with_Trauma.pdf

---

[1] All URLs are accessible as of June 17, 2015.

- National Child Traumatic Stress Network's *After the Hurricane: Helping Young Children Heal*, available at http://www.nctsnet.org/nctsn_assets/pdfs/edu_materials/Helping_Young_Children_ Heal.pdf
- Traumatic Loss Coalitions for Youth's *Helping Children Cope in the Aftermath of Hurricane Sandy*, available at http://www.spanadvocacy.org/sites/g/files/g524681/f/files/HelpingChildren CopeinAftermathofHurricane.pdf
- National Voluntary Organizations Active in Disaster's (VOAD's) *Spiritual Care Guidelines*, available at http://www.nvoad.org/resource-center

DISASTER CASE MANAGEMENT

- FEMA's *Disaster Case Management: Program Guidance*, a program that provides assistance in accessing disaster-specific federal benefits, available at http://www.fema.gov/media-library-data/20130726-1908-25045-2403/dcm_pg_final_3_8_13.pdf
- National VOAD's *Tools for State VOADs to Prepare for Disaster Case Management*, available at http://www.nvoad.org/wp-content/uploads/2014/05/tools_for_state_voads_to_prepare_for_dcm_-_ draft_-_2012.pdf
- HHS's Concept of Operations for Immediate Disaster Case Management at https://www.acf.hhs. gov/sites/default/files/ohsepr/immediate_dcm_concept_of_operations_conops_october_2012_508_ compliant.pdf

HEALTH CARE SYSTEM RECOVERY

- Harvard School of Public Health and the Commonwealth of Massachusetts Department of Public Health's *Essential Functions and Considerations for Hospital Recovery*, available at https://cdn1.sph. harvard.edu/wp-content/uploads/sites/1608/2014/09/HSPH-Emergency-Preparedness-Response-Exercise-Program_Hospital-Recovery.pdf
- USA Center for Rural Public Health Preparedness at Texas A&M University's *Partnering to Achieve Rural Emergency Preparedness: A Workbook for Healthcare Providers in Rural Communities*, available at http://www.cidrap.umn.edu/sites/default/files/public/php/318/318_workbook.pdf

MEASURING AND ASSESSING COMMUNITY HEALTH STATUS

- Community Commons' Community Health Needs Assessment toolkit, a platform that aids hospitals and other organizations working to understand a community's health needs and improve overall health and well-being, available at http://assessment.communitycommons.org/CHNA
- Mobilizing for Action through Planning and Partnerships (MAPP), a framework using a six-phase process (organizing, visioning, assessments, strategic issues, goals/strategies, and action cycle) to enable communities to prioritize and address public health issues, available at http://www.naccho. org/topics/infrastructure/mapp/framework/index.cfm
- County Health Rankings (Robert Wood Johnson Foundation and University of Wisconsin), an annual measurement of health factors for each county in each state in the country, available at http://www.countyhealthrankings.org
- America's Health Rankings®, a state-by-state assessment of the nation's health, available at http:// www.americashealthrankings.org/about/annual
- The Sustainable Communities Index's (SCI's) set of methods to measure the environmental, economic, and social conditions of cities and neighborhoods that affect human health, available at http://www. sustainablecommunitiesindex.org

- Health Resources and Services Administration's (HRSA's) Health Professional Shortage Area scores, which assess baseline needs and help develop disaster plans, available at http://www.hrsa.gov/shortage/find.html

MODEL POST-DISASTER RECOVERY PLANS AND PLANNING GUIDES

- APA's *Planning for Post-Disaster Recovery: Next Generation*, available at https://www.planning.org/pas/reports/pdf/PAS_576.pdf
- Florida Department of Community Affairs and Florida Division of Emergency Management's *Post-Disaster Redevelopment Plan: A Guide for Florida Communities*, available at http://www.floridadisaster.org/recovery/documents/Post%20Disaster%20Redevelopment%20Planning%20Guidebook%20Lo.pdf
- Hillsborough County's *Post-Disaster Redevelopment Plan*, available at http://www.hillsboroughcounty.org/index.aspx?nid=1795
- Pinellas County's *Post-Disaster Redevelopment Plan*, available at http://www.tbrpc.org/tampabaydisaster/pinellaspdrp/pdf/doc/PinellasPDRP_June2012.pdf
- Fairfax County's *Pre-Disaster Recovery Plan*, available at http://www.fairfaxcounty.gov/oem/pdrp/pdrp-complete-doc-march2012.pdf
- Belfer Center's *Lessons from Katrina: How a Community Can Spearhead Successful Disaster Recovery,* which uses the Broadmoor neighborhood's redevelopment as the model for a community-driven planning process, available at http://belfercenter.ksg.harvard.edu/publication/17815/lessons_from_katrina.html

PLANNING FOR VULNERABLE POPULATIONS, INCLUDING CHILDREN

- The Centers for Disease Control and Prevention's (CDC's) *Public Health Workbook to Define, Locate, and Reach Special, Vulnerable, and At-risk Populations in an Emergency*, available at http://www.bt.cdc.gov/workbook/pdf/ph_workbookfinal.pdf
- RAND's *Enhancing Public Health Emergency Preparedness for Special Needs Populations: A Toolkit for State and Local Planning and Response*, available at http://www.rand.org/pubs/technical_reports/TR681.html
- RAND's Special Needs Populations Mapping for Public Health Preparedness, a Web-based mapping tool that public health agencies can use to locate vulnerable populations in their communities, available at http://www.rand.org/health/projects/special-needs-populations-mapping
- ASTHO and CDC planning guidance for at-risk populations during a pandemic, available at http://www.astho.org/Programs/Infectious-Disease/At-Risk-Populations
- Administration for Children and Families' (ACF's) *Children and Youth Task Force in Disasters: Guidelines for Development*, available at http://www.acf.hhs.gov/sites/default/files/ohsepr/childrens_task_force_development_web.pdf
- New Jersey Department of Children and Families' *Sheltering Guidelines for Children and Families*, available at http://nj.gov/dcf/home/Sheltering%20Guidance%20for%20Children%20and%20Families.pdf

POST-DISASTER RECOVERY TOOLS

- FEMA's Community Recovery Management Toolkit, "a compilation of guidance, case studies, tools, and training to assist local communities in managing long-term recovery following a disaster," available at http://www.fema.gov/national-disaster-recovery-framework/community-recovery-management-toolkit

- Coordinated Assistance Network (CAN), which allows information sharing among multiple disaster relief organizations, available at http://www.can.org/images/CommunityIntro.pdf
- National VOAD's *Long Term Recovery Guide*, available at http://www.nvoad.org/wp-content/uploads/2014/05/long_term_recovery_guide_-_final_2012.pdf
- AARP's Disaster Recovery Toolkit, which provides policy information, tools, and resources for building more livable communities after disasters, available at http://www.aarp.org/livable-communities/tool-kits-resources/info-2015/disaster-recovery-tool-kit.html

PROMOTING INDIVIDUAL AND COMMUNITY PREPAREDNESS

- FEMA's *Are You Ready?: An In-depth Guide to Citizen Preparedness*, available at http://www.fema.gov/pdf/areyouready/areyouready_full.pdf
- SF72, an emergency preparedness program developed by the San Francisco Department of Emergency Management that emphasizes increasing social connectedness, available at http://www.sf72.org/home
- National VOAD, a forum where member organizations share information and resources to promote community resiliency and to provide support to people affected by disasters, available at http://www.nvoad.org/resource-center

WORKER AND HOMEOWNER HEALTH PROTECTION RESOURCES

- The National Clearinghouse for Worker Safety and Health Training, available at http://tools.niehs.nih.gov/wetp/index.cfm
- U.S. Department of Housing and Urban Development resources on post-disaster housing repair and restoration, available at http://portal.hud.gov/hudportal/HUD?src=/program_offices/healthy_homes/disasterrecovery

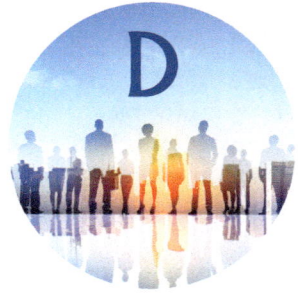

Measures and Tools for Healthy Communities

The following measures and tools have been or could be used to evaluate recovery progress toward healthier communities after disasters.

AMERICA'S HEALTH RANKINGS®

America's Health Rankings® is an "annual assessment of the nation's health on a state-by-state basis." It is a collaborative partnership between United Health Foundation, the American Public Health Association and Partnership for Prevention™, which together created the Scientific Advisory Committee that recommends improvements that will maintain the value of the comparative, longitudinal information that is collected and measured. The ranking system is based off of the World Health Organization holistic definition of health. American's Health Rankings® has been measuring states' population health for the past 25 years, making it the longest-running complete annual assessment of the nation's overall population health (America's Health Rankings®, 2014).

America's Health Rankings® analyzes two types of measures—determinants and outcomes. The health determinants, such as air pollution and underemployment rate, account for 75 percent of the overall score and are divided into groups: behaviors; community and environmental conditions; public and health policies; and clinical care. The remaining 25 percent of the overall score are health outcomes. The system combines 27 individual core measures and 22 supplemental measures from each of these areas and merges them into one comprehensive view of the overall population health of a state. The report is ranked from 1-50, with each state being ranked against others by their health determinants score and health outcomes score. For a state to improve its health rank, focus must be on improving the determinants of health. Recently added in 2013 was a Senior Report that focuses on the population health of citizens 65 years old and above. The goal of these rankings is to stimulate conversations and actions in communities to improve the health of the state as well as the nation (America's Health Rankings®, 2014).

COUNTY HEALTH RANKINGS

The annual County Health Rankings measures health factors for nearly every county in the United States and then ranks them for each state. It is a partnership between the Robert Wood Johnson Foundation and the University of Wisconsin Population Health Institute (County Health Rankings, 2010). Community leaders can use the ranking system to assess baseline health status, prioritize, and organize community action plans before a disaster to inform post-disaster redevelopment planning.

The annual County Health Rankings reveals how factors such as where we live, learn, work, and play impacts health. As part of this process, County Health Rankings compiles county-health measures from national data sources (e.g., the American Community Survey and the Federal Bureau of Investigation's Uniform Crime Reporting). These measures are then standardized and combined to produce rankings within states.

Included to encourage improvements in community and county health is an action plan called *Roadmaps to Health* that will help guide community members in the development of a healthier community. The continuous Action Cycle provides information and action steps (listed below) for each community role and how it fits into the cycle as a whole.

- Work Together
- Assess Needs and Resources
- Focus on What's Important
- Choose Effective Policies and Programs
- Act on What's Important
- Evaluate Actions
- Communicate (County Health Rankings, 2013)

The County Rankings are designed to help each county understand its own unique health needs and to implement programs and policies that will improve the overall population health of the county, which will improve the overall health of the state and the nation.

SUSTAINABLE COMMUNITIES INDEX

The Sustainable Communities Index (SCI) is a set of methods to measure environmental, economic, and social conditions of cities and neighborhoods (SCI, 2014b). The conditions that SCI measures, including housing, transportation, civic engagement, education, and health systems, all affect human health (SCI, 2014b). The SCI does not provide data for each community; rather it provides a list of health objectives, the indicators of that objective, and the specific methods to measure the indicators. For example, one objective is "Increase park, open space and recreation facilities" (SCI, 2014e). The indicators of this objective are recreational area score, recreation facility access, and community garden access (SCI, 2014e). Recreation facility access is measured by calculating the number of people living within ¼ mile of a community recreational facility, then dividing that number of people by the total number of people in the neighborhood (SCI, 2014d). This measurement—the percentage of people who live within ¼ mile of a facility—is used as an indicator of how well a community is achieving the objective to "Increase park, open space, and recreation facilities." Using these tools, a city can measure how and where the community needs improvement and use the data to guide policy, planning, and development (SCI, 2014b).

The development of SCI began with the Eastern Neighborhoods Community Health Impact Assessment (ENCHIA), created by the San Francisco Department of Public Health (SFDPH) to assess the health impact of the intense development happening in San Francisco in the early 2000s (SCI, 2014c). The experience with ENCHIA led to the development of the Healthy Development Measurement Tool (HDMT), which was designed to support evidence-based and health-oriented planning for development projects (SCI, 2014c). Over the next several years, the HDMT was applied to planning projects in San Francisco, as well as adapted for use in cities including Denver, Colorado, Philadelphia, Pennsylvania, and Geneva, Switzerland (SCI, 2014c). In 2012, the Sustainable Communities Index was launched, building on the experiences with ENCHIA and HDMT (SCI, 2014c).

The SCI and its predecessors have been used in both large and small communities to guide planning for projects ranging from the location of a new preschool in Bernal Heights, California, to recovery after a hurricane in Galveston, Texas (SCI, 2014a). After Hurricane Ike, Galveston was faced with the challenge of rebuilding housing and neighborhoods; one of the hardest-hit neighborhoods contained the majority of all public housing. This rebuilding gave Galveston the opportunity "to make housing and neighborhood development choices that promote a healthier future" (Nolen et al., 2014, p. 4). The SCI was adapted for the local context of Galveston, and through a community engagement process, 23 indicators were chosen (Nolen et al., 2014). Indicators were chosen based on their link to health outcomes, especially for low-income residents. Indicators included, for example:

- Proximity to parks and recreational facilities
- Proximity to elementary schools
- Proximity to health care services
- Density of stores selling alcohol
- Presence of environmental hazards (Nolen et al., 2014)

The indicators were divided into neighborhood-level, block-level, and unit-level (Nolen et al., 2014). Data on these indicators were collected and analyzed and then used to develop recommendations on how to rebuild Galveston in a way that mitigates health-harming conditions and encourages choices that have a positive impact on health (Nolen et al., 2014).

HEALTHY COMMUNITIES TRANSFORMATION INITIATIVE

The U.S. Department of Housing and Urban Development (HUD) has recently launched the Healthy Communities Transformation Initiative (HCTI) and is in the process of developing two key tools for the initiative: the Healthy Communities Index (HCI) and the Healthy Communities Assessment Tool (HCAT). The goal of the HCTI, and its associated tools, is to help local communities "assess the physical, social, and economic roots of community health" and to use this assessment to inform evidence-based policies, planning, and development (HUD, 2014).

The HCI will be comprised of standardized healthy community indicators chosen based on their link to health outcomes, ease of measurability, and relationship to established national public health objectives. The indicators will cover topics ranging from housing to employment to social participation. These indicators can be used to assess the baseline status of a community's health and then to track progress as the community moves forward. The HCI indicators will form the basis for the HCAT, which will facilitate the use of the indicators and also feature tools to help communities select and prioritize objectives. For example, the HCAT may include a guideline of recommended health targets, or provide sample policies designed to improve community health (HUD, 2014).

LIVABILITY INDEX

The AARP Public Policy Institute developed and launched the Livability Index in April 2015. The Livability Index measures the livability of a community based on individual preferences, objective indicators, and policy interventions. Users can search the index by address, ZIP Code, or community. The index will generate an overall score as well as a score for seven major livability categories: housing, neighborhood, environment, health, transportation, engagement, and opportunity. Through this effort, AARP is working to identify what is considered a "livable" community by the 50+ population; provide a framework for local and state changes in policy, planning, and investment; inform residents about what it means to be a livable community, thereby allowing them to make informed choices; and encourage participation in community change. The Livability Index serves as a Web-based tool, integrating mapping technology, preference survey results, quantitative measures, and public policies. It also incorporates nationally available data to yield a better understanding of the needs of the older adult population (AARP, 2015).

SOCIAL VULNERABILITY INDEX

Developed in 2003 by Cutter et al., the Social Vulnerability Index (SVI) is "intended to spatially identify socially vulnerable populations, to help more completely understand the risk of hazards to these populations, and to aid in mitigating, preparing for, responding to, and recovering from that risk" (Flanagan et al., 2011, p. 16). The Social Vulnerability Index has four domains: socioeconomic status, household composition and disability, minority status and language, and housing and transportation. The source of data for this model is 15 census variables from the 2000 U.S. Census of Population and Housing at the census tract or "community" level. For each community in the nation, the SVI toolkit provides an SVI value for each of the 15 census variables, each of the four domains, and an overall SVI. Also included in the report were flags, representing a percentile ranking of 90 or higher for each of the variables and domains as well as the total flags for each tract (Flanagan et al., 2011).

The Social Vulnerability Index can be used during all phases of a disaster to inform decision making. The SVI was used after Hurricane Katrina, for example, to understand the impact of the disaster and recovery progress in New Orleans. Areas with socioeconomically vulnerable populations were found to have recovered more slowly from heavy flood damage than those without socioeconomically vulnerable populations. By using the Social Vulnerability Index, state and local agencies may better identify vulnerable populations, allowing disaster recovery decision makers to better target and support community-based disaster mitigation and preparedness (Flanagan et al., 2011).

REFERENCES

AARP. 2015. *Livability index.* https://livabilityindex.aarp.org/livability-defined (accessed June 17, 2015).

America's Health Rankings®. 2014. *About the annual report.* http://www.americashealthrankings.org/about/annual (accessed December 4, 2014).

County Health Rankings. 2010. *Our approach.* http://www.countyhealthrankings.org/our-approach (accessed December 1, 2014).

County Health Rankings. 2013. *Action center.* http://www.countyhealthrankings.org/roadmaps/action-center (accessed December 4, 2014).

Cutter, S. L., B. J. Boruff, and W. L. Shirley. 2003. Social vulnerability to environmental hazards. *Social Science Quarterly* 84(2):242-261.

Flanagan, B. E., E. W. Gregory, E. J. Hallisey, J. L. Heitgerd, and B. Lewis. 2011. A social vulnerability index for disaster management. *Journal of Homeland Security and Emergency Management* 8(1).

HUD (U.S. Department of Housing and Urban Development). 2014. *HUD Healthy Communities Transformation Initiative.* http://healthyhousingsolutions.com/wp-content/uploads/2014/11/HUD_HCTI_project_overview_FINAL.pdf (accessed June 17, 2015).

Nolen, L., J. Prochaska, M. Rushing, E. Fuller, J. E. Dills, R. Buschmann, C. Miller, S. Tarlekar, H. Avey, E. Ruel, and D. Oakley. 2014. *Improving health through housing and neighborhood development in Galveston, Texas: Use of health impact assessment to develop planning tools and coordinated community action.* http://www.pewtrusts.org/en/~/media/Assets/External-Sites/Health-Impact-Project/GalvestonHIAFinalSummaryReport1 (accessed December 4, 2014).

SCI (Sustainable Communities Index). 2014a. *Case studies.* http://www.sustainablecommunitiesindex.org/case_studies.php (accessed October 20, 2014).

SCI. 2014b. *Frequent questions.* http://www.sustainablecommunitiesindex.org/webpages/view/46 (accessed October 20, 2014).

SCI. 2014c. *History.* http://www.sustainablecommunitiesindex.org/webpages/view/47 (accessed October 20, 2014).

SCI. 2014d. *Indicator PR.3.B recreation facility access.* http://www.sustainablecommunitiesindex.org/indicators/view/92 (accessed October 20, 2014).

SCI. 2014e. *Measures.* http://www.sustainablecommunitiesindex.org/indicators (accessed October 20, 2014).

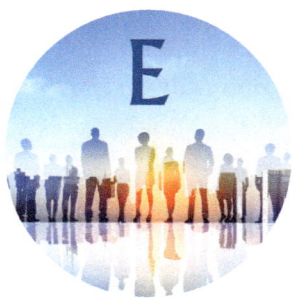

Committee-Identified Research Needs

OVERARCHING RESEARCH NEEDS

- What are the facilitators and barriers to a Health in All Policies approach in the disaster recovery context?
- How does integration of health improvement plans with comprehensive plans and pre-disaster recovery plans prior to a disaster support a healthy community approach to disaster recovery?
- What are the optimal organizational arrangements at state and local levels under the structure of the National Disaster Recovery Framework (NDRF) that would facilitate coordination across sectors, including the often separate health and social services domains?
- What strategies can be used to better integrate the ongoing collaborative initiatives that occur in nearly all communities under the rubric of community development and human services transformation into NDRF-driven organizational and governance structures for recovery?
- What measurement methodology and core set of metrics would enable communities to evaluate the effects of recovery activities on health outcomes and adjust strategic approaches as needed in the context of a learning system? What is the evidence for return on investment?
- How can aligning grant guidance and technical assistance support a more coordinated federal effort to promote recovery planning and the incorporation of a community-derived healthy, resilient, and sustainable community?

PUBLIC HEALTH RECOVERY

- For those with chronic health problems exacerbated by the effects of disasters, what are the stages of exacerbation? How can identifying persons that are at highest risk for most rapid deterioration assist in prioritization of limited resources during recovery?

HEALTH CARE RECOVERY

- How can team-based and community-based care approaches that emerge after a disaster be sustained?

- What is the effect of the Patient Protection and Affordable Care Act on health care system recovery approaches?
- How can health care coalitions be optimally leveraged to better integrate health care leadership into recovery planning and operations?
- What are the long-term impacts on health when access to care is disrupted?

BEHAVIORAL HEALTH RECOVERY

- What is the effectiveness of interventions that are currently commonly employed for psychosocial support, including psychological first aid, crisis counseling, and psychoeducation? How does the population-based Crisis Counseling Assistance and Training Program (CCP) model compare to other models (e.g., exposure-based model)?
- What is the effectiveness of current counselor training programs?
- How can interventions be better matched to specific target groups, including vulnerable populations such as children?
- What is the effect of strengthening social networks on incidence of post-disaster behavioral health disorders?

SOCIAL SERVICES RECOVERY

- How does early identification of and support for vulnerable populations reduce long-term psychological consequences or long-term recovery needs?
- How can the social services system maintain a healthy workforce and optimize its utilization after disaster? What percentage of workers can an agency expect to lose as a result of trauma, loss, burnout, or family needs?
- What training do event-based volunteers need to be able to support the social services system? What types of tasks are appropriate for volunteers? How can faith-based and other nongovernmental organizations be mobilized in pre-disaster recovery planning?
- What strategies can be promoted to better facilitate information sharing among social services providers at all levels during and after disasters?
- What are the long-term impacts to beneficiaries of government assistance and their families when a disaster causes disruptions in benefits?

PLACE-BASED STRATEGIES FOR RECOVERY

- How do high levels of collaboration at the local level among the community development and health and social services sectors to examine problems holistically translate to better post-disaster recovery?
- How does the built environment impact social cohesion, behavioral health, and well-being, and how can this knowledge be transformed into resilience-building strategies?
- What are the best ways to incorporate healthy community outcomes into transportation planning? Are there best practices for educating both internal and external stakeholders on this?
- What risk-based strategies can be employed during recovery planning to reduce physical, psychological, economic, and social consequences of future disasters?

HEALTHY HOUSING RECOVERY

- What evidence is available demonstrating improved health and well-being outcomes resulting from a collaborative approach to housing recovery that integrates design, social/behavioral, and health perspectives?

- How can temporary housing strategies be designed to improve social connectedness and associated impacts on health?
- How does investment in post-disaster housing reconstruction that complies with green and healthy housing building standards translate to a return on investment in long-term health outcomes?
- What are the key barriers to adoption of green building standards for post-disaster housing reconstruction?

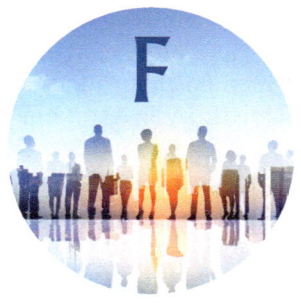

Key to Select Terms Used to Describe Primary Actors and Key Partners in Chapter 5–10 Checklists

Across jurisdictions there is great variability in the agencies and organizations that have roles in disaster recovery, their organizational structures, and the terms used to describe them. The checklists in Chapters 5–10 of this report identify primary actors and key partners for a series of pre-event, short-term, and intermediate- to long-term recovery priorities. Although it is not feasible to capture all possible relevant organizations (and synonyms for those organizations), the intent of this appendix is to expand on select terms used to describe actors and partners identified in the checklists to stimulate thinking about the stakeholders that the committee believes communities should consider engaging in the specified disaster recovery priorities. In some cases, organizations may fall under more than one actor/partner category.

Child Care Organizations: This category encompasses organizations and professionals from a number of sectors that focus on addressing the needs of children, including but not limited to public and private providers of early education and child care services (including Head Start programs, home-based child care providers, and camps), child welfare authorities, social services, and family violence prevention services.

Community- and Faith-Based Organizations: This category encompasses faith-based and other nonprofit community organizations that provide community members with a range of services, including but not limited to shelter, food and nutritional assistance, financial support, transportation assistance, legal assistance, housing assistance, workforce training, youth and adult education and literacy support, child care and senior services, cultural development, and health services, including behavioral health services. Such organizations may also include charities, foundations and philanthropies, church groups, professional associations, academic organizations, neighborhood associations, youth organizations (e.g., Boy Scouts of America, Girl Scouts of the USA, Boys and Girls Clubs of America), and advocacy groups for at-risk populations such as those living with disabilities and the homeless.

Community Data Centers: This category refers to local or regional governmental and nongovernmental organizations (e.g., the Greater New Orleans Community Data Center) that collect and disseminate community-level data, including but not limited to population- and demographic-level data, crime rates, real estate sales, and economic and health indicators.

Community Development Organizations: This category encompasses governmental, nongovernmental (e.g., community development corporations), and private organizations (e.g., banks, real estate investors) that work to transform impoverished, blighted neighborhoods and improve quality of life and economic security for low- and middle-income individuals by investing in affordable housing, workforce development, and access to community services and amenities (e.g., child care centers, health clinics, grocery stores, public transit, recreational facilities, and charter schools).

Disaster Relief Organizations: This category includes those faith-based and other nongovernmental organizations involved in disaster planning, response, mitigation, and recovery. These organizations can be local (e.g., Community Organizations Active in Disasters, Volunteer Organizations Active in Disasters, long-term recovery committees) or national (e.g., National Voluntary Organizations Active in Disaster, Catholic Charities, the American Red Cross) in scope.

Education System: This category encompasses public and private providers of education, including schools, administration, and educators at the primary and secondary (K–12), as well as post-secondary (colleges and universities), levels. Also included are providers of early childhood education (e.g., preschools, Head Start programs), vocational and technical training institutions, school boards and state boards of education, accreditation authorities, and adult and childhood education and literacy support programs.

Elected Officials and Community Leaders: This category encompasses elected and public officials in local, state, and federal governments who have responsibility for providing leadership in community strategic planning and emergency management (i.e., governors, mayors, city managers and council members, emergency managers, disaster recovery coordinators). This category also encompasses unelected community leaders, including those that foster collaboration and teamwork throughout the community, such as members of neighborhood councils and leaders from business, education, or the faith community.

Health and Medical System Partners: This category encompasses a wide range of private for-profit, nonprofit, and governmental (local, state, and federal) entities involved in the delivery of health care, including but not limited to health care coalitions, hospitals, clinics, networks of outpatient providers (e.g., private primary and specialty care providers), occupational health professionals, surgical and procedure centers, long-term care facilities, home health care and hospice, emergency medical services, behavioral health services, community and large chain pharmacies, and walk-in health services. Also included are those facilitators of health care spanning financial (payers), health information and communication technology, diagnostics, and logistics (e.g., supply chain, transportation) fields, as well as nongovernmental public health partners such as academic public health professionals, local health coalitions and health advocacy groups, and public health professional organizations.

Urban and Regional Planning Agencies: This category encompasses governmental, academic, private, and nonprofit organizations providing urban and regional planning services. Regional planning agencies such as Metropolitan Planning Organizations and Regional Planning Commissions operate at the substate level.

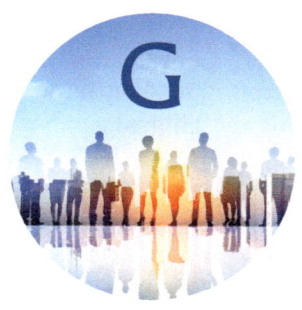

Public Committee Meeting Agendas

Held by the Committee on Post-Disaster Recovery of a Community's
Public Health, Medical, and Social Services
(November 2013-October 2014)

MEETING ONE: November 25, 2013
National Academy of Sciences Keck Building
500 Fifth Street, NW, Washington, DC 20001

AGENDA

11:00 a.m.   Welcome and Introductions

                  REED TUCKSON, *Committee Chair*
                  Managing Director
                  Tuckson Health Connections, LLC

11:15 a.m.   Background and Charge to the Committee

                  NICOLE LURIE
                  Assistant Secretary for Preparedness and Response
                  U.S. Department of Health and Human Services

11:45 a.m.   Panel Discussion with Sponsors

                  ANGELA McGOWAN (*via teleconference*)
                  Senior Program Officer
                  Robert Wood Johnson Foundation

ESMERALDA PEREIRA
Deputy Director for Recovery Coordination
Office of the Assistant Secretary for Preparedness and Response
U.S. Department of Health and Human Services

WARREN FRIEDMAN
Senior Advisor to the Director
Office of Healthy Homes and Lead Hazard Control
U.S. Department of Housing and Urban Development

AARON EAGAN (*via teleconference*)
Senior Program Manager
National Center for Occupational Health and Infection Control
Office of Public Health
Veterans Health Administration

1:00 p.m.	LUNCH
2:00 p.m.	National Disaster Recovery Framework

ALEX AMPARO
Deputy Assistant Administrator, Recovery Directorate
Federal Emergency Management Agency
U.S. Department of Homeland Security

2:45 p.m.	The Katrina Experience: Considerations for Health System Recovery

KAREN DESALVO
Health Commissioner and Senior Health Policy Advisor to the Mayor
City of New Orleans

3:30 p.m.	Public Comment Period
3:45 p.m.	ADJOURN OPEN SESSION

MEETING TWO: FEBRUARY 3, 2014
National Academy of Sciences Building
2101 Constitution Avenue, NW, Washington, DC 20418

AGENDA

8:00 a.m.   Welcome and Meeting Objectives

                 REED TUCKSON, *Committee Chair*
                 Tuckson Health Connections, LLC

8:15 a.m.   Health Considerations During Short-Term, Intermediate, and Long-Term Recovery

                 IRWIN REDLENER
                 Director, National Center for Disaster Preparedness
                 Earth Institute, Columbia University

8:35 a.m.   Discussion with Committee

8:45 a.m.   Public Health Panel Presentations

                 HOWARD ZUCKER
                 First Deputy Commissioner of Health
                 New York State Health Department

                 BRUCE CLEMENTS
                 Director, Public Health Preparedness
                 Texas Department of State Health Services

                 DOUGLAS BEARDSLEY (*via teleconference*)
                 Director, Johnson County Public Health
                 Iowa City, Iowa

9:30 a.m.   Discussion with Committee

10:00 a.m.   Medical System Panel Presentations

                 LEWIS GOLDFRANK
                 Director of Emergency Medicine
                 Bellevue Hospital Center and New York University Hospitals

                 SCOTT MATIN (*by phone*)
                 Vice President of Clinical & Business Services
                 Monmouth Ocean Hospital Service Corporation

                 BETTY PFEFFERBAUM
                 Chair, Department of Psychiatry
                 College of Medicine
                 University of Oklahoma Health Sciences Center

DOUGLAS WALKER
Clinical Director
Mercy Family Center

10:50 a.m.   Discussion with Committee

11:20 a.m.   BREAK

11:30 a.m.   Social Services Panel Presentations

CDR JONATHAN WHITE
Deputy Director
Office of Human Services Emergency Preparedness Response
Administration on Children and Families

KIMBERLY BURGO
Senior Director of Disaster Response Operations
Catholic Charities

LISA BROWN
Associate Professor, School of Aging Studies
University of South Florida

12:15 p.m.   Discussion with Committee

12:45 p.m.   LUNCH

1:45 p.m.   Community Planning Panel Presentations

ROBERT OLSHANSKY
Professor of Urban and Regional Planning
University of Illinois at Urbana-Champaign

JAMES SCHWAB
Senior Research Associate
American Planning Association

GAVIN SMITH
Department of City and Regional Planning
University of North Carolina at Chapel Hill

2:30 p.m.   Discussion with Committee

3:00 p.m.   Housing Panel Presentations

TENNILLE SMITH PARKER
Acting Director/Assistant Director
Disaster Recovery and Special Issues
Division Office of Block Grant Assistance
U.S. Department of Housing and Urban Development

THOMAS PHILLIPS
Principal Scientist
Healthy Building Research

3:30 p.m.   Discussion with Committee

3:50 p.m.   BREAK

4:00 p.m.   Transportation and Infrastructure Panel Presentations

HERBY LISSADE
Chief, Office of Emergency Management
California Department of Transportation

KAREN DURHAM-AGUILERA
Director, Contingency Operations and Office of Homeland Security
U.S. Army Corps of Engineers

CAPT LYNN SLEPSKI
Senior Public Health Advisor
Office of Intelligence, Security and Emergency Response
Office of the Secretary of Transportation
U.S. Department of Transportation

4:45 p.m.   Discussion with Committee

5:15 p.m.   ADJOURN

MEETING THREE: April 28-29, 2014
The National Academy of Sciences Keck Building
500 Fifth Street, NW, Washington, DC 20001

AGENDA

April 28, 2014

8:00 a.m.   Welcome and Meeting Objectives

REED TUCKSON, *Committee Chair*
Tuckson Health Connections, LLC

8:15 a.m.   Coordination Among Federal Recovery Support Functions

ESMERALDA PEREIRA
Deputy Director for Recovery Coordination
Office of the Assistant Secretary for Preparedness and Response
U.S. Department of Health and Human Services

MYRA SHIRD
Program Specialist, Community Planning and Capacity Building Branch
Recovery Directorate
Federal Emergency Management Agency
U.S. Department of Homeland Security

KAREN ZHANG
National Coordinator-Natural and Cultural Resource Recovery
U.S. Department of the Interior

RENA HOLLAND
Office of Disaster Management and National Security,
U.S. Department of Housing and Urban Development

WARREN FRIEDMAN
Senior Advisor to the Director
Office of Healthy Homes and Lead Hazard Control
U.S. Department of Housing and Urban Development

RADM STEVEN SMITH
Director, Office of Disaster Planning
U.S. Small Business Administration

ADHIR KACKAR
Acting Director of Operations,
Office of Sustainable Communities
U.S. Environmental Protection Agency

9:45 a.m.   BREAK

10:00 a.m.   Coordination Among State and Local Government Agencies

                BRUCE LOCKWOOD
                President
                International Association of Emergency Managers

                UMAIR SHAH
                Executive Director
                Harris County Public Health & Environmental Services
                Board Member, National Association of City and County Health Officials

                THOMAS WIECZOREK
                Director, Center for Public Safety Management
                International City/County Management Association

                KAREN HOWARD AND STEVEN LONG (*via teleconference*)
                Department of Neighborhood and Development Services
                City of Iowa City

12:30 p.m.   LUNCH

1:30 p.m.   Considerations for Community Health in Disaster Recovery

                ANITA CHANDRA
                Senior Policy Researcher
                Director, Behavioral and Policy Sciences Department Faculty Member
                Pardee RAND Graduate School, RAND Corporation

3:30 p.m.   BREAK

3:45 p.m.   Role of Public Information in Health Systems Recovery

                EMILY KNEARL
                Health Risk Communications
                Division of Public Health
                Delaware Department of Health and Social Services

4:15 p.m.   Community Experiences with Social Media during Recovery

                REBECCA AND GENEVIEVE WILLIAMS
                Joplin Tornado Info

4:45 p.m.   Harnessing Digital Information to Inform Recovery Efforts

                WENDY HARMAN
                Director of Information Management and Situational Awareness
                American Red Cross

5:15 p.m.   Public Comment Period

5:30 p.m.   ADJOURN

April 29, 2014

8:30 a.m.   Education and Training Opportunities in Long-Term Community Recovery:
                 Preliminary Observations from the Field

                 LAUREN WALSH
                 Senior Research Associate
                 National Center for Disaster Medicine and Public Health

                 KENNETH SCHOR
                 Acting Director
                 National Center for Disaster Medicine and Public Health

9:30 a.m.   ADJOURN OPEN SESSION

MEETING FOUR: June 13, 2014
The National Academy of Sciences Keck Building
500 5th St., NW, Washington, DC 20001

AGENDA

9:00 a.m.   Welcome and Introductions

Reed Tuckson, *Committee Chair*
Managing Director
Tuckson Health Connections, LLC

9:15 a.m.   Investing in Health: Pre- and Post-Disaster Experiences from Oklahoma City

Mick Cornett
Mayor
Oklahoma City, OK

10:00 a.m.   A Health in All Policies Approach to Disaster Recovery: Lessons from Galveston

Alexandra Nolen
Director, Center to Eliminate Health Disparities
Associate Executive Director, Coordinating Center for Global Health
University of Texas Medical Branch

11:30 a.m.   ADJOURN OPEN SESSION

MEETING FIVE: August 14, 2014
WebEx (Teleconference) Meeting

Agenda

12:00 p.m.   Welcome and Introductions

REED TUCKSON, *Committee Chair*

12:10 p.m.   SAMHSA Perspectives on Behavioral Health Recovery Challenges

PAMELA S. HYDE (presenter)
Administrator
Substance Abuse and Mental Health Services Agency
U.S. Department of Health and Human Services

ANNE MATTHEWS-YOUNES
Director, Division of Prevention, Traumatic Stress and Special Programs
Substance Abuse and Mental Health Services Agency
U.S. Department of Health and Human Services

TERRI SPEAR
Emergency Coordinator
Office of Policy, Planning and Innovation
Substance Abuse and Mental Health Services Agency
U.S. Department of Health and Human Services

MARYANN ROBINSON
Branch Chief
Emergency Mental Health & Traumatic Stress Services Branch
Division of Prevention, Traumatic Stress and Special Programs
Substance Abuse and Mental Health Services Agency
U.S. Department of Health and Human Services

MARYANN ROBINSON
Branch Chief
Emergency Mental Health & Traumatic Stress Services Branch
Division of Prevention, Traumatic Stress and Special Programs
Substance Abuse and Mental Health Services Agency
U.S. Department of Health and Human Services

12:40 p.m.   Perspectives on Behavioral Health Recovery Challenges from the Field

JACK HERRMANN
Senior Advisor & Chief for Public Health Preparedness
National Association of County and City Health Officials

NAOMI PAGET
Disaster Spiritual Care Area Advisor
American Red Cross

1:00 p.m.   Discussion with Committee

2:00 p.m.   ADJOURN OPEN SESSION

MEETING SIX: October 2, 2014
WebEx (Teleconference) Meeting

AGENDA

3:00 p.m.   PHEP Grantees' Use of Funds to Improve Health in Communities Post-Disaster

CHRISTA-MARIE SINGLETON
Senior Medical Advisor
Centers for Disease Control and Prevention

4:00 p.m.   ADJOURN

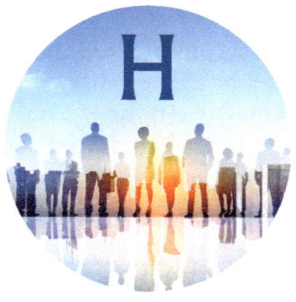

Committee Biosketches

Reed V. Tuckson, M.D., FACP (*Chair*) is Managing Director at Tuckson Health Connections, LLC. Most recently, he served as Executive Vice President and Chief of Medical Affairs at UnitedHealth Group. Formerly, he served as: Senior Vice President for Professional Standards at the American Medical Association; President of the Charles R. Drew University of Medicine and Science; Senior Vice President for Programs at the March of Dimes Birth Defects Foundation; and Commissioner of Public Health for the District of Columbia. Dr. Tuckson is an active member of the Institute of Medicine of the National Academy of Sciences, serving on, or chairing, several boards and committees. He is also active on the Advisory Committee to the Director of the National Institutes of Health and serves on the Boards of Cell Therapeutics, Inc., Howard University, and the American Telemedicine Association among others. He has past service on cabinet level advisory committees concerned with health reform, infant mortality, children's health, violence, and radiation testing. Dr. Tuckson is a graduate of Howard University and Georgetown University School of Medicine. He completed Internal Medicine Residency and Fellowship Programs at the Hospital of the University of Pennsylvania.

Daniel P. Aldrich, Ph.D., M.A., is an Associate Professor of Political Science, University Faculty Scholar, and Director of Asian Studies at Purdue University. Dr. Aldrich recently completed a Fulbright research fellowship in the University of Tokyo's Economics Department for 2012-2013 and served as an American Association for the Advancement of Science fellow at United States Agency for International Development (USAID) from 2011-2012. He has previously been a Visiting Scholar at the University of Tokyo's Law Faculty in Japan, an Advanced Research Fellow at Harvard University's Program on U.S.-Japan Relations, a Visiting Researcher at Centre Américain, Sciences Po in Paris, France, and a Visiting Professor at the Tata Institute for Disaster Management in Mumbai, India. He is a board member of the journals *Asian Politics and Policy* and *Risk Hazards and Crisis in Public Policy* and is a Mansfield U.S. Japan Network for the Future alumnus. He is the section organizer for the American Political Science Association's Disasters and Crises Related Group. His research interests include post-disaster recovery, the siting of controversial facilities, the interaction between civil society and the state, and the socialization of women and men through experience. He has published more than 30 peer-reviewed articles, along with more than 60 book chapters, articles, book reviews, and op-eds for general audiences in five main areas: disaster recovery, controversial facility siting, countering violent extremism, fieldwork practices, and sex differences in political behavior. Dr. Aldrich's first book, *Site Fights: Divisive Facilities and Civil Society in Japan and the West*, was published by Cornell University Press in the spring of 2008. His second book, *Building Resilience: Social Capital in Disaster Recovery*, was published in the summer of 2012 by the University of Chicago Press. He earned a B.A. in Asian Studies and Japanese from the University of North Carolina at Chapel Hill, an M.A. in Asian Studies from the University of California, Berkeley, and an M.A. and a Ph.D. in Political Science from Harvard University.

Steven Blessing, M.A., is Chief of the Emergency Medical Services and Preparedness Section at the Delaware Division of Public Health. He worked in various positions within Delaware State Division of Public Health since 1994. Prior to becoming Section Chief, Mr. Blessing was the Delaware State Emergency Medical Services Director from 2002-2010, and before that he was the Delaware State Paramedic Administrator. Mr. Blessing is a Past President of the National Association of State Emergency Medical Services Officials (NASEMSO), and he is a member of numerous committees dealing with public health and preparedness. Mr. Blessing received his M.A. in Business from Webster University in St. Louis, Missouri, and a B.A. in Political Science from the University of Delaware.

Lynn Britton, M.B.A., is the President and Chief Executive Officer of Mercy Health (Mercy), a position he assumed in January 2009, after serving as Senior Vice President since 2004. Mr. Britton has been with Mercy for more than 20 years, serving as Vice President for Mercy's supply chain operating division, Resource Optimization and Innovation (ROI), from 2000 to 2004. Following his service to ROI, he led Mercy in the design and implementation of the comprehensive electronic health record across medical practices for 1,900 integrated physicians and 30 hospitals. Mr. Britton holds an M.A. in business from Oklahoma City University and a B.A. in Accounting from Abilene Christian University.

Harry L. Brown, Ph.D., is Senior Vice President of Community Planning and Initiatives at United Way of Central Alabama, where he has worked since 1983. In this role, he is responsible for strategic planning, grants management, and development of community-based programs in financial literacy, transportation, community development, and other areas. Previously, he was Director of the Social Work Program at Talledega College and, before that, Senior Planner in the Jefferson County, Alabama, Office of Senior Citizens Activities. His work in disaster recovery has encompassed the Birmingham EF-5 tornado in 1998, Hurricane Katrina in 2005, and the Alabama EF-5 and EF-4 tornadoes of 2011 and 2012. Dr. Brown was the chair of the Long Term Recovery Committee for these three disasters. He received his Ph.D. in Social Work from Tulane University.

Terry L. Cline, Ph.D., is the Commissioner of Health for Oklahoma, a position he has held since June 2009. In February 2011, he was appointed to serve concurrently as Oklahoma's Cabinet Secretary of Health and Human Services. Prior to his role in Oklahoma, Dr. Cline completed a post as Health Attaché at the U.S. Embassy in Baghdad, Iraq, where he advised the U.S. Ambassador, the Iraqi Minister of Health, and the U.S. Department of Health and Human Services on health-related challenges in Iraq. Dr. Cline served in this capacity under the Administrations of both President George W. Bush and President Barack Obama. Previously, Dr. Cline served as Administrator for the Substance Abuse and Mental Health Services Administration from 2006-2008. From 2001-2006, he served as Oklahoma's Commissioner of the Department of Mental Health and Substance Abuse Services. Dr. Cline has also served as a local provider through an earlier post as the Clinical Director of the Cambridge Youth Guidance Center in Cambridge, Massachusetts, and as a Staff Psychologist at McLean Hospital in Belmont, Massachusetts. In addition, his professional history includes a 6-year appointment as a Clinical Instructor in the Department of Psychiatry at Harvard Medical School and Chairman of the governing board for a Harvard teaching hospital in Cambridge. Dr. Cline attended the University of Oklahoma where he earned a B.A. in Psychology. He received both an M.A. and a Ph.D. in Clinical Psychology from Oklahoma State University.

Lawrence Deyton, M.D., M.S.P.H., is a Clinical Professor of Medicine at George Washington University's (GWU's) School of Medicine and Health Sciences and a Professor of Health Policy at GWU's School of Public Health and Health Services. He previously served as the Director of the Center for Tobacco Products (CTP) at the U.S. Food and Drug Administration (FDA). Dr. Deyton was appointed as the FDA's first director of the CTP shortly after the passage of the Family Smoking Prevention and Tobacco Control Act in 2009. Prior to joining the FDA, Dr. Deyton was the Chief Public Health and Environmental Hazards Officer for the U.S. Department of Veterans Affairs (VA), where he oversaw VA's public health programs, including emergency preparedness and response of VA's health system. Dr. Deyton served for 11 years in leadership positions in the National Institute of Allergy and Infectious Diseases at the National Institutes of Health, 6 years in the Office of the Assistant Secretary for Health at the U.S. Department of Health and Human Services, and as a legislative aide with the House of Representatives Subcommittee on Health and the Environment in the 1970s. Dr. Deyton was a founder of the Whitman Walker Clinic, now a community-based AIDS service organization in Washington, DC, in 1978. He earned his M.D. from GWU, his M.S.P.H. at the Harvard School of Public Health, and completed his undergraduate work at the University of Kansas. In 2011, Dr. Deyton was a finalist for the prestigious Samuel J. Heyman Service to America Medal for his outstanding contributions to the health, safety, and well-being of Americans.

Alisa Diggs, M.P.H., PA-c, serves as the Clinical Advisor for Cities Readiness Initiative activities in Maricopa County, Arizona, the fourth most populous county in the United States, and he is the former Maricopa County Department of Public Health Program Manager for the Office of Preparedness and Response. Ms. Diggs led in the design and implementation of the Medical Coordination Center, a regional, Medical Multi-Agency Coordination Center, and envisioned and initiated planning for regional Alternate Care System (ACS) to address medical surge capacity during disasters. Ms. Diggs is the primary liaison between the department and Emergency Management, Homeland Security, Law Enforcement, Fire and Emergency Medical Service agencies across the jurisdiction, and she coordinates activities between the department and the regions' health care delivery (hospitals, clinics, urgent care centers, surgical centers) agencies. Prior to the public health preparedness assignment Ms. Diggs developed a vector-borne and zoonotic disease program within the Office of Epidemiology, including disease-specific protocols and procedures and recruitment/training of a team of investigators and analysts. Before committing to a career in public health, Ms. Diggs practiced as a physician assistant in internal medicine, family practice and emergency room/urgent care services in nonprofit, for-profit, and government environments. As an undergraduate, Ms. Diggs gained hands-on experience working in a clinical laboratory and as an Emergency Medical Technician. Ms. Diggs has co-authored several papers and posters and presented on a variety of topics such as vector-borne diseases, infectious disease outbreaks, medical countermeasure deployment, and the development of a Medical Coordination Center for disaster response. Ms. Diggs is currently detailed to the National Counterterrorism Center in the National Capitol Region. Her assignment on the Joint Counterterrorism Assessment Team involves engagement with key federal agencies to develop mechanisms to enhance the sharing of intelligence with state, local, tribal, and private-sector partners within the Healthcare and Public Health Sector. Ms. Diggs received her M.A. in Public Health at the University of Arizona and completed her B.S. in Physician Assistant Studies at the City College of New York.

Dennis Dura began his career in the emergency management field in 1981 as a volunteer coordinator in his home township's emergency management program. He turned this experience and training into a consulting career working on off-site emergency plans for nuclear power plants and the jurisdictions around the nation. In 1988, Mr. Dura joined the American Red Cross and became a volunteer Disaster Consultant in New Jersey. This volunteer work lead to paid positions in the organization as Manager of Disaster Services in St. Louis, Director of Disaster Preparedness in Chicago, and Disaster Preparedness Specialist in New Jersey. In 1997, after years in the nongovernmental organization side of the field, he joined the New Jersey State Police, Office of Emergency Management (NJOEM). Mr. Dura progressed through the ranks in NJOEM and served in numerous positions, such as Operations Officer and Hurricane Preparedness

Officer. Much of his work at NJOEM specialized in human services issues such as mass care, individual assistance, and volunteer and donations management. As part of state government's response to the 9/11 attack, he served on a specialized inter-governmental team to establish the Family Assistance Center at Liberty State Park. In 2003 he joined the New Jersey Department of Human Services. His focus was on human service emergency management issues such as developing the Department's Community Emergency Response Team, Business/Continuity of Operations planning and preparedness and a concentration on Mass Care/Emergency Assistance and Individual Assistance. In 2007 Mr. Dura left state government and accepted a position with the American Radio Relay League (ARRL), the national association for amateur radio as their first Emergency Preparedness & Response Manager to improve amateur radio capabilities in disaster responses. In 2010, Mr. Dura returned to the American Red Cross in Washington, DC, as a Liaison Officer to FEMA Headquarters. In March 2012, Mr. Dura came back to New Jersey and the Department of Human Services, Office of Emergency Management as an Assistant Director. In October 2012, when Superstorm Sandy struck New Jersey, Mr. Dura took a lead in Mass Care operations until activities at the State EOC subsided. His work transitioned to the FEMA-State Joint Field Office to close out mass care and transition to a lead role in Individual Assistance. In February, his assignment for Sandy at the Joint Field Office was heading up the Task Force on the close out of the Temporary Housing Assistance (TSA) program. Mr. Dura is also engaged with several emergency management consulting firms across the United States applying the mass care/human services emergency management expertise to all levels of government. Mr. Dura holds a B.S. in Criminal Justice from The College of New Jersey. He is a Certified Business Resilience Manager and is a member of numerous professional emergency management organizations. He has conducted numerous assessments of emergency management programs around the United States as an Emergency Management Accreditation Program (EMAP) Assessor. He holds an FCC Extra Class Amateur Radio License.

J. Barry Hokanson, AICP, is Principal at PLN Associates in Illinois. Mr. Hokanson has more than 45 years of urban planning experience with agencies in California, Illinois, Iowa, Kansas, and Texas, with responsibility for environmental and development regulations, building codes, transportation planning, strategic planning, community development, stormwater and flood plain management, decision-support technology, facilities management systems, emergency response planning, and post-disaster recovery planning in both urban and suburban areas. He has managed large staff groups in city and county governments, including extensive interaction with elected and appointed officials. Prior to work as a subcontractor in the Federal Emergency Management Agency's (FEMA's) long-term community recovery program for Louisiana, Texas, Tennessee, and New York (2005 to 2013), Mr. Hokanson held executive and consulting positions in regions such as Chicago, Dallas, and Kansas City. He is active in professional organizations and is a member of the American Planning Association, American Institute of Certified Planners, Natural Hazard Mitigation Association, and Urban and Regional Information Systems Association. He holds an M.A. in Urban and Regional Planning from the University of Iowa.

David E. Jacobs, Ph.D., M.S., is the Director of Research at the National Center for Healthy Housing in the United States. He previously worked at the U.S. Department of Housing and Urban Development as Director of the Office of Healthy Homes and Lead Hazard Control, where he was responsible for policy development, grants management, enforcement, public education and training, and research. He also was responsible for helping to plan part of the Department's Continuity of Operations Plan. He wrote the first federal interagency strategy on childhood lead poisoning prevention in the United States. He also conceived and won congressional support for the U.S. Healthy Homes initiative in 1999. He has testified before Congress and other legislative bodies on many occasions and has numerous scientific peer-reviewed publications on building science, health outcomes of green healthy housing construction and rehabilitation, childhood lead poisoning prevention, and other topics. He was responsible for commissioning an Institute of Medicine report on ethical considerations in housing intervention research. Dr. Jacobs is currently an

Adjunct Associate Professor at the School of Public Health at the University of Illinois at Chicago and a Faculty Associate at the Johns Hopkins Bloomberg School of Public Health.

Agnes Leshner, M.A., has been the Director of Montgomery County Maryland's Child Welfare Services for more than 25 years. Her staff provides a large variety of services to children and families, including investigations of reported child abuse and neglect, family preservation, kinship care, foster care, adoption, and foster home finding. Many of the cases require immediate attention, court involvement, and coordination with community resources. Previously, Ms. Leshner served as the Director of Research, Development and Training for the Montgomery County Department of Social Services. Before coming to the County, Ms. Leshner spent many years as the Director of a Partial Hospitalization program for severely mentally ill adults at Geisinger Mental Health Center in central Pennsylvania. She received a B.A. in Psychology from the University of Windsor, Canada, and an M.A. in Psychology from Bucknell University. Ms. Leshner is a trained family therapist through the Philadelphia Child Guidance Clinic. Throughout her tenure in Montgomery County, Ms. Leshner has focused on developing partnerships with other agencies and service providers. She has been recognized formally through awards from agencies concerned with housing, mental health services, and child protection, and from a variety of community commissions and task forces.

Robert S. Ogilvie, Ph.D., is the Director of SPUR Oakland. Previously, he served as the Vice President for Strategic Engagement at ChangeLab Solutions. Over the past 20 years he has worked extensively in community development and planning to help improve low- and middle-income neighborhoods. Prior to joining ChangeLab Solutions, he served as a faculty member in the Department of City and Regional Planning at the University of California, Berkeley; as a consultant to city and county governments, non-profit organizations, and neighborhood activists; and as Director of Volunteers at the Partnership for the Homeless in New York City. He is the author of *Voluntarism, Community Life, and the American Ethic* (Indiana University Press, 2004), co-author of *Opening School Grounds to the Community After Hours: A Toolkit on Joint Use,* and editor of *Community Development Approaches to Improving Public Health* (Routledge, 2012). Dr. Igilvie co-leads the California Convergence Joint Use Policy Task Force and is a member of the Editorial Board of Community Development: Journal of the Community Development Society. He is also a member of the National Advisory Committee of the Robert Wood Johnson Foundation's Public Health Law Research Program, and he serves on the steering committee of the Strategic Alliance for Healthy Food and Activity Environments. Dr. Ogilvie is a member of the American Planning Association, the American Public Health Association, the California Redevelopment Association, the San Francisco Planning and Urban Research Association, and the Urban Land Institute. He holds a Ph.D. in Political Science from Columbia University.

Richard Reed, M.S.W., is Senior Vice President, Disaster Cycle Services at the American Red Cross. In this role, he leads the development and execution of programs that help Americans prevent, prepare for, and respond to disasters nationwide. He led a comprehensive organizational assessment of all American Red Cross preparedness, response, and recovery programs which resulted in revamped processes to improve service delivery in disasters small and large. Prior to taking the role at Red Cross, Mr. Reed was at the White House, serving as Deputy Assistant to the President for Homeland Security. He led the development of national policy related to resilience, transborder security, and community partnerships. With an experienced team of more than 30 senior professionals, Mr. Reed covered a broad and deep homeland security portfolio that includes all-hazards preparedness, individual and community partnerships and resilience, critical infrastructure protection and resilience, domestic incident management, continuity of government, national exercises, transportation security (aviation, maritime, and ground), piracy, information sharing, border security, and immigration. His prior White House tenure included service as Special Assistant to the President for Homeland Security and Director for Continuity (2006-2009) and Special Assistant to the President and Senior Director for Resilience Policy (2009-2012). Mr. Reed's federal service exceeds 20 years, with positions in the U.S. Department of Veterans Affairs, the Federal Emergency

Management Agency, and the General Services Administration. He is known for his adept leadership of the U.S. government interagency through disasters and emergencies of all types, including the 2009 H1N1 pandemic, Haiti earthquake (during which he was deployed), the BP Deepwater Horizon oil spill, the Fukushima earthquake, tsunami, and nuclear emergency, and countless domestic natural disasters, including hurricanes, tornados, and flooding. In addition, he has been instrumental in the development of national policy on a range of matters, including continuity of government, national preparedness, critical infrastructure security and resilience, national security and emergency preparedness communications, medical countermeasures following a biological attack, cyber security, border security, and immigration. Mr. Reed has bachelor's degrees from Indiana University and Purdue University, and an M.A. in Social Work from Indiana University.

Richard Serino has spent more than 40 years in public service. During this time he provided extensive leadership on emergency management and emergency medical and homeland security at local, state, federal, and international levels. Mr. Serino is currently a Distinguished Visiting Fellow at Harvard School of Public Health, National Preparedness Leadership Initiative. Mr. Serino was appointed by President Obama and confirmed by the Senate as the Federal Emergency Management Agency's eighth Deputy Administrator in October 2009 and served until 2014. In this role, he also served as the Chief Operating Officer (COO) of the agency with more than a $25 billion budget. Prior to his appointment as Deputy Administrator, he spent 36 years at Boston EMS where he rose through the ranks to become Chief. He also served as the Assistant Director of the Boston Public Health Commission. Mr. Serino responded to over 60 national disasters while at the Federal Emergency Management Agency (FEMA) and during Hurricane Sandy, he was the lead federal area commander for New York and New Jersey. Mr. Serino was also on scene at the Boston Marathon bombings as the U.S. Department of Homeland Security senior official. A sampling of federally declared disasters Mr. Serino responded to include flooding in Colorado, Georgia, North Dakota, and New England; the wildfires in Colorado and Texas; tornadoes in Alabama, Georgia, Joplin, Missouri, and Mississippi; tsunami destruction in the American Samoa; and hurricane stricken areas from Hurricanes Isaac, Irene, and Earl. Mr. Serino briefed the President of the United States on a number of disasters and briefed and traveled with Vice President Biden to a number of affected communities to survey the destruction. Mr. Serino refocused FEMA to establish "Whole Community" as a foundational concept for how business is done at FEMA and across the emergency management team. He expanded relationships with new and existing partners spanning the public, private, nonprofit, and faith based communities. Mr. Serino helped develop FEMA's number 1 priority for the next 4 years—to "Be Survivor Centric in Mission and Program Delivery." FEMA will reorient its activities and improve its programs to be survivor centric, ensuring that FEMA supports the delivery of services are focused on easing the experience of survivors—as individuals, neighborhoods, and communities. These two strategic initiatives helped reorient the culture of emergency management. In putting survivors of a disaster first, Mr. Serino remodeled what response looks like by making survivors the key part of a centralized and integrated response. As the Agency's COO, Mr. Serino fundamentally changed how FEMA operates. He created administrative improvements that were focused on emphasizing financial accountability, created FEMA Stat, which improved the use of analytics to drive decisions, advanced the workforce training and engagement, and fostered a culture of innovation. Under Mr. Serino's leadership, FEMA started initiatives such as FEMA Corps and the FEMA Think Tank, created a new Disaster Workforce, and led Workplace Transformation. Mr. Serino instituted a culture of innovation that led to the development of several successful changes and programs, including the National Think Tank. The Think Tank is a transparent way for citizens to speak directly to government leadership and offer their input and ideas. The monthly calls portion of the Think Tank have not just trended globally on Twitter, but have also given the "Whole of Community" a voice directly to leadership. Additionally, Mr. Serino created and developed FEMA Corps, which has launched an innovative partnership to establish a FEMA-devoted unit of 1,600 service corps members within AmeriCorps National Civilian Community Corps (NCCC) solely devoted to disaster preparedness, response, and recovery. His leadership took FEMA Corps from idea to implementation in nine months. FEMA Corps is a presidentially recognized model program of national service that provides 18- to 24-year-olds with an opportunity to serve their country during disasters. When the program is at full operational capability, and in an average disaster year, there will be an expected savings of approximately $60 million in 1 year. During his tenure at Boston EMS he transformed it to one of the best and nationally recognized EMS systems in the country. He bolstered the city's response plans for major emergencies, including chemical, biological, and radiological attacks. He also led citywide planning for H1N1 influenza. Mr. Serino served as an Incident Commander for more than 35 mass casualty incidents and for all of Boston's major planned events, including the Boston Marathon, Boston's Fourth of July celebration, First Night, and the 2004 Democratic National Convention, a national special security event. Mr. Serino has received more than 35 local, national, and international awards for heroism, public service, and innovation; including Harvard University National Public Leadership Institute's "Leader of the Year"; nationally recognized as an Innovator in EMS with the "Innovators in EMS Award" and Boston's highest Public Service award, "Henry L. Shattuck Public Service Award." Mr. Serino published more than 10 articles, including "Emergency Medical Consequence Planning and Management for National Special Security Events After September 11: Boston: 2004," Disaster Medicine and Public Health Preparedness, August 2008, and "In a Moment's Notice: Surge Capacity for Terrorist Bombings," U.S. Department of Health and Human Services, Centers for Disease Control and Prevention, April 2007. Mr. Serino attended Harvard University's Kennedy School of Government Senior Executives in State and Local Government program in 2000, completed the Kennedy School's National Preparedness Leadership Initiative in 2005, and graduated from the Executive Leadership Program, Center for Homeland Defense and Security at the Naval Postgraduate School.

Ciro Ugarte, M.D., a Peruvian national, began his professional career working in general practice in the highlands of Cusco, Peru. In 1987, Dr. Ugarte was appointed as Director of Norms, Regional Director, and later as Deputy Director General at the National Institute of Occupational Health in Peru. In late 1988, he was appointed as Executive Director and Director General of the Ministry of Health of Peru, a position he held until 1999. During this period he also served as: Permanent Member of the National Committee of the Peruvian Red Cross Society; Official Representative of the Peruvian Government to the International Committee of the Red Cross; consultant for Latin America of the Office of U.S. Foreign Disaster Assistance (OFDA/USAID); Professor at the School of Medicine of the National University of San Marcos and at the National School of Public Health of Peru; member of the United Nations Disaster Assessment and Coordination Team (UNDAC), and President of the Peruvian Society of Emergency Medicine. Dr. Ugarte started working for the Pan American Health Organization/World Health Organization (PAHO/WHO) as a consultant in Honduras, where he coordinated the United Nations Interagency Team for Disaster Reduction. In 2000 he was appointed as Sub-regional Advisor for South America in Ecuador and in 2002 as Regional Advisor based in Washington, DC. In 2014 he was appointed as Director of the Emergency Preparedness and Disaster Relief Department of PAHO/WHO. Dr. Ugarte has extensive experience in emergency preparedness and disaster relief. He coordinated the implementation of public health measures and provision of health care and recovery at national and international levels in cases of earthquakes, severe floods, volcanic eruptions, landslides, hazardous materials incidents, armed conflicts, terrorist attacks, taking of hostages, epidemics, pandemics, and others. He is the author of numerous publications and articles on vulnerability reduction in health facilities, hospital disaster planning, outbreaks and epidemics preparedness and response, health impact of earthquakes, damage and needs assessment, national contingency planning, safe hospitals, and others.

Linda Usdin, Dr.P.H., is the President of swamplily llc. In this capacity, she has helped match the strategic interests of philanthropic organizations with the needs and capacity of local nonprofits and governmental agencies in diverse areas, such as homelessness, early child care, leadership development, and transparency and accountability in governance. In the past 6 years, she has worked with the Ford, the Open Society, the Conrad N. Hilton, the Louisiana Disaster Recovery, and the Greater New Orleans foundations. During the past 15 years, Dr. Usdin has worked for local and national foundations as a program development and evaluation consultant. In addition, she has taught courses on building community engagement in public health efforts for the South Central Public Health Leadership Institute, the Centers for Disease Control and Prevention, and Tulane University School of Public Health and Tropical Medicine, and has facilitated strategic planning processes for groups such as the City of New Orleans, National Network of Public Health Institutes, and Montefiore Medical Center in the Bronx. She currently holds a position as Adjunct Faculty at Tulane University School of Public Health and Tropical Medicine. Dr. Usdin graduated magna cum laude with a B.A. in Psychology from Duke University, has an M.A. in Public Health from the University of California, Berkeley, and a Dr.PH. from the international health department at Tulane School of Public Health and Tropical Medicine.

Printed by Printforce, United Kingdom